HANDBOOK

OF CURRENT

HEALTH &

MEDICINE

HANDBOOK

OF CURRENT

HEALTH &

MEDICINE

BRYAN BUNCH

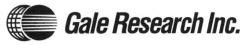

Gale Research Inc.

An International Thomson Publishing Company

NEW YORK • LONDON • BONN • BOSTON • DETROIT • MADRID
MELBOURNE • MEXICO CITY • PARIS • SINGAPORE • TOKYO
TORONTO • WASHINGTON • ALBANY NY • BELMONT CA • CINCINNATI OH

MAI *33 3 3897*✓

BRYAN BUNCH
Obituaries by Sally Bunch
Copyedited by Andrea Gacki

Gale Research Inc. Staff

Christine B. Jeryan, Denise Kasinec, and Jim Edwards, *Project Coordinators*

Paul Lewon, Kyung-Sun Lim, Jacqueline Longe, Zoran Minderović, Donna Olendorf, Bridget Travers, Sheila Walencewicz, *Assisting Editors*

Mary Beth Trimper, *Production Director*
Catherine Kemp, *Production Assistant*

Cynthia Baldwin, *Art Director*
Mark Howell, *Cover Design*

Jeffrey Muhr, *Editorial Technical Support*

ISSN 1078-9707
ISBN 0-8103-9551-7

Printed in the United States of America.
Published simultaneously in the United Kingdom by Gale Research International Limited (An affiliated company of Gale Research Inc.)

10 9 8 7 6 5 4 3 2 1

I(T)P™ Gale Research Inc., an International Thomson Publishing Company.
ITP logo is a trademark under license.

Contents

B942h

FERTILITY, PREGNANCY, AND BIRTH

CHILDHOOD AND GROWTH

ENVIRONMENTAL HAZARDS

MENTAL HEALTH

NEW TOOLS IN MEDICINE

AGING AND DEATH

APPENDICES   589

INDEX   623

HOW TO USE THIS BOOK

Handbook of Current Health and Medicine is designed to provide easy access to information on major developments in health and medicine that occurred during the early 1990s. It also presents background for interpreting these developments and serves as an up-to-date handbook of basic health information. Data included have been chosen to cover facts that are frequently needed while reading or writing about health issues. The same data also form an essential aid to understanding new health and medical devices, experiments, and theories.

As the following plan for the book indicates, *Handbook of Current Health and Medicine* is designed so that it can be read from start to finish—perhaps with some skimming or skipping of the tabular material—to obtain an overview of health and medicine in the early 1990s. Many readers, however, will prefer to treat *Handbook of Current Health and Medicine* like a magazine, browsing among articles that are of particular interest to them. In either case, the structure and content of the book make it a reference work to which one can return again and again.

Plan of the Book

The book begins with an introduction describing the current state of the medical enterprise. Following that, 11 broad subject areas are covered in an order that to some degree parallels the life of a human being:

Genetics—inheritance from the parents
Conception, development, and birth
Childhood health and diseases
Wellness—diet, exercise, smoking, alcohol, and other drugs
Differing health problems for women and men
Environment and health
Mind and body
Viruses, bacteria, and other parasites
Heart disease, cancer, autoimmunity, and other chronic conditions
Treatment, from diagnosis to surgery and drugs
Old age and death

The book concludes with several appendices devoted to data that are likely to be referred to frequently and that are common to all the main subject areas.

Within each broad subject area, the same basic plan is followed:

State of the Subject   Each subject-area section begins with an article on the state of that subject in the early 1990s.

Timetable of the Subject   This is followed by a historical timetable through 1989 consisting of short entries describing major developments in the subject area in chronological order. The timetables are designed both for easy reference and so that the reader can develop a feel for how a subject has evolved.

Sections   The bulk of the book consists of articles on medical developments of 1990, 1991, 1992, and 1993. The individual articles are grouped into several sections on a given theme. For example, the "Genes and Medicine" subject area contains three sections after the timetable: "New Developments in Genetic Science" is concerned with the general progress of genetics as that science affects health and medicine; "Genes and Chromosomes as a Cause of Disease" relates discoveries of specific genes that not only cause hereditary diseases but sometimes predispose a person to chronic diseases that have other causes; and "Gene Therapy" relates to use of genetics in treatment of disease.

Articles   Within each section, individual topics are covered in one or more articles. For example, "Gene Therapy" contains separate articles that deal with the following topics: the use of genetic engineering in the pioneering experiments with an uncommon hereditary disease, ADA deficiency; the most common hereditary disease in the U.S., cystic fibrosis; a series of different approaches toward using genetic engineering to treat cancer, which is only partly a hereditary disease; and finally other unrelated new developments in gene therapy, in one of the frequent UPDATE sections. Articles are labeled UPDATE to indicate that they summarize recent gains in a specific area that is currently very active.

Set-Off Background Material   An important feature within many articles is background material that is set off from the body of the article. The main focus of this book is on current health and medicine, but some readers may not have the prerequisite knowledge to understand new technical developments. Sometimes a simple glossary is all that is needed to clarify an article or a table. Other times it may be a paragraph or two that briefly describe the history of a key development.

Science periodicals or yearbooks, which constitute the most accessible source of current scientific and technological information outside of this book, either omit such background material or incorporate it into the body of articles. *Handbook of Current Health and Medicine* is unique in allowing the reader a choice.

Tables, Charts, and Lists of Useful Data   Most tables that have to do with a particular subject matter are grouped at the end of the broad subject sections. Sometimes, when it is particularly useful with regard to a specific article, a table is included in or immediately follows the article. Every effort has been made to include the most useful data in considerable detail.

References   Articles conclude with a listing of periodical references and suggestions for additional reading. For the most part, development outpaces book publishing and the progress of the early 1990s, outside of this volume, can be found only in magazines and newspapers. The magazines listed are commonly available in general libraries in the United States. Medical journals are excluded as too technical. The only newspaper listed is the *New York Times,* because of both its great accessibility across most of the United States and its extensive coverage. There is special emphasis on three widely read weekly journals, *Science, Science News,* and *Nature.* Both *Science* and *Nature* cover most events of interest with explanations for the general reader and also publish much original research. *Science News* provides good coverage of current health and medicine in short, fact-filled articles. Most other periodicals listed are monthlies, bimonthlies, or quarterlies that tend to provide scanty accounts of current medical developments several months after they occur. Detailed articles often are devoted to long-term trends. Nevertheless, magazines such as *Scientific American* or *Discover* constitute a second tier of additional reading. Oddly, there is no reliable magazine concerning the science of health and medicine directed toward the general reader, although there are several popular magazines on health themes.

Purpose of *Handbook of Current Health and Medicine*

The most important function of *Handbook of Current Health and Medicine* is to serve as a basic source of facts about new developments in health and medicine. While there are much larger encyclopedias of health and medicine available, as well as large handbooks for specific subject areas, *Handbook of Current Health and Medicine* is a relatively small, accessible reference that cuts across all sciences and is up-to-date in a way that standard references cannot manage.

As we approach the twenty-first century, health and medicine continue to develop at an exponential rate. It is possible to keep up with new investigations and theories by reading a large number of periodicals each month but, because scientific and technological developments often unfold over the course of months or years, periodicals often present such information in a fragmented manner and without overview. *Handbook of Current Health and Medicine* is able to summarize developments that have taken place over an extended period of time. New developments are the focus of the book, and all subject areas of health and medicine are included.

Who Needs This Book

Everyone who regularly uses current scientific data that span several fields or that cover a particular subject needs *Handbook of Current Health and Medicine.* Chief among these people are reference librarians, health and medicine writers and reporters, and health teachers. Additionally, the information in this book can help anyone take steps to improve his or her health and to become knowledgeable about the treatment offered by a physician or hospital.

The State of Medicine

THE STATE OF HEALTH AND MEDICINE TODAY

Modern science has transformed medicine in the twentieth century, and the century is not even over. This book begins with 1990 and covers the early 1990s, so it may be helpful in thinking about the state of health and medicine today to go back to remember what its state was a hundred years ago.

In 1890 the germ theory of disease was still a new idea. Surgeons were just beginning to put on rubber gloves, but they had yet to don the surgical mask. Although general anesthetics were in use in industrialized parts of the world, local anesthesia would be introduced that year. X rays were five years in the future, and artificial radioactivity would be discovered soon after. Genetics was rediscovered and became known in 1900. No one had imaged a virus, and it was not certain that such a thing could exist. Blood transfusions and vitamins also go back to the first years of the twentieth century.

Fifty years after 1890 and before 1990, the first antibiotics were being developed. Machines such as the heart-lung machine and kidney dialysis machine—artificial organs that worked outside the body—were being introduced to medicine. During World War II Oswald Avery and his coworkers demonstrated that DNA is the chemical basis of genetics. The next year fluoridation of water supplies started.

When we come to the 1990s, we find it quite probable that medical practice is changing at least as much as it did in the early 1940s and possibly as much as in the 1890s and early years of the century.

For one thing, knowledge of genetics has increased exponentially; the complete genetic map for humans is just around the corner and few doubt that it will be completed. It is clear that the genetics of the 1990s has the power to change medicine as much as the discoveries of X rays and vitamins almost a century ago. The idea of causing the cells of a person to behave in a more desirable way by permanently changing them and their descendants has already reached early fulfillment.

Another area where recent advances are making everything different, although with roots that are decades old, is in fertility, conception, and treatment of the fetus. And after the baby is born, parents learn new ways to handle feeding and sleep in hopes of avoiding Sudden Infant Death Syndrome (SIDS) as well as problems later in life.

Many breakthroughs in diet and other wellness issues have been heralded, including several in the 1990s. From a vantage point one hundred years in the future, the 1990s may be seen as the decade when eating practices were defined so that diet enhanced health and longevity. Such late twentieth-century devices as dentures will be viewed with even more amusement than the young already do today.

After nearly three thousand years of Western civilization, the health of women is finally becoming an issue that men, as well as women, take seriously. Although hysteria and fainting may have been replaced by hypoglycemia and anorexia as "female complaints," the early 1990s may be the turning point in which women's health studies are merged with those of men so that both sexes get equal attention. In this field, "separate but equal" makes sense, for women's bodies and men's bodies truly are different.

Psychiatry is about a hundred years old in anything like its modern form, but it seems about to enter a new phase that will be far more biological than any in the past. As millions smooth out their lives with Prozac and related compounds, it remains unclear whether medicated minds are better or worse off than unmedicated minds. Earlier psychoactive drugs have eventually been found to pose as many problems as solutions. Yet it seems clear that the vastly increased knowledge of how the brain works will lead to further chemical fixes for mental problems.

Progress is also rapid in areas of public health that have increasingly caused general and political concern: the environment; accidental death; and infectious diseases. Governments around the world and the United Nations and other international agencies intervene more and more in these three areas, with considerable benefit to individuals. The breakdown of communism and the Soviet Union has started the process of environmental change in eastern Europe and northern Asia, regions that were not part of the otherwise worldwide movement until recently. New international covenants will also make it easier for developing countries to progress in environmental protection and control of infectious diseases.

Unfortunately, not all infectious disease responds to public health measures (vaccination, quarantine, sanitation, improved nutrition, and widespread treatment programs). New diseases continue to appear and some old diseases mutate and become widespread again. Although the overall improvement in the control of most infectious diseases is expected to continue, AIDS continues to be a problem because of its methods of transmission and the lack of any cure once HIV infection takes hold.

Because of the century of progress against environmental and infectious disease, the main killers in most of the world (the industrial nations and China) today are circulatory diseases and cancer. Progress on this front has been limited in effect, but great in understanding. It was not very long ago that the cause of cancer was uncertain, for example. Today the causes have been traced to the genes as well as the viruses and other environmental stimuli that affect the genes. Heart disease is actually declining in the West, probably as a result of adopting a diet that is more like that of the East. Still, heart disease and cancer remain as major challenges for the next hundred years.

In diagnosis, monoclonal antibodies are making a contribution, although they have not so far lived up to their initial promise. Almost routine use of CT scans and MRI scans in the U.S. may be having an impact on health, but no one has produced a definitive study showing that this is the case. Diagnosis by way of genetics is the new kid on the block, and, as is often the case, is viewed with considerable suspicion; nevertheless, while worries about ethics are real, it is clear that one way or another genes will be used in determining the cause of disease.

Once the cause of a disorder has been established, treatment may vary. Surgery is becoming more and more "high tech." Cells and even body parts (such as capillaries) are tiny, so microsurgical techniques are used more and more. Minimizing the entry incision into the body is now possible for many common surgical procedures, resulting in what is often called "band-aid surgery." And lasers are everywhere, reattaching retinas, burning spinal discs, sealing off hernias, and on and on. Drugs are more and more sophisticated, although often the new genetically engineered drugs fail to work or have serious, unexpected side effects. The limited success of the artificial kidney (that is, dialysis) has saved or extended productively millions of lives in the past fifty years; similar devices for other organs appear to be at hand, making a partly bionic person more feasible.

Bionic or not, delaying death remains possible, but preventing it is not. As medical science becomes increasingly successful in controlling disease and improving health, more people are living long enough to develop the problems of age. Increasingly the question of when to stop treatment and let people die is becoming a major ethical problem for medicine. And that ethical problem is not the only one, as the new medicine enters the new millennium.

Ethical Issues of New Medicine

Ethics for doctors was a problem even in ancient times—hence, medical laws in the Code of Hammurabi that detail penalties for surgeons causing death or blindness and the Hippocratic Oath's promise not to use medicine to cause injury. Today medicine and other treatments are much more powerful, resulting in ethical issues that are more subtle.

One of the main ethical problems facing the new medicine is whether or not to use powerful tools, developed to prevent or treat what we perceive as defects, to rearrange the bodies or minds of people who are in the normal range. Although the ethical problems are not resolved, doctors around the U.S. are already prescribing artificial growth hormone to short normal children and powerful mood-elevating drugs to sad or troubled adults.

In the case of the growth hormone, it is not now known for sure whether providing additional hormone to a child whose body already makes a normal supply will increase adult height. An early genetic experiment in which the gene for human growth hormone was given to a rat did produce a giant, so there is reason to suspect that additional hormone might cause children of normal, but short, parents to become taller. The U.S. National Institutes of Health is conducting a controversial study— suspended largely for ethical issues in 1992, but restarted the next year—to find out what happens to short normal children who receive the hormone. However, critics say that even if tall adults result, the whole idea is wrong. The hormone is also very expensive at present. Is it worth $20,000-a-year for a boy who would have been 5 feet tall to become—perhaps a hundred thousand dollars later—6 feet tall? Some doctors think that it is, because short people suffer disadvantages in a generally taller society.

Health and Medicine in Developing Countries

Anyone in the U.S. who habitually reads obituary pages in the newspaper will notice that heart attacks and cancer are the major causes of death. Although these *are* the major causes of death in the U.S., they do not reflect the world health situation. Around the world, death from infectious diseases and parasites is more common than death from heart disease, strokes, and cancer combined. Some rates are not that different between the U.S. and the world as a whole—notably deaths from external causes (that is, accidents, homicides, and suicides). Other rates differ wildly, with about nine times as many deaths per 100,000 from perinatal, or birth-related, causes around the world as in the U.S. Most people know that these differences result from higher levels of poverty in other parts of the world. The rate of death from infectious disease and the rate of infant mortality in developing countries contribute to higher worldwide rates of infant mortality and infectious disease deaths.

On July 9, 1993 the World Bank reported that health gains in developing countries have brought world health much closer to that of the industrialized West than in 1960. The study, "Investing in Health," showed that this improvement in health was proceeding much more rapidly than any improvement in wealth. The World Bank is interested in this issue because it expects to disburse about a billion dollars for health-related projects in 1995, three times 1990 expenditure.

In the period covered by the study, 1960 to 1990, life expectancy at birth in the nations identified by the World Bank as developing rose from 46 years to 63 years, largely as a result of such public health measures as immunization and improvements in sanitation. In 1990 the number of children who die before their fifth birthday in developing countries is a third of what it was in 1960. In addition to childhood immunization, a large part of this improvement can be traced to oral rehydration, an inexpensive and effective treatment for the diarrhea that is a major immediate cause of death in a number of infectious diseases.

But everyone agrees that the health of children in developing countries can still be greatly improved. Some major steps began in September 1990, the end year for the World Bank statistics, when 149 nations met at the United Nations for the World Summit for Children, sponsored by UNICEF. Goals were set for the year 2000 and the individual nations then established detailed plans toward meeting those goals, which included such specifics as the complete elimination of tetanus in newborns and vitamin-A deficiency in children; the near elimination of polio and death from measles; universal iodization of salt; and access to clean water. These individual goals aim to reduce infant mortality by a third and maternal death rates and malnutrition in children by a half. Many of the specific steps proposed are the same as those that the World Bank plans to support.

Good Health in China Based on Children and Poverty

Since the advent of communism, the Chinese government has set different priorities in health care from those in the West, and, for the Chinese situation, these priorities have been very successful. Despite the traditional Chinese reverence for their elders, it is in the West that huge amounts of health-care dollars are spent on the last six months of life; in China the emphasis is on prenatal care and healthy children. As a result, the infant mortality rate in cities and large towns is comparable to that in the West, and about 85 percent of all infants are vaccinated against the common childhood diseases in their first year of life. Taken as whole, infant mortality is a bit more than 30 per 1000 in China, still three times the rate in the U.S. and Europe, but two-thirds that of Mexico, half that of Brazil, and almost of quarter of that of India, the other great Asian mainland state. Better prenatal care also reduces the death rate from complications of pregnancy and giving birth. In China prenatal care would be even more nearly universal if some pregnant women did not avoid doctors after the first successful birth out of the not unreasonable fear that they would be pressured into an abortion as a result of China's strict population-control policies.

Because infant mortality and childhood diseases have a strong effect on overall life expectancy, life expectancy in China is about 70, nearly as high as in the industrialized West (about 75) and ten years higher than that of India. Overall, about five percent of China's gross national product (GNP) goes for health care, as opposed to about 15 percent in the U.S. in 1994.

Some of the credit for China's relative success can be attributed to the lifestyle of most of its citizens. People who cannot afford automobiles get more exercise and have fewer fatal accidents; people who cannot afford red meat generally eat a lower-cholesterol, lower-fat diet; and people who have little money are less likely to be killed in the course of a robbery. It is thought that rising incomes will destroy some of this health advantage.

Health and Medicine in the U.S.

Health care became a dominant political issue in the U.S. in the early 1990s in part because President Bill Clinton pushed hard for changes in the way health care was financed. Americans across the nation already knew that health-care economics had gotten out of hand. The cost of health care was rising faster than nearly every other segment of the economy. Furthermore, most health insurance in the U.S. had become tied to employment, and the nation's overall employment situation was changing rapidly and for the worse for many in the middle class. As a result, while only 13 percent of employed persons missed a month or more of health-insurance coverage between February 1990 and September 1992 according to the latest available U.S. Census Bureau figures, 38 percent of the unemployed had a similar (and often longer) gap during that time. Overall, 25 percent of all Americans were without health insurance for at least a month. At any given time in the early 1990s, about 39 million Americans (17 percent of the population) lacked health coverage.

The cost of health care in the U.S. is documented through 1991 and has been estimated by the Metropolitan Life Insurance Company for 1992-1994. U.S. Department of Commerce estimates are slightly higher, reaching a total of $1060.5 million by 1994.

COST OF HEALTH CARE

Year	Total cost in millions	Percent increase by year
1970	$74.4	—
1975	$132.9	12.4%
1980	$250.1	13.5%
1985	$422.6	11.0%
1990	$675.0	9.8%
1991	$751.8	11.4%
1992	$828.0	10.1%
1993	$910.0	9.9%
1994	$995.0	9.3%

Broadly speaking, the Consumer Price Index rose about 40 percent from the early 1980s to 1992, while in the same ten-year period, the cost of health care rose about 160 percent, or four times as much. Similarly, health care was less than ten percent of the U.S. gross national product at the start of the 1980s, but had reached nearly 15 percent of the gross national product in 1994.

What did that money buy? A U.S. Commerce Department spokesperson claimed that insurance overhead, as opposed to the actual cost of care, accounts for nearly 25 percent of all spending on health care. Figured another way, hospital costs (not including nursing homes) accounted for almost 40 percent, physicians and dentists for somewhat more than 20 percent, and drugs and medical equipment for almost 10 percent (in this accounting, the money spent for insurance overhead is included as part of the amount spent).

Health Maintenance Organizations (HMOs) are often thought to be one way to control costs. In an HMO, a fixed fee is paid for health care annually and teams of health care workers are provided to make it happen. From 1987 to 1992 the number of Americans enrolled in HMOs rose from 29.3 million (in 662 HMOs) to 41.4 million (in only 544 HMOs). At the same time, the profits from running an HMO rose faster than any other health-related business. Figures are difficult to come by, but there is no clear-cut evidence that the HMOs actually do control costs better than other ways of paying for health insurance.

Germany Experiments with Drugs

Germany has a health-care plan that is very similar to the combination of insurer alliances and employer support proposed by U.S. President Bill Clinton. Most Germans belong to such alliances, sharing the cost of insurance equally with employers. Doctors and pharmacies are reimbursed directly from the alliances, not through the patient, much the way that a hospital in the U.S. is normally reimbursed directly by an insurer when the patient is insured.

As in other Western nations, the cost of health care in Germany has increased much faster than the inflation rate. Starting on January 1, 1993 the German government instituted a new plan to control one of the fast-rising costs, the cost of drugs. Specifically, it took two steps: one mandates the prices paid by the alliances for specific drugs; the other puts a cap on total spending on drugs. In U.S. dollars, the cap is $15 billion per year.

To make this plan work, the actual cap was based on a combination of physicians' fees and drug expenses. Any amount over $15 billion spent for drugs was deducted proportionally from physicians' fees. The cap figure was $1.5 billion less than spending on drugs in 1992, so something had to give.

The result was a change in the amount and type of medicine prescribed by German doctors. Physicians stopped prescribing expensive "name-brand" drugs and switched their patients to generics. In some cases, where there are several possible treatments for a condition (for example, beta blockers, calcium blockers, ACE inhibitors, and other drugs for treating high blood pressure), physicians avoided the higher-cost drugs. Some patients were unhappy and searched around for a doctor who would prescribe the specific drug they were used to or that they had some reason to believe would work better.

The new policy did have the intended result—the overall cost of drugs dropped dramatically. Figures were not available early in 1994, but it seems likely that the cost of drugs in 1993 was more than $2 billion below the $15 billion cap. The sales of generic drugs also shot up dramatically. Pharmaceutical companies claim that the manufacturers that invest the most in research on new drugs were hit hardest and that all drug makers will lose money, even the companies specializing in generics who face stiff competition from each other. An industry survey backed up claims that profits were way down, research expenditures had been cut, and employees were being fired. Government records, however, showed that few jobs were actually lost. Indeed, the larger companies that also spend the most on research sell as much of 80 percent of their volume outside of Germany, reducing the impact of spending reductions in Germany considerably.

(Periodical References and Additional Reading: *New York Times* 4-14-91, p I-1; *New York Times* 7-7-93, p A6; *New York Times* 10-3-93, p I-21; *New York Times* 11-23-93, p D1; *New York Times* 12-29-93, p A12; *Discover* 1-94, p 83; *Statistical Bulletin* 1/3-94, p 30; *New York Times* 3-29-94, p D23)

TIMETABLE OF MEDICINE AND HEALTH TO 1990

2500 BC   Traditional date for Huang Ti, the third Emperor of China, who, among other accomplishments, is credited with the *Nei Ching* ("The Yellow Emperor's Classic of Internal Medicine"); it is a collection describing medical practice in terms of yin and yang and the five "elements"—fire, earth, metal, water, and wood.

1000 BC   About this time, the Israelites compile the Law of Moses, which includes strict diet laws, rules for hygiene, how to deal with hemophilia, and how to sterilize a house in case of "leprosy" (possibly the disease we know as syphilis).

40 BC   The *Ayurveda* is compiled; it becomes the basic Hindu medical treatise.

1130   Scholars in Toledo begin translating the works of Arabic scientist Avicenna [born Bukhara, Uzbekistan, 980; died Hamadan, Iran, June 1037] into Latin; these cover almost every aspect of health and medicine.

1284   Mamluk Sultan Qalawin builds Mansuri Maristan in Cairo, the most sophisticated medical center of its time, with separate wards for fevers, eye diseases, surgery, dysentery, and mental illness.

1473   The first complete Latin edition of the Avicenna's *Canon of Medicine* is printed in Milan.

1518   The Royal College of Physicians in London is established.

1662   Johann Baptista van Helmont [born Brussels, Belgium, January 12, 1580; died Brussels, December 30, 1635 or 1644] publishes *Oriatrike* (Physic Refined), which becomes very popular.

1666   Physician Thomas Sydenham, "the English Hippocrates," [born Wynford Eagle, England, September 10, 1624; died London, December 29, 1689] publishes *Methodus Curandi Febres*; in this and other books, he advocates the use of opium to relieve pain, chinchona bark (quinine) to relieve malaria, and iron to relieve anemia.

1754   The University of Halle (Germany) graduates the first female M.D.

1763   The first American medical society is founded in New London, Connecticut.

1765   John Morgan [born Philadelphia, Pennsylvania, June 10, 1735; died Philadelphia, October 15, 1789] founds the first medical school in America at the College of Pennsylvania.

1810   *Organon of Rational Healing* by Christian Friedrich Samuel Hahnemann [born Meissen, Germany, April 10, 1755; died Paris, July 2, 1843] introduces homeopathy.

1966   Henry Beecher of Massachusetts General Hospital in Boston Massachusetts criticizes 22 published medical studies for poor ethical practices in research on living patients; his report leads to a complete revamping of ethics guidelines for medical research.

1975   Nevada becomes the first state in the U.S. to regulate acupuncture; its Board of Chinese Medicine develops the required examination to be licensed to practice acupuncture in the state.

RACE AND HEALTH

The U.S. Declaration of Independence states that "all men are created equal," which we interpret to mean "all men and women are equal at birth." When it comes to health, however, there are considerable differences among broad classes of people and between males and females (*See* "The State of Health by Gender," p 211). In addition to very different health care for the rich and poor and apparent lack of concern for women in the male medical establishment, there are also inborn differences—created ones if you will. It is not always easy, however, to sort out the health "endowed by our Creator" from the effects of differing life styles, economic conditions, and societal influences.

The concept of "race" has had so many different meanings that many anthropologists today would say that the word itself is meaningless. There is considerable evidence to support this point of view about race. In ordinary discourse, however, people today recognize that broad groups sharing certain inherited physical characteristics can be recognized and certain of these are designated as races. Thus, people in the U.S. speak of the black race to identify people with a suite of characteristics inherited from African ancestors and speak of the white race for those in which characteristics of European ancestors are predominant. Similarly, certain Asian-Americans or peoples of indigenous ancestry (often termed Native Americans) are also identified as races. We recognize that this distinction may at times be artificial and that one "race" shades into the other, but medical and income statistics are frequently grouped on the basis of this classification scheme. Such statistics form the basis of much of the following discussion.

Health in Persons of African Descent

It has long been known that African-Americans, especially males, have a greater incidence of high blood pressure than Americans of European descent. A similar statistical imbalance between the two races in the U.S. exists for diabetes. These racial differences are not necessarily inborn, although they may be. The case for causation is not proved either way, but the effects of the differences become factors in other diseases as well. High blood pressure, for example, influences heart disease, although other factors are almost certainly involved.

Deaths from heart disease are higher in the U.S. among blacks than among whites. A study of cardiac arrests in Chicago released on August 26, 1993 showed that blacks in their 30s were more than twice as likely as whites of the same age to have a heart attack; blacks of all ages were more likely than similarly aged whites to undergo sudden heart stoppage. This research, conducted by Lance B. Becker and coworkers at the University of Chicago, followed 6451 heart attacks outside of hospital settings that occurred in Chicago in 1987 and 1988.

One reason to suspect that race alone is not the cause of differences is that death rates from specific diseases change separately for each race over time. But the disparity in rates has declined in the past 20 years. Perhaps the change in overall death rates for heart disease in blacks and whites results more from a change in the age profile of the races than from differences in health or health care.

Changes in death rates within a race can vary enormously. In 1950, for example, the death rate for cancer was lower among black males than among white males, but since then the black-male rate has risen about 80 percent while the white-male death rate from cancer has risen only 20 percent. During the same period, the death rates for both black and white females fell slightly. Since the genetic make-up of the populations involved has not varied significantly during that period, such rate changes are suspected to be socioeconomic or environmental. In some cases, differing medical treatment is a factor, but this difference is not always a direct result of racism. Poverty is often involved. A corollary to poverty may also be involved; while 11 percent of white Americans in 1992 lacked medical insurance, the figure was 21 percent for blacks and an astonishing 32 percent for those identifying themselves as Hispanics.

Treatment consequences can also vary. A study by Kristen Kjerulff of the University of Maryland School of Medicine and coworkers published in the November 1993 issue of *Obstetrics and Gynecology* showed that women of African-American descent who had hysterectomies in Maryland between 1986 and 1991 were 2.7 times as likely as matched white women to be hospitalized for more than ten days after the operation, only in part because of a 1.4 times greater rate of such complications as infection. Furthermore, the death rate for the black patients in the study was 3.1 times that of white patients after age, severity of other medical conditions, and treatment were taken into account.

Major reports in 1991 and 1992 identified some of the factors involved in the differences between African-Americans and other Americans for kidney transplants, cancer, and heart bypasses. In the 1990s, blacks received proportionally fewer kidney transplants than their high rate of kidney disease warrants; black men and women had higher cancer rates than whites; and African-Americans underwent heart-bypass operations a little more than a quarter as often as whites did, despite higher death rates among blacks from heart disease.

Kidney disease.   A study conducted for the American Society of Transplant Physicians by Martin G. White, Gabriel M. Danovitch, and other specialists in kidney transplant published in the January 31, 1991 *New England Journal of Medicine* found that blacks in the U.S. experienced 28 percent of the serious kidney disease diagnosed—very high for only 12 percent of the overall U.S. population—but only received 21 percent of the kidney transplants. Serious kidney disease as defined in the study requires either lifetime kidney dialysis or a transplant. Furthermore, black transplant recipients had a survival rate for the transplanted kidney that was only about 90 percent of the rate for white recipients.

The most likely cause for this disparity is the difference in the sizes of the black and white population in the U.S. and differences in attitude toward and knowledge of kidney transplants. Since 7 out of 8 Americans are not black, if all other factors were equal, only 1 out of 8 donated organs would come from blacks. All other factors are not equal, however, and only 1 out of 12 kidneys donated for transplant comes from blacks.

Like all organ transplants, kidney transplants are successful in part because of genetic compatibility between the donor and the recipient; this is why transplants from close relatives are generally more successful. Since black and whites are less likely to be closely related to each other than whites and whites or blacks and blacks are, it is more difficult to get good matches between kidneys donated by whites and potential black recipients. If the matches are not so good, the transplants fail more often. And, as noted above, African-Americans are less likely to have health insurance that will cover the cost of a transplant operation.

Not only is there less knowledge of kidney transplants in the black community, but also blacks are more likely to belong to religions that discourage organ transplants or to have developed a distrust of the medical system in general.

Cancer.   Another study, published in the April 17, 1991 *Journal of the National Cancer Institute*, claims that all of the higher incidence of cancer in African-Americans is attributable to poverty, not race. Claudia R. Baquet and coworkers from the U.S. National Cancer Institute adjusted the data from the 1980 census to equalize such socioeconomic factors as population density, education, and income. The adjusted figures showed no significant difference in overall cancer rates for blacks and whites in the study regions around Atlanta, Georgia; Detroit, Michigan; and San Francisco-Oakland, California. Unadjusted statistics show black cancer rates six to ten percent higher than whites. Thus, the disparity is in the different socioeconomic status of blacks and whites in those regions.

Despite the resemblance in cancer incidence rates between black and whites, the U.S. National Cancer Institute reports that black cancer patients die 35 percent more frequently from cancer than whites do.

Specific types of cancer did show differences between the races even after adjustment, but whites had higher rates for some cancers and black rates were higher for others. Persons of European descent were found to have a higher risk of breast, rectal, and lung cancer, while African-Americans were more likely to develop stomach, cervical, or prostate cancer. African-Americans are thought to have the world's highest rate of prostate cancer and the death rate is twice that of white Americans. Currently, colorectal cancer is rising in blacks and becoming less common among persons of European descent in the U.S.

Some diseases of blood cells, including cancers as well as other diseases, can only be treated successfully by bone marrow transplants. The lack of donors of African-American descent makes it more difficult to find matching bone marrow, for although the donor and recipient do not have to be of the same race, matches within races are more common than interracial ones. Less than two percent of the recipients of bone marrow through the National Marrow Donor Program are black, mainly because of poor matches.

Heart disease. Just as treatment for kidney disease varies by race, so does the treatment for heart disease. A study published on March 19, 1992 in the *Journal of the American Medical Association* and written by Arthur J. Hartz of the Medical College of Wisconsin and others revealed that black patients on Medicare undergo heart bypass operations a fourth as often as white Medicare patients. Again, the apparent reasons for the disparity are complex and not the simple racism or even poverty that one might suspect as the cause. For example, the higher rate of heart disease among blacks is thought to be due to high blood pressure; but the kind of heart disease commonly caused by high blood pressure is not a type that can be treated with bypass surgery. Furthermore, by using the 86,463 Medicare patients who underwent bypass surgery in 1986 as the sample, the study virtually eliminated poverty as a possible cause of different rates; Medicare pays most bills for the operation. Because most people over the age of 65 use Medicare and because older people are more likely to have heart disease, the study covered about half all of the heart bypass operations in the U.S. for that year.

Similar results for heart disease were obtained in a study reported on August 26, 1993 in the *New England Journal of Medicine* that also used a population in which finances were effectively eliminated as a cause of disparity. Jeff Whittle and coworkers at the Pittsburgh Department of Veterans Affairs Medical Center reviewed the records of 428,300 patients in Veterans Affairs hospitals from 1987 to 1991. They found the same three-to-one disparity in heart bypass operations (1 black patient for each 4 persons receiving bypasses means that 3 times as many whites as blacks get the operation). Furthermore, white patients were treated with balloon angioplasty twice as often as blacks. There was a less dramatic, but still significant, ratio of more than three to two for angiograms, a cardiac diagnostic procedure.

With poverty eliminated as a factor and race per se perhaps not much involved, what causes the disparity? For some reason either African Americans seek such operations less often or else the doctors they use schedule the operations less often. In the rural South, where the disparity in heart treatments among Medicare patients reaches seven to one, it is thought likely that poor education of both patient and physician may be a part of the picture. Some cardiologists believe that fear of operations may be involved, especially among black men. Technical reasons include the possibility that health problems other than heart disease may make such procedures as bypass operations or angioplasty too risky for black patients more often than for whites. More research is needed, however, to establish the cause.

Although connections were not directly made, the study of heart attacks in Chicago also showed that whites were more than three times as likely as blacks to survive a heart attack outside a hospital.

Other Differences between Races

For many of the major causes of death in 1992, the rates were lowest for persons identifying themselves as Asian Americans. Native Americans (Indians) had the highest rate of suicide and motor-vehicle-related deaths, very likely a result of the high rate of alcoholism in this population.

(Periodical References and Additional Reading: *New York Times* 2-1-91; *New York Times* 4-7-91; *New York Times* 3-18-93, p B6; *New York Times* 8-25-91, p B8; *New York Times* 9-16-93, p A16; *New York Times* 11-16-93, p C10; *Scientific American* 1-94, p 130; *Scientific American* 4-94, p 72)

Alternative Medicine UPDATE

Alternatives to standard Western-style medicine are widely used around the world, including the U.S. and Europe. Among the therapies most Western physicians label "alternative medicine" are the following:

Acupuncture: ancient Chinese method of stimulating specific nerve centers at various points on the body, often with thin needles

Alternative drugs: compounds such as laetrile whose claims are not accepted by orthodox physicians

Biofeedback: use of conditioning techniques to empower the control specific body responses, such as blood pressure

Chiropractic: manipulation of the spine to improve health

Electromagnetism: mostly use of electric or magnetic fields to promote bone growth, but sometimes used for other purposes (MRI, the diagnostic use of magnetism, is mainstream medicine, not alternative)

Herbal medicine: use of natural substances close to their original form, primarily dried plants tissues, to promote healing or wellness

Homeopathy: treatment of illness through the use of very powerful drugs in very small amounts

Meditation: relaxation techniques as well as imaging techniques to promote general or specific control of mind over body

Osteopathy: manipulation of various bones and joints to cure disease conditions of various types, not just in the bones or joints

Ozone therapy: the gas ozone, an activated form of oxygen, is introduced into the immune system to kill germs and to strengthen the immune system

Self-help groups: organizations such as Alcoholics Anonymous or Weight Watchers that promote better health by encouraging people with similar problems to provide therapy for each other

Touch therapy: touching sick people to make them well

A study showed that people in the U.S. spent about $13.7 billion on alternative medicine, despite the fact that most health insurance plans will not reimburse patients for most treatments. Using criteria that include most of the therapies listed above, the study, conducted by David M. Eisenberg of Beth Israel Hospital and Harvard Medical School along with several coworkers, was published in the January 28, 1993 *New England Journal of Medicine*. It reported on a telephone survey of 1539 adults. The authors estimated that 34 percent of Americans used at least one form of alternative medicine in 1990. About ten percent of those surveyed had visited a practitioner, as opposed to being in a self-help group or administering self medication (such as herbs). The list of ailments for which they saw practitioners— backaches, anxiety, allergies, and chronic pain—suggests that most respondents went to a chiropractor or acupuncturist. Of those visiting a practitioner, 72 percent failed to tell their regular medical physician that they had done so.

Despite the popularity of many of the alternative medical treatments in the U.S. and around the world, many conventional physicians were unhappy with a U.S. National Institutes of Health (NIH) decision to institute an Office of Alternative Medicine. Congress established the new office in 1992; Joe Jacobs was named director and the office opened in 1993. Its goal is to support research in alternative medicine by specific grants, just as is done by other NIH offices. The 1993 budget was $2 million, not a great deal by NIH standards. The total 1993 NIH budget was $10.3 billion, a few billion less than the amount spent on alternative medicine in 1990.

Some NIH alternative medicine studies were underway before the advent of the new office, including a study by the National Institute of Drug Abuse of acupuncture as a treatment for addiction. Other studies are investigating the use of transcendental meditation as a treatment for high blood pressure.

(Periodical References and Additional Reading: *New York Times* 1-10-93, p I-1; *New York Times* 1-28-93, p A12; *New York Times* 3-6-93, p 26)

Genes and Medicine

THE STATE OF GENETIC MEDICINE

Of all the areas of human progress in the last decade of the twentieth century, the application of genetic ideas to medicine is proceeding fastest. Major new experiments are undertaken around the world, often yielding successes that no one expected to come for years or even for generations. Keeping up at all with genetic medicine is very difficult, and keeping up with the absolute latest is impossible, for the latest advance is replaced by some new miracle even as one tries to grasp the subtleties of the current wonder.

On November 17, 1993 the American Medical Association took an important step toward conveying the leap in genetic therapy to the medical profession, if not the general public. It arranged to have more than 150 articles appear on the same day in the 11 medical journals it publishes. These articles demonstrated that the genetic revolution is here and there can be no turning back. Innocence lost cannot be regained, even as ethical issues become more complex and subtle.

A month later, in another dramatic development, a team of French researchers headed by Daniel Cohen of the Centre d'Etude du Polymorphisme Humain in Paris announced the first comprehensive map of all the human chromosomes. The "map" consists of the locations of some 2000 genetic markers and about 33,000 types of living yeast cells, each with a particular segment of a human chromosome engineered into it. A worker interested in a particular segment of a chromosome can order the segment with a marker on it from the French group. Although this is a far cry from the complete map of every gene that is under development, it is an important step along the way. Even before this, somewhat more detailed maps had been published for chromosome 21 and for the Y chromosome.

It is useful to characterize the new developments in genetic medicine under three main headings: basic genetic science that has immediate or long-range medical applications; specific discoveries of how some alleles of genes result in defects that hamper the lives of humans in whom such genes are expressed; and the use of genetic engineering techniques to alleviate, prevent, or cure disease. Another important series of genetic advances, the application to diagnoses, followed by conventional treatment if needed, is considered in more detail in the section of *Handbook of Current Health and Medicine* that deals with diagnosis, beginning on page 469.

Background

Most cells contain recognizable small pairs of bodies called *chromosomes*. Each chromosome consists primarily of a large molecule of *deoxyribonucleic acid (DNA)*, which has the structure of a ladder that has been twisted. When chromosomes double, the DNA untwists and each new chromosome gets one of the uprights of the ladder. Each of the two uprights is then used to build a new chromosome that, barring mistakes, is exactly like the original before the doubling.

Mitosis is the name for the process in which each upright of the DNA ladder unwinds, separates from its mirror image, and then builds a new chromosome with two uprights. Mitosis results in two identical chromosomes where once there was one. Then the cell has twice as many chromosomes as it needs or that would be good for it, so it divides in two. The result is two identical cells, called daughter cells. If all goes well, each daughter cell is exactly like its parent insofar as DNA is concerned. All cells have undergone mitosis somewhere along the way, since each organism starts with a single cell and every cell is the daughter, usually many generations removed, of that original cell.

Although each chromosome doubles in normal cell division, in the division that produces egg or sperm cells for animals or plants the chromosome pairs separate instead of doubling. *Meiosis* is a different process of chromosome separation that occurs only in cells that give rise to ova (eggs) and sperm. It is more complex than mitosis. As a result of meiosis, four nonidentical daughter cells are produced, each with half the chromosomes of the original cell. If all has gone well, each daughter cell contains one and only one member of the original pairs. If all has not gone well, serious genetic disease can result in offspring. In one of the early stages of meiosis, parts of DNA molecules are sometimes exchanged between members of a pair of chromosomes, so the resulting chromosome in the daughter cell may not be exactly like either original chromosome in the parent.

A mnemonic device can help differentiate between mitosis and meiosis. Think of the cell that divides asexually as *it*, as in mITosis, while the sexual one, mEiosis, has an *e*, just like *sEx*.

By the 1940s it was already apparent that mitosis and meiosis are used to transmit hereditary characteristics from one cell to its daughters, although the role of DNA and the mechanism involved were not understood until the 1950s. Since such characteristics are expressed in the cells and ultimately in the whole organism, the DNA can be said to control cell development as well as heredity.

Each upright of the DNA twisted ladder, or *double helix* to use a more technical name, carries the information needed for this process in the form of strings of four different subunits called *nucleotides.*, which consist of a part of the upright of the ladder attached to a "half rung" called a *base*. It is the bases that are different. The bases are adenine, thymine, guanine, and cytosine, usually abbreviated to A, T, G, and C. Although each DNA molecule contains the same four bases, the number and arrangement varies enormously. It is the exact arrangement that is preserved when a chromosome doubles itself.

A sequence of bases, usually hundreds of bases long or even thousands of bases long in some cases, that is a single unit of heredity is called a *gene*. The average gene has about 1500 bases. To understand exactly what a gene does, it is necessary to have a clearer understanding of what a protein is than the common understanding of proteins as one of the six nutrients people require.

The work and structure of all cells is mainly carried out by or consists of a group of highly variable complex polymerized chemicals called *proteins*. "Highly variable complex polymerized" means that protein molecules are very large structures built from a moderate number of chemical building blocks that interact with each other to produce effective shapes. Each protein is constructed from combinations of 20-some subunits called *amino acids*. The information in the sequence of bases in DNA called a gene is a method of describing each protein to elements in the cell that then use that information to assemble the giant molecules. Nearly every combination of three of the four bases A, T, G, and C identifies exactly one amino acid. DNA is such a large molecule that the average chromosome can describe tens of thousands of proteins. Since each sequence of bases describing exactly one protein is a gene, the 23 pairs of human chromosomes carry the information for about a hundred thousand genes. Not all of these genes are active at any one time, but mechanisms based ultimately in the DNA turn genes on and off as needed. Indeed, in addition to the genes, the DNA of plants and animals contains long sequences of bases that seem to do nothing.

Recall that the definition of *protein* uses the phrase "highly variable." Substitution of one or two amino acids in a protein may or may not affect the way it works in the body. The same is true of the loss or addition of a few amino acids. Genes that are mainly alike, but not exactly the same, produce slightly different proteins or, in some cases, fail to produce a protein at all. The different forms of a gene that occupy a particular locus on a chromosome are called *alleles*. Originally alleles were recognized on the basis of large dichotomies in organisms, such as the difference between smooth and wrinkled pea seeds. A more modern view is that alleles are similar sequences of DNA that produce different forms of a given protein if they succeed in producing a protein—sometimes the differences between DNA sequences cause the gene to fail completely. Thus, instead of there being two different forms of a gene, there may be as many as 30 or 40 that occur relatively often and 300 or 400 that occur rarely. There could theoretically be hundreds or thousands of different alleles for a complex gene.

A gene by itself does not do anything. It is a record of information, like a file on a computer disk drive. You need a complex machine to turn the magnetic patterns on a disk drive into words or pictures on a screen. Think of proteins as the equivalent of words and pictures if the gene is the equivalent of bits recorded magnetically on a disk drive.

Involved every step of the way in the production of proteins from the genetic information, and sometimes acting for itself alone, is *ribonucleic acid (RNA)*, a polymer made from four different bases that are strung out along a backbone made from a simple sugar and phosphoric acid. The four bases are like those of DNA except that thymine (T) is replaced with the similar base uracil (U), so the four bases of RNA are cytosine (C), guanine (G), adenine (A), and uracil.

In a simplified view of how a protein is made, the main actors are various forms of RNA. The first step is *transcription,* in which a type of RNA called messenger RNA forms along the DNA and matches it base for base—that is, each C on the DNA matches a G on the RNA and vice versa while each A on the DNA matches a U on RNA and each T on DNA matches an A on RNA. Thus the RNA is just like the complementary strand of DNA except for the substitution of U for T. The messenger RNA then moves to a ribosome, a complex with some proteins, where the second process, *translation*, takes place. In the ribosome, the messenger RNA is pulled through the ribosome one codon at a time (a *codon* is a pattern of three bases such as ACC or UAU that represents a single amino acid or the beginning or end of a gene). As each codon passes through, it is matched with a small molecule of RNA called a transfer RNA. The transfer RNA has brought along an amino acid from among those that are just floating around in the cell waiting to be picked up by a transfer RNA. Twenty-odd special proteins match the appropriate transfer RNA and amino acid. The transfer RNAs drop off their amino acids in the ribosome, where they are added one at a time to the new protein chain that is forming there. When a stop codon is reached, the protein chain pops out and the messenger RNA leaves the ribosome.

Note that the above description is simplified. One simplification is that all the action of most of the already existing proteins that make this process take place has been omitted. Left to itself, DNA does nothing and RNA, versatile as it is, does not do much. A group of proteins is there to assemble the RNA on the DNA template to begin with, for example. This group is called a *transcription factor* or *transcription machine*. Its main component is a protein called RNA polymerase. Another group of about 80 proteins operates the ribosome.

Another simplification is that something needs to turn the gene on in the first place so that the various steps toward protein synthesis can take place. This is a different gene that encodes a different protein. Similarly, a third gene and concomitant protein is needed to turn the whole process off.

Other simplifications include leaving out the process of *methylization* in which chemicals called methyl groups are attached to the messenger RNA to protect parts of it from special chemicals designed to cut it to pieces; and omitting the processing that removes "junk" parts of RNA before it reaches the ribosome (for organisms other than bacteria, there is generally more junk than functioning RNA).

The hypothesis that each gene makes (through several steps involving RNA) one protein and that each protein stems from a single gene goes back to 1941, when very little was understood about the physical nature of genes. At that time proteins were moderately well understood. By 1953 Frederick Sanger was able, in a heroic effort, to analyze completely for the first time the structure of a fairly small protein, insulin. That was the same year that James Watson and Francis Crick deduced the structure of DNA, the key step in unraveling the physical basis of genetics. Within a few years, the principal action had shifted from studying proteins to studying genes. The genetic code was deciphered and machines were developed that could find the sequence of bases on DNA that make up the code. This advance removed a big part of the difficult biochemical problem of describing the structures of proteins and replaced it with the largely solved problem of deciphering a gene.

Knowledge of the genetic code and resulting protein allows the tools of *genetic engineering* to be applied. Genetic engineering is any practice in which genes are deliberately altered in living cells. At one end of the spectrum it consists of modifying a gene in a bacterium or yeast to produce a protein that would be difficult to obtain in another way. At the other end it consists of altering the genetic structure of a sexually reproducing animal so that some of its offspring also carry and express the same gene. In between are such techniques as inserting cells with modified genes into an individual, either temporarily or so that they are incorporated into tissues or organs permanently. The proteins produced by genetic engineering range from replacements for a protein missing or damaged as a result of a hereditary disease to proteins specifically intended to cause the immune system to attack and destroy specific cells.

Genetic engineering had its tentative beginning in 1973. In 1975 there were six laboratories in the United States and a few outside the United States that conducted genetic engineering. By the early 1990s the practice was almost commonplace. Even some high schools were performing genetic engineering experiments as part of the curriculum.

The diseases involved, that is the genetic disorders, number more than a thousand. By the end of 1993 about 40 of these diseases have been traced to the gene responsible and many others have been located on a particular sections of a given chromosome.

Much of the basic research that may eventually have medical impact is highly technical; scientists are still trying to find the complete pathway from a string of codons in DNA to a moderately complex expressed trait, such as hair color. The more they find, however, the more difficult the problems seem. When Gregor Mendel experimented with peas, he was able to find very simple expressions of either/or genes. Plants were either tall or short, but not of an intermediate height. Seeds were either smooth or wrinkled.

No known human gene is as simple as the pea genes in Mendel's experiments (indeed, there is some evidence that the pea genes were not that simple either, so Mendel doctored his data to make his point better). Scientists do not know how to class a human population into tall and short, for instance, and to predict on the basis of the parental genes what the heights of the children might be.

When it comes to disease, the picture is just as complicated. Researchers originally believed that since one gene produced a single protein, understanding the protein would explain all the effects of a defective gene. This has not worked in most cases because the situation is normally complicated by:

1. different alleles of the gene producing different versions of the protein;

2. the protein producing different effects in one place in the body from the effects in another;

3. different versions of the protein interacting with other gene products in unexpected ways;

4. the timing of the gene being turned on or off being affected by which alleles of the gene are present on the two chromosomes in the pair;

5. the effects of different alleles of genes other than the one responsible for producing the given protein;

6. interactions with the environment; and

7. probably other factors that have not been revealed yet.

The result of these complications is that diagnosis, including prenatal diagnosis, and treatment are not nearly so simple as people once believed. People who carry two copies of an allele that in others produces disease symptoms may not have the disease expressed; or, one symptom of a disease syndrome may be expressed in some case, while other symptoms fail to appear. There are apparently as many as 350 alleles of

MUTANT, MISSING, DEFECTIVE, OR
JUST PLAIN DIFFERENT GENES

Articles in the popular press and even some scientific writings often refer to a disease as being caused by a "defective" or a "missing" gene. One headline in a popular article in 1993 referred to a "mutant" gene. The article itself concerned the discovery by Richard B. Weinberg of the Bowman Gray School of Medicine at Wake Forest University and coworkers, reported in November 1993, of a gene that seems to prevent cholesterol in food from becoming low-density lipoprotein (LDL) in the blood. Since LDL is nick-named "bad cholesterol" for its presumed involvement in heart disease, possession of such a gene would seem to be a benefit. Despite this apparent advantage, the report, besides calling the gene "mutant," also calls it "flawed."

The "mutant" gene appears in 15 percent of the population in places like the U.S. where a high-fat diet is common, although the version that fails to convert dietary cholesterol into LDL is rarer in parts of the world where people normally eat a low-fat diet. This is reminiscent of the statistics for sickle-cell anemia, a gene carried by 20 percent or more of the population in parts of Africa, but of very low frequency, if present at all, in cool regions of the world. In the case of the sickle-cell gene, the trade-off between a less effective form of hemoglobin in some individuals with sickle-cell disease and protection from malaria in many carriers of the sickle-cell trait is well known.

Another helpful mutant gene was discovered in the small Italian village of Limone (pop. 996 in 1992) in 1982. This gene apparently originated in the marriage of a couple in 1644. Because of the isolation of the village, 44 of the residents still possess the gene, which enables its protein product, called A-1 (like the sauce), to bind and release fat molecules faster, preventing cholesterol from building up in the arteries.

Probably the genes that reduce LDL or cholesterol build-up are called "mutant" to avoid the much more common "defective." The hemoglobin gene in sickle-cell anemia, along with many other genes involved in conditions that are classed as diseases, is often called defective. The hemoglobin or other protein produced by a gene is often called defective as well. In most cases the label defective is used because the main function recognized for the gene is performed badly or not at all as a result of changes in the DNA code. The "mutant" gene produces a protein that is only one amino-acid different from that produced by nonmutant genes.

Perhaps even more alarming than a mutant or a defective gene is a "missing" gene. A gene is missing if a significant stretch of DNA somehow does not make it into an egg or a sperm, although the corresponding gene of the paired chromosome is normally present, covering somewhat for the missing gene. In most cases, however, a "missing" gene is not completely missing, just inactive or ineffective for one reason or another. A gene could be perceived as missing if another gene that is supposed to turn on the apparently missing one fails to do so. Often, however, especially in the popular press, a person is identified as missing the gene that makes a particular protein when in truth the gene is present, it is turned on, and it makes a form of the protein that fails to accomplish some important task.

Geneticists experimentally create so-called "knock-out mice," in which a specific gene is "knocked out." The gene is not missing, as a hole is knocked out in manufacturing a switch box; instead it is knocked out as in boxing—put to sleep, permanently in this case. Instead of removing one gene from the DNA, a disruptive stretch of DNA is added to the gene.

Small differences in DNA sequences do not always result in genes that appear to be missing or defective. Often two different gene alleles make different forms of a protein that both function. If the two proteins appear to function equally well, the difference between the genes is called *neutral*. There is a considerable range from a pair of neutral genes to alleles in which one produces an effective gene and the other fails to produce a protein of any kind. In between are pairs of alleles with almost every possible kind of difference.

Thus, genes are seldom if ever truly missing and a particular allele can only be termed defective in terms of what people expect of it. In that sense, a gene that causes dietary cholesterol to become serum LDL is defective, even when it is present in 85 percent or more of the population. The allele that fails to produce this effect is the desirable gene. The same is true with the gene for the mutant A-1 protein. But most gene products accomplish more than a single task. From an evolutionary point of view, the version of the gene that is common in all populations and nearly universal in many of them probably has functions that tend to keep organisms alive or at least allow them to reproduce. Otherwise, since it is not a neutral gene, it would tend to be eliminated by natural selection, except in isolated populations such as a small village in the Italian mountains.

Indeed, one way to characterize the difference between alleles is to say that the common type is the "wild type." This is a bias-free description that does not imply that the wild type is better than the altered (not "domestic") gene.

It is almost always more accurate to speak or write of different alleles instead of mutant, missing, or defective genes. When an allele causes a recognizable suite of undesirable functioning, such as the alleles identified with muscular dystrophy, cystic fibrosis, Tay-Sachs disease, or colorectal cancer, a writer finds it difficult not to call the allele defective.

---

the gene involved in cystic fibrosis, 30 for Tay-Sachs disease, and 17 for Lesch-Nyhan syndrome.

Michael Kaback, who deals in genetic counseling at the University of California at San Diego, summarized the current state of genetic medicine as a good example of "the smarter you get, the less you know."

Genetic Screening

Knowing that the location of a gene is near a particular marker on a particular chromosome means that it is fairly easy to determine whether or not a particular allele is present. Searching for alleles connected with a disease or disease in general is called *genetic screening*. It becomes even more effective when the exact gene has been sequenced, since the gene can be recovered separately and analyzed to see which allele is present.

In modern times, newborns are routinely screened for various defects, ranging from poorly developed organs to chemical imbalances. On a state-by-state basis, screening for specific hereditary defects is mandatory. Until the rise of genetic engineering, the only defects that could be located in this way were those manifest at birth, either by observation of effects or measurement of enzyme levels.

More recently, genetic screening has been extended. It can now be done before birth using ultrasound, amniocentesis, chorionic villus sampling, and percutaneous umbilical blood sampling. Screening for hereditary diseases that do not produce noticeable symptoms until a person is older, perhaps only a few months older or perhaps when the person is as much as 30 years older, is also possible. In some prenatal screening and most screening for conditions that develop well after birth, genes are examined for harmful alleles.

Although such extension might appear noncontroversial, little in the realm of genetics happens without ethical questions being asked. On November 4, 1993, a panel of geneticists, pediatricians, genetic counselors, ethicists, and lawyers representing the Institute of Medicine of the U.S. National Academy of Sciences weighed in on the side of limiting genetic screening of newborns and fetuses. Their report, "Assessing Genetic Risks: Implication for Health and Social Policy," argued against testing for hereditary diseases known to be incurable at the time of the test, such as Duchenne muscular dystrophy. The panel argued that knowing that the disease, which usually causes death by the time the victim reaches his 20s, is present does nothing for the person being screened. The panel did not, however, call for a ban on genetic screening; they voted in favor of voluntary screening instead of the mandatory screening already the law in several states. They also felt that tests should be discouraged unless the tests lead to improved treatment of the person being tested. The panel was also concerned that employers or health insurers might use genetic screening of adults to discriminate against people genetically disposed toward a particular disease.

Some members of the panel disagreed with the conclusions regarding screening of newborns, pointing out in additional views submitted with the report that when quick treatment can mitigate or even reverse the course of the disease, mandatory screening can result in speedier care, such as putting a baby on a special diet or administering special supplements. Quick action can prevent permanent brain damage in the case of phenylketonuria (for which mandatory screening preceded genetic engineering) or hypothyroidism, and improves survival in the case of cystic fibrosis.

Often a single allele in a pair can produce a defective protein only if paired with another allele of exactly the same variety. One common disease for which this is true is sickle-cell anemia, which is caused by such a recessive gene. The person with one sickle-cell gene in the pair does not develop a serious illness, but a person with two sickle-cell genes does. Thus, the person with one sickle-cell gene is a *carrier*, who can transmit the full-blown disease to a child provided that the child's other parent also provides a sickle-cell gene. The Institute of Medicine report also argued against telling parents that their child is a carrier of a hereditary disease, although some panel members noted that the mother might want to know to make future reproductive choices.

This controversy is all about testing babies after they are born. Prenatal testing, with the possibility of elective abortion, is even more controversial. Opponents denounce the general practice of abortion to prevent diseases such as Duchenne muscular dystrophy or thalassemia as eugenics, but individual parents and doctors who make the decisions on a case by case basis are more likely pragmatists than eugenicists. For those diseases, and many others, a short and painful life is the best that can be forecast today.

But, as pointed out by Richard Horton, North American editor of the medical journal *Lancet,* the situation is even less obvious for diseases with longer life expectancies or with a late onset. He asks about the value of 25 years of life to a person with cystic fibrosis or, even more dramatically, 60 years of life before the onset of late-onset Alzheimer's disease. In between, there is Huntington's disease, which often has no noticeable symptoms until a person is in his or her 30s and then may cause 10 to 20 years of misery before death.

Furthermore, such testing is coming earlier and earlier, making abortion easier to contemplate. Since 1992 some "test tube" babies have been born after their genes were screened in a Petri dish before *in vitro* fertilization.

In New York City and Israel a group of Orthodox Jews have taken the issue to an earlier stage than prenatal testing, counseling young people on which partners are genetically dangerous to marry if healthy children are a goal. The program, known as Dor Yeshorim (Hebrew for "generation of the righteous"), began in 1983 as a response to Tay-Sachs disease, a hundred times more prevalent in Jews from central Europe than among the rest of the world. In this Jewish population, known as Ashkenazi, Tay-Sachs births are ten times as common as cystic fibrosis, the most common genetic disorder of European-descended non-Jews. Thousands of prospective couples have paid for tests in the Dor Yeshorim program, and hundreds of engagements have been terminated for genetic incompatibility.

The founder of the Dor Yeshorim program and his wife had four of their ten children die from Tay-Sachs disease, a devastating ailment that begins when a baby is about six months old and quickly progresses, leading invariably to death at an early age, usually within three years. Nearly every genetic ethicist cites Tay-Sachs disease as the clearest case in which genetic screening prevents much suffering with little to be said against it. Ashkenazi Jews also have a long tradition of partly arranged marriages, so couples seem less likely to rebel against restrictions, especially self-imposed as these are, on their freedom of choice.

As more and more destructive gene alleles have been identified, Dor Yeshorim has added two more hereditary diseases to its testing program—cystic fibrosis and Gaucher's disease. These are more problematical, since many different alleles and possibly additional genes are involved in cystic fibrosis and Gaucher's disease. (The most common type of Gaucher's disease may lead to anemia, bone pain, and enlarged liver or spleen. It usually shows no symptoms until about the age of 45 and even then it is controllable, although only with an expensive drug, Ceredase.)

The centers in Brooklyn, New York and Jerusalem are also planning to add Canavan's disease, which is similar in its age onset and prognosis for early death to Tay-Sachs disease, to Dor Yeshorim as soon as a genetic test for it becomes available.

The discovery of location of the gene for Canavan's disease was announced in early October 1993.

Cloning and Pre-implant Testing

Just how early an embryo can be tested so that those showing undesirable genes can be culled became clear when the first product of such a process was born, as reported in the September 9, 1992 issue of the *New England Journal of Medicine*. Alan H. Handyside of Hammersmith Hospital in London and coworkers along with the parents had chosen among six fertilized ova on the basis of genetic tests. Two of the six were implanted and the other four not used.

The main criteria used for acceptance or rejection of the fertilized ova was a test for the presence of a disease-causing allele of the CFTR gene that produces cystic fibrosis. Since 1992 doctors have come to realize that the cystic fibrosis picture is far more complicated than a "good gene, bad gene" situation, but that was not at issue in this case. (*See also* "Cystic Fibrosis and Viral Gene Delivery," p 70.) Happily, the girl born as a result of the tests is free of the disease.

Three couples, including the girl's parents, contributed fertilized ova to the experiment in hopes of obtaining disease-free offspring. One couple was only able to obtain an analysis of a single fertilized ovum, which was found to have two copies of the disease-causing allele. They elected not to have an untestable fertilized ovum or the one with the two undesirable genes implanted. Another couple chose two of five fertilized ova for implantation based on the results of the genetic tests, but the woman did not become pregnant.

In addition to the ethical problems involved, such testing makes an already costly procedure even more expensive. All the many concerns about expensive procedures are further complicated by the fact that treatment for persons with hereditary diseases can be even more expensive than embryo implantation and testing.

Although no implants have been tried, the whole ethical puzzle becomes even more difficult with the advent of artificial twinning for humans. In this form of producing twins, sometimes called "cloning," an embryo that is still a cluster of cells on a petri dish is broken apart. At that early stage in development, each part can continue normal development. While so far as is known, no one has then proceeded to implant the twins in one or two prospective mothers, there appears to be no technical impediment to the success of such a procedure. (*See also* "Don't Call It Cloning," p 93.)

Combining embryo cloning with genetic testing of the embryo would have given two of the couples involved in the Hammersmith procedures an additional chance for a child that did not have even one copy of the disease-causing allele. Each couple had only one embryo for which both copies of the gene were alleles believed not to cause the disease. With cloning, that embryo could have been separated into several copies and each copy implanted. As it happened, however, without cloning, each of the two couples also chose to have an insurance embryo that would have grown into a carrier of the disease if implantation had been successful for that embryo.

The whole issue may also become more immediate with the imminent development of microelectronic gene analyzers and amplifiers, which are expected to speed up DNA analysis greatly and also to reduce costs significantly. The new technology is based on shaping automatic chemical devices on silicon wafers with lasers, the same technology already in use in manufacturing the most advanced chips for computers.

(Periodical references and further reading: *New York Times* 8-28-92, p C1; *New York Times* 8-13-92, p A7; *Harvard Health Letter* 3-93, p 3; *Science* 6-4-93, p 1422; *New York Times* 9-24-93, p A1; *Science* 11-12-93, p 984; *New York Times* 11-16-93, p C1; *Science* 10-22-93, p 533; *Science* 10-29-93, p 674; *Science News* 11-20-93, p 325; *New York Times* 11-5-93, p A20; *Science* 11-12-93, p 984; *New York Times* 11-17-93, p C17; *Science News* 11-20-93, p 325; *New York Times* 11-29-93, p A16; *Science* 11-19-93, p 1212; *New York Times* 12-7-93, p A1; *New York Times* 12-16-93, p A1; *Scientific American* 1-94, p 149; *Time* 1-17-94, p 46)

TIMETABLE OF GENETICS TO 1990

12,000 BC   The dog is the first animal to be domesticated, a process that probably results from genetic modification of wolves.

9000 BC   The first plant, a form of wheat, and also the first farm animals, goats and sheep, are domesticated in the Near East around this time; domestication is a process that results in the genetic modification of wild plants and animals to make them more suitable for human use; after this time domestication of various plants and animals occurs at various sites around the world.

1865   Gregor Mendel [born Heizendorf, Silesia, July 22, 1822; died Brünn, Bohemia, January 6, 1884] publishes his theories of genetics in the obscure *Transactions of the Brünn Natural History Society;* he is the first to demonstrate, in experiments on pea plants, that genes come in pairs and can have two forms; he postulates dominant and recessive genes.

1883   Francis Galton's [born Birmingham, England, February 16, 1822; died Haslemere, England, January 17, 1911] *Enquiries into Human Faculty* introduces the term *eugenics* and suggests that human beings can be improved by selective breeding.

1900   During this year, Hugo Marie De Vries [born Haarlem, Netherlands, February 16, 1848; died Lunteren, Netherlands, July 20, 1888], Karl Franz Joseph Correns [born Munich, Germany, September 19, 1864; died Berlin, February 14, 1933], and Erich Tschermak von Seysenegg [born Vienna, Austria, November 12, 1871; died Vienna, October 11, 1962] independently rediscover Gregor Mendel's work on genetics, which had been ignored for 40 years.

1901   The journal *Biometrika*, in which psychologists support the idea of eugenics, is founded.

1905   Clarence McClung finds that female mammals have two X chromosomes and that males have an X paired with a Y.

1907   Thomas Hunt Morgan [born Lexington, Kentucky, September 25, 1866; died Pasadena, California, December 4, 1945] starts experiments with the fruit fly *Drosophila melanogaster* that establish that the units of heredity are located in cells on small bodies called chromosomes.

1909   Wilhelm Johannsen [born Copenhagen, Denmark, February 3, 1857; died Copenhagen, November 11, 1927] coins the word *gene* to describe the unit of heredity.

1910   Thomas Hunt Morgan discovers that some genes in fruit flies are linked to a particular sex; in *D. melanogaster* a white-eyed mutation appears in males only.

1911   Thomas Hunt Morgan starts mapping genes in the fruit fly to particular chromosomes.

1918   The number of human chromosomes per cell is counted (incorrectly) for the first time; Herbert M. Evans counts 48.

1934   In Norway, the hereditary disease phenylketonuria is recognized; it produces a characteristic mental retardation.

1936   Andrei Nikolaevitch Belozersky isolates deoxyribonucleic acid (DNA) for the first time.

1941   George Wells Beadle [born Wahoo, Nebraska, October 22, 1903; died Pomona, California, June 9, 1989] and Edward Lawrie Tatum [born Boulder, Colorado, December 14, 1909; died New York, November 5, 1975] theorize that each enzyme is controlled by a single gene.

1944   Oswald Theodore Avery [born Halifax, Canada, October 21, 1877; died Nashville, Tennessee, February 20, 1955], Colin MacLeod, and Maclyn McCarthy determine that DNA in chromosomes is the repository of genes; genes had been generally believed to be proteins prior to this discovery.

1953   James Watson [born Chicago, Illinois, April 6, 1928] and Francis Crick [born Northampton, England, June 8, 1918] determine the structure of DNA, the basis of heredity; DNA is a double helix that carries genetic information in combinations of four different nucleotides that form the strands of the helix.

1954   J. Lin Tjio and Albert Levan show that humans have 46 chromosomes arranged in 23 pairs, rather than 48 as was previously believed.

1959   Scientists establish that the chromosome known as Y confers maleness in humans; a human with two X chromosomes will normally be female, although there can be exceptions if male genes cross over.

David A. Hungerford [born Brockton, Massachusetts, May 7, 1927; died 1993] and Peter C. Nowell [born Philadelphia, Pennsylvania, February 8, 1928] discover that the blood cancer chronic granulocytic leukemia is linked to a specific change visible on chromosome 22, the first direct evidence that chromosomes, and by implication genes, are involved in causing cancer.

Jérôme Lejeune [born Montrouge, France, June 13, 1926; died Paris, April 3, 1994] discovers that an extra chromosome is the cause of Down's syndrome.

1960   W. R. Centerwall proposes that phenylketonuria symptoms of mental retardation can be prevented by restricting individuals with the disease to a diet free of the amino acid phenylalinine.

1961   Marshall Nirenberg [born New York, April 10, 1927] and J. H. Matthaei of the U.S. National Institutes of Health learn to read one of the "letters" of the genetic code when they find that a combination of three uracil bases in a row (UUU—called a *codon*) in ribonucleic acid (RNA) codes for the amino acid phenylalinine.

1967   Charles Yanofsky [New York, April 17, 1925] is the first to prove that the sequence of codons in a gene determines exactly the sequence of amino acids in the protein that is the gene product.

1968   Werner Arber [born Granichen, Switzerland, June 3, 1929] discovers restriction enzymes, a class of proteins that will make genetic engineering possible.

David Zipser [born New York, May 31, 1937] discovers the meaning of the last remaining undeciphered codon of the genetic code in RNA, the pattern uracil-guanine-adenine (UGA) that means "stop making this protein."

1969   Jonathan Beckwith [born Cambridge, Massachusetts, December 25, 1935] and coworkers are the first to isolate a single gene.

Roger Donahue is the first to map a human gene to a chromosome other than the X and Y chromosomes; it is the gene for the "Duffy" blood type.

1970   Har Gobin Khorana [born Raipur, India, January 9, 1922] and coworkers produce the first artificial gene.

Howard Temin [born Philadelphia, Pennsylvania, December 10, 1934] and David Baltimore [born New York, March 7, 1938] discover the enzyme that causes RNA to be transcribed to DNA, a key step in the development of genetic engineering.

1973   Stanley N. Cohen [born Perth Amboy, New Jersey, February 17, 1935] and Herbert W. Boyer [born Pittsburgh, Pennsylvania, July 10, 1936] succeed in putting a specific gene into a bacterium, the first instance of true genetic engineering.

1977   Phillip A. Sharp [born Falmouth, Kentucky, June 6, 1944] and, independently, Richard J. Roberts [born Derby, England, September 6, 1943], and coworkers discover that DNA in organisms more complex than bacteria contains long stretches of apparently meaningless material that is not part of any gene; the sequence of noncoding nucleotides is labeled an *intron*.

1978   David Botstein [born Zurich, Switzerland, September 8, 1942], Ronald W. Davis [born Marda, Illinois, July 17, 1941], and Mark H. Skolnick [born Temple, Texas, January 28, 1946] propose at a conference in April that DNA sequencing can be used to develop gene markers for various genetic diseases.

1979   Human insulin is synthesized by genetic engineering methods.

Arnold J. Levine [born Brooklyn, New York, July 30, 1939] of Princeton University and David Lane of the Molecular Research Council in Cambridge, England, discover a protein involved in cancer in monkeys that they name p53 and locate the gene that produces the protein; the p53 gene is later discovered to be key to the development of many forms of cancer in humans.

1980   The pharmaceutical firm Eli Lilly starts the production and testing of human insulin, using genetically altered bacteria; the insulin can be used by diabetics that are allergic to insulin obtained from animals.

Martin Cline and coworkers transfer genes from one mouse to another and succeed in having the gene function in the new organism.

The successful production of human interferon in bacteria is announced by Charles Weissmann of the University of Geneva.

1981   The genetic code for the hepatitis B surface antigen is found, opening up the possibility of a bioengineered vaccine.

At Ohio University in Athens, Ohio scientists transfer genes from other organisms into mice for the first time.

1982   The U.S. Food and Drug Administration grants approval to Eli Lilly & Company to market human insulin produced by bacteria, the first commercial product of genetic engineering.

The Swedish firm Kabivitrum produces synthetic growth hormone using genetically engineered bacteria.

1983   Scientists show that a protein produced by genetically engineered yeast can protect chimpanzees against hepatitis B.

1984   Workers at the New York State Department of Health develop a genetically modified vaccinia virus that protects animals against hepatitis B, herpes simplex, and influenza.

The first clinical trials of a vaccine against hepatitis B produced by yeast that has been given genes for a surface molecule of the hepatitis virus start on June 1.

David, known as "the boy in the bubble" because he lived for 12 years in a plastic bubble to protect against diseases, dies; he lived in the bubble because he was a victim of the genetic condition known as Severe Combined Immunodeficiency Disease (SCID), which results in an ineffective immune system; an attempt to correct his SCID with donated bone marrow failed to take, and death followed soon after.

1985   The U.S. Food and Drug Administration in October approves marketing growth hormone manufactured by bacteria, the second drug produced by genetic engineering (after human insulin) to be sold in the United States.

1986   The U.S. Food and Drug Administration in July approves a hepatitis B vaccine made by yeast, the first vaccine to be approved for humans that is produced by genetic engineering.

The first genetically altered virus (for herpes in swine) is marketed and the first field trials of a genetically altered plant begin.

Louis Kunkel [born New York, October 13, 1949] and coworkers discover the gene that is defective in Duchenne muscular dystrophy, a common, fatal form of the disease.

1987   Experimental vaccination of foxes against rabies begins in Belgium, using baits containing a vaccine created by genetic engineering and dropped from helicopters; the experiment is successful and leads to a large-scale vaccination campaign.

1988   Rudolf Jaenisch and coworkers announce on March 10 that they have succeeded in implanting the gene for a hereditary disease of humans in mice; this opens the way to study such diseases more easily and leads to improved treatment.

1989   In September, Francis Collins, Lap-Chee Tsui, and coworkers find and make copies of the gene that causes most cystic fibrosis.

W. French Anderson [born Tulsa, Oklahoma, December 31, 1936], Michael Blaese [born Minneapolis, Minnesota, February 16, 1939], and Kenneth W. Culver use genetic engineering to tag cells called tumor-infiltrating lymphocytes and inject them into cancer patients; while the primary purpose is to trace the movement of the lymphocytes through the body, this is the first introduction of cells altered by genetic engineering into humans.

NEW DEVELOPMENTS IN GENETIC SCIENCE

FINDING GENES FASTER

The physical means by which biologists unravel genetic mechanisms are complex and clever. In most cases, the methods used are more mysterious to the nonscientist than the results obtained. People accept that a gene has been found and that it codes for a particular protein without having a clear notion of what has been done to locate or to analyze the gene.

The intellectual task is called "decoding." The process is akin to taking a long message written with only four symbols repeated in an ever-changing pattern page after page with no breaks and finding which parts represent discrete letters and which combinations of run-together letters are words. Furthermore, when the words are located, they are in a different language and need to be translated. Faced with such a task, the cryptographer and the biologist utilize many of the same methods.

In the case of gene location, many of the important functional parts of the code have been known for years—the codes used to start and stop a gene, for example. Still, the message is not written on sheets of paper or available in any visible way. Not only must the code be broken, but also ways to observe the "letters"—the codons, as they are called—need to be found. Mostly this is accomplished by chemical means. Although the methods employed are vastly more complex than the analytical chemistry you may recall from high school, the means and observables are not all that different.

One of the first steps in the chemical process of decoding is to split the message into fragments. A chemical can be used to break the message at specific locations. The resulting fragments can be separated from each other by weight or by electrical activity.

Because genes are biochemicals, biological activity of various types can also be used to locate particular sequences of codons. The double-helix structure of DNA is famous. When the two strands of a fragmented helix are separated and then the single-strand fragments allowed to re-mingle, natural affinities link mirror image strands. Once a known sequence is obtained as a single strand, it can be used to pick out its mirror image from a soup of fragments. The fragments do not have to match exactly, but sequences that are similar will cling to each other at the places that are the mirror images. Since 1981, much of the process of chemically finding sequences of bases in DNA has been increasingly automated. Despite automation, the search for a specific sequence often involves many false trails and is quite time consuming.

A new technique for scanning DNA to find matches, developed by Patrick O. Brown of Stanford University Medical Center and coworkers, was described in the May 1993 issue of *Nature Genetics*. After fragments are allowed to re-link, enzymes destroy all but perfect matches. If DNA fragments from two individuals are mixed together, the stretches that they have in common can be located quickly. This is much faster than previous methods that involved a lot of partial matches and inference. So far, however, the new technique, called Genomic Mismatch Scanning or GMS, has only been completely successful on yeast, although preliminary trials with human DNA have been encouraging.

(Periodical References and Additional Reading: *Science News* 5-8-93, p 294)

PATENTING GENES

To the layperson the idea that human genes can be patented is patently absurd. Will scientists next will want to patent the human elbow or eye? Nevertheless, in the United States patent applications were prepared by the thousands in 1991-92 for something approximating human genes.

The U.S. Patent and Trademark Office (PTO) received a patent application for 347 gene fragments from the U.S. National Institutes of Health (NIH) in the fall of 1991. In February 1992 the NIH filed for patents on another 2375 fragments. In the fall of 1992, the NIH added an additional 3400 fragments, bringing the total to 6122 pieces of DNA. Others had filed for patents on genes earlier and more continue to do so. Within a few years, according to one estimate, patent applications will have been filed for every one of the approximately 100,000 genes in the human genome. Although all these applications were initially rejected by the PTO, the U.S. Health and Human Services Department has continued to press for patent recognition.

NIH Files for Patents on the Brain's DNA

In June 1991 J. Craig Venter, then of the U.S. National Institute of Neurological Disorders and Stroke, announced that his project for locating and sequencing the bases on all human genes expressed in the brain would patent its results as the project proceeded. Many scientists strongly objected. James Watson, then director of the Human Genome Project, led the critics by saying that "virtually any monkey" could do the kind of work Venter and his group were doing. Most critics believed that the work failed to meet the U.S. patent law requirements that the work be new, nonobvious, and useful—especially the nonobvious and useful criteria. The methods Venter's group used are common to much of genetic research and the applications are at this point unknown.

When Venter's group first made its scientific intentions plain in an article in the June 21, 1991 issue of *Science,* a few thousand human genes had been sequenced by various scientists and listed in a central repository called GenBank. The first Venter report noted that although his group was finding a lot of junk, they also had located a couple of hundred pieces of genes that controlled something unknown in human brains. Venter's project came to the attention of patent attorney Max Hensley, who proposed to the NIH Office of Technology Transfer office that the pieces be patented to protect them from unauthorized use by commercial companies. The idea was passed on to Venter, who filed for patents not only for the 347 "expressed sequence tags," or base sequences of complementary DNA (cDNA) that can used as probes, but also for the entire (but still unknown) gene sequence incorporating the tags and for

TAGS AND FISHING FOR GENES

The actual "devices" for which the NIH patent applications were filed are sequences of what is known as *complementary DNA* (cDNA) from clones of human brain genes and other human genes. First, messenger RNA is collected from human brain tissue, with each molecule a template created from a specific gene. A new DNA strand is formed on each molecule of the messenger RNA, which is called complementary DNA since it is the complement, found by matching bases, of the messenger RNA; otherwise, cDNA is exactly the same as any single-stranded DNA. The sequence of bases in cDNA can be read by a gene scanning machine, although it takes time. A sequence of about 350 to 500 bases from a gene is enough, however, to be likely to be unique to that gene. Such a tag can then be synthesized in other automatic machines. The tag can be made easy to retrieve by labeling it with a radioactive tracer or in some other way. The synthetic cDNA tag can then be used as a baited hook to fish for entire gene.

This is not necessarily easy. Some of the expressed sequence tags are very short, perhaps only 6 or 7 codons long. Such a short sequence of codons may be a part of many genes. Longer tags are more useful. Despite the difficulties, the method has sometimes been successful in finding a specific gene.

Even after a gene is located, its function must be determined. Until recently, at least most patents for naturally occurring substances described the function rather than the chemical composition. The Harvard patent on protein GP120, issued in 1988, did not give a specific sequence of amino acids, for example.

the expressed protein—although he dropped the application for the protein after the first applications were rejected. Commentators differ on whether any or all of the remaining claims will be granted by the PTO; the legal maneuvering is expected to take years.

Policy Responses and Other Consequences

Other branches of the U.S. government are also involved in the dispute. The NIH Office of Technology Transfer, headed by Reid Adler, has been the main backer of gene patenting. In November 1991 the White House Office of Science and Technology Policy joined the fracas; they announced that a policy on patenting genes would be delineated early in 1992. In December 1992, however, the PTO rejected the NIH bid. But early in 1993 the NIH submitted a revised application.

The U.S. Congress has asked its own Office of Technology Assessment (OTA) to study the situation and report to Congress by spring 1994. OTA hearings in July 1993 brought scientists from around the world to testify, all of them opposed to even the concept of patenting genes or tags for genes.

In the meantime, various other attempts to patent genes are winding up in the courts. In October 1992, for example, C. Thomas Caskey of the Howard Hughes

Medical Institute at Baylor College of Medicine identified and cloned one of the genes that regulate normal development of the brain and filed for a patent in hopes of producing a commercial test that could be used to prevent the birth of children with defects in that gene. But it has since been established that six of the expressed sequence tags that the NIH is trying to patent are part of the Caskey gene, clouding Caskey's application and possibly delaying development of the genetic screening test.

The NIH support for the concept of patenting has led genetic researchers throughout the U.S. to file for patents on their own work. Venter himself left the NIH at midnight on July 13, 1992 to become a leader in the most active group, a private venture named the Institute for Genomic Research with a commercial arm called Human Genome Sciences that is allied with the pharmaceutical firm SmithKline Beecham. Venter took most of his staff with him, about 30 researchers. Although the number of patent applications filed by the new Venter operation has not been revealed, workers there claim to be finding several hundred tags each day, mostly of DNA from the human brain.

Although the various commercial patent applications are also on hold, they are not being ignored. For example, one of the groups working on the gene in which a defect causes Duchenne muscular dystrophy applied for a patent on it. The rights to the patent application were then sold to a commercial biotechnology firm. While the NIH applications were not involved and the PTO has not granted the patent, the mere application for a patent has led to threats of lawsuits by the biotechnology firm. In turn, the threat of legal action is disrupting some research on muscular dystrophy.

Despite objections to gene patenting by most scientists outside the U.S., some commercial operations have fewer doubts. The Sagami Chemical Research Institute in Japan (a commercial firm, despite the name) filed for patents on 70 stretches of DNA in April 1993. Government operations are not immune to the lure of patents either. Britain's Medical Research Council filed for patents on more than a thousand tags in August 1992, claiming the filing was a defensive action in response to the NIH. In both France and Britain, government applications were withdrawn after official reconsideration. At the end of 1993, a number of European professional societies and charities devoted to particular diseases had, to one degree or another, announced opposition to gene patenting. Some would ban patenting of tags but permit patenting of genes, while others would ban patenting of tags and whole genes, but permit patenting of tests, devices, drugs, and procedures that incorporate particular genes.

TIMETABLE OF GENE PATENTS

1789	The United States enacts its first patent law.
1949	Because of an increase in patent applications involving specific organisms, the U.S. Patent and Trademark Office (PTO) requires that an example of the actual organism be submitted along with the patent.
1969	Jonathan Beckwirth and coworkers are the first to isolate a single gene; it is the bacterial gene for a step in the metabolism of sugar.
1970	Har Gobind Khorana and coworkers at the University of Wisconsin announce the first complete synthesis of a gene, the gene for analine-transfer RNA; although previous workers had synthesized genes using natural genes as templates, this gene was assembled directly from its chemical components.

The PTO extends patent protection to plant seeds.

1976   Khorana and coworkers announce construction of the first completely functional synthetic gene along with its regulators.

1980   The U.S. Supreme Court rules that a microbe developed by Ananda K. Chakrabarty for General Electric to use in oil cleanup can be patented, allowing the first patent for microorganisms produced by people.

Stanley N. Cohen of Stanford University and Herbert W. Boyer of the University of California at San Francisco receive the first patent issued for a method of genetic engineering; royalties on the patent go to their universities, which applied for the patent in 1974 along with an application for a patent on the results of using the technique.

1981   Bio Logicals of Toronto, Ontario, announces that the first fast and inexpensive gene synthesizer, a device for automatically assembling DNA or RNA sequences to order, will go on sale.

1984   On August 28 Cohen and Boyer's patent on recombinant DNA molecules containing foreign genes in bacteria (plasmids), applied for in 1974, is granted; a request for the use of recombinant DNA molecules in yeasts is put off for later decision.

1985   PTO grants a patent for a genetically engineered species of maize (corn), the first patent for a eukaryote (higher life form).

1986   The U.S. Department of Agriculture grants the Biologics Corporation of Omaha, Nebraska the world's first license to market a living organism produced by genetic engineering; it is a virus used as a vaccine to prevent herpes in swine.

The U.S. Federal Technology Transfer Act becomes law; some interpret this law to mean that any human genes found by U.S. researchers must be patented.

Leroy Hood and coworkers at CalTech announce development of an automated device that can determine the sequence of 10,000 bases along a DNA molecule in a 24-hour period.

1987   On April 21 the PTO extends patent protection to all animals except humans; humans are deemed not eligible for patenting because of the Thirteenth Amendment to the U.S. Constitution, which forbids slavery; unanswered is the question of how much of the human genome need be involved to invoke the Thirteenth Amendment.

The Board of Patent Appeals and Interferences rules that sterile genetically engineered oysters that grow to be especially plump can be patented.

More than 6000 patents related to genetic engineering are pending before the PTO, including patents for 21 genetically engineered animals.

Researchers from MIT and Collaborative Research, Inc., announce that they have mapped over 400 markers that can be used to identify human genes.

The U.S. Department of Energy announces that its goal is to map the human genome.

1988   On February 16 the PTO issues a patent to Harvard University for commercial use of the naturally occurring protein Gp120, patentable because Harvard isolated the protein, a part of the HIV virus, in 1984.

On April 12 the PTO issues patent No. 4,736,866 to Harvard Medical School for a mouse developed by Philip Leder and Timothy Y. Stewart by genetic engineering; it is the first U.S. patent issued for a vertebrate.

The U.S. National Institutes of Health (NIH) take the lead in mapping the human genome with James D. Watson as head of the Human Genome Project.

1991   In June Craig Venter of the NIH files for patents on 347 sequences of complementary DNA (cDNA), effectively parts of genes, from the human brain; his research group has used an automated process to find the sequence of bases in these fragments of cDNA, which were obtained from commercial sources of brain clones of cDNA.

1992   In August the PTO rejects an NIH application for patents on gene fragments; the application now includes more than 6000 fragments.

(Periodical References and Additional Reading: *New York Times* 7-28-92, p C1; *New York Times* 9-6-92, p IV-12; *New York Times* 10-8-92, p B26; *New York Times* 2-3-94, p A1; *Science News* 9-4-93, p 154; *Nature* 12-2-93, p 391)

DIETARY CORRECTIONS FOR GENETIC DISEASES

Many rules of inorganic chemistry do not apply to the complex chemicals made by living organisms. Although one water molecule is the same as any other water molecule, a protein from one organism is generally different than a protein from another organism, even one of the same species. Furthermore, an individual organism can produce more than one type of a given protein.

One of the best known examples of two types of a protein from an individual is hemoglobin (see also "Pigs and Other Animals Become More Human," p 47). Before birth, many mammals, including humans, produce a more effective form of hemoglobin, one that outcompetes the mother's hemoglobin. This insures that the fetus gets plenty of oxygen during development. A few months after birth, the body stops making the fetal form of hemoglobin, and an entirely different gene is switched on to make the normal adult form. Exactly why the gene for the fetal form is switched off and the one for the adult form is switched on is not known at this time, although it is likely that the fetal form is more "costly" in some way.

For some people, the fetal form is not switched off completely, however. As early as the 1970s physicians observed that some people continue to make and use fetal hemoglobin in some of their blood cells even as adults. This was first observed in people with sickle-cell anemia, a genetic disease characterized by malformed hemoglobin. Fetal hemoglobin is produced by a different gene from regular hemoglobin. Thus, defects in the genes that cause sickle-cell anemia or beta thalassemia do not affect the gene that produces fetal hemoglobin. Those anemic individuals whose fetal hemoglobin gene fails to shut down exhibit much milder symptoms of the disease, since at least some of their red blood cells contain effective fetal hemoglobin.

Genes do not switch off arbitrarily. Something triggers genes to shut off or to switch back on. In 1987 Susan P. Perrine of Children's Hospital Oakland (California) Research Institute and coworkers observed that a chemical in the blood of diabetic mothers delays the fetal hemoglobin shut-off. Perrine and her colleagues studied the switching mechanism and reached the conclusion that a common food additive, butyrate, is similar enough to the chemical in the diabetic mothers to warrant testing. Initial tests were run on three patients with sickle-cell anemia and three patients with beta thalassemia. By January 14, 1993 the team could report in the *New England Journal of Medicine* that butyrate, given by injection, resulted in significant increases in fetal hemoglobin and no consequential side effects in the six patients in the study. A planned second round of tests will use oral butyrate and a larger group of patients.

The same journal also carried a report from a team using drugs to increase fetal hemoglobin in anemias. A combination of a powerful anticancer drug that blocks DNA reproduction and a growth factor for red blood cells also increased concentrations of fetal hemoglobin, but the treatment posed the risk of serious side effects.

(Periodical References and Further Reading: *New York Times* 1-14-93; *Science News* 1-23-94, p 52)

GENETICALLY ENGINEERED FOODS

Early in 1994 the first genetically engineered foods were expected to go on the market, although genetic engineering had already become a part of food production. As early as 1987, plants with altered genes began field trials in real fields. Since then, more than 500 such trials have been conducted and the first fruits, literally, to reach the public will be a tomato and a squash. If the food companies have their way, these will be followed by virus-resistant cantaloupes, herbicide-resistant soybeans, high-starch potatoes, and almost 60 other genetically engineered products already in development and testing.

Although none of the field trials identified any problems and the U.S. Food and Drug Administration declared on May 26, 1992 that genetically engineered food would be treated as safe, the Union of Concerned Scientists produced a report on December 20, 1993 called "Perils Amidst the Promises" that asked the U.S. government to postpone commercial introduction of genetically engineered plants until further tests are made. The chief scientists who generated the report, Margaret G. Mellon and Jane Rissler, objected primarily to the use of plant viruses to introduce new genes into the crops; they felt this might result in changes in the viruses that could lead to epidemics. Furthermore, they were concerned that genetically altered plants could spread as weeds more readily than natural plants, despite a careful trial in England of genetically altered oilseed rape, the source of canola oil, that showed no such tendencies.

Other food products based on genetic engineering also entered the marketplace during the early 1990s, but these were based on bacteria or yeast, not on plants.

Cheese with a Genetic Twist

When a calf drinks milk from its mother, a specialized hormone in the calf's stomach causes the milk to form soft, nutritious curds. Long ago, farmers found that the stomach lining had this same effect even after it was removed from the animal. Calves slaughtered for veal provided the stomachs. The linings were removed, salted, and dried. People then soaked the linings in warm water to obtain the active substance, called rennet. A couple of tablespoons of rennet turns a gallon of milk into a soft cheese (like cottage cheese), which can then be processed into hard cheese of various kinds. Other kinds of rennet were also found, including rennet from the plant called lady's bed straw, used primarily for making cheese for strict lacto-vegetarians.

The key ingredient in rennet is a hormone called renin. In the 1980s agricultural scientists located the gene for renin, reproduced ("cloned") it, and inserted it into bacteria. By 1990 Pfizer Inc. won approval from the U.S. Food and Drug Administration (FDA) to market this genetically engineered renin. For some reason, this particular alteration of food production techniques with genetic engineering failed to draw protests.

Milk from Genetically Encouraged Cows

Scientists studying cattle long ago found the hormone that encourages cows to produce milk to feed their calves. Much earlier than that discovery, farmers developed a series of practices that encourage cows to produce milk in much larger amounts than even a pair of calves need and to continue to do so long after the calves have been slaughtered or weaned. This was accomplished by millennia of selection for milk production and a program of mating the cows with bulls each year. Both forms of breeding result in greater milk production as a result of an increase in the milk-production hormone. Scientists who isolated this hormone named it bovine somatotropin, or BST.

When genetic engineering was developed, starting in the 1980s, researchers located the gene for BST. Eventually the BST gene was inserted into bacteria so that the hormone could be produced in quantity. Tests showed that, if injected in cows once every two weeks, it works just like the natural hormone and increases milk production even further. In a herd of cattle, average milk production from cows given additional BST rises about 10 percent and for some cows the increase may be as much as 20 percent.

Studies have detected no rise in BST in milk, although the milk is not identical to milk from untreated cows. The main difference is an elevation in a protein called insulin-like growth factor 1 (IGF-1). Scientists are not concerned by higher levels of IGF-1 because this protein is inactivated by digestive enzymes and in milk processing.

Many people object to the use of BST to increase milk production for other reasons as well: first, simply because it is another instance of genetic engineering applied to food; second, because it might cause some harm to cattle; and third, and most relevant economically, milk production in the U.S. is too high already. Farmers frequently dump milk and the U.S. government absorbs some of the excess production by buying and storing large quantities of cheese and butter—occasionally distributing the excess to the poor. The U.S. Congressional Budget Office estimates that increased milk production as a result of BST use will cost the U.S. subsidy program an additional $15 million a year.

The main known side effect for cows of this increased milk production is an occasional rash on the udder called mastitis. Mastitis is common among cows that are heavy milk producers. There is some concern that such a rash might cause farmers to use more antibiotics; the antibiotics could then find their way into the milk, resulting in a decreased ability of the antibiotics to cure infection in people who drank the milk.

Despite such objections, the FDA, after nine years of review, granted approval on

November 5, 1993 to Monsanto Corporation to begin selling BST under the brand name Posilac as of February 4, 1994. The milk from cows using Posilac will not be labeled in any way, however. Monsanto must monitor the milk for at least two years to make certain that it does not contain increased levels of antibiotics. Three other companies are also seeking FDA approval for their brands of BST. On the other side, further protests are planned in hopes of getting the Monsanto permission rescinded. Meanwhile, food scientists are preparing to seek approval for PST (porcine somatotropin), which is expected to reduce fat levels in pigs to amazingly low levels.

New Tomatoes in Town

Calgene Inc. led the way with the first complete, genetically engineered food, its Flavr Savr tomato. This tomato is genetically engineered to be harvested at a later stage of ripeness than is usual for commercially grown tomatoes. As every backyard gardener knows, tomatoes only develop their characteristic flavor when they ripen on the vine, but supermarket tomatoes are picked green and chemically ripened, so they don't taste as good as vine-ripened tomatoes. The Flavr Savr may or may not taste better than other supermarket tomatoes; the slow ripening is also intended to give the tomato a longer shelf life.

The Flavr Savr is the first genetically engineered food to be approved for marketing by the U.S. Department of Agriculture (USDA), but failed to reach stores until 1994 because it lacked similar approval from the FDA. Calgene asked the FDA on January 5, 1993 to approve the marker gene the corporation used to locate genetically altered tomato cells as a food additive. The marker gene is a bacterial gene called *kan(r)*, which provides resistance to the antibiotic kanamycin.

A key to the development of plant genetics is the ability to grow whole plants from single cells. Bacteria that infect plant cells are used to introduce the genes for long shelf life and flavor retention into cultures of single cells. The same bacteria also carry the gene for resistance to kanamycin. Not every cell in the culture is infected, but the ones that are can be separated from the ones that are not by killing the uninfected cells with the antibiotic. The other cells are then further cultured to produce plants that can be grown in fields. These plants will eventually produce fruit with the desired characteristics. Without the marker gene, it is impossible to know which plants have the desirable fruit characteristics.

The principal objection to the *kan(r)* gene is that it might reduce the effectiveness of kanamycin or the related antibiotic neomycin in attacking human disease. Such an effect has not been demonstrated, but critics see this as a theoretical possibility. The principal opposition comes from activist and author Jeremy Rifkin, but in 1992 his concerns were echoed in a petition signed by 1500 U.S. chefs who threatened to boycott the new tomato and similar genetically altered foods.

The Flavr Savr tomato was financed largely by the Campbell Soup Company. In 1993 the company responded to protests by announcing that they have no plans to market the tomato in any form, while denying that consumer protests had anything to do with their announcement or decision.

On November 26, 1993 scientists from Cornell University announced that they had located the allele of a gene in tomatoes that causes its possessors to resist speck, a bacterial disease caused by *Pseudomonas syringae*. Speck causes leaves to drop from the plant, reducing yield and, if sufficiently severe, causing plant death. The Cornell team, headed by Steven Tanksley, also demonstrated that they could insert the allele into plants that did not have it, and thereby confer resistance. Since this is an allele of a naturally occurring tomato gene involved in communication between cells, there is little reason to expect protests against tomatoes grown from plants genetically engineered to be resistant.

(Periodical References and Additional Reading: *New York Times* 5-26-92, p A1; *New York Times* 5-27-92, p A16; *Discover* 1-93, p 44; *New York Times* 1-6-93, p D4; *New York Times* 6-22-93, p C4; *New York Times* 8-3-93, p 4; *New York Times* 11-6-93, p A1; *New York Times* 11-17-93, p C17; *New York Times* 11-26-93, p A25; *New York Times* 12-21-93, p A23)

THE GAY GENE

In the past, some psychologists traced a son's homosexuality to his mother. Now there is a glimmer of genetic evidence that a mother's genes may contribute to male homosexuality. A study directed by Dean A. Hamer of the U.S. National Cancer Institute reveals evidence for a so-called "gay gene" on the X chromosome.

Hamer's group studied 114 men who were strict homosexuals and their close male relatives. They found that the brothers, maternal uncles, and maternal male cousins of these 114 men had higher rates of homosexuality than the rate for the general public (which the Hamer group took to be two percent, using a definition of exclusive male homosexuality). This kind of distribution is consistent with a gene on the X chromosome, a chromosome that both sons and daughters obtain from their mothers.

Genes are not transmitted in isolation. Stretches of DNA that are passed along contain the gene and a bit near the gene. This bit may or may not contain an easily identified marker. Hamer and his coworkers showed that when X chromosomes from homosexual brothers and their male relatives are compared, the same set of five

---

WHAT BASIS IS THERE FOR ESTIMATING THE NUMBER OF GAY MEN?

In 1992, studies in England and France each found that 1.4 percent of the male population is exclusively homosexual. A much more famous figure of 10 percent, found by Alfred Kinsey and coworkers in 1948, included bisexuals. Kinsey's figure for exclusive homosexuals was four percent, but the population he surveyed is widely believed to contain a higher percentage than normal of homosexuals. In 1993 Koray Tanfer and coworkers at the Battelle Human Affairs Research Center interviewed 3000 men about their sex lives, of whom about 30 said they had been exclusively homosexual for the past ten years. About 40 more said they had some male and some female partners. Based on these figures, the Hamer study's use of two percent for strict male homosexuality is conservative in the context of the research, which looked for an excess over the background level of exclusive male homosexuality.

HOW THE "FEMALE" X CHROMOSOME CAUSES MALES TO BE THE WAY THEY ARE

When chromosomes are pictured in biology or medical textbooks, the pairs are easy to recognize and the individual chromosomes are quite clear. This is far from the case in real life, since the chromosomes— mostly DNA on a protein substructure—are all tangled up in the nucleus of the cell most of the time. They are so hard to separate and to count that from 1918 until 1954, scientists believed that there were 48 chromosomes in 24 pairs, although the correct number is 46 in 23 pairs.

Most of those pairs in the textbook pictures are nearly twins. But there is one mismatch shown. The X chromosome is Arnold Schwarzenegger, while its partner Y is Danny DeVito. Different species of animals use different genetic systems to produce males and females, but the XY system is the one that humans use. The giant X and tiny Y indicate that the chromosomes shown in the picture are from a male. A similar picture of the chromosomes of a human female shows all the pairs as nearly alike, since women have two X chromosomes and no Y.

There are no pictures of human chromosomes representing a person with two Y chromosomes and no X chromosomes. Many of the essential functions of cells and development are directed by genes on the X chromosome. Without at least one X chromosome, an embryo cannot survive until birth.

If the Y chromosome has some genes for general cell functions or development beyond directing the growth into maleness, they have not yet been found. The Y chromosome comes stripped down for just the one goal, which is why it is so much smaller than X or than other chromosomes.

Genes on a pair of chromosomes are usually matched. A gene that produces a given protein is found on each chromosome in the pair, although the protein may be subtly or even greatly different as a product of each of the two genes. The genes that produce versions of the same protein are called *alleles.*

Some vital proteins have their production directed by alleles found on the X chromosome. For a female, with two X chromosomes, there are two alleles, each directing the same or two very similar proteins. A male, with one X and one Y, has only a single allele of the gene.

Suppose one X chromosome contains an allele that directs production of a version of a protein that fails to accomplish its expected task in cells. A female has another X chromosome that probably produces a version of the protein that is effective. Thus, for most females, the protein's job will get done. For males, however, a gene for a defective protein on the X chromosome has no back-up, since males have only one X chromosome. The protein will be defective and the job will not get done.

A mother, being female, has two X chromosomes. A son inherits one of those X chromosomes along with a Y chromosome from his father. If one of the mother's X chromosomes has a "bad" gene, her son has a 50 percent chance of inheriting it. Thus, a hereditary disease that is carried by the mother on an X chromosome is only expressed in her sons, not her daughters. Furthermore, since other genes come on pairs of chromosomes, hereditary diseases carried by the X chromosomes are relatively common. For the other chromosome pairs, if there is an unfortunate allele on one chromosome, it is likely to be masked by the more effective allele on the other chromosome.

---

markers appear on more than three-fourths of the chromosomes. This result suggests that a gene located among those markers is a factor in the development of homosexuality. If so, it is one of about a hundred genes found on that stretch of the X chromosome. The search is complicated by the lack of an understanding of how a single protein might influence something as complex as sexual behavior. The only viable clue is a slight brain difference in the hypothalamus found in 1991.

In the past, similar methods have appeared to identify genes for alcoholism, depression, and schizophrenia. Critics are quick to point out that these findings were not confirmed by other studies.

Two separate twin studies, one by J. Michael Bailey of Northwestern University in Evanston, Illinois and the other by Richard C. Pillard of Boston University School of Medicine, provide further evidence of a possible hereditary basis for homosexuality. The first study, announced in December 1991, involved 161 homosexual men in varying genetic closeness to their brothers (identical twins, fraternal twins, adopted brothers, making a total of 335 men in the study) while the second, announced in the summer of 1992, investigated about 300 homosexual women. Both studies had similar findings. Both twins were gay in about 50 percent of the identical twins studied. Both twins were gay in less than 25 percent of the fraternal twins studied. And, even fewer gay pairs were found among the adopted siblings. While the data are not in dispute, the interpretation is—other factors may account for that concordance of homosexual twins for example.

If one assumes that only four percent of the total population of male humans are homosexual, these results would imply that genes account for half of male homosexuality. Non-twin biological brothers were not questioned, but the interviews with the primary group revealed 9.2 percent of the brothers to be homosexual, a figure so low as to cast doubt on the idea that there is a genetic component to homosexuality.

In an interview with *Science*, Bailey offered explanations of these results after the first study. He believes that genes influence development of the INAH-3 region in the brain, leading ultimately to a predisposition toward homosexuality. Bailey stated that he assumes that the basis of homosexuality is biological, with half coming from heredity and the other half from other environmental and random biological factors. It is difficult to find reliable studies showing an environmental influence on sexual orientation. The results by Bailey and Pillard were published in *Archives of General Psychiatry*.

(Periodical References and Additional Reading: *Discover* 1-93, p 55; *New York Times* 3-12-93, p A11; *Scientific American* 6-93, p 122; *Science* 7-16-93, pp 291, 321; *Science News* 7-17-93, p 37; *Discover* 1-94, pp 70, 71)

ANIMAL MODELS FOR HUMAN DISEASES

Biologists have gained great insights into the operation of genes by creating mice in which a targeted gene is "knocked out." A disruptive stretch of DNA is added to the gene at the embryo stage, preferably in the middle of the gene. The added DNA is typically a codon that says "terminate making this protein." It interferes with the gene sufficiently so that no active protein is produced. When the procedure has been successful for several mice, knocking out the same gene in each, the adult "knock-out" mice can be bred with each other or other suitable mice to start a line that inherits this "knocked out" gene.

The point of the procedure is to create mice that mimic the human diseases resulting when an allele of a gene either produces no protein or produces a protein that fails to accomplish its task in the interactions of the cells and proteins in the body. As of the end of 1993 mice produced by this procedure can be used as models for a form of thalassemia, Lesch-Nyhan syndrome, Duchenne muscular dystrophy, sickle-cell anemia, Gaucher's disease, and cystic fibrosis.

Animal models for human diseases also have been created by adding a human gene to the animal, instead of knocking out an animal gene. For example, researchers interested in such arthritic and inflammatory diseases as spinal arthritis and psoriasis believed that a protein called HLA-B27 contributed to or marked the disease. They inserted the pair of human genes that together produce this protein into rats. The rats that expressed the genes and produced the protein developed inflammatory arthritic symptoms, while their siblings that failed to produce HLA-B27 also failed to develop the arthritic symptoms.

Scientists are also able to make synthetic versions of genes and then insert the synthetic gene into animals to model human diseases or simply to see if the synthetic gene will produce the protein it is supposed to make. A particularly useful technique developed by several groups of researchers in 1993 builds a chromosome in yeast (a Yeast Artificial Chromosome, or YAC) before inserting it into a mouse embryo. The growing mice incorporate the YAC and express the gene by manufacturing the protein. Later generations of mice will contain some that express the YAC in every cell and some that do not. Inbreeding can then be used to develop a pure line of mice that produce specified human proteins. It is not even necessary to isolate the gene; a YAC can be made with a large segment of human DNA that is known to contain the desired gene.

Genetically altered animal models can be patented; the first such patent was awarded in 1988 to the Harvard Mouse. This mouse is genetically engineered to grow malignant tumors and is used in cancer studies. The Ohio Mouse, a second patented mouse, has the human gene for interferon inserted. This mouse continually manufactures human interferon, which makes it resistant to viral infections. Although the gene was inserted into the mouse line by injecting the embryo with the human gene, the line patented now reproduces by normal inbreeding.

Treatment of Mice with Genetic Diseases

Among the virtues of using lines of mice that mimic human hereditary diseases is that treatment ideas can be tested in mice before human trials are begun. Such mouse tests are, however, often more successful than subsequent human trials, probably because "wild" humans are more complex than specially bred lines of mice.

Shiverer mice are bred to have a genetic disease. When embryos of shiverer mice are provided with the wild-type gene, the embryos can grow into mice that do not have the disease. Other genetic diseases in mouse lines have been successfully cured by the use of genes treated in various ways. In all these cases, of course, the parent mice are not cured, only some of their offspring. Using the same methods, offspring lacking predisposition to a disease (such as diabetes) have been produced from lines into which the predisposition was previously introduced. Mice that have the gene for the protein dystrophin knocked out or altered develop a mouse version of muscular dystrophy. A line of dystrophic mice can, however, be switched to a healthy line by inserting the correct version of the gene into embryos of the knock-out mice.

More useful for humans are treatments that can change the genes of an individual who has a genetic disease or genetic predisposition so that he or she becomes healthy or is protected against a disease. Such treatments have been accomplished in mice, especially with regard to cancer. One successful method uses cells that seek out tumors and destroy them. Jeffrey S. Chamberlain of the University of Michigan, who led his team to success in 1993 in inserting a new dystrophin gene into mouse embryos, has suggested that the same gene could be inserted in muscles using a viral

---

WILD MICE, NAKED MICE, AND MORE

Unlike wild humans, wild mice are not necessarily less civilized or more unruly than other mice. Naked mice are not used in immune experiments because it would slow down the experiment to remove the clothes from other mice. Shiverer mice have a genetic disease, not just a cold cage.

Biologists use the term *wild* or *wild-type* to characterize natural populations, whether or not the creatures involved live in the woods or in cages. A domestic dog that lives in a pack in the woods is not wild in this sense, since it has been genetically altered by domestication. Populations of mice, even if they have been kept in cages for generations, are wild if they have continually bred with mice introduced from natural populations. By extension, geneticists often refer to populations of semidomesticated animals, such as white laboratory rats, as wild so long as the animals have not been bred for a particular purpose.

Mice are "naked" when their immune systems have been destroyed by breeding. Such mice are useful because they do not mount an immune response to grafts from other mice or even from other species.

Mouse lines bred for specific purposes often have technical names of the R2D2 variety, but sometimes a line is known for a specific characteristic, such as shivering or dancing. Shiverer mice have been bred with the gene for the basic protein in the covering of nerves knocked out. They get their name because they are subject to tremors and convulsions.

---

vector. Using this technique, muscular dystrophy could be cured in an individual born with the disease, not just in an embryo. If such a vector is developed, it almost certainly will be tried in mice before it is used in humans.

(Periodical References and Additional Reading: *New York Times* 11-30-90; *New York Times* 3-31-93, p C3; *Science* 10-22-93, p 533)

PIGS AND OTHER ANIMALS BECOME MORE HUMAN

Medical students studying the development of humans from conception to birth usually work with pig embryos because they are so similar to human embryos. Pigs share a number of traits with humans—little body hair, similar size, similar diet, considerable intelligence, and so forth. Some years ago a science-fiction writer exploited this resemblance in a short story about a scientist who proved that humans are more closely related to pigs than to great apes. The scientist was disowned by the biological community because no one wanted to be related to pigs. Yesterday's science fiction often becomes today's science, although in the case of pigs, the tale has a twist.

Pigs Make Human Blood

On June 16, 1991 officials of DNX Inc., a biotechnology company in Princeton New Jersey, announced the development of a successful technique to insert functioning human hemoglobin genes into pigs. About 15 percent of the genetically altered pig's blood cells contain human hemoglobin. The aim is to harvest a key ingredient for a blood substitute for humans that will be immunologically neutral. A supply of such a blood substitute will enable humans of any blood type to accept safe and effective transfusions of the substitute in place of somewhat risky and often scarce donated blood. DNX officials stated that it will be at least five years, if all goes well, before such a substitute can be developed and tested in humans. Other workers in the field have commented that some kind of blood substitute will be commercially available soon after the mid-1990s.

Even if a blood substitute becomes available, it will not replace the need for human blood in many applications. The substitute will be used primarily when there is a sudden great demand (as in wartime or other disasters) or a need for a rare blood type that cannot be met in other ways. Any blood substitute, especially one produced in part by genetic engineering, is expected to be much more costly than donated or purchased human blood, although DNX officials predict that costs will be comparable when all factors, such as the expense of tissue typing procedures, are taken into account.

DNX has experimented with pigs for some years. In the 1980s, the company received a lot of adverse publicity (under the name Embryogen) when pigs injected with growth hormone became crippled. The hemoglobin experiments involved hundreds of pigs and pig embryos. The two human genes that control hemoglobin production were inserted into pig embryos that were then implanted in sows. By 1991 three pigs, each of which produces about one human hemoglobin molecule for

---

Background

Hemoglobin in mammals is a protein that carries oxygen from place to place in the body. In its natural state it is packaged in the erythrocytes (red blood cells). The red blood cells are not, however, necessary for hemoglobin to accomplish its task; they primarily function as decay-resistant packaging. Free hemoglobin released in the blood only lasts a few hours, but packed into erythrocytes it can persist for a couple of weeks. The erythrocyte packages have no other direct purpose, but they are covered with various antigens. These antigens are the primary cause of different blood groups.

---

each six pig hemoglobin molecules, had been created. Experiments in breeding the genetically altered pigs have not been reported, but there seems to be no theoretical reason why such breeding would fail. If breeding is successful, the supply of cheap genetically altered pigs could reach several million animals within a few years.

Free hemoglobin (naked hemoglobin not encased in red blood cells) is quickly destroyed in living systems, so free hemoglobin needs to be administered continually until enough red blood cells have been made by the body. It is thought that free hemoglobin can be preserved by freeze drying or freezing for longer periods than whole red blood cells survive under refrigeration. This theory is far from proven. Efforts to preserve pure human hemoglobin outside of cells have so far failed in human trials, probably because antigens from the red blood cells contaminate the hemoglobin.

Although hemoglobin from other mammals is almost the same as human hemoglobin, almost is not good enough. Purified cow hemoglobin has been tested in humans without success. The Somatogen company is producing and testing human hemoglobin with genetically engineered bacteria, but there are fears that bacterial toxins will make these efforts fail.

Pigs Make Human Organs

In 1993 DNX was one of two groups to announce another success with gene transfers into pigs. This time, the two groups transplanted genes for complement supressor, a part of the human immune system, into pigs. Complement supressor keeps the human immune system from launching a major attack on its own organs. When foreign cells appear in the body (such as bacteria or parasites), however, they are not usually equipped with human complement suppressor. Complement is produced in the blood in great amounts in response to the foreign cell, where it punches holes in the cell membrane. Its presence also stimulates other parts of the immune system to attack the foreign cells.

Organ transplants are particularly sensitive to complement reaction. Despite tissue typing that matches transplanted organs as closely as possible to the recipient's tissue, the recipient's immune system often attacks organs from other humans as foreign. About a third of all kidney transplants, for example, fail as a result of this reaction, even when other immune reactions have been successfully countered by cyclosporine or other treatments. When organ transplants from another species into humans have been tried, the results have been uniformly disastrous, largely because of the complement reaction. It is believed that organs from another species might function in humans if the complement reaction could be suppressed.

John Logan of DNX Corporation and David White from Cambridge University in England both reported in October 1993 that their teams succeeded in inserting human suppressor genes in pig embryos, which then produced the suppressor molecules on cells in the growing pigs. The next step in this research is expected to be transplantation of organs from pigs into primates other than humans. If this is successful, organs from the genetically altered pigs will be transplanted into humans. Success is far from assured, however, for the immune system has many ways to defend the body. Suppressing the complement reaction might not be sufficient to protect pig organs from attack by some other part of the immune system.

Whether used to supply hemoglobin or organs, genetically altered pigs may become part of your life in the future. Farmers have the capacity to produce an almost unlimited supply of pigs by regular breeding methods. Once a breeding stock of genetically altered pigs becomes available, the overall supply should rise quickly to meet any conceivable demand.

Other Animal Innovations

In the Netherlands, Genpharm International has developed a bull that carries the genes for a human protein called lactoferin. Lactoferin is found in human milk; when consumed by infants, it inhibits bacterial growth and promotes retention of iron. (There is not much iron in milk itself, so when ordinary human or cow milk forms the main part of an infant's diet, iron retention is important to prevent anemia.) Bulls, of course, do not produce milk. The gene for lactoferin is dominant, however, so cows impregnated by the bull produce the lactoferin-laced milk. Genpharm hopes to patent the bull and to sell either the lactoferin separately to add to formula or to sell the milk directly for use in formula. Another company, Genzyme, is also developing animals that produce human proteins in milk, although Genzyme is working with goats instead of cattle. Genpharm is also developing mice that produce human antibodies to use in fighting specific diseases.

(Periodical References and Further Reading: *New York Times* 6-16-91, p I1; *New York Times* 7-8-92, p D5; *New York Times* 2-3-93, p A1; *New York Times* 10-19-93, p C3; *Time* 1-17-94, p 46)

GENES AND CHROMOSOMES AS A CAUSE OF DISEASE

THREE-BASE REPEATS:
FRAGILE X, HUNTINGTON'S DISEASE, AND MORE

It is like a stuck key on a compppppppppputer. The same letter of the genetic code repeats over and over. Just as the intended product of keyboarding, a word, is altered or made nonfunctioning by the repetition from a stuck key, the protein product of a gene is similarly altered and damaged by the repeated code. In particular, a three-base code that signifies a single amino acid is the kind of repeat that causes the problem. First encountered early in 1991 in the gene for an uncommon hereditary disease known as spinobulbar muscular atrophy (also known as Kennedy's disease), such repeated codes are now known to be found in the genes at the root of at least four other hereditary disorders.

The cause of the gene repeats is not known, but it is thought that they can occur both in meiosis (resulting in development of an individual in which the gene with the repetitions is present in every cell) and in mitosis (leading to a cell line that has the gene repeats). In the first case, the number of repetitions of the three-bases tends to increase from generation to generation. In the second case, repeats can develop later in life and the individual will have some cell lines with no extra repetitions, some with a few extra, and perhaps cell lines with many repetitions.

A connection between three-base repeats and colon cancer emerged in 1993, when genetic analysis of colon tumors revealed that different cells from a single tumor often had long stretches of three-base repeats in various places. The possible cause for this effect is that the cancer itself causes poor copying of DNA from cell to cell, resulting in the repetition of short DNA units as many as a thousand times in some cells. Meanwhile, another tumor cell from the same cancer may show fewer repeats or none at all.

Fragile X and Mental Retardation

In the May 31, 1991 issue of *Cell*, Stephen T. Warren of Emery University School of Medicine and coworkers announced the discovery of the genetic cause of the second most common form (after Down's syndrome) of mental retardation in boys. Like many other hereditary conditions, fragile-X syndrome occurs most often in males (*see also* "The Gay Gene," p 42), although it also can affect females.

The hereditary defect is called fragile-X syndrome because the X chromosome in affected persons appears under the microscope to be thinned almost to breaking. The gene has been named *FMR-1* and its protein product FMRP, although evidence suggests that FMRP is actually produced as at least four different proteins. Possibly the process of making FMRP from the *FMR-1* gene results in assembling the same protein elements in four or more different ways. Research leading to these conclusions was

Background

Fragile-X syndrome accounts for an estimated five to ten percent of the cases of mental retardation in the U.S., occurring in about one out of every 1250 men and about half as often in women. Many individuals with the syndrome are hyperactive in addition to having some degree of mental retardation. The degree of retardation can range from barely noticeable learning disabilities to impaired speech. About 20 percent of males displaying the typical "fragile" deformation of the X chromosome show no symptoms whatsoever and are normal with regard to all the fragile-X symptoms. The symptoms of the disease lead researchers to believe that the protein FMRP produced by the fragile-X gene is somehow involved in the transmission of signals between nerve cells in the brain.

conducted by a large team from Erasmus University in Rotterdam and published in the June 24, 1993 *Nature*.

Although located at the easily observed "fragile" spot, the gene itself proved to be very difficult to separate from the rest of the chromosome. Other researchers were very close to success just before Warren's group isolated it. Warren's group located the gene by analyzing families in which the fragile-X allele of *FMR-1* appeared and by forming hybrids between hamster and human cells, a method that aids in isolating the human genes from the hamster genes.

When found, the fragile-X gene showed a large number of repetitions of the three-base (trinucleotide) codon for argine (CGG). Later analysis revealed, however, that the large number of CGG repeats does not result in a protein that has a long chain of argine amino bases. Instead, when the normal number is exceeded in the string of CGG repeats—the normal number is less than about 50 repeats—the gene fails to make any protein at all. Some alleles have been found in which there are as many as 1500 repeats.

Myotonic Dystrophy and Kennedy's Disease

Duchenne muscular dystrophy, which appears in childhood, has captured many headlines in the past decade because it was among the first hereditary diseases for which the genetic cause was found. A different hereditary disease, myotonic dystrophy, is the most common form of muscular dystrophy in adults, however, striking about one in 8000 persons. In the February 6, 1992 *Nature*, three teams of researchers announced the discovery of the location of the gene for myotonic dystrophy. Furthermore, because of changes in the weight of the protein product of the gene from person to person, they suspected that the alleles that cause the disease include multiple repeats of DNA. Later research showed that myotonic muscular dystrophy is also caused by a three-base repeat in the gene, which is located on the long arm of chromosome 19. The normal gene contains from five to 37 repeats of the three-base codon CTG. Persons with myotonic dystrophy have been found with 44 to 3000 CTG repeats.

Spinobulbar muscular atrophy or Kennedy's disease was the first genetic defect found to be caused by three-base repeats. In Kennedy's disease, the three-base repeat is CAG, which normally is a repeating part of the gene for an androgen receptor. In normal cases, the number of CAG repeats ranges from 11 to 31. The allele that causes the disease typically has 40 to 60 repeats, making the normal and disease-causing alleles fairly close in size. Perhaps for this reason, it is possible to produce this genetic disorder in mice—the only one of the human disorders caused by triplet repeats that has an animal model. In fact, no natural animal gene has ever been observed to have a trinucleotide repeat that varies the way human genes do. All animals studied do have sections in genes that include repeating segments, but these sections stay essentially the same from individual to individual.

Unlike Kennedy's disease, the repeating segments for fragile-X and myotonic dystrophy are not actually on the gene, but are near one end or the other in the noncoding section of DNA. Since the repeating section is not actually on the gene for those disorders, it is far from clear how the repeat affects the health of the individual. There are generally many more repeats for fragile-X or myotonic dystrophy than for Kennedy's disease, which may be a clue.

Huntington's Disease: The Search Continues

As soon as it became clear that specific genes could be identified, one of the most sought-after was the allele that causes Huntington's disease. The story of the successful search for the location of the gene is well known to those who follow medical research. The sequel to that discovery is a continuing tale, for unlocking the secrets of the gene itself and its action has proven to be more difficult than finding the location of the gene in the first place.

After ten years of research, the gene was isolated in the spring of 1993. The discovery, by a cooperative known as the Huntington's Disease Collaborative Re-

Background

Huntington's disease is also known as Huntington's chorea since one of the most noticeable symptoms of the late stages of the disease is a characteristic suite of movements (*chorea* is the Greek word for "dance"). The uncontrolled hand darting, lurching, and head bobbing that characterize Huntington's disease result from destruction of two small regions of the basal ganglia called the putamen and the caudate nucleus. These brain regions control movement of the "voluntary" muscles. Before the disease reaches this stage symptoms may include irritability, sleeplessness, lack of concentration, and loss of memory. Often during early stages the person with Huntington's disease develops antisocial behaviors, including alcoholism, which can complicate diagnosis unless the disease is suspected because other family members have it.

It is easy to think of Huntington's disease as rare, but it is not. Estimates are that one out of 10,000 persons carries the Huntington's dominant allele of gene. In the U.S., about 30,000 persons are afflicted and 150,000 others are considered at risk. Usually the disease symptoms do not begin to develop until the individual carrying the gene is an adult and often the disease takes decades to progress to the point of causing death.

search Group, was announced in the March 26 issue of *Cell*. The gene was found on chromosome 4 near the marker that was previously used to determine which members of a family known to harbor the gene will develop the illness. Although credit is given to the Collaborative Group, the actual team that completed the task was led by James Gusella of Massachusetts General Hospital, and included Marcy MacDonald, Mabel Duyao, and Christine Ambrose.

Knowing the exact structure of the gene has not yet been sufficient to illuminate the gene's function or to indicate why it fails as a person with some forms of the gene grows older. It is clear, however, that the Huntington's disease allele differs from the normal gene in the number of three-base repeats it carries. One of the three-base codons in the gene, the codon CAG for the amino acid glutamine, is repeated, not just once, but over and over. Such a CAG repeat in the gene occurs in everyone, but individuals with 9 to 37 repeats do not develop Huntington's disease, while those with more than 37 repetitions do develop the disease. Furthermore, the number of repeats is connected in some way to the age of onset of the disease—persons who have more repetitions, perhaps as many as 121, develop symptoms earlier than those with fewer repetitions.

There are many unresolved puzzles about the trinucleotide repeats in Huntington's disease. The number of repetitions in the gene found in DNA from the sperm cells of a man with Huntington's disease varied oddly from one cell to another. Body cells, however, all had the same number of repeats in the allele. As with the other three-base repeats, if the genes of several generations are compared, later generations seem to have more repetitions than earlier ones.

The search for the function of the gene is complicated. Although Huntington's disease damages the central nervous system, the gene itself normally seems to operate—make its gene product—in every cell of the body according to research directed by Francis S. Collins of the U.S. National Center for Human Genome Research. It appears that an allele with a trinucleotide repeat greater than 37 can still do its job or at least cause no damage in most cells. But neurons, especially the neurons in the part of the brain called the basal ganglia, are destroyed.

Ataxias

The word *ataxia* refers to any loss of muscular coordination, but the rare hereditary diseases known as spinocerebellar ataxias can progress to the loss of the ability to breathe or to swallow, leading eventually to death. In July 1993, Huda Y. Zoghbi of Baylor College of Medicine in Houston, Texas, Harry T. Orr of the University of Minnesota, and coworkers found that one of the spinocerebellar ataxias is among the hereditary diseases caused by an allele that contains extra three-base repeats. These CAG repeats, the three-base sequence implicated in Kennedy's and Huntington's diseases, are located on a gene found on chromosome 6. As with other defects caused by such repetitions, the ataxia symptoms are worse and the disease develops earlier in individuals with more repeats, which can vary from about 40 to 80 CAG repetitions. The number of repeats may vary from parent to child, with more occurring in later generations of the same family. Persons with fewer than 36 CAG repeats do not have the ataxia.

About the same time, researchers in Japan and an international team working with Cuban and French families identified the genes for two other ataxias. Although the three ataxia genes are located on three different chromosomes, the familiar pattern of increased severity in later generations suggests that the other two ataxias may also be caused by three-base repeats.

(Periodical References and Further Reading: *New York Times* 2-14-91, p B14; *New York Times* 5-30-91, p A1; *Science News* 6-8-91, p 359; *Science News* 2-15-92, p 102; *New York Times* 3-24-93, p A1; *Science* 4-2-93, p 28; *New York Times* 5-11-93, p C3; *Science* 6-4-93, p 1422; *Nature* 6-24-93, p 722; *Science News* 7-10-93, p 20; *Science* 10-29-93, p 674; *New York Times* 11-2-93, p C3; *Discover* 12-93, p 98)

GENES FOR CANCER

Among the great successes of the explosion of knowledge of genetics since 1953 has been the discovery of the genetic bases of cancer. Since several forms of cancer are considered different diseases, it is not surprising that different genes are implicated in the cancers that attack different types of tissue. At the same time, it appears that most of the time cancer initiation is a process of two or more steps. While one gene readies a cell for transformation into a malignancy, the action of one or more other genes is often required before the transformation becomes complete. Thus, possession of a "cancer gene" typically predisposes the possessor to a cancer initiated by the gene, the gene does not by itself cause disease. One gene is often associated with a given type of cancer, while another gene involved in the process is general to a number of cancer types.

Neurofibromatosis, 1 and 2

Neurofibromatoses are basically characterized by a proliferation of tumors in the nervous system. The tumors are not malignant and therefore are not cancers, but the cause of neurofibromatosis is genetically similar to that of most cancers. Two different types are recognized, since the genes causing the diseases are mapped to different chromosomes. The identification of the gene *NF1* from chromosome 17 in 1990 was one of the first breakthroughs in tying a given gene to a specific type of tumor. Type 1 neurofibromatosis is the more common type, occurring in 1 out of 3000 individuals. Three years later, two different teams were each able to sequence the gene *NF2* from chromosome 22. This gene predisposes a person to the much less common neurofibromatosis type 2, which only occurs in 1 out of 37,000 individuals.

The *p53* Switch

Machines designed by humans are usually straightforward. A switch, for example, turns on a light or a motor directly by completing a circuit; if a gauge regulates operation of a part of a machine, such as steam pressure, the gauge is designed to shut off a switch or to open a valve. But sometimes the increase in pressure causes the gauge to take several actions at once; it may shut off a switch to the heater, open a valve to let off excess steam, and close another switch to cause a warning light to shine. Nature's designs for genes are most often of this latter kind; when one gene is turned on by something in its environment, it manufactures a gene product that then affects several other parts of the organism.

A machine that operates via several levels of action is so foreign to the way humans normally design mechanisms that people find such machines to be funny; this sort of humor is exploited in the famous cartoons of Rube Goldberg, whose name has entered the language to describe an unwieldy, poorly designed device. A Rube Goldberg alarm clock might work as follows: morning sunlight is focused onto a piece of paper, setting the paper on fire; the heat warms the bottom of a gerbil's cage, waking the gerbil; the gerbil does its morning exercises in a wheel, causing the wheel to rotate; a belt from the wheel drives a series of gears that knock a bucket of water off a high perch; the water falls on a lever that lifts one side of the bed; the sleeper is rolled out of bed and wakes up. Although people find such Rube Goldberg devices humorous, genes very often work this way. Scientists sometimes call these pathways cascades.

One of the first genes found to be implicated in cancer is one called *p53*. It was discovered in 1979 in animal viruses that cause cancer. Although the animal viruses do not cause cancer in humans, in 1990 an allele of *p53* was identified as the defect that causes the rare Li-Fraumeni syndrome in humans, a syndrome that increases susceptibility to sarcomas and breast cancer. In 1992 separate studies at Massachusetts General Hospital Cancer Center and Massachusetts Eye and Ear Infirmary found that versions of the gene might account for up to one percent of all cancers in children and young adults. Since then, one form or another of the *p53* gene has been observed in somewhat more than half of all cancer cells examined for it. Research on the mechanisms of the gene *p53* was so intense in 1993 that the protein it produces, known as p53 (genes are usually written in italics, while proteins are given in roman type), became *Science* magazine's "Molecule of the Year" for 1993.

The *p53* gene is now known to be a means for regulating cell growth. Bert Vogelstein at Johns Hopkins and coworkers, and, independently, Stephen Elledge, Wade Harper, and coworkers at Baylor College of Medicine, announced in the November 1993 *Cell* that the *p53* gene regulates the operations of a second gene, named either *WAF1* or *CIP1*. (Another group at Baylor also discovered the gene's specific function but published its results later.) *WAF1* or *CIP1* retards cell growth, probably by counteracting the production of genes that produce cyclin-dependent kinases, which tend to promote cell growth. The products of all the genes involved are thought to have other functions in addition to the ones concerned with cell growth.

In short, one effect of a defective form of *p53* is that it leaves the *WAF1* (or *CIP1*) gene uncontrolled, which probably results in the *WAF1* (*CIP1*) gene allowing other genes to produce substances that encourage cells to grow. Thus, ineffective *p53* contributes to the uncontrolled cell growth that is the main distinguishing characteristic of cancer.

The first indication that *p53* might be involved in human cancer occurred in the early 1980s when Bert Vogelstein observed that colon cancer tissue samples often showed damage to the part of chromosome 17 where the *p53* gene resides. In the early 1990s researchers found the *p53* gene displaying a number of other connections to cancer. The first clue was the previously mentioned discovery of the role of an allele of *p53* at the root of Li-Fraumeni syndrome. This discovery then led Stephen H. Friend of Massachusetts General Hospital in Boston and coworkers to demonstrate that a fairly common allele of *p53* predisposes persons to breast cancer or other specific cancers. In 1991 one type of damage to the gene was found to be caused by the cancer-causing mold product aflatoxin, which is implicated in liver cancer. Other researchers found that additional environmental chemicals linked to cancer also specifically damage the *p53* gene.

The Ras Pathway

Genes such as *p53* are sometimes called *oncogenes,* because they are involved in cancer (*onco* means tumor in Greek), or *proto-oncogenes* in recognition of the fact that the most common alleles of oncogenes have a normal function in the body and do not cause disease. Along with *p53*, one of the first proto-oncogenes to be discovered, *ras,* became much better understood in the first part of the 1990s. The gene *ras* was among the 20-odd proto-oncogenes recognized in the late 1970s and early 1980s. (Hundreds of cancer-related genes have now been identified.) By 1983 a damaged *ras* gene was found in lung cancer cells but not in other cells, among the most dramatic early research connecting genes to cancer.

Determination of the method by which *ras* affects the genes for cell growth, known as the Ras pathway, was a major breakthrough shared by several groups in 1993. Scientists were excited by the discoveries because unraveling how *ras* works appeared to be a key to a number of gene functions. The potential clinical implications of the discovery are significant as well. The much-studied cellular messenger known as cyclic AMP was shown to interrupt growth promotion fostered by the Ras pathway. This suggests that finding a way to increase the amount of cyclic AMP in a cancer cell may turn off growth, limiting the cancer or even changing the cells back to normal.

Colorectal Cancer Genes

Since the mid-1960s, physicians have known that members of some families carry an allele that enhances the likelihood of several varieties of cancer, of which colorectal is the most common. A key to investigating inheritance of this gene, known as the hereditary nonpolyposis colorectal cancer gene or HNPCC gene, was the location of very large families in which the gene occurs. Such large families are necessary to provide a sufficient number of cases of gene expression.

A team including Bert Vogelstein (of the *p53* gene—see above) and Stanley R. Hamilton of Johns Hopkins University School of Medicine, Albert de la Chapelle of the University of Helsinki in Finland, and coworkers studied two such families from opposite ends of the earth, New Zealand and Canada. The researchers reported in the May 7, 1993 issue of *Science* that they had located the gene involved on a short stretch of chromosome 2 and that the HNPCC gene seems to cause its damage by directing other genes of various sorts to repeat unnecessarily and destructively short sequences of DNA bases. Furthermore, the same kind of repeats are frequently found in colorectal cancers even when there is no family history of the HNPCC gene. This gene is thought to be involved in as many as 22,000 cases of colon cancer in the U.S. every year and perhaps as many as a million Americans carry the defective allele. About 55,000 deaths annually are caused by one or another forms of colon cancer in the U.S., and knowledge about the HNPCC gene and its mechanisms is expected to contribute to understanding and detecting various forms of colon cancer.

The discovery that DNA repeats are common in colon cancer was confirmed in an independent study conducted by a group led by Stephen N. Thibodeau of the Mayo Clinic. This study revealed that 25 cancers out of 90 examined contained the repeated DNA stretches of the HNPCC gene. Repeats in a different gene were also found to be involved in some cases of colorectal cancer by another group (see "Fragment repeats" below).

The actual gene was found and announced in December 1993 by two different groups of researchers. The first group, Richard D. Kolodner of the Dana-Farber Cancer Institute in Boston, Richard Fishel of the University of Vermont Medical School in Burlington, and six coworkers, recognized that they were studying a protein in yeast with the same functions as the then unknown HNPCC gene in humans. In yeast, the gene produces a protein called MSH2 that checks for incorrect matches in DNA replication in mitosis, calling other proteins into action to correct any errors located. Kolodner, Fishel, and coworkers then looked for the gene on human chromosome 2 and found it. Their report was published in the December 3 *Cell.* Bert Volgelstein and 24 coworkers isolated the same gene as a continuation of their work with HNPCC, and *Cell* carried their report on December 17, although the results were announced at the same time as the Kolodner-Fishel report. One result of two groups identifying the gene at essentially the same time is to leave the question of the gene's name somewhat up in the air. Prior work with the gene in yeast may result in a final name of *MSH2* for the HNPCC gene.

It is thought that further work will lead to a blood test that will reveal the presence of the allele. Persons with the allele will than be encouraged to have frequent follow-up examinations. Colorectal cancer is one of the most treatable cancers if located in its early stages. Some of the other cancers thought to be caused by the gene are less amenable to treatment, but are also less common.

The search for *the* colorectal cancer gene has resulted in the identification of a number of different genes as the cause of this disease. In March 1991 a gene called *MCC* (for mutated colon cancer) was identified and touted as the colorectal cancer gene. Five months later the trumpets sounded for *APC* (for adenomatous polyposis coli), thought to be the first gene in a chain leading to colorectal cancer. Both of these genes are located on chromosome 5, while the HNPCC gene is found on chromosome 2.

The gene *APC* does cause a rare form of colon cancer that results from a condition named familial adenomatous polyposis, so named because it "runs in families" and is characterized by many polyps (polyposis), resembling warts (adenomatous), in the colon. Discovery of the gene led to a diagnostic procedure for the disease announced in the *New England Journal of Medicine* by Kenneth W. Kinzler and Steven M. Powell of the Johns Hopkins University School of Medicine Center in Baltimore,

Maryland on December 30, 1993. It is hoped that a similar blood test to detect the HNPCC gene will be developed very soon. If applied to the entire population, the two tests together could detect about 16 percent of all colon cancers before they start.

Suppressor Genes, Off and On

Wilm's tumor occurs when an individual acquires two copies of a defective gene. (The normal function of this gene is, so far, poorly understood by scientists.) If a person is born with one normal gene and one defective gene, he or she often develops malformations of the urinary tract or genitals. If the normal gene later stops producing its correct gene product for some reason, the person develops an uncontrolled growth of kidney tissue that is called Wilm's tumor. Usually such tumors develop in children around the age of three or four. Fortunately, a combination of chemotherapy and radiation nearly always destroys the tumor and permits normal kidney development.

The specific gene involved was identified by David Housman of MIT in 1990. Since then, scientists have been able to experiment with a mouse version of the gene.

Background

From the time of the ancient Greeks until the 1980s the causes of cancer were very poorly understood. The explanations varied with the expectations of the age, ranging from evil spells in primitive societies to environmental causes in the ecologically conscious 1970s. The environment as a factor in cancer was first suggested as early as 1775. By 1910 the newly discovered viruses were proposed as the cause. Two other late-nineteenth-century discoveries—X rays and radioactivity—were eventually found to cause cancer as well.

Despite the essential correctness of the view that cancer can result from exposure to chemicals in the environment, from radiation exposure (whether from radium or from the Sun), or from infection by specific viral agents, the precise mechanisms at work were far from clear. Furthermore, some kinds of cancer seemed to "run in families," while other cancers were apparently affected by mental stress. Finally, in 1967, K.D. Zang and H. Singer identified a specific change in a chromosome found in a tumor.

All of these theories began to make sense when biologists discovered how DNA and various proteins directed by DNA control cell growth. It was first determined that malfunctions of certain specific genes resulted in uncontrolled growth of cancer. Later it was demonstrated that these genes are the ones that direct normal growth.

In some cases, the gene is damaged by something in the environment, such as a chemical or radiation. A virus can also damage a gene while directing the DNA in the cell to make copies of the virus. Some research suggests that a gene from hepatitis B virus causes cancer whenever it is expressed in liver cells. A particular allele of a gene might regulate growth badly even when undamaged or might be especially susceptible to damage. Thus, all the previously proposed causes of cancer, except for evil spells, can be understood as manifestations of a damaged gene or an ineffective allele of a gene.

Jordan A. Kreidberg, Rudolf Jaenisch, and coworkers at Whitehead Institute for Biomedical Researcher in Cambridge, Massachusetts, have created mice in which one or both alleles of the Wilm's gene are "knocked out" of the genome. They reported in the August 27, 1993 *Cell* that mice lacking both copies of the gene fail to develop kidneys at all. Mice with one copy of the gene develop normally, not even showing the defects that humans with one ineffective allele encounter. So far, there has been no way to "knock out" the other copy of the gene after the kidney has developed, so a mouse model for Wilm's tumors has not yet been created.

Current cancer theory suggests that genes like the Wilm's gene are tumor suppressors that ordinarily regulate growth. Ineffective versions do not so much encourage cancer growth as permit it. The research with mice suggests that, in the case of the Wilm's gene at least, the same gene must actively promote growth at early stages and then prohibit growth later on. Given the complexity of biological systems, such a pattern is not only possible, but typical.

Another tumor suppressor gene was located in 1993. A large group of scientists, working long-distance but together, at the National Cancer Institute in the U.S., Cambridge University in England, and the Centre d'Etude du Polymorphisme Humain in France identified the gene that, when it malfunctions, causes von Hippel-Landau disease. This syndrome predisposes a person to cancer of the kidney or another location in the body, including the eye and the brain. Approximately 1 in 36,000 persons has the syndrome, which typically results in death in middle age from one of the various cancers.

THREE WAYS TO MAKE CANCER

Biologists have identified three ways that a gene, often working in concert with other genes, can cause cellular mechanisms to go awry and produce one of the diseases we collectively call cancer.

Proto-oncogenes: Genes that promote growth can be transmitted in forms that cause unceasing growth or they can be damaged in ways that produce the same result. Sometimes these genes are called oncogenes because of their connection with cancer. However, undamaged versions of the genes do not cause cancer, but rather perform vital cell functions.

Anti-oncogenes: Many of the proto-oncogenes are controlled by other genes. When these genes, sometimes called tumor suppressor genes (although they also control normal growth), are present as in ineffective alleles or damaged forms, unrestricted cell growth results.

A bad transcription gene: In 1993 a new cancer-causing mechanism was discovered. A gene was identified that increases the number of repeats in repeated DNA sequences at various points of the cell. In many cases, the repeated sections interfere with the common proteins produced by affected genes in ways that lead to tumor production. Apparently the gene, found in both yeast and in human families with an inherited predisposition toward colon cancer, is involved in mitosis. If the allele of the gene fails to transcribe repeated sections faithfully, cancer can result. In addition to colorectal cancer, the gene is thought to have a role in cancers of the kidney, ovary, and lining of the uterus.

Fragment Repeats

The same cancer-related gene can have many different alleles. Each allele that causes cancer may lead to the same or similar cancers. The variations in alleles occur when different bases in the gene are affected or when the same base or group of bases is either deleted, substituted for, or repeated. The same cancer can result from different variations because each one inactivates the same gene product.

In the August 19, 1993 *New England Journal of Medicine*, Theodore G. Krontris of Tufts University School of Medicine in Boston and coworkers described the varied effects caused by repetition of a single 28-base fragment of the gene HRAS-1—one of the genes that controls cell division and differentiation. The fragment is generally repeated in all versions of the gene, with about 94 percent of people studied having one of four alleles in which the number of repeats seems to be normal—that is, no known cancers result for these numbers of repeats. The remaining 6 percent of the people studied have alleles in which the unusual number of repetitions seems to be connected with cancers. The August 19 report states that slightly less than one in ten breast, bladder, or colorectal cancers occur in patients with the unusual alleles of the HRAS-1 gene.

SUMMARY OF KNOWN TUMOR TYPES CAUSED BY DOMINANT GENES

In these familial syndromes, a gene inherited as one allele in a pair has been located on a particular chromosome. In some cases the gene itself has also been located and sequenced.

Hereditary predisposition	Chromosome Location	Gene Found?	Gene Class
Basal cell skin cancers (Gorlin syndrome)	9	No	
Colorectal cancers (adenomatous polyposis)	5	Yes, *APC*	Anti-Oncogene
(non-polyposis)	2	Yes, HNPCC gene or *MSH2*	Bad transcription
Early-onset breast cancer	17	No	
Glandular cancers (Type 1 endocrine neoplasia)	11	No	
(Type 2 endocrine neoplasia)	10	No	
Kidney cancers (Wilm's tumor)	11	Yes, *WT1*	Anti-Oncogene
Li-Fraumeni syndrome (several cancer types)	17	Yes, *p53*	Anti-Oncogene
Melanoma (a skin cancer)	9	No	
Neurofibromatosis (Type 1)	17	Yes, *NF1*	Anti-Oncogene
(Type 2)	22	Yes, *NF2*	Anti-Oncogene
Retinoblastoma (eyes, bones)	13	Yes, *Rb*	Anti-Oncogene
Thyroid carcinoma; pheochromocytoma		Yes, *RET*	Anti-Oncogene
von Hippel-Landau syndrome (several cancer types)	3	Yes, *VHL*	Anti-Oncogene

(Periodical References and Additional Reading: *New York Times* 11-30-90, p A1; *New York Times* 4-23-91, p C1; *New York Times* 5-24-91, p A16; *New York Times* 8-9-91; *Harvard Health Letter* 3-92, p 4; *Discover* 1-93, p 89; *Science* 5-7-93, pp 751, 810, 812, 816; *Science News* 5-8-93, p 292; *New York Times* 5-11-93, p C3; *Science* 5-28-93, pp 1235, 1317; *New York Times* 6-6-93, p A1; *Nature* 6-10-93, pp 495, 515; *New York Times* 8-31-93, p C3; *Science News* 9-4-93, p 148; *Science* 9-10-93, p 1385; *Science News* 9-18-93, p 189; *Science* 11-12-93, p 988; *New York Times* 11-23-93, p C6; *Scientific American* 12-93, p 47; *New York Times* 12-3-93, p A1; *Time* 12-3-93, p 58; *Science* 12-10-93, pp 1644, 1645, 1667, 1731, 1734; *Science* 12-24-93, pp 1953, 1958, 1980; *New York Times* 12-30-93, p A12; *Harvard Health Letter* 3-94, p 3)

GENES FOR ALCOHOLISM?

Millions of people around the world believe that alcoholism is a disease. Among its symptoms are tolerance for large amounts of alcohol, although that tolerance often decreases with age. Furthermore, people with the disease of alcoholism—known as alcoholics—are often unable to stop drinking alcohol so long as it is available. Once an alcoholic is exposed to alcohol, even in small amounts, uncontrolled drinking may begin.

Physicians and other researchers have long tried to tie alcoholism to a specific genetic defect. Despite a vast body of anecdotal evidence, especially concerning people who develop the symptoms associated with alcoholism from their first exposure to alcohol, often early in childhood, hard evidence that holds up over time has been lacking. One report of twins raised apart shows that children of alcoholics raised in nonalcoholic families still become alcoholic, while another reaches the opposite conclusion. The results of the best twin studies vary widely from showing no genetic contribution to suggesting about 3/5 heredity blended with 2/5 other causes. A study linking alcoholism to other substance abuse and to severe depression showed that adopted children of depressed parents show no increase in that cluster of symptoms, while close relatives of the depressed parents are more likely to show the symptoms than the population at large.

Here are some of the most recent results:

One Gene That May or May Not Be It

Most researchers expect to find a genetic basis for alcoholism. The U.S. National Institute of Alcohol Abuse and Alcoholism (NIAAA), for example, has a separate section on genetic studies. But identification of a specific gene has been very difficult.

The first study to identify a particular gene with alcoholism was conducted by Kenneth Blum of the University of Texas Health Sciences Center in San Antonio and Ernest P. Nobel of the University of California in Los Angeles; it was reported in the *Journal of the American Medical Association* on April 18, 1990. They found that 69 percent of the persons they studied who died as a direct result of alcoholism shared the same allele of the dopamine D2 receptor gene on chromosome 11, as compared with 20 percent of a matched sample from people identified as non-alcoholics. The gene codes for a protein that transports the neurotransmitter dopamine, thought to play a major role in the human pleasure mechanism, into nerve cells (*see also* "The

Ubiquity of NO in Life," p 305). The dopamine system has been suspected of involvement in alcoholism and other addictions for a number of years. Follow-up studies by the same researchers with living alcoholics also found a high percentage of them have this allele of the dopamine D2 receptor gene.

Within the year, the NIAAA announced in the same journal that the Blum-Nobel study had *not* been confirmed by its own division of genetics. The NIAAA study, conducted by Annabel M. Bolos and coworkers, looked at 40 unrelated alcoholics, 127 persons identified as non-alcoholics, and 14 members of two large families known to be disposed toward alcoholism. The suspect allele did not appear in significantly high percentages in the alcoholics and the predisposed families; slightly more than a third of the alcoholics and slightly less than a third of the controls had the allele. A second study, in 1991, by Joel Gelernter of the Veterans Administration Medical Center in West Haven, Connecticut, agreed with the NIAAA results, as did several other later studies.

There may be some alcoholics influenced by the allele identified by Blum and Nobel, especially since the populations included in these studies differed greatly in the type of alcoholism displayed. Later studies by Blum and Nobel and by others, and even a reanalysis of the NIAAA data, continue to show an association between the gene and severe alcoholism, with little evidence for the gene in the case of mild or moderate alcoholism. Furthermore, a separate study connected a different D2 allele, known as B1, to addiction of all kinds, including alcoholism. Despite these possibilities, most researchers in the field think that the gene for alcoholism, if it exists, remains to be found.

Rat Receptors

A strain of rats with a low tolerance for alcohol has been bred. Known as ANTs (alcohol non-tolerants, nothing to do with the well-known insects), the rats have a point mutation in the gene for the GABA neurotransmitter receptor. In addition to low alcohol tolerance, demonstrated by loss of coordination and reflexes, the rats also show abnormal reactions to the tranquilizer diazepam (Valium). Diazepam and alcohol act on the same receptors. Although the rat discovery might be interpreted as a technical confirmation of a gene for alcoholism, it is not clear what the connection might be with human conditions. Indeed, it is not entirely proven that the mutation directly accounts for the changes in the rats' tolerance to alcohol.

(Periodical References and Further Reading: *New York Times* 12-26-90; *Science News* 1-12-91, p 29; *Science News* 6-1-91, p 351; *Science News* 9-21-92, p 190; *Science News* 11-14-92, p 332; *New York Times* 1-5-93, p C3; *Nature* 1-28-93, pp 302, 356; *Science News* 1-30-93, p 70; *Science News* 4-21-93, p 246; *Scientific American* 7-93, p 122)

OTHER GENETIC DISEASES

The genes responsible for hereditary diseases are gradually being located, although the connection between a specific allele of a gene and a recognized disorder is often much looser than expected. Connections can range from a vague predisposition toward alcoholism, addiction, or obesity; through genetic patterns associated to one degree or another with diseases long recognized to have some hereditary basis, such as type II diabetes; to a sharply defined lack of a specific enzyme as in hemophilia.

The diabetes linkage announced in the *New England Journal of Medicine* in January 1993 illustrates some of the difficulty in making a specific connection. Although diabetes comes in several forms and may be the result of immune-system reactions that may or may not be triggered by viral infections, it also "runs in families." Thus, there is some genetic link, especially for the type II form, also known as non-insulin-dependent or adult-onset diabetes. When Leif C. Groop and coworkers at the Helsinki University Hospital in Finland studied the genetic makeup of 107 people with type II diabetes, comparing them to 164 controls, the Finnish doctors found that gene allele for sugar storage was different in 30 percent of the people with type II diabetes but this same difference occurred in only 8 percent of the controls. Despite the difference in the gene, however, sugar storage mechanisms are the same in those with the diabetes-associated allele and those with the more common wild-type allele. Thus, although there is a statistically significant connection, it is not very significant and the effect, if any, is obscure. Perhaps the sugar-storage gene is simply located on the chromosome near the spot where a more effective diabetes gene resides so that the true diabetes gene tends to be inherited along with the sugar-storage gene.

Hereditary ALS

On January 1, 1993, James O. McNamara of the Duke University Medical Center and coworkers announced the discovery of a suspicious gene in a region of chromosome 21 known from family studies to be involved in hereditary amyotrophic lateral sclerosis (ALS), a genetic disorder with the same symptoms as the much more common disease of unknown origin that is often referred to as Lou Gehrig's disease. In addition to the two forms of ALS, there is a another poorly understood disease in this class that is endemic to the island of Guam, but is mysteriously disappearing from the island today. Location of the gene for the hereditary disease provides several clues that may apply to ordinary ALS and the Guam disease and possibly to other related muscle disorders.

McNamara's announcement was slightly premature. Two months later, a large team of researchers led by Robert Brown Jr. of Massachusetts General Hospital and Robert Horvitz of Massachusetts Institute of Technology announced the correct location and function of the gene involved in the March 4, 1993 *Nature*.

In both hereditary ALS and the Guam disease, evidence points to the neurotransmitter glutamate as a possible culprit. A chemical mimicking glutamate is implicated in the Guam disease and the McNamara team found that the suspicious gene codes for part of the glutamate receptor on nerve cells. It was previously known from *in vitro* studies that high levels of glutamate cause calcium to build up in cells. Eventually the overdose of calcium kills the nerve cells. McNamara thinks that the allele of the gene that occurs in individuals with hereditary ALS causes the receptor to take a bit too much calcium into the nerve cells, resulting, after many years, in cell death.

This may be the ultimate result, but the actual gene encodes a familiar protein known as Cu/Xn-binding superoxide dismutase (SOD1 — to differentiate it from two other superoxide dismutase proteins). The basic task of SOD1 is to free the cytoplasm that makes up most of the interior of cells from free radicals. Free radicals are loose cannons, including oxygen molecules with electric charges, that produce highly reactive molecules that can interfere with normal working of the cells. The other two varieties of SOD accomplish the same task in mitochondria and in spaces between cells. Because the evidence points to high calcium ion concentrations inside cells as the actual cause of cell death, a shortage of SOD1 may allow free radicals to damage calcium ion channels that pump the ions out of the interiors of cells. Thus, even though McNamara had the wrong gene, he may have had the right idea. Investigators also hope that this knowledge will lead to ways to treat the much more common non-hereditary form of ALS.

Menkes' Syndrome and Wilson's Disease

In January 1993 three separate teams of researchers reported locating on the X chromosome the gene responsible for proper copper transport across the cell membrane and into the cell. The gene, named *MNK* in reference to the hereditary disease Menkes' syndrome, resembles a bacterial gene known to be involved in transporting copper across cell membranes. The immediate clinical benefit will be quicker diagnoses of babies born with the syndrome. Injections of copper solutions, if started early enough in life, prevent the mental retardation, seizures, and other symptoms of Menkes' disease. Like other genetic diseases linked to the X chromosome, Menkes' syndrome mainly attacks males.

The location of the *MNK* gene quickly led to the discovery of another copper-transport gene that is also involved in a hereditary disease. Wilson's disease is caused by copper that builds up in the brain, causing symptoms similar to schizophrenia, and the liver, causing death by early adolescence. A group led by T. Conrad Gilliam of Columbia University had previously located the Wilson's disease gene on chromosome 13. When the discovery of *MNK* was announced, Gilliam hoped that the gene he was looking for would be similar to *MNK*. He discussed this theory with Rudolph Tanzi of Massachusetts General Hospital, who, as it turned out, had found such a gene on chromosome 13 as a result of an entirely different research program. By the time of the 1993 World Congress on Psychiatric Genetics in New Orleans in October 1993, Gilliam was able to announce that the gene for Wilson's disease had been identified.

Adult Leukemia

In the February 12, 1993 issue of *Science* two reports linked adult leukemia, a disease characterized by the uncontrolled growth of leukocytes (white blood cells), with a gene that encodes one of two regulatory proteins for interferon. Working with humans, Cheryl L. Willman of the University of New Mexico School of Medicine and coworkers showed that an insufficiency of the protein can be implicated in leukemia. The gene for the protein in humans is located on a stretch of chromosome 5 known to be ineffective in many leukemia patients. Apparently both alleles of the gene must function correctly for the protein to be produced in normal amounts, so the tendency toward adult leukemia can be passed on from either parent.

Working with mouse cells *in vitro*, Hirashi Harada, Motoo Kitagawa, and coworkers from Osaka University in Japan showed that too much of the other regulatory protein for interferon resulted in excessive cell growth of the type found in leukemia. But if the same factor that Willman found in short supply in humans with leukemia is present in normal amounts in the mice, then the mouse cells no longer make too much of the second regulatory protein. Thus, the Japanese work also indicates that an ineffective form of the gene for the protein Willman found might predispose a person for leukemia.

Canavan's Disease

In the October 1993 issue of *Nature Genetics*, Reuben Matalon of the Research Institute of Miami Children's Hospital in Florida and coworkers reported that they had cloned the gene underlying Canavan's disease, unraveled its code, and located both the allele that produces 85 percent of the cases of this hereditary disease and a different allele that causes another 7 percent of the cases. While the gene is made from thousands of bases, a change in just one of these is the most common cause of the disease.

Canavan's disease has been recognized for 60 years, but not until 1988 did anyone grasp the mechanism of its devastating course—babies born with the defect cannot sit, walk, or talk and most die before the age of five. These symptoms occur because the myelin insulation around nerve cells is ineffective. The person who unraveled the causes of the disease was the same Reuben Matalon who found the gene five years later. He and his coworkers discovered that in Canavan's disease a key biochemical reaction in nerve cells stops at one point in the chain of chemical reactions. The chemical at that point in the reaction (N-acetyl-L-aspartic acid, or NAA) is not modified by the appropriate enzyme, so it builds up in the cells. NAA is not degraded because the necessary enzyme is not produced by the ineffective gene that is responsible for Canavan's disease. Matalon's work will immediately result in quicker diagnosis of the disease, and also will make possible better genetic counseling for couples at risk because of their ethnic background (Jews from Eastern Europe and their descendants).

Late-Onset Alzheimer's Disease

Even though the mechanisms that cause Alzheimer's disease, a progressive loss of mental faculties that most often occurs late in life, are not well understood, a gene allele that predisposes a person to the disease has been located. This discovery was announced in the August 13, 1993 *Science* by a team of researchers from Duke University Medical Center that included Margaret A. Pericak-Vance, Ann M. Saunders, Allen D. Roses, Warren J. Strittmatter, Guy Salvesen, John Gilbert, P.C. Gaskell, Mark Alberts, Elizabeth H. Corder, and Donald E. Schmechel. The allele is called apoE4 and about 2 to 3 percent of humans are thought to bear two copies of this allele, putting them at risk for developing Alzheimer's late in life. (*See also* "Alzheimer's Disease," p 456.) Even people with a single copy of the allele have a considerably greater risk of developing the disease and also develop it earlier than those with a different allele.

The gene, on chromosome 19, codes for an important protein, designated apolipoprotein E, that transports cholesterol through the bloodstream. There are several alleles, of which apoE2, apoE3, and apoE4 are relatively common; most people have apoE3 (90 percent with one copy and 60 percent with two).

In addition to the common variety of Alzheimer's associated with apoE4, there are at least three rare types of the disease (or, more accurately, types of disease that are clinically identical to Alzheimer's, despite a somewhat different cause) that are hereditary in a stronger form. Two of these have been linked to unknown genes on different chromosomes. In 1990, John Hardy and coworkers at St. Mary's Hospital Medical School in London found that a gene on chromosome 21 has an allele that produces the characteristic brain deposits found in Alzheimer's. A form of Alzheimer's associated with families known as the "Volga Germans" (descended from Germans who moved to the shores of the Volga River in the eighteenth century) has not been associated with any particular chromosome so far, although it is clearly a hereditary form of the disease. Another gene, on chromosome 14, is linked to a familial early-onset variety of the disease.

Hemophilia A

Hemophilia comes in two forms, A and B. Type A, in which blood-clotting Factor VIII is missing, is more common than type B, in which the missing protein is Factor IX. In the early 1980s researchers identified the gene involved in hemophilia A, a gene that in its normal form produces Factor VIII. It was not until 1993, however, that researchers were able to explain the genetic defect in hemophilia A. The defect turned out to be a reversed segment of the gene for Factor VIII. The gene, located near the tip of the X chromosome, can undergo an interchange of sections, a form of recombination, when the chromosome tip flips and temporarily forms a loop. The inverted portion was not detected previously because whole molecules of DNA are always broken into small sections for study and identification. Although some of the small segments of the gene were flipped around, the chemical tests could not detect this. The same bases were there in the same order and, for a small section, there was no way to tell which end was the start and which the conclusion. The gene with the reversed segment is unable to produce Factor VIII. RNA attempts to transcribe the defective gene, but the transcription stops when it reaches the reversed segment. Consequently, no Factor VIII is produced and a severe form of hemophilia results.

This mechanism was discovered by Francesco Gianelli at Guy's Hospital in London. Gianelli tried to use RNA to copy the Factor VII gene, but he got two separate RNA pieces instead of the one long piece expected. An explanation for this result, based upon an inverted segment, was proposed in November 1993 by Jane Gitschier of the University of California in San Francisco and Haig H. Kazazian, Jr., of Johns Hopkins University in Baltimore, Maryland. While understanding the cause is unlikely to affect the treatment of hemophilia A, it will enable researchers for the first time to identify this form of hemophilia by examining DNA. Thus, it may have some application in genetic counseling.

MAJOR HEREDITARY DISEASES

Disease	Location of gene	Description
ADA deficiency	Chromosome 20	A form of Severe Combined Imunodeficiency Deficiency Disease (SCID); defective immune system results in early death from infections
Adrenoleukodystrophy	X chromosome	Known as ALD or "Lorenzo's Oil Disease"
Alzheimer's disease	Chromosome 14* Chromosome 19 Chromosome 21*	Degeneration of brain cells leads to loss of memory and eventually to death
Amyloidosis	Chromosome 18	Accumulation of an insoluble protein in tissues
Amyotrophic lateral sclerosis*	Chromosome 21	Known as ALS or Lou Gehrig's Disease; results in destruction of nerves; invariably fatal
Canavan's disease	Chromosome ???	Chemical buildup in cells results in death before age of five; more common among Ashkenazi Jews
Cystic fibrosis	Chromosome 7	Mucus in lungs most often leads to death from infection, but output of pancreas and male reproductive system are also affected
Familial hypercholesterolemia	Chromosome 19	Extremely high cholesterol levels often lead to early heart disease
Familial polyposis of colon	Chromosome 5	Polyps develop in colon and frequently lead to colorectal cancer
Gaucher's disease	Chromosome 1	Deficiency in an essential enzyme leading to accumulation of harmful lipids; most common among Ashkenazi Jews
Hemochromatosis	Chromosome 6	Abnormally high absorption of iron leads to buildup of iron in tissues
Hemophilia (A & B)	X chromosome	Lack of a blood clotting factor (different in A and B forms of disease)
Huntington's disease	Chromosome 4	Nerve cell degeneration affecting behavior; symptoms appear in adults and lead to death
Menkes' syndrome	X chromosome	Improper copper transport into cells
Multiple exsotoses*	Chromosome 8	Disorder of bone and cartilage
Muscular dystrophy	X chromosome	Both the Duchenne and Becker types cause progressive deterioration of muscles
Myotonic dystrophy	Chromosome 19	Symptoms same as muscular dystrophy, but strikes adults
Phenylketonuria	Chromosome 12	Known as PKU; enzyme for metabolizing the amino acid phenylalanine is missing, leading to buildup of acid and mental retardation
Polycystic kidney disease	Chromosome 16	Causes renal failure as a result of cysts in kidneys

Disease	Location of gene	Description
Retinitis pigmentosa	Chromosome 3	Progressive degeneration of the retina, leading to blindness
Sickle cell anemia	Chromosome 11	Red blood cells deformed; they carry less oxygen and tend to clump in arterioles and capillaries
Spinocerebellar ataxia	Chromosome 6	Nerves in brain and spinal cord are destroyed, impairing coordination
Tay-Sachs disease	Chromosome 15	Disorder of lipid metabolism that causes death in early childhood; especially common among Ashkenazi Jews and some French-Canadians
Wilson's disease	Chromosome 13	Various mutations in the gene that makes a copper transport protein result in copper's building up in the brain and liver

* Hereditary forms only. Similar symptoms result in a more common disease of the same name with no known cause.

(Periodical References and Further Reading: *New York Times* 10-23-92, p A16; *Science* 10-23-92, pp 550, 668; *Science News* 1-2-93, p 5; *Science News* 1-9-93, p 30; *New York Times* 1-12-93, p C3; *Nature* 3-4-93, pp 20, 59; *Science* 3-5-93, p 1393; *New York Times* 5-6-93, p A1; *Science* 8-13-93, pp 828, 921; *Science* 8-20-93, pp 986, 1047; *New York Times* 10-5-93, p C1; *Nature* 10-7-93, p 590; *Science News* 10-9-93, p 234; *Science* 10-15-93, p 333; *Scientific American* 11-93, p 28; *New York Times* 11-2-93, p C8; *New York Times* 11-29-93, p A16; *Time* 1-17-94, p 46)

GENE THERAPY

GENE THERAPY: THE ADA EXPERIMENTS

Gene therapy refers to any medical procedure in which modified genes are introduced into the cells of victims of disease. Although gene therapies exist for other than hereditary diseases, the most controversial and potentially important use of the technique is for the treatment of hereditary diseases.

The First Experiment

In September 1990 the first true gene therapy to be officially sanctioned and provided for a human patient began in a four-year-old American girl with ADA deficiency. Weekly doses of a synthetic replacement enzyme called PEG-ADA (polyethylene glycol-conjugated ADA) kept the patient fairly healthy until the gene therapy began.

The gene therapy consisted of the following steps:

1. Some of the girl's blood was withdrawn.

2. T-cells, white blood cells that normally produce the ADA enzyme, were removed from the blood and grown in cultures until there were a large number of them.

3. A virus bearing an effective allele of the ADA gene was used to transduce (infect) the T cells.

4. Nearly a billion of the T cells, many of which were now producing ADA, were transfused into the girl's bloodstream.

5. This same treatment was repeated every few weeks.

This treatment was judged successful. Within three months the patient's white-blood-cell count was within the normal range and her immune system was capable of mounting a defense against foreign proteins for the first time. The increase in white cell count was only partly the direct result of the transfusions of T cells. The patient was found to have ten times as many T cells as had been transfused, indicating that her system was producing and retaining more T cells on its own. Soon her immune system was able to respond to such challenges as a skin test for tetanus, fighting the tiny bit of the tetanus bacterium and producing an angry red welt where the patch test was administered. Her parents even started taking her to a shopping mall. After a year, the girl was able to enter kindergarten as a regular student, a very different situation than the famous "boy in a bubble," who had a similar immune-system defect.

Other Experimental Treatments

In January 1991, a nine-year-old girl with ADA deficiency began gene therapy using the same method; the results in this case have also been positive. Encouraged by the U.S. experience, researchers have used a similar treatment with a five-year-old boy in Milan, Italy (since March 1992), and a ten-year-old girl in Bethesda, Maryland (since May 1993). The results are not uniformly positive, however. Some immune functions have not developed in the first two U.S. patients. The researchers are planning to

Background

ADA-deficiency disease is caused by ineffective alleles of the gene that produces the enzyme adenosine deaminase (ADA). ADA helps break down products of normal metabolism that in their whole form are toxic to parts of the immune system. When ADA fails to accomplish this task, the toxic residues accumulate in bone marrow and the thymus, the two main places where cells of the immune system grow and develop. Toxic residues there prevent lymphocytes from making new DNA molecules, so they cannot undergo mitosis. The result is that fewer T and B cells are present to defend against infection.

One form of ADA-deficiency results in so few T and B cells that it is called SCID for Severe Combined Immunodeficiency Disease (SCID). SCID can sometimes be cured by transplanting bone marrow from a healthy sibling into the patient whose cells do not produce ADA. If the bone marrow is sufficiently compatible, the transplant will cure the disease, but for the most famous SCID case, David, the "boy in the bubble," the transplant was unknowingly accompanied by a virus that killed David. (The gene for David's form of SCID was located after his 1984 death and reported in April 1993; it was an allele of the interleukin-2 receptor gene that fails to produce the receptor, resulting in few or no T cells reaching maturity.)

change the mix of T cells somewhat in hopes of obtaining the missing immune responses. The treatment is also very expensive—about $100,000 a year.

Carly Todd, an English one-year-old with ADA deficiency, underwent a different kind of gene therapy. In this case, the attempt has been made to alter genetically the stem cells in her bone marrow, the cells that normally produce blood cells. If successful, such a treatment will allow her body to produce its own T cells with an effective ADA gene. Similar therapies using altered stem cells were attempted on newborns Andrew Gobea (by Donald B. Kohn at Childrens Hospital in Los Angeles CA on May 14, 1993) and Zachary Riggens (by Diana Wera at the University of California Medical Center at San Francisco Medical Center on May 17, 1993). The stem cells in these cases were obtained from blood from the babies' umbilical cords, which, like bone marrow, normally contains stem cells. Early reports on the stem-cell approach suggest that the British experiment was not successful. No announcement has been made regarding the two newborn babies as of mid-January 1994.

(Periodical References and Further Reading: *New York Times* 12-14-90, p A24; *New York Times Magazine* 3-31-91, p 31; *New York Times* 7-28-91; *Science* 5-8-92, p 808; *New York Times* 4-9-93, p A18; *New York Times* 5-18-93, p C10; *Nature* 7-1-93, p 8; *Scientific American* 9-93, p 65; *Time* 1-17-94, p 46)

CYSTIC FIBROSIS AND VIRAL GENE DELIVERY

Four years after discovery of the gene whose alleles cause cystic fibrosis (in September 1989), and slightly more than a year after trials in mice, doctors were able to insert effective copies of the gene into a human being. After measuring the new gene's

Background

Among descendants of Europeans in the U.S., cystic fibrosis affects one individual in about 2500 births. About 30,000 Americans have cystic fibrosis, although genetic screening has revealed that many more of the suspect alleles are found in the population than even that incidence suggests. One study found 11 percent of the persons tested had peculiar alleles of the CFTR gene.

Cystic fibrosis was first recognized as a separate disease in 1938. The classic symptoms of this disease range from unusually salty sweat to a defective pancreas caused by blockage of its output. Cystic fibrosis may clog the pancreas early in development, even before birth. Lack of the digestive enzymes produced by the pancreas results in poor nutrition unless compensated for by dietary changes and supplements or replacements for the missing enzymes. Since 1968 it has been known that another common effect of cystic fibrosis is failure of development of the vas deferens, the tube that in human males carries sperm to the penis.

The effects of cystic fibrosis on the lungs are often lethal, however. Before antibiotics, most children with cystic fibrosis died in infancy because of pulmonary infections. The high frequency of infection results from the inability of the hairlike cilia, impeded by the thick mucus, to move bacteria or other invaders out of the lungs, as they normally do by producing outward-bound waves in ordinary mucus.

In addition to the experimental genetic treatments for the disease, various other treatments for cystic fibrosis have been developed in recent years, resulting in an increase in life expectancy from childhood to the 20s or 30s. These treatments include administration of pancreatic enzymes to improve digestion and antibiotics to protect against bacteria, as well as special exercises to improve breathing and attention to a proper diet. As a result, the median age of survival is now 29.

The relationship of alleles of the gene to the disease is extremely complex. More than 350 different alleles of the gene had been found by the end of 1993. As a result, many persons have inherited two different alleles from each parent, with varying results. Even when two copies of either of one of the alleles would cause cystic fibrosis, the pair of different alleles can sometimes fail to do so. Studies show that only five to ten percent of the normal amount of CFTR will prevent most symptoms of cystic fibrosis.

Other pairs of alleles of the gene can produce some symptoms of the disease, but not all, resulting in diseases recognized as infertility from loss of the vas deferens, as asthma (a form often complicated by allergic bronchopulmonary aspergillosis), or as bronchitis (a form called chronic pseudomonas bronchitis) instead of as cystic fibrosis. Many researchers think that the evidence points to involvement of alleles of different genes as well. If so, the other gene may influence the expression of the CFTR gene.

output of the protein normally missing in victims of the disorder, success of the experiment was announced in the October 22, 1993 issue of *Cell* by Michael J. Welsh of the University of Iowa College of Medicine and his coworkers. Although the effective version of the gene functioned in a human, it did not provide a cure for cystic fibrosis because it produced the protein in the wrong place in the body. Specifically, Welsh and coworkers used inactivated cold viruses (technically, adenoviruses) to carry the gene into the nasal passages where it was integrated into the cells lining those passages. Even so, the viral genes were not expected to become a part of the reproducing cells, so the cure would not be permanent.

In cystic fibrosis, mucus causes the most problems in the lungs and pancreas, not in the nose. The missing or defective protein is a chloride channel that transports chloride ions and water through cell membranes. It is called CFTR, meaning Cystic Fibrosis Transmembrane Conductance Regulator. Without the channel CFTR provides, the normal mucus that lines the lungs (and nasal passages) loses water and becomes thick and viscous, clogging the passageways. The viscous mucus not only interferes with breathing, but provides a fertile environment for infections, which eventually cause death. Animal experiments suggest that if as many as ten percent of the cells in the lining of the lungs have an effective CFTR gene, the mucus buildup can be stopped.

October 1993 produced a wealth of other genetics-related research on cystic fibrosis. An earlier experiment, started on April 17, 1993 by Ronald Crystal of New York Hospital-Cornell Medical Center and coworkers, also used adenoviruses, which were squirted into the lungs as well as into nasal passages. One of the three initial volunteers developed inflammation and a spot on a lung, so that experiment was terminated short of its planned number of nine human volunteers. Crystal was also planning to use the nasal passages (and a lower dose of viruses) in further experiments to insure that patients were not harmed. At the North American Cystic Fibrosis Conference in October 1993, Crystal reported that the patients treated in his genetic therapy experiments showed improvements in the flow of chloride channels.

CFTR is not the only promising gene product for the treatment of cystic fibrosis. Richard C. Boucher of the University of North Carolina at Chapel Hill and coworkers reported in the October 15, 1993 *Science* that mice with symptoms of cystic fibrosis have an additional chloride channel based on uridine 5'-triphosphate (UTP). Provision of UTP by genetic engineering or other means may alleviate the mucus problem in humans. The concept behind this therapy is similar to the production of fetal hemoglobin to alleviate sickle-cell anemia.

Another study, by Yiping Yang of the University of Pennsylvania Medical Center in Philadelphia and reported in the October 15 *Proceedings of the National Academy of Sciences,* showed that, in many cases, defective CFTR from a different allele of the gene will still function if it reaches the correct place in the cell. This allele causes the CFTR to stay in the interior of the cell instead of poking through the cell membrane. Modifying the protein to which the defective CFTR sticks is another possible approach to treating the disease.

Using Genetics to Prevent Conception

In 1992 doctors in the U.K. used the genetic information then available about the CFTR gene to select the ovum (egg) to be used in *in vitro* fertilization for a couple carrying a defective allele of the gene. After several ova were fertilized in a Petri dish, DNA from each ovum was sampled. Eggs that were deemed free of defective versions of the gene were then implanted in the mother. About nine months later a child was born that was free of the disease.

Since that time more than 15 similar successes have been recorded worldwide, sometimes for cystic fibrosis and sometimes for other genetic defects. The method is extremely expensive, however, on top of the already high cost of *in vitro* fertilization, so it is unlikely to become widespread.

Attacking DNA for Medicinal Purposes

Genentech, Inc., known mainly for producing drugs by changing an organism's DNA so that the organism produces the desired drug, introduced an effective treatment for cystic fibrosis in 1993 that uses DNA more directly in the patient. The medicine, produced by Genentech's normal genetic engineering, is called recombinant human deoxyribonuclease, or rhDNase. The idea behind the drug is that the enzyme deoxyribonuclease, which breaks down DNA, will thereby thin the mucus in the lungs of cystic fibrosis patients. While this is far from the cure that genetic engineering may yet produce, the new drug is an important aid in keeping people with cystic fibrosis healthy. Patients inhale rhDNase with an atomizer, which takes it directly to the lungs.

Alpha-1-antitrypsin-deficiency Emphysema

As early as April 1991, Ronald Crystal demonstrated the promise of his method for introducing genes into lungs with experiments in rats using a different gene, one in which some alleles cause another common inherited disorder of humans, alpha-1-antitrypsin-deficiency. This deficiency results in the hardening of the air sacs in the lungs, producing the symptoms called emphysema. This hereditary form of emphysema is a third more common than cystic fibrosis in the U.S., but it does not result in symptoms until persons born with the genetic flaw reach their 30s or 40s. Emphysema in this form invariably leads to an early death.

Crystal was able to demonstrate that rats produced human alpha-1-antitrypsin in their lungs after being infected with an adenovirus to which the corrected gene was attached. Later he used the same technique with the CFTR gene, first on rats and then on monkeys before the attempt with humans.

(Periodical References and Additional Reading: *New York Times* 4-23-91; *Science* 5-8-92, p 774; *New York Times* 8-22-92, p 9; *New York Times* 9-2-92, p D5; *New York Times* 12-4-92, p A28; *New York Times* 4-20-93, p C5; *New York Times* 10-15-93, p A24; *Science News* 10-23-93, p 260; *New York Times* 11-16-93, p C1; *Harvard Health Letter*, 3-94, p 3)

GENES AGAINST CANCER

The knowledge that cancer, no matter what initiates it, is ultimately a disease of the genes strongly suggests that a genetic cure be sought for it. For tumors, however, replacing the cancer with cells in which the genetic defects—usually multiple—have been corrected makes no sense; it is better just to remove the tumor when possible. But genetic engineering can be used against tumors in other ways.

The First Experiment

The first experiment in treating cancer with genetically altered cells began on January 29, 1991. Two melanoma patients received some of their own immune cells that had been strengthened by transduction (that is, infection) with the gene that produces the protein called tumor necrosis factor. Tumor necrosis factor, as its name suggests, causes cancer cells to die. The type of cells used in the experiment, tumor-infiltrating lymphocytes, are white blood cells that previous experiments showed actively seek out cancers and invade them. The experiment was conducted by a team headed by Steven A. Rosenberg of the U.S. National Cancer Institute.

The test was undertaken with some concern for the patients, although neither patient was expected to live more than about four months without some form of dramatic intervention. The U.S. Food and Drug Administration became involved because they feared, based on earlier attempts to use injected tumor necrosis factor to treat cancer, that the toxic protein would itself become the cause of death. Rosenberg was able to allay fears somewhat by agreeing to begin with very small numbers of genetically engineered cells and only increasing the number administered very slowly.

By July, after nearly seven months of therapy, the patients were still alive and new patients were being recruited for the experiment, with two additional ones added before July 18, 1991. At that point, however, the very low doses of genetically engineered cells, which had not caused any toxic problems, were suspected to be too low to produce much tumor necrosis factor. Indeed, it was not clear if the introduced cells were producing any of the deadly protein at all.

Aiming to Increase Specific Proteins

A year later, Clemma A. Hewitt became the first person to receive a different gene therapy approved for "compassionate use" in a terminally ill patient. The treatment used genetically altered tumor cells from the patient's own brain tumor. The altered cells produced interleukin 2, a substance that promotes growth and activity of the leukocytes called T cells. It was hoped that the leukocytes would then attack and destroy not only the altered cells, but also other tumor cells displaying the same antigens. Unlike the earlier melanoma experiments, this technique was essentially unproven. The doctors treating Mrs. Hewitt, Ivor Royston and Robert Sobol of the San Diego Regional Cancer Center, successfully argued that she would certainly die soon without such treatment.

At first the treatment seemed to be working. After a half year or more her condition seemed to have stabilized. Because all cancers occasionally go into a remission or a period of no growth, however, the evidence for improvement was only suggestive and not conclusive. Then Mrs. Hewitt's condition began to deteriorate and she died in October 93 from the effects of the cancer.

A similar approach had a different result in experiments with mice, as reported by

Michael Feldman of the Weizmann Institute of Science in Israel and coworkers in the February 15 *Journal of Immunology*. Mice specially bred to have rapidly spreading cancer were used. Tumors were removed from these mice and a gene to make one type of interferon was inserted into the tumor cells. Mice that received the interferon genes did not develop new tumors, but untreated mice did. The complete success of this experiment was striking.

Another successful experiment with mice adds the gene for a protein called granulocyte-macrophage colony-stimulating factor (GMCSF) to cells removed from a kidney tumor, and then reintroduces the genetically engineered cells into the mouse's body. The altered tumor cells stimulate the immune system to attack and destroy all tumor cells, not just the ones with the new gene. Trials on humans were just getting started at the end of 1993.

A similar experiment, with a different mechanism, has been successful with rats. On January 1, 1993 Mark L. Tykocinski and coworkers at Case Western Reserve University announced in *Science* that another form of genetically altered tumor cell could act as a "vaccine" against the tumor. When reinjected, the altered cells turn on the immune system, which proceeds to destroy the cancer. Their research involved rats with the brain cancer glioblastoma. Specifically, Tykocinski and his colleagues knocked out the gene for insulin-like growth factor in rat tumor cells. When reinjected into rats, the immune system perceived the altered cells as foreign, so it mounted an attack against them. The unaltered cancer cells remaining in the rats were also attacked.

Preventing Drug Damage

Much of the recent success against cancer has come from chemotherapy, but patients can be more devastated by the treatment than by the cancer. Taxol, for example, is effective against ovarian cancer, but it so suppresses the immune system that more than two or three courses of treatment can result in death from infection or internal bleeding caused by lack of immune function. As a result, many patients are forced to end Taxol treatments before growth of the cancer is arrested.

Albert B. Deisseroth of the University of Texas is investigating an experimental treatment to solve this problem by inserting a gene called *MDR* (for multiple-drug resistance) into white blood cells. If the treatment works, the immune system should develop enough resistance to Taxol that chemotherapy treatment of the cancer can be extended. As with many other genetic studies, this approach has been successful in mice. Differences in the human immune system, however, mean that success with mice is no guarantee of success with cancer patients.

Increasing Drug Damage

The opposite idea is behind an approach to treating brain cancer by genetic engineering. Kenneth W. Culver of Iowa Methodist Medical Center and Edward H. Oldfield of the U.S. National Institutes of Health demonstrated in 1992 that they could treat rats with terminal brain cancer by inserting herpes simplex genes into the tumors and then using an antiherpes drug, ganciclovir, to kill the infected tumor cells. In rat trials, not only were the infected cells killed by the drug, but also other cells near them (for unknown reasons). Human trials began in December 1992, but results are not yet known. Work with human brains is expected to be more difficult than studies of rat brains.

Blocking the Gene Product

If a physician knows that an allele of a gene or a damaged version of the gene is part of a genetic chain causing cancer, treatment can consist of blocking the gene product instead of the gene itself. This approach is under investigation by Dennis J. Slamon of the University of California in Los Angeles and, independently, by Mark I. Greene of the University of Pennsylvania. Human trials began with safety testing in 1993. Both doctors are working with the proto-oncogene *neu* and its protein, called P185. Greene was a member of the team that discovered *neu* in the 1980s. Since then *neu* has been implicated in about 30 percent of human breast cancer cases.

The treatment under investigation uses monoclonal antibodies that attack P185. Overproduction of P185 by versions of *neu* is part of the chain leading to cancer. Although the *neu* gene will continue to produce too much P185, the antibodies are intended to remove the protein from circulation in the blood, preventing cancer and possibly causing already existing cancers to stop growing or spreading to other locations in the body.

Greene has already tested the antibody treatment in a mouse model, where it delayed the appearance of cancer in most of the malignancy-prone mice and prevented it altogether in about half the mice. Such experiments are often more successful in mice than in humans, however, because mouse-derived antibodies are used in each case. While such antibodies present no problems for mice, the human immune system quickly rejects mouse-derived antibodies.

Injecting Genes into Tumors

While other researchers have taken cells from the body, altered their genes, and returned them to do battle with cancer, Gary J. Nabel of the Howard Hughes Medical Institute at the University of Michigan and coworkers have taken a more direct approach. They encased in fatty envelopes genes that produce a protein known to cause the immune system to attack cells and "mailed" the genes to the cells. The "mailing" was more like a broadcast, however, since these "envelopes" are not addressed to particular cells.

Cell membranes are composed of fats called lipids and, like most semi-liquid fats, these membranes will merge with other fatty globules that touch them. Genes inserted into the lipid envelopes often are found inside the cell membrane, and therefore inside the cell, after such a merger. The envelopes, known as liposomes, are directly injected into the cancer, and the gene carried by the liposome is incorporated into about 5 percent of the tumor cells, where it becomes activated and starts producing its protein product. The gene used in the experiment makes the protein HLA-B7. Among its virtues for fighting cancer is its effect on nearby cells. When a

Background

Liposomes have long been touted as a drug delivery system, but have so far failed to live up to their promise. For use in delivering genes, they have both advantages and disadvantages over the more common method of using partly inactivated viruses.

The viruses contain specific mechanisms that transport DNA into targeted cells and are nature's way of getting foreign DNA into the working chromosome. But scientists worry that viruses could somehow become reactivated inside the body and cause serious illnesses. Furthermore, one of the specialties of the immune system is the ability to root out and destroy foreign viruses, although it is not always as successful at the task as one would wish.

Liposomes are mere chemicals, not almost-living organisms. Although they do not seek out particular cells, they are less likely to be attacked by the immune system and are completely unable to become active carriers of an infectious disease.

cancer cell begins producing additional HLA-B7, the immune system attacks any cells in the vicinity, since it homes in on the protein, which is a powerful antigen.

None of the five patients in the experiment previously had the gene for HLA-B7, so its production, observed in all five, demonstrated that the technique worked. All patients had late-stage melanomas that had failed to respond to earlier treatment. Two of the patients showed some immune response, although only a few cells were producing the protein. One of the patients even experienced tumor loss at one injection site and regression at others, although he was not cured completely. Another injected tumor did not respond at all. The trial showed gene expression without toxic effects, a primary goal of the research.

The researchers are enthusiastic about the possible applications of this new treatment and plan more trials. They are altering their procedures in hopes of reaching more of the cells with the injected genes. Several biotechnology companies are also developing variants of direct DNA injection into the body with the expectation that some DNA will lodge in places in the cells where the genes will function. These efforts include treatments for other diseases in addition to cancer, including cystic fibrosis, muscle wasting diseases, and infections.

Diagnosis and Staging Conventional Treatment

Even if cancer is treated with such conventional therapies as surgery, radiation, or chemotherapy, genetic engineering still has a role to play. Pathologists at present identify cancer cells by such physical means as shape or structure, but such visual evidence is not always completely reliable. Some cancers, such as those affecting white blood cells (leukemias), are not made evident by changes in shape or structure. However, a pathologist can use genetic engineering to determine if the cells are cancerous much more reliably, especially when genetic means are combined with the older architectural methods. If a particular genetic defect that is known to cause cancer is suspected, tests can be even more specific.

When cancer is found, genetic engineering can continue to aid in treatment. The same cell identification techniques can be used to determine the spread of the disease by examining cells in various parts of affected or possibly affected organs. The tests also can be used to determine the effectiveness of a treatment, and can do so faster, enabling quicker responses, which might include increasing or decreasing chemo-therapy, for instance.

(Periodical References and Additional Reading: *New York Times* 1-30-91, p A1; *New York Times* 7-18-91; *New York Times* 9-16-92, p A20; *New York Times* 1-1-93, p A18; *New York Times Magazine* 3-31-91, p 31; *New York Times* 4-6-93, p C6; *Scientific American* 10-93, p 16; *New York Times* 10-23-93, p 10; *New York Times* 11-17-93, p C17; *Scientific American* 12-93, p 18; *New York Times* 12-1-93, p B10; *Science News* 12-4-93, p 372; *Time* 1-17-94, p 46)

Human Gene Therapy UPDATE

Gene therapy for human diseases has gone from science-fiction in the 1970s, through the first clumsy experiment in the 1980s, to partially successful experimental trials in the early 1990s. By the end of 1993 more than 50 trials were underway to implant working genes to correct defects in about 160 human patients. Animal research expected to lead to human therapy for other disorders was even more active. Active gene therapy experiments were conducted for a number of genetic diseases including ADA (*see* "Gene Therapy: The ADA Experiments," p 69), cystic fibrosis (*see* "Cystic Fibrosis and Viral Gene Delivery," p 70), hemophilia, muscular dystrophy, familial hypercholesterolemia, sickle-cell anemia, and thalassemia. In addition, gene therapy was also being tested against cancer (*see* "Genes against Cancer," p 73) and AIDS. An experiment using gene therapy to treat Parkinson's disease is in the planning stage.

Genetic defects are involved in more than two percent of live births. Opponents of gene therapy say that extraordinary means are not needed for such rare hereditary diseases. However, that ratio looms much larger when translated into one baby out of every 50 born. From this perspective, the potential for gene therapy is great.

Among the problems genetic engineers face is the diversity of hereditary disease. The number of disorders that can be traced to alleles of specific genes is enormous — if many alleles were not lethal before birth, the total number of possible hereditary diseases would be on the order of the number of genes, often estimated as 100,000. Furthermore, different alleles of the same gene may have different effects. This has been studied most for cystic fibrosis, where different combinations of alleles cause the severity of the disease to vary. Such variable effects have also been found in Tay-Sachs disease; some apparently lethal combinations of alleles fail entirely to produce Tay-Sachs symptoms.

Given this wide range of possibilities, doctors have chosen to give the first officially sanctioned genetic therapy to patients with ADA-deficiency, a syndrome so rare that there are only about 25 living examples of it worldwide at any given time (see also "Gene Therapy: The ADA Experiments," p 69). Furthermore, the syndrome is already treatable with weekly doses of an effective drug. Why not start instead at the top with a disease such as sickle-cell anemia that affects large number of people and that is not greatly helped by treatments available in present-day clinical practice?

Familial Hypercholesterolemia

In June 1992 a 29-year-old woman from Quebec became the first person to be treated for a hereditary condition in which cholesterol builds up throughout the body, usually causing an early death from a heart attack. Although people think of cholesterol from dietary sources when they attempt to reduce blood cholesterol levels, in actuality most of the cholesterol in the body is produced in the liver. The young woman, who suffers from familial hypercholesterolemia, has a liver that produces far too much cholesterol.

This excess cholesterol is the result of a protein that controls the production of cholesterol. The protein is called the low-density lipoprotein (LDL) receptor; LDL, often called "bad cholesterol," is the kind that causes the clogging of arteries that results in heart disease or stroke. If there is not enough of the receptor, LDL fails to be taken into cells, where it is used to build cell membranes. Instead, it builds up in the blood, where it causes trouble.

The liver is one of the few parts of a human body that can rebuild itself after trauma of various kinds. (The evolutionary reason is thought to be connected to the liver's role in removing toxic materials from the blood; damage caused by the toxins must be repaired, so repairable livers confer a selective advantage.) Since the LDL-receptor gene is expressed by liver cells and the liver can recover from damage, the usually tricky part of getting the gene to where it will do its work is simpler in this case. About 15 percent of the liver is removed surgically and an effective form of the LDL-receptor gene is added to the liver cells. The cells are then reinserted into the liver by putting them into the blood just before it enters the liver at the portal vein.

James M. Wilson of the University of Michigan Medical School in Ann Arbor successfully performed this operation on the young woman from Quebec. A biopsy a few months later showed that the new LDL receptor genes were active in the regrown liver. Furthermore, the effect on the LDL in the blood was dramatic. Cholesterol concentrations dropped from 20 to 40 percent without drugs (which, in any case, had been ineffective without the LDL receptors). It is believed that drugs can be used to produce even lower levels of cholesterol now that the receptor is functioning.

Preliminary results for this first patient were sufficiently encouraging that Dr. Wilson was given permission by the Recombinant DNA Advisory Committee of the U.S. National Institutes of Health to try the same procedure on four additional patients. Two persons received the new genes at the University of Michigan in 1993 and the other two were treated at the University of Pennsylvania early in 1994.

Hemophilia B

Among the other diseases likely to be amenable to gene therapy is hemophilia, an ancient disease that is mentioned in the Bible. Although the public correctly understands hemophilia as a genetic disorder in which blood fails to clot, the victim's problem in most cases is not external bleeding caused by cuts or scrapes; it is internal bleeding at joints that causes great pain and interferes with proper growth, as well as other internal bleeding that can be life threatening.

Hemophilia B results from one of several alleles of a gene on the X chromosome. These ineffective alleles result in failure to produce useful or active amounts of a protein involved in blood clotting, a protein known today as factor IX, although sometimes labeled plasma thromboplastin (PTC). In the twentieth century, medicine has progressed from a total inability to treat hemophilia B; to treatment with blood transfusions; to supplying the missing factor IX from donated blood; to using heat-treated factor IX to prevent spread of AIDS and hepatitis; to using genetically engineered factor IX. Now, near the end of the century, doctors will soon be able to introduce new genes into a person with hemophilia B that will permanently cure the disease with no further injections and without the enormous expense of genetically engineered factor IX. A genetic cure accomplished by transplanting genes has already been effective in a mouse; this research was carried out by Inder Verma of the Salk Institute for Biological Studies in La Jolla, California, in 1991.

As is usually the case, the progression from mouse to human is not necessarily straightforward. In this case, the therapy was next tried in dogs. On October 1, 1993, *Science* reported the partial success of gene therapy on three dogs bred to have hemophilia B. The team of researchers included Mark A. Kay, Savio L.C. Woo, Steven Rothenberg, and Milton Finegold from Baylor College of Medicine in Houston, Texas; Charles N. Landen, Dwight A. Bellinger, M.S. Read, and Kenneth M. Brinkhous from the University of North Carolina; and Arthur R. Thompson from Puget Sound Blood Center. Large parts (about two-thirds) of the livers from four specially bred Chapel Hill dogs (one dog died as a result) were removed and the blood entering the liver was infused with a genetically altered virus in hopes that the virus would infect the regenerating liver cells. Some of the infected liver cells did begin producing factor IX, which none of these liver cells had produced before. The factor IX reduced clotting time to about one-half to one-third of what it had been before the therapy (from about 45 minutes to about 15 minutes in the most successful case). Although this is still two to three times as long as it takes a normal dog's blood to clot, it represents significant progress. Furthermore, as time went on, the level of clotting persisted (the report was issued after a nine-month observation period).

Surprisingly, very little factor IX was produced, especially considering the large change in clotting time. The amount of factor IX in the treated dogs' blood was still only about 0.1 percent of the amount in the blood of normal dogs. Low levels of factor IX in humans have been clinically shown to benefit the patient. A difference between one percent of normal factor IX and 1.5 percent is enough to make the difference between a serious disease and a minor annoyance.

Further work will continue with dogs before this therapy is attempted on humans. This research work will investigate better ways to introduce the gene into cells in the body, possibly by using a more effective virus. Other groups have been working with cells infected by a virus outside the body. They then transplant cells that are already producing factor IX into the body. This therapeutic technique has the advantage of not involving a dangerous liver operation.

About 13,000 people in the U.S. have hemophilia, of which about 11,000 have hemophilia A and 2,000 have hemophilia B. The Somatix Therapy Corporation of

Alameda, California, with the aid of Inder Varma, is working to develop a gene therapy for hemophilia A. (For more on hemophilia A, *see* "Other Genetic Diseases," p 62.)

(Periodical References and Further Reading: *New York Times* 12-8-92, p C3; *Science* 10-1-93, pp 29, 117; *Science News* 10-2-93, p 215; *New York Times* 10-15-93, p A24; *New York Times* 11-17-93, p C17; *Scientific American* 12-93, p 18; *Harvard Health Letter*, 3-94, p 2)

Fertility, Pregnancy, and Birth

THE STATE OF OBSTETRIC MEDICINE AND FERTILITY

The beginning of life is also the beginning of health progress and problems. Not only is each individual birth a health challenge, but births in the aggregate can result in population growth, which can lead to famine, pollution, and spread of infectious disease.

Unexpected Fertility Declines in Developing Countries

Concern with population changes is certainly not new, but recently in the West there has been more concern about declines in fertility than population growth (see the Environment section, which begins on p 241). Since World War II, however, wild, unchecked population growth has been a phenomenon of developing countries, especially those in Latin America and Sub-Sahara Africa. Experts in the past believed the dichotomy between low birth rates in industrialized nations and high ones in nonindustrialized ones was a direct result of industrialization itself. This phenomenon was called "demographic transition." Since it appeared industrialization was proceeding slowly or not at all in many developing nations, sociologists once expected rapid population growth in developing countries to continue indefinitely.

The World Fertility Surveys of 1972 and 1985 and a continuing survey since 1985 have provided the first evidence of what is really happening to population in developing countries. Surprisingly, fertility is declining and the surveys predict further declines. Apparently industrialization is not the force behind lower fertility rates after all. Contraception, especially sterilization, has made the difference.

The surveys use as one of their main measures a number called the "total fertility rate," which is simply the number of babies an average woman between the ages of 15 and 44 would have if she continued to have babies at the same rate she was when surveyed. By that measure, nearly all of the more than 30 nations included in the survey showed a sharp decline in fertility between the 1970s and the early 1990s. (Since different years are available for different nations, it is not meaningful to combine the results.) For example, in Colombia, the total fertility rate was 4.7 children per woman in 1976 and only 2.8 in 1990. This decline is now attributed to the use of family planning by 38 percent of all women of childbearing age in developing countries around the world. Of these, 80 percent use modern methods of contraception as the means to family planning, most commonly voluntary female sterilization.

Furthermore, based on responses to the question posed to women, "Do you want to have more children," it appears the decline is not over. In 1991 Charles Westoff of Princeton University in New Jersey predicted that by 1996 total fertility rates will decline by ten percent in Africa and by 13 percent in Latin America. If all women who want family planning services were to gain access to them, the studies suggest the population growth rate in the developing world, now about 2.3 percent per year, would be reduced to about 1.6 percent per year.

Trends in Industrial States

In the U.S. and other modern industrial states, the extremes of the pregnancy and birth spectrum coexist, and to some degree, different populations of prospective mothers view the respective extremes as desirable.

At one extreme is the well-known legend of the peasant woman working in the field who gives birth alone and continues working as if this were a minor interruption. While no one necessarily wants to return to such days, there continues to be a segment of prospective motherhood that, knowing birth is a natural process, wishes pregnancy and birth to be as unaided as possible. Conception is accomplished in the old-fashioned way, usually without even the benefit of a thermometer; activities in pregnancy continue as always except perhaps for avoiding alcohol, tobacco, or other drugs and walking a bit more; birth is attended by a midwife, while the mother gives birth without chemical inducements or even minor surgery; and breast feeding follows. Furthermore, although they do not necessarily undergo the pregnancy as just described, many modern women, like the mythical peasant, go back to work in as short a time as possible—sometimes just days.

The other extreme begins with chemical inducements for the prospective mother to release ova (eggs) and continues with *in vitro* fertilization followed by embryo implantation to get the baby-to-be on the way. Pregnancy is closely monitored with ultrasound, amniocentesis, and other means of testing. If problems develop, the difficulties may be corrected with fetal surgery or other fetal intervention—or the pregnancy may be terminated and another attempt made later. The baby is removed by caesarean section and may be transferred if needed to a life-support system for a few days.

Most pregnancies fall in between these two extremes. Good statistics are hard to come by, but it appears the trend toward more natural childbirth took place in the 1960s and 1970s, and since then technological approaches have gradually become more common. This change is due in part to the relatively recent development of new techniques. The moderately low-tech caesarean is now performed in nearly one birth in four in the U.S., a rate considered high even by the American College of Obstetricians and Gynecologists. (The U.S. Centers for Disease Control and Prevention thinks that the rate of caesareans should be closer to one in seven.)

Ethical Issues

Although there are ethical issues surrounding the natural approach to childbirth, most of them are very old news. But new technology has spawned a host of ethical concerns spanning conception through birth, concerns that remain contentious and unresolved. Most are handled in more detail in subsequent articles, but it may be helpful to list this set of issues in one place:

- How early in life should birth control information or equipment be given to persons? For example, should condoms be given to teenagers?
- Does human life begin at conception, implantation of the embryo in the uterus, when the fetus could survive outside the body, or at birth? How would this change if at all for *in vitro* fertilization? (*See* "Encouraging Conception and Pregnancy," p 90, for a discussion of *in vitro* techniques.)
- Should abortion be legal in the U.S. (or elsewhere)? Under what circumstances?
- Should abortion be made easier and simpler, as with an abortion pill?
- Is it unethical to discard unused embryos or ova in the process of *in vitro* fertilization?
- Who has the right to control the use of embryos when a couple is divorced?
- How long should frozen embryos be kept? (There are tens of thousands already stored in the U.S. alone.)
- Should embryos be tested genetically before implant and discarded if not suitable? How does one define "unsuitable"?
- Should embryos be "cloned" so that couples may keep another embryo twin in a frozen stage until they find out how the other twin develops? (*See* "Don't Call It 'Cloning'," p 93.)
- Should frozen embryos be maintained in order to produce potential organ donors if a sibling of the embryo needs a donor later in life?
- Can fetal tissue from abortions, spontaneous or otherwise, be used in transplants to cure such illnesses as diabetes or Parkinson's disease without encouraging abortion for the purpose of providing the tissue? Does that matter?
- Should women in their 50s and even 60s be technologically enabled to give birth?

These issues have been debated hotly and sometimes violently—doctors at abortion clinics have been shot over some of these issues. The most inflammatory issues, however, appear to be abortion itself and distribution of birth control methods to young persons. The other concerns have preoccupied specialists in ethics and physicians who have to deal with specific situations, but are less of an issue to the general public.

(Periodical References and Additional Reading: *New York Times* 6-2-92, p A1; *New York Times* 6-5-92, p A10; *New York Times* 4-23-93, p A16; *Scientific American* 12-93, p 60; *New York Times* 12-28-93, p A1; *New York Times* 1-2-94, p IV-5)

STAGES BEFORE BIRTH

There is a rich vocabulary describing conception, development, and birth, not all of it suitable for use in a book intended for the general public. Not everyone agrees on the meaning of all of the words, however; several different definitions of *embryo* are used, for instance. Here is a quick checklist of most of the relevant terms that are used in this chapter.

abortion: Abortion was a medical term long before it became a political issue. In theory, although not always in medical speech, expulsion of a fetus before the end of the 12th week of pregnancy is an abortion, while expulsion between the 12th and the 24th week is a miscarriage; after the 24th week, the term *stillbirth* is used if the baby is born dead. As popular speech has developed, however, the word *abortion* has come to mean any termination of pregnancy as a result of intentional medical intervention, while *miscarriage* or *stillbirth* have come to refer to terminations without medical intervention. In the following discussion, the more popular language is used.

conception: Technically, conception is the same as fertilization, but as generally used by medical workers, conception is thought to occur when the embryo becomes implanted. Figuring a pregnancy from the date of conception, however, is done from the suspected time of fertilization, while the dates often used for length of a pregnancy begin with the last menstrual date, which is easier to establish.

embryo: A fertilized ovum, or zygote, divides into a pair of joined cells, becoming the smallest possible embryo in *in vitro* fertilization. At this stage, however, the small group of cells is also called a blastocyst (and the cells are called blastomeres) by more careful writers. When a mammalian blastocyst implants itself in the uterus wall, it is definitely an embryo, although during *in vitro* fertilization or storage before implantation, a bundle of cells that has grown to a number of cells (32, usually) which would make it a candidate for implantation is also called an embryo. After implantation in the uterus, the growing cell mass continues to be known as an embryo for several weeks. Some writers wait until cells begin to differentiate to use the term *embryo*. When the shape of the new individual begins to emerge and organs develop, the term *fetus* is introduced, after which it is a fetus until birth.

fertilization: The joining of a sperm and an ovum to form a cell that can develop into an individual.

fetus: For vertebrates that have live births rather than external eggs (these include some fish and reptiles and most mammals), a fetus is the developing animal between the embryo stage and birth. In humans, an implanted embryo graduates to a fetus after five, eight, nine, or 12 weeks depending on which expert you consult.

implant, implantation: The process of a fertilized cell or groups of cells attaching itself to the wall of the uterus (womb) in a placental mammal (does not usually occur in marsupials). This step is necessary for normal development.

***in vitro* fertilization:**   Often called "test tube" fertilization, the *in vitro* process is usually accomplished by placing semen containing sperm in a shallow laboratory container (a Petri dish) along with several ova. Zygotes that are formed are moved to other Petri dishes containing growing media until the developing and dividing cells form an embryo large enough for implantation. In a newer technique, sperm may be directly injected into ova.

miscarriage: *See* abortion, above.

ovum, ova: Technically, the ovum (plural, ova) is any cell produced by meiosis (sexual cell reproduction) that under appropriate circumstances can grow into a new individual of the species, whether animal or plant. For ordinary sexual reproduction, the ovum starts out lacking half the chromosomes needed for growth, which it obtains by merging with another cell, called a sperm. The common term *egg* is often used for the human ovum, since an ovum corresponds in function to the unfertilized egg of a bird or reptile.

semen: A thick liquid produced by male animals as a transport medium for sperm; often used to mean the sperm that are in the semen as well.

sperm: In animals or plants, a mobile cell produced by meiosis (sexual cell division) that contains half of the chromosomes needed to cause an ovum to begin developing into an individual.

zygote: When an ovum (egg) of a sexual reproducer, whether plant or animal, has been fertilized by a sperm, the single cell that results is a zygote.

TIMETABLE OF FERTILITY, PREGNANCY, AND BIRTH TO 1990

2000 BC	Contraceptives are introduced in Egypt.
1500	Jakob Nufer of Switzerland performs the first recorded caesarean section operation on a living woman, his wife; however, the mother dies as a result of the procedure.
1700	Bernardino Rammazzini's *De morbis artificum* is the first systematic treatment of occupational disorders; the author concludes that more nuns than married women develop breast cancer, possibly for reasons related to pregnancy and lactation.
1721	Jean Palfyn introduces the use of obstetric forceps for facilitating birth.
1752	William Smellie's *Treatise on Midwifery* is the first scientific approach to obstetrics.
1774	*Anatomy of the Human Gravid Uterus* by William Hunter [born Lanarkshire, Scotland, May 23, 1718; died London, England, March 30, 1783] is his greatest work in anatomy and contains 24 masterpieces of anatomical illustration.
1861	Rudolf Albert von Kölliker [born Zurich, Switzerland, July 6, 1817; died Würzburg, Bavaria, November 2, 1905] is among the first to interpret the development of the embryo in terms of cell theory.
1867	Emeline Brigham patents a pessary, described on the application as a womb supporter, but clearly intended for contraception (then illegal).
1901	In Russia, a practical technique for artificial insemination of farm animals is introduced.

1917   Margaret Sanger [born Corning, New York, September 14, 1883; died Tucson, Arizona, September 6, 1966] and M. C. Stopes [born Surrey, England, October 15, 1880; died Dorking, England, October 2, 1958] write about birth control.

1933   Grantley Dick-Read [born Beccles, England, January 26, 1890; died June 1959] writes *Natural Childbirth*, advocating exercises and procedures for childbirth without drugs.

1950   Embryos are transplanted in cattle for the first time.

1951   The birth control pill, which combines estrogen and progesterone to prevent ovulation, is invented.

1952   British doctor Douglas Bevis [born 1888] develops amniocentesis, a method of examining the genetic heritage and health status of a fetus while it is still in the womb.

1956   Birth control pills are used in a large-scale test conducted by John Rock [born Marlborough, Massachusetts, March 24, 1890; died Peterborough, New Hampshire, December 4, 1984] and Gregory Pincus [born Woodbine, New Jersey, April 9, 1903; died Boston, Massachusetts, August 22, 1967] in Puerto Rico.

1961   Jack Lippes [born Buffalo, New York, February 19, 1924] introduces an inert plastic IUD (intrauterine device) for birth control.

1965   The U.S. Supreme Court in a seven to two decision written by Justice William O. Douglas [born Maine, Minnesota, October 16, 1898; died January 19, 1980] resolves the case of *Griswold v. Connecticut,* in which Estelle Griswold [born 1900?; died 1981] of the Planned Parenthood League had been convicted of violating a Connecticut statute against supplying birth control information to married persons, by declaring the Connecticut law to be a violation of a constitutionally guaranteed right of privacy in marriage.

1967   Clomiphene is introduced to increase fertility; it also results in an increase in multiple births.

1968   English researchers report in April that oral contraceptives can cause blood clots in susceptible women.

1969   The British physiologist Robert G. Edwards and the surgeon Patrick C. Steptoe [born Oxford, England, June 9, 1913; died Canterbury, England, March 21, 1988] perform the first successful fertilization *in vitro* of a human ovum; the first baby (nicknamed a "test-tube baby") resulting from this technique is born in England in 1978.

1971   Studies suggest that diethylstilbestrol (DES), a synthetic hormone sometimes prescribed to expectant mothers to lower the risk of miscarriage, also predisposes daughters born from the medicated pregnancy to higher risk of cancer or other malformations of the reproductive tract.

1972   It is demonstrated that giving coricosteroids to pregnant women who are in premature labor about 24 hours before they are to give birth speeds maturation of the fetal lungs and blood vessels in the baby, reducing such complications as respiratory distress syndrome and bleeding in the brain.

1973   U.S. Supreme Court Justice Harry A. Blackmun [born Nashville, Illinois, November 12, 1908] writes the majority decision in *Roe v. Wade,* which essentially makes abortion legal throughout the U.S.

1978   The first human baby conceived outside the body: Louise Joy Brown, called the "test-tube baby," is born to Lesley Brown in the United Kingdom; in a technique developed by Robert G. Edwards and Patrick C. Steptoe, the ovum is extracted from the mother to be inseminated in a Petri dish, and then reimplanted.

1979   Danish scientist Steen Willadsen develops the first embryo clones of a mammal, artificially twinning a sheep embryo by separating it into two viable cells, each of which when implanted in a ewe produces the birth of a lamb.

1980   Use of the drug diethylstilbestrol (DES), prescribed as an aid to prevent miscarriages, is stopped after the realization that children born to mothers who took DES are susceptible to cancers and other problems in the reproductive tract.

1983   John Buster and Maria Bustillo of the Harbor-UCLA Medical Center in Torrance, California, perform the first successful human embryo transfers.

Fernand Daffos [born Neuvic, Coreze, France, October 27, 1947] is the first doctor to use fetal blood taken by a needle through the umbilical cord for diagnosis of disease in the fetus, a test called Percutaneous Umbilical Blood Sampling (PUBS).

1984   Surgeon William H. Clewall of the University of Colorado Health Sciences Center at Denver performs the first successful surgery on a fetus before birth.

1986   The U.S. Food and Drug Administration bans the import of abortion-causing drug RU 486.

1988   RU 486, also called the abortion pill, developed by Etienne-Emile Baulieu [born Strasbourg, France, December 12, 1926], is introduced in general use in France; it induces an abortion up to seven weeks after fertilization by blocking receptors for the production of the hormone progesterone.

1990   U.S. medical doctor Ronald Baker patents a noninvasive monitor for monitoring fetal heartbeats; the transducer detecting the heartbeats consists of thin sheets of piezopolymer made of polyvinylidene difluoride.

FERTILITY

ENCOURAGING CONCEPTION AND PREGNANCY

In 1935 after three years of marriage, a St. Louis woman with a history that included an earlier tubal pregnancy complained to a specialist in conception that she seemed unable to become pregnant. The doctor's advice? Eat more lettuce. In this case, the prescription worked.

Medical practice became a lot more sophisticated in the next 40 years. When John and Lesley Brown of Oldham, England, found that their union was not fertile, their doctors, Patrick C. Steptoe and Robert G. Edwards, recognized that Mrs. Brown's problem was blocked Fallopian tubes. Drs. Steptoe and Edwards decided to try for the 71st time the process that became known as test-tube fertilization (although it takes place in a glass Petri dish and is more properly called *in vitro* fertilization). The attempt with the Browns was a success, and Louise—the first "test-tube baby"—was born July 25, 1978. Since then, the Browns with the aid of the same method produced Louise's baby sister Natalie; and about 20,000 other children around the world have been born through 1992 as a result of similar procedures.

In the U.S. about 14 percent per attempt of all couples who try *in vitro* fertilization succeed in having a baby. In the United Kingdom it is even lower—12.5 percent.

The U.S. Public Health Service estimates that about 2.3 million married couples in the U.S. are unable to conceive after 12 months of unprotected intercourse or are known to be infertile for other reasons. Since there are about 55 million married couples in the U.S., this is a rate of approximately four percent. Put another way, according to these criteria about one in 25 couples cannot have children. A different source claims that twice as many women in the U.S. (five million in all) are infertile, but in this case couples are not being measured.

Diagnosing Blocked Tubes

Of the infertile women in the U.S., about 40 percent are thought to suffer from blocked Fallopian tubes, usually as a result of a prior infection that caused scar tissue to form in the very thin tubes. Until recently the only way to be certain that this condition was the cause of infertility and, in some cases, to locate a place where a blockage could be surgically eliminated was a procedure in which a chemical opaque to X rays is inserted in the tube and its progress through the tube followed with X rays. About 125,000 of such procedures, called hysterosalpingrograms (HSG), are performed worldwide each year. These are not entirely accurate, however, and must take place in an operating room environment, often with anesthesia.

Since 1992, Imagyn Medical Inc. of Laguna Niguel, California has been marketing a new method (not approved in the U.S. yet) called transcervical falloposcopy, which cleverly uses a balloon to open a channel through the tube from which the interior can be observed with optical fibers and displayed on a television monitor. The procedure is considered less invasive than HSG.

A Trail of Ethical Questions

Although some critics at the time felt that the test-tube conception was unethical, most doctors and people desiring parenthood felt that the *in vitro* method was simply aiding a natural process and no more unethical than taking a vitamin pill or attaching an artificial leg. Since the 1970s, however, the methods of producing conception and improving chances of a safe delivery after unorthodox fertility rites have improved greatly, and the ethical questions have become much more complex.

For example, since 1991 some doctors have tested embryos still in the Petri dish for serious chromosomal or genetic disorders such as Down's syndrome, Tay-Sachs Disease, or sickle-cell anemia. These disorders all have well-known risk factors, so such tests can be used when appropriate and skipped when there is no particular reason to suspect a problem. But in the early 1990s many other specific genes have been located that are involved in hereditary diseases, sometimes only as a predisposition. Should doctors, as a *Washington Post* report on future practice has it, "fertilize a dozen eggs, test each embryo for a battery of genetic traits and then begin pregnancy with the one they like best," or would that lead to a homogeneous and dull population of lookalikes, as in some science-fiction novels?

Another set of questions arises from the treatment of embryos that are not implanted. Few feel that the unused embryos should simply be discarded. First of all, until the mother has successfully delivered a baby, the embryos are usually saved by freezing in liquid nitrogen. That way, a second or third attempt at an implant can be made if earlier ones fail. But freezing in liquid nitrogen is so effective that it appears that the embryos can be kept indefinitely, so after the wanted baby is born, the issue of disposal appears. If the couple thinks that they might want another baby in a few years, the embryos remain frozen. If not, one possibility is to donate the unused embryo either to a couple whose infertility problem requires a donated embryo or to a research project using embryos. But many couples want to keep their options open as long as possible, so most embryos stay frozen indefinitely. The actual number of frozen embryos worldwide is not available, but preliminary evidence from the U.S. suggests that it is well over a hundred thousand.

Furthermore, although fertility clinics now have learned to get couples to sign a pre-freezing agreement, custody battles over the embryos are not uncommon. In at least one case in 1992 an ex-husband was able to block his ex-wife's access to their frozen embryo; when he won custody after a four and a half year court struggle, he had the seven frozen embryos destroyed.

Improved Fertilization

The least controversial part of the new fertility science is the basic technique pioneered by Steptoe and Edwards. As their 70 failures before a success demonstrate, *in vitro* fertilization is an art. In 1991, for example, there were 22,000 attempts to fertilize human ova (eggs) in a Petri dish in the U.S., but only about 3300 mothers became pregnant as a result. Although some who worry about the rate of population growth or who think the procedure interferes with God's plan would like to replace all *in vitro* fertilization with adoption of children born naturally to families that cannot care for them, most observers would like to see the success rate improved.

One difficulty has been that instead of a simple mechanical condition like Mrs. Brown's blocked tubes, the husband's sperm is often the problem. Sperm counts may be low, or the sperm themselves may be defective, having little motility (ability to move) for example. In Belgium, André C. Van Steirteghem of Brussels Free University decided to inject single sperm into ova, even though similar attempts with animals have failed. (Nearly all fertility-improvement methods were adopted by cattle breeders long before they were used on humans.) Amazingly, human sperm can fertilize ova by injection even though no success has been reported with other species. By the end of 1993, Dr. Steirteghem had produced over 300 pregnancies (and, of them, over 100 healthy babies) as a result of *in vitro* microinjection of sperm. In 1993 the technique began to be successfully used in the U.S.

Grandmothers (and Older Women) Become Mothers

One unexpected extension of the basic techniques of *in vitro* fertilization has been the ability of women previously thought to be beyond child-bearing age to conceive. Although no one has matched the feat of the biblical Abraham's wife Sarah, who produced Isaac when she was 90, the number of women in their 50s who became pregnant in the early 1990s was at least in the dozens. By the end of 1993, it appeared the record age for modern times was 61, the age at which Rossana Dalla Corte gave birth in Rome in mid-1994. But the record may be a greater age already, since many of the doctors and mothers involved do not seek publicity.

The first reports concerned women in their 40s. On September 9, 1992, Mark V. Sauer at the University of Southern California in Los Angeles reported in the *Journal of the American Medical Association* that 65 women between the ages of 40 and 52 who had been implanted with embryos from *in vitro* fertilization were as successful in giving birth as women under the age of 40. The catch was that the ova (eggs) of the embryos carried by the older women were donated by younger women. Similar research discussed in the same report demonstrated that in cases in which 57 women over 40 used their own ova, the women had only 25 percent of the success rate of the women who had been implanted with donated ova. A preliminary study by Sauer reported in 1990 used only seven women and had suggested that the use of young women's ova would be successful—four of those postmenopausal women had given birth. Sauer's theory is that the reason older women seldom become pregnant has much to do with the age of the ovum and little connection to the age of the uterus.

Encouraged, Sauer and his group went on to work with still older women, and were able to report in the February 6, 1993 *Lancet* that a group of 14 women in their fifties had a 50 percent success rate (apparently, three pregnant women had yet to give birth at the time of the report) with ova from younger women.

A week later the first of the new family possibilities came to light when news broke that a 53-year-old woman in Orchard Park, New York, had given birth to her own grandson on December 28, 1992. When her daughter-in-law was unable to become pregnant as a result of a hysterectomy, Geraldine Wesolowski agreed to become a surrogate mother. All went well and Matthew Wesolowski became a fertility first.

(Periodical References and Additional Reading: *Citizen-Register* 1-1-91; *Science News* 9-12-92, p 165; *New York Times* 12-20-92, p III-9; *Science News* 2-13-93, p 100; *Science* 5-14-93, p 932;

New York Times 6-2-93, p A1; *New York Times* 6-5-93, p A10; *New York Times* 6-16-93, p A18; *New York Times* 8-11-93, p C11; *New York Times* 10-4-93, p A18; *New York Times* 10-26-93, p A15; *New York Times* 12-28-93, p A1; *New York Times* 1-2-94, p IV-5)

DON'T CALL IT "CLONING"

Among the "Andy-Warhol-15-minutes-of-fame" winners in the 1990s were Jerry Hall and Robert Stillman of George Washington University Medical Center in Washington, D.C. They made headlines and late-night television monologues by announcing that they were the first to "clone" a human. This is not to say that they succeeded in taking the genes from one adult human and growing an identical new human from them, which is what biologists mean by cloning. Instead they showed that a human embryo at a very early stage, at least two but not more than eight cells can be split into two parts that will continue to divide and grow after separation. (In this discussion, the word *embryo* is used with the meaning given it in most fertility clinics, where it describes any small cluster of cells that result from a fertilized ovum before implantation.) This is not a major technical feat. Scientists and veterinarians have accomplished as much with sheep and cattle many times since Steen Willadsen of the Institute of Animal Physiology in Cambridge, England, first accomplished the feat for sheep, which was announced in the January 12, 1979 *Nature*. Although Hall and Stillman called their experiment "cloning," critics point out that the practice, carried out to maximize useful genes in cattle, is really "twinning" that has been artificially induced. It is also called "embryo cloning," but not unmodified "cloning"; only in *in vitro* fertilization is the mass of cells that was cloned called an embryo.

Hall and Stillman described their work for the first time on October 13, 1993 at the annual meeting of the American Fertility Society, but they received little notice from fellow fertility experts. When an article on the subject was about to appear in *Science,* the widely read journal of the American Association for the Advancement of Science, reporters got wind of the technique and put it on the front pages. A press conference by Hall and Stillman no doubt helped in the publicity.

For now at least, the most likely application of artificial twinning in humans, if ethical questions are put aside, would be improvement of the chance that one of the twin embryos would survive to birth and provide a couple with a child. Ethical questions for that application are not a problem to most people, but other applications might be troublesome to some. For example: Should couples be allowed to keep an embryo twin in a frozen state until they find out how the other twin develops? Some have suggested that such a frozen embryo could be maintained as a potential organ donor if the embryo's twin needs an organ. A more likely use might be to improve genetic testing of an embryo by testing its embryo clone in destructive ways.

The Hall-Stillman research separated 17 embryos with two, four, or eight cells and then helped the individual cells grow on an agar-covered plate. Where they obtained the human embryos for the experiment and what finally happened to them after twinning and so forth is not mysterious. They used uncommon ova that had been fertilized by more than one sperm cell, which makes the embryos unsuitable for implanting. Although cells from the four-or eight-cell stage stopped dividing too soon for implantation, the cells from the eight two-cell embryos could have been implanted in a uterus of a prospective mother. But Hall, Stillman, and their coworkers considered that stage the conclusion of their experiment. Furthermore, because of the source of the embryos, even the cells that were still dividing were thought incapable of successful maturation. After the experiment, the "clones" were disposed of by the same procedures as in any failed *in vitro* case.

Artificial twinning of humans was made possible by the earlier work of Hall with Sandra Yee. In 1991 they developed a way to make separated embryo cells form a protective coat similar to the one that must be dissolved or otherwise removed before an embryo can be separated into individual cells.

(Periodical References and Additional Reading: *New York Times* 10-24-93, p A1; *New York Times* 10-26-93, p A1; *Science* 10-29-93, p 652; *Science News* 10-30-93, p 276; *Discover* 1-94, p 84; *Science News* 2-5-94, p 92)

EMBRYO CLONING, STEP BY STEP

First of all, it helps to clarify the somewhat confusing nomenclature surrounding cloning. Cloning in the strict sense of the word is using a body cell (as opposed to an egg cell) from an adult to produce a genetically identical copy of the adult. This has never been accomplished for any mammal. The Hall-Stillman method, described below, is sometimes called "twin cloning," although "embryo cloning" is likely to become the accepted name for the procedure. A better technical name would be something like "blastocyst cloning," although some scientists might prefer to avoid the word *cloning* altogether and say "blastomere separation." The words *blastocyst* and *blastomere* are defined below.

When an ovum (egg) of a sexual reproducer, whether plant or animal, has been fertilized by a sperm, the single cell that results is a zygote, but the zygote soon divides into a pair of joined cells. In humans, this happens about 30 hours after fertilization. At this stage, the cell cluster that most fertility clinics call an embryo is properly called a blastocyst (and the cells are called blastomeres). After six or seven days, the still dividing human blastocyst normally implants itself in the uterus wall and all agree to call it an embryo. In humans, an implanted embryo graduates to a fetus, with discernable organs, after several weeks.

To produce twins or multiple copies, the outside membrane of the blastocyst, called the zona pellucida, must be removed, which is done by dissolving the membrane with the enzyme pronase. Then the blastocyst can be separated into individual cells, which are maintained in a special growing medium free from calcium ions. After separation, however, in the Hall-Yee method the cells are moved to a seaweed derivative that contains sodium (Na) alginate, which causes each cell to form its own artificial zona pellucida. Within that artificial membrane, the cells begin to form a new blastocyst and are moved into an ordinary agar culture medium.

If the cells divide five times after the separation, producing a blastocyst with 32 cells, the cell mass is ready to be implanted in a human uterus. It was at this stage that Hall and Stillman ended their experiment. Only copies produced begun by twinning after the first division reached this stage, however. Copies started at later stages soon stopped dividing.

DISCOURAGING CONCEPTION

In the U.S. there are about 3.5 million unintended pregnancies each year, despite the availability of various forms of family planning, discussed below. Indeed, it is thought that 95 percent of all American women use some form of family planning.

Nearly all "family planning" is actually birth control, which in other words is conception prevention. The ancient Egyptians are said to have used a barrier device that corresponds to the modern diaphragm and spermicidal jelly combination. A controversial new book claims that somewhat less ancient Greeks had an herb, now extinct from overharvesting, that prevented pregnancy; this was like a "morning after" pill, although it was generally taken immediately after intercourse instead of the next day. Other, somewhat less effective herbs were used until the rise of the modern physician, who paid no attention to the folk medicine. Various forms of condoms were used in more recent times and basically continue today, although for strict conception prevention with no concern for disease prevention, other devices have proven more popular. Some of these devices are new in the 1990s; others are new in the U.S. during this time; and even the old methods have been studied anew. This section presents the latest developments in modern birth control. Figures on effectiveness of the various birth control methods are those released by the Alan Guttmacher Institute, unless noted.

Don't Use Anything

Although the normal rate of pregnancies caused by unprotected intercourse is about 85 percent per year, this rate can be reduced to about 14 to 16 percent a year simply by avoiding periods when the woman is especially fertile. (The American Medical Association reports a rate of 25 percent.)

Officially called natural family planning, but most often known as "the rhythm method" because periods of relative "safe" intercourse alternate with periods of high fertility, this method obtains results comparable to practical experience with most barrier devices when the rhythm method is followed carefully. It is most effective when practiced in conjunction with daily temperature readings and cervical mucus inspections for the woman, which help to pinpoint fertile periods (temperature rises slightly at ovulation and mucus thins). Intercourse two days after ovulation and before the start of the next period is least likely to result in conception. It is also possible to calculate that a period of higher probability for conception will occur between about 18 and 11 days before the end of a menstrual cycle, but this calendar method is fraught with possibilities for error.

Use One Time Only

The condom, a barrier device for males that covers the penis during intercourse and is intended to keep semen in its interior, has never been a very satisfactory birth control device. But AIDS, the incurable, deadly sexually transmitted disease, has brought the condom back as a recommendation for all sex with anyone who might possibly transmit the disease. Thus, despite leaks, slippage, and undesirable aesthetics, the male condom is still widely used.

Among the condom's drawbacks is that the person most responsible for seeing that the device is used and who most often is in charge of purchase and installation at an appropriate moment is *not* the person who becomes pregnant if the condom is not used or is used improperly.

In Britain, Chartex International developed their alternative to this situation, and named it Femidon. Femidon was already in use in several European countries when on May 10, 1993 the U.S. Food and Drug Administration (FDA) approved it. In the U.S., however, the device will be officially known as "Reality." Unofficially, this vaginal pouch is known to everyone as the "female condom." It is a polyurethane sheath about six-and-a-half inches long with a pair of flexible rings to hold it in place.

Although the FDA approved Reality, it was careful not to encourage use of the female condom. For one thing, Reality's pregnancy rate is estimated to be about 21 to 26 percent a year, compared to about 15 percent for the familiar latex male condom. (Some male condoms are made from other substances, but latex is by far the most effective version.) Also, polyurethane is not the proven protection against AIDS that latex is, although the U.S. Centers for Disease Control and Prevention report that laboratory tests suggest the female condom is a good barrier when properly used.

On the other hand, a pregnancy rate of approximately 20 percent is a distinct improvement over the unprotected rate of 85 percent a year, so those who do not want to use any of the other means available for birth control might wish to turn to the female condom. Most users feel that it is more pleasurable in use than the male version.

Reuse As Needed

Although the female condom is new, for many years women have had a variety of barrier devices to prevent sperm from entering the cervix and causing pregnancy. These include jellies, creams, or foams that kill sperm (spermicides), which must be applied before intercourse in order to be effective; a device to cover the opening to the uterus by blocking the end of the vagina, called a diaphragm, which must be correctly inserted and left in place for at least six hours after intercourse to be effective; and a smaller device called a cervical cap that fits snugly over the cervix, the opening to the uterus. The two rubber barriers are intended to be used in conjunction with a spermicide, and vice-versa, as the following annual pregnancy rates demonstrate: spermicides alone: 25 percent (AMA figures); diaphragm alone: 14 to 16 percent; cervical cap alone: 18 percent; diaphragm or cervical cap plus spermicide: 3 percent (AMA figure). One study released at the beginning of 1991, however, found that spermicides used with diaphragms or with condoms contributed to urinary tract infections. Contradictory studies released about the same time also showed that all barrier contraceptives might be linked to preeclampsia or are not linked to that condition, sometimes called by its former name of toxemia.

Instead of barrier methods of birth control, women can use small devices that a physician inserts into the uterus which prevent implantation, although no one is certain exactly why or how these interuterine devices (IUDs) work. Some IUDs use a substance such as copper or progesten to enhance their anti-conception effects, and these need to be replaced every year or two. Others rely on mechanical means only and are normally checked and replaced after about five years.

The IUD received a great deal of unfavorable publicity in the U.S. throughout the 1980s because one form, the Dalkon Shield, was shown in several studies to raise the risk of pelvic infection significantly. Although a study released in April 1991 attempted to clear the Dalkon Shield of the charges, the damage has already been done to the reputation of IUDs in the U.S. Although IUDs continue to be popular throughout the world, especially in China, they are rarely used in the U.S. Indeed, nearly all forms of IUD have been withdrawn from the U.S. market. Despite the concerns about pelvic infection, many doctors recognize that the IUD is a particularly effective form of birth control, with an annual pregnancy rate from 1 to 2 percent, which is better than other mechanical devices.

Take the Morning After

Although RU 486 is primarily known as an abortion inducer, it can also be used to prevent implantation. The American Society of Obstetricians and Gynecologists declared that pregnancy begins with implantation, a definition most abortion proponents reject. By that definition, prevention of implantation is not abortion. A drug that is administered after intercourse and before implantation is generally known as a "morning after" pill, although typical "morning after" remedies can be used up to 72 hours after intercourse. The report on the morning after use of RU 486 comes from a Scottish study in October 1992.

Although it is not generally known, ordinary birth control pills (see below) are regularly used as morning after pills by emergency rooms and college health clinics. The procedure is to take two birth control pills, wait twelve hours, and take two more. Medical supervision is strongly suggested, as this procedure produces considerable nausea and vomiting.

The Agency for International Development defines pregnancy as fertilization, not as implantation, so by that definition, morning after pills work by causing very early abortions. The same is true for birth control pills.

Take Every Morning for 21 Days

The typical birth control pill is a combination of two groups of hormones, which are often named as if each consisted of a single chemical: estrogen and progesterone. Estrogen includes such components as estradiol, estriol, and estrone, which are separate chemicals. The general class of hormones that are called progesterone consists of several hormones called progestogens, including progestins. Many doctors or writers use the terms indiscriminantly, however. Pills are typically taken for 21 days and then discontinued for a week, during which a menstrual period occurs. The effect of the hormones is to keep the ovum from being released from the ovary, preventing conception as a result. For such combination pills, the annual pregnancy rate ranges from 0.1 percent for perfect compliance with all the requirements for use to 6 percent for the average person taking average care. Although the best pregnancy rate is 0.1

percent per year for the combination pills, it is 0.5 percent per year or greater for progestin-only pills, sometimes called mini-pills.

The virtue of the mini-pills is that they are less likely to cause high blood pressure or other complications, for which the risk is increased by estrogen. Although these side effects of combination pills are not considered serious for women under the age of 30, they may pose problems for older women.

In 1993 Darcey V. Spicer, Malcom C. Pike, and coworkers from the University of Southern California reported in *Conception* on a two-year trial of an entirely different approach to birth control pills. Instead of a combination of estrogen and progesterone, they used a gonadotropin-releasing hormone to induce artificial menopause. Other hormones, including small amounts of estrogen, a brief regime of progesterone, and some androgens, are used to relieve the menopause by inducing four menstrual periods a year and to counter some of the negative effects of the artificial menopause, such as bone thinning and hot flashes. The reason for such a complex routine is to prevent the changes estrogen and progesterone induce, changes that encourage cancers of the breasts, ovaries, or endometrium. As a side benefit, the new regime lowers LDL ("bad") cholesterol and prevents PMS (pre-menstrual syndrome). It is too early to tell whether or not the desired reduction in cancer will result. Besides, until some better delivery method is developed other than the present combination of injections and occasional pills, the method will remain experimental.

Although no similar pill has been developed for men, once-a-week injections of a testosterone derivative have been shown to eliminate sperm, which return to normal levels a few months after stopping injections. If the injections could be less frequent, this might be a viable method.

Works for Months

On October 29, 1992, rather late by the reckonings of many, the FDA approved an injectable drug for women that prevents conception for three months after each injection. Depo-Provera, the trade name for medroxyprogesterone acetate, had long been used elsewhere in the world. Since its introduction in 1969 about 30 million women had given it a try, with about nine million still using it in 1992.

Depo-Provera is a synthetic form of progesterone that forms tiny crystals. When injected into a muscle, the crystals gradually dissolve, allowing the synthetic progesterone to enter the bloodstream and interfere with the menstrual cycle and therefore with pregnancy. The annual pregnancy rate is 0.3 percent for full compliance with the sequence of injections, and only 0.4 percent for the average user.

Depo-Provera took such a long time to reach the U.S. because of concerns that it might promote breast cancer and osteoporosis. Its manufacturer, Upjohn, is continuing research on osteoporosis, but nevertheless began to market the injections in the U.S. on January 12, 1993. In Canada, however, the Health Protection Branch remained concerned about the drug and its possible effects on cancer and bones. The Branch turned down Upjohn's application on June 2, 1993.

A couple of days later, the World Health Organization (WHO), which had helped millions gain access to Depo-Provera, endorsed two different injectable drugs that do not disrupt the menstrual cycle and do not cause as much weight gain or other side effects as Depo-Provera. Because they are intended to keep the menstrual cycle on track, the drugs, Cyclofem and Mesigyna, have to be injected monthly instead of just four times a year. Each drug is a combination of estrogen and progesterone. WHO's committee also announced that their studies showed that Depo-Provera did not encourage development of either breast or cervical cancer.

Other injectable, once-a-month drugs are available in China and in Latin America, but WHO did not think these drugs as effective as Cyclofem or Mesigyna, which prevented 99.6 percent of 10,000 women in clinical trials from becoming pregnant. Pregnancy becomes possible again two or three months after stopping the injections.

An experimental vaccine against sperm, tested so far only in mice, was announced on November 1, 1993 by Roy Curtiss of Washington University in St. Louis, Missouri. Unlike Depo-Provera, the vaccine, genetically engineered from the bacterium that causes salmonella, can be given to males as well as females. The effects might last several months. Another idea has been to vaccinate men against hormones that are on the chain of sperm production, a process that has actually been tried on humans by the Indian National Institute of Immunology in New Delhi.

Works for Five Years

On December 10, 1990, the FDA approved a birth control implant that had already been approved in 16 countries worldwide and used by 355,000 women, some for over ten years. Called Norplant in the U.S., the implant consists of six matchstick-sized silicone rubber tubes containing levonorgestrel, a synthetic version of the hormone progestogen (a progestin) that is also used in several birth control pill formulations. The implant slowly releases the drug around the clock, preventing conception for five years at a time, probably by inhibiting ovulation and blocking sperm by thickening cervical mucus. When conception is desired, the implant, inserted under the skin in an upper arm, can be removed and fertility resumes immediately. Implants can also be replaced after each five-year interval of effectiveness. The main side effect is menstrual irregularities. The pregnancy rate per year is 0.2 percent among users, about the same as sterilization, according to the Population Council, but the Alan Guttmacher Institute reports a much lower rate of 0.04 percent for compliance with the requirements of Norplant and only 0.05 percent for average use. The Guttmacher Institute figures suggest that Norplant is the most effective birth control available.

Norplant became available in the U.S. in February 1991 and was used by over 875,000 American women by the end of 1993. Norplant also became a political issue quickly because the device could be implanted without a woman's permission—a judge ordered a woman on welfare whom he thought became pregnant too often to be implanted with Norplant—and because the Baltimore school system began planning to provide Norplant to its students. A major barrier to increased use of the contraceptive was that the cost of the implant was kept artificially high, which according to a spokesperson for its American manufacturer was to prevent its becoming known as a device for poor people. In the U.S. the implant, which is thought to cost about $16 to manufacture, sold in 1993 for $355 not including the doctor's fee for implantation. In some countries the cost of the device is as low as $23, and outside the U.S. the highest price is $120. The U.S. manufacturer had by the end of 1993 distributed the implant free to about 13,000 poor women and said that it would lower the price to public clinics by some unspecified amount in December 1995.

A device that works much like Norplant is a ring that releases the same or similar hormones which can be inserted in the vagina. An advantage of the ring, which is undergoing tests in various countries (but not the U.S.), is that not even minor surgery is required.

Works Forever

For about 15 percent of the men over 40 in the U.S., the birth control method of choice is an operation developed over 100 years ago that consists of sealing off the two tubes that carry sperm from the testes to the outside world. The simple operation—it only takes about half an hour to perform—is called a vasectomy, and it results in sterility after the period of time needed for stored sperm to be eliminated. The annual pregnancy rate for a vasectomy is 0.1 percent; attempts to restore fertility are successful about half the time. About half a million American men obtain vasectomies every year. Vasectomy seems to be popular, however, only in nations with a seemingly strong Anglo-Saxon heritage such as the U.S., Britain, or Australia and in China, India, and South Korea. It is not at all popular in Latin cultures or in most developing countries.

Although no direct side effects are evident—including no diminution of sexual performance or drive—vasectomy has been occasionally accused of subtle ill effects on health, ranging from kidney stones to testicular cancer. But studies connecting vasectomy to atherosclerosis in the 1970s were later refuted, and studies in 1989 and 1993 showing an increase in prostate cancer rates are suspect because so many men develop prostate cancer in any case (about one in 11, mostly in old age) that statistical connections are hard to prove. In 1992, researchers from Oxford University, and in 1993, researchers from Harvard Medical School compared the health histories of tens of thousands of men who had or did not have vasectomies. The comparisons showed none of the expected side effects; men with vasectomies actually had a lower risk of heart disease or stroke.

The corresponding operation for women is a more complex surgical task called tubal ligation, popularly called "getting your tubes tied." This method of blocking the output of the Fallopian tubes is somewhat more common in the U.S. than vasectomy, although it is even less reversible; about 650,000 women a year opt for this form of sterilization. It is even more popular in developing countries, where tubal ligation is often the most common form of birth control. The annual pregnancy rate for tubal ligation is 0.2 percent and it has not been connected with any side effects, although it is a riskier procedure than vasectomy because of the need to use a general anesthesia.

(Periodical References and Additional Reading: *New York Times* 12-7-90; *New York Times* 12-11-90, p A1; *New York Times* 4-15-91, p A1; *New York Times* 10-11-92, p IV-2; *New York Times* 10-30-92, p A1; *New York Times* 11-8-92, p IV-6; *New York Times* 12-11-92, p A32; *New York*

Times 1-13-93, p D4; *New York Times* 2-17-93, p C12; *Science News* 2-20-93, p 116; *New York Times* 2-21-93, p IV-2; *Scientific American* 4-93, p 18; *New York Times* 4-28-93, p A13; *New York Times* 5-11-93, p C5; *New York Times* 6-3-93, p D2; *New York Times* 6-6-93, p 20; *Harvard Health Letter* 8-83, p 5; *Nature* 9-2-93, p 15; *New York Times* 11-2-93, p C9; *New York Times* 11-11-93, p B12; *New York Times* 12-15-93, p B1; *Archaeology* 3/4-94, p 29)

PREGNANCY

TERMINATING PREGNANCY

Legal abortion was virtually nonexistent in the United States until the late 1960s, when several states broadened the grounds upon which abortions could be obtained. By 1972, after such populous states as New York had enacted much less restrictive abortion laws, the number of legal abortions exceeded a half million. Soon, after the *Roe v. Wade* decision favoring legal abortion, the number more than doubled. Since then, the absolute number of abortions in the U.S. has continued to rise rather slowly.

More surprising, the ratio of the number of legal abortions to the number of live births declined throughout the 1980s in the U.S. Depending upon the point of view of the writer or speaker, different reasons were put forth for the decline. Some felt that anti-abortion political movements and religious pronouncements were causing legal abortions to decline. Others thought that the decline resulted from what Martha Farnsworth Riche, director of the Population Reference Bureau, referred to as "closing the gap between wanted and unwanted pregnancies." Increased promotion of birth control, especially the encouragement of condoms as a method of reducing sexually transmitted diseases, could also have resulted in a lower abortion rate. Birth control could also count for a small drop in the percentage of abortions to unmarried women. The larger rise in the percentage of abortions to nonwhite women is more difficult to explain.

The latest data on American abortions is a 1990 report. A report released on December 19, 1992 by the U.S. Centers for Disease Control put the total number of abortions in 1990 as 344 abortions per 1000 live births, for a total number in the U.S. in 1990 of about 1.4 million. The total number was slightly higher than in 1980, however, reflecting increases in population.

An analysis of official statistics, released by the Alan Guttmacher Institute in 1994, gives the following rates of induced abortions in women between the ages of 15 and 49 in selected countries (years vary somewhat from country to country, but most were in the mid 1980s).

PERCENTAGES OF
INDUCED ABORTIONS

Former Soviet Union	18.1%
Cuba	5.8%
Peru	5.2%
Chile	4.5%
Dominican Republic	4.4%
Brazil	3.7%
Colombia	3.4%
United States	2.7%

Mexico	2.3%
England and Wales	2.7%
Canada	1.2%
The Netherlands	0.5%

Despite the decline in the U.S. abortion rate, opposition to medically induced abortions continues unabated. The most striking event in the early 1990s was the March 10, 1993 murder of a doctor by an abortion protester as the doctor, David Gunn, approached the rear entrance of his abortion clinic in Pensacola, Florida. Dr. Gunn was shot in the back by abortion protester Michael F. Griffen. A number of anti-abortion workers interviewed after learning of the killing were ambivalent about whether murder under the circumstances might be permissible. Other acts of violence increased. Arson was used against clinics 12 times in 1992, compared to four uses of arson in 1990.

RU 486 Update

RU 486 is the drug mifespristone and when used correctly, it safely induces abortions. In use in France, Britain, Sweden, and China where it has been taken safely by well over 100,000 women, it was banned in the U.S. from 1986 to 1993. So far, the drug has been effective in inducing abortion about 96 percent of the time. It has been involved in one death, although in that case the drug itself was not the cause of death. Furthermore, RU 486 can be used as a "morning-after" pill, preventing implantation of a fertilized egg when taken within 72 hours after intercourse, as revealed in a study by Anna Glasier and coworkers at the University of Edinburgh (published in the October 8, 1992 *New England Journal of Medicine*).

On July 24, 1992 the U.S. Supreme Court refused to order the return of 12 RU 486 pills to Leona Benten; the pills had been confiscated on July 1, 1992 by customs officials because they were on the U.S. Food and Drug Import-alert list. When the pills were confiscated and she lost the lawsuit, Ms. Benten changed her plans and obtained a conventional abortion.

In January 1993, however, U.S. President Bill Clinton fulfilled campaign promises by taking steps toward lifting the ban. The struggle over the drug moved into a new phase, although it was far from over.

On February 24, 1993 David A. Kessler, U.S. Commissioner of Food and Drugs, announced that the Roussel-Uclaf subsidiary of Hoechst A.G.—Roussel-Uclaf is the "RU" of RU 486—was willing to discuss marketing the drug in the U.S., a change of its earlier policy. Roussel told Kessler that they wanted large-scale clinical tests in the U.S. before the drug could be approved, partly to be certain that the drug, which works well in France, Britain, and Sweden, would also be safe and effective in the U.S. The tests would also familiarize U.S. doctors with the drug in a situation where Roussel had a large amount of control. But even after such tests, Roussel did not want to distribute the drug.

On March 17, 1993 Roussel-Uclaf announced that a then unnamed U.S. research

Background

RU 486 is a steroid that acts by blocking the hormone progesterone, which means that it is classed as an antiprogestin. Without that hormone, the maternal blood supply to the fetus or embryo fails and the fetus or embryo is expelled from the uterus. In practice, a second drug, a prostaglandin, is injected to increase the strength of the uterine contractions, insuring that the dead fetus or embryo is flushed out. It was the prostaglandin that caused the one death associated with RU 486. However, a group of French researchers reported in the May 26, 1993 *New England Journal of Medicine* that the injections could be replaced by administering an oral drug, misoprostol (American trade name Cytotec), which is similar to a prostaglandin. In addition to the RU 486, women take from one to three misoprostol tablets to increase the blood flow.

If taken within nine weeks after the last menstrual period, RU 486 and the prostaglandin have been found to be effective in inducing abortion 96 percent of the time. The main side effect is heavy bleeding as the fetus or embryo is expelled. About one woman in a thousand needs a blood transfusion because of the loss of blood.

As a "morning-after" pill to prevent implantation, one 600-milligram dose of RU 486 within 72 hours after intercourse is all that is required.

group would test the abortion drug in the U.S. Two weeks later, on April 1, 1993, the Abortion Rights Mobilization group (ARM) stated at a press conference that they had recruited scientists to chemically copy RU 486 and test their version of the pill. ARM also said that they had obtained Chinese copies of RU 486 for their tests. Tests of the two copied pills would be conducted on about 100 women primarily to make certain that the copies were safe to use. Later ARM revealed that they planned to use a provision in New York State law that would make tests within the state legal. This would require action by the New York State Board of Pharmacy, which had not occurred by early 1994.

By October 1993 it was clear that the Roussel-Uclaf plan for U.S. testing was stagnant, largely because the drug manufacturer was reluctant to go ahead with the tests because of continued fear of litigation and potential boycotts. In November, however, Etienne-Emile Baulieu, the developer of the RU 486 pill, said that he had a preliminary agreement to set up his own firm to make and sell the pill in the U.S. when it obtains FDA approval.

Later in November 1993 the FDA announced approval of small-scale tests on RU 486, but only tests for the treatment of breast cancer, not for use in inducing abortion. Previously the FDA had allowed three patients to use the pill for breast cancer and also allowed one man to use the drug to treat brain cancer. Results were mixed. RU 486 is already considered to be an effective treatment for the rare Cushing's disease, an overproduction of hormones by the adrenal gland.

(Periodical references and additional reading: *New York Times* 1-10-91; *New York Times* 7-2-92, p A12; *New York Times* 7-6-92, p A16; *New York Times* 7-15-92, p A1; *New York Times* 7-16-92, p A18; *New York Times* 7-17-92, p A21; *New York Times* 7-18-92, p 1; *New York Times* 7-30-92, p A22; *New York Times* 10-8-92, p A1; *New York Times* 12-19-92, p 9; *New York*

Times 2-25-93, p A1; *New York Times* 2-11-93, p A1; *New York Times* 3-19-93, p A12; *New York Times* 5-27-93, p B9; *New York Times* 10-13-93, p A17; *New York Times* 11-15-93, p A12; *New York Times* 4-12-94, p C5)

A BETTER PREGNANCY

Despite the advances in fertility research and a vastly improved understanding of development from a fertilized egg to a free-living human being, much about conception and pregnancy occurs according to its own timetable. When using natural means of fertilization, even with the help of temperature studies to monitor fertility levels, it is not certain why conception occurs sometimes and fails in others. The same is more true of artificial fertilization than is usually realized, except by disappointed couples hoping to become parents and the doctors treating them.

Repeated Miscarriages

After conception, the progress of pregnancy is heavily influenced by factors that science understands only vaguely. Approximately one million reported pregnancies each year in the U.S. fail to come to term because of natural causes, most often as a result of miscarriages in the first three months of pregnancy. Perhaps as many as 40 percent of the miscarriages are due to genetic defects in the fetus. Many others occur as a result of maternal problems ranging from sexually transmitted diseases to hormonal deficiencies. In some cases such problems lead to a series of miscarriages. The cause for many other miscarriages remains unknown, and very often the subsequent pregnancy successfully comes to term.

A particular problem, however, concerns about one in 600 couples who suffer three or more miscarriages in a row for causes that until recently have been unknown. Today, however, a growing number of doctors believe that the cause of such miscarriages is found in the immune system and that the problem can often be corrected. Such doctors claim success rates ranging from two-thirds to more than four-fifths of the couples treated. Despite such claims, the mystery of birth is such that many successes occur with no treatment, so it is difficult to establish that the treatment produced the effect. Usually such difficulties are resolved in double-blind studies combined with statistical analysis, but such objective evidence is hard to come by when a natural, usually happy event such as a successful pregnancy is the subject instead of the more common medical problem of a serious disease.

The theory behind the most common treatments for repeated miscarriage is that the normal protection the fetus receives from mother's immune system has somehow failed. The fetal immunity does not come because the mother's immune system recognized the fetus as part of her body; instead, the fetus must mount a protective barrier in the form of antibodies against antibodies to protect itself. Therefore, doctors try to strengthen the blocking system by administering gamma globin, a mixture of many kinds of antibodies, or by using immune system cells from the father or from unrelated persons to stimulate the blocking antibodies.

Another immunity problem that causes repeated miscarriages is a class of antibodies that can cause blood clots. When these are found in the mother, low-dose aspirin and other anticoagulants or immune-suppressing drugs have proven helpful.

A Conflict of Interest

In the early 1990s a number of evolutionary biologists reinterpreted pregnancy as a conflict of interest between two forces, the developing fetus and the mother. For example, since the fetus has only half the mother's genes, it is in the interest of the mother to miscarry if all is not going well either with the fetus or with herself. The mother can then start a more satisfactory pregnancy or start again at a more convenient time. But the fetus has 100 percent of its own genes, so it wants to continue at all costs.

Some common complications of pregnancy can be explained in this way, including high blood pressure (preeclampsia) and gestational diabetes. Since it is in the fetal interest to have as much blood as possible flow through the placenta, the fetus should release hormones that increase blood pressure. Similarly, it is in the interest of the mother to hang on to sugar she needs for energy, but the fetus also wants the sugar. At first the mother produces less insulin so that less sugar is metabolized. Then the fetus produces a hormone that blocks the action of insulin and causes the mother to increase the supply of insulin. If all goes well, the two sides reach a balance. If not, the mother may end up with gestational diabetes, which can later turn into permanent type II diabetes. Both these explanations were developed by David Haig, an evolutionary biologist at Harvard University.

Margie Profet of the University of California at Berkeley also invokes evolution to explain changes during pregnancy. She believes that the nausea and distaste for many foods early in pregnancy—usually called "morning sickness," although it generally occurs all day—is a result of a mechanism derived from evolution and designed to protect the fetus from toxic compounds in food, compounds that the mother can tolerate but that the very young fetus cannot. Later in development, when the fetus is less vulnerable, the nausea goes away. Support for Profet's theory comes from several studies that show mothers with little or no morning sickness have two to three times as many miscarriages as those with nausea. This suggests that perhaps some of these miscarriages result from toxins in food.

Although most doctors believe that morning sickness persists through the first 13 weeks of pregnancy in most cases, at least one expert finds that the average length of nausea is 17.3 weeks. While for many this is a minor complication of pregnancy, the latest figures (covering 1989) from the National Center for Health Statistics show that 55,000 pregnant women were hospitalized from complications of vomiting. Surveys suggest that some women have such bad morning sickness that they opt for an abortion.

Building Better Babies

Mothers can often greatly improve their chances of delivering a healthy baby by monitoring their own actions. These ought to include such common-sense measures as quitting such habits as drinking alcohol, smoking tobacco, and using drugs other than those overseen by a physician (and perhaps being even a bit reluctant to use those). Good nutrition, with a special emphasis on folacin (*See* "Vitamin UPDATE," p 160), is essential.

Here are some more specific study results to consider:

Alcohol: Heavy drinking during early pregnancy causes about 5000 cases of fetal alcohol syndrome in the U.S. each year and contributes to less severe effects in another 35,000 cases according to the U.S. National Council on Alcoholism and Drug Dependence.

Aspirin: Although there is considerable evidence that aspirin in small doses helps pregnant women escape high blood pressure (*See* "New Uses for Aspirin," p 527), at least one study, published in the October 21, 1993 *New England Journal of Medicine*, reported otherwise. It showed that the risk of the placenta separating from the uterus, which can be life-threatening for both mother and child, is higher for mothers taking even low doses of aspirin, especially when aspirin is used later in the pregnancy. Certainly, aspirin should not be taken without a physician's recommendation.

Bacteria: Many women (15 to 40 percent of healthy women) are infected with group B streptococcus bacteria with no ill effects, which is also true for most babies born with the bacterium found on their skins. But for the estimated one in 40 babies born to women carrying the bacterium who become internally infected, it is a different story. In the U.S. alone, about 2000 of such infants die each year, and many others suffer permanent damage to the brain or other organs. Thus, on November 5, 1992 the American Academy of Pediatrics called for screening of pregnant women for the group B streptococcus, which can then be eliminated with antibiotics administered just before birth, because babies become infected in the birth canal if at all.

Chemicals: In 1992, studies revealed that the glycol ethers used in making semiconductor circuits (chips), some aerospace manufacture, and some printing operations cause a slight but significant increase in the risk of miscarriage. Steps have since been taken to eliminate usage of these particular chemicals, but all chemicals used in manufacturing should be viewed with caution.

Coffee: Not all news is bad. The February 3, 1993 *Journal of the American Medical Association* contained a report that reanalyzed some older data and found that drinking fewer than three cups of coffee a day caused no increase in miscarriages or growth retardation in the fetus.

Hot tubs and saunas: An analysis of 22,762 births published in the August 19, 1994 *Journal of the American Medical Association* found that heat exposure during the first two months of pregnancy led to increased risk of spina bifida or brain damage. Specifically, the statistics, which were based on the small numbers of birth defects found in the study, indicated that women with no known heat exposure during pregnancy experienced a rate of 1.8 per thousand birth defects in their infants; the rate went up to 3.4 per thousand for women who had high fevers during early pregnancy; it increased to 5.4 among the 367 who reported using saunas; and was 5.6 among the 1,254 hot-tub users. Hot tubs and saunas already carry warnings against use by pregnant women.

Viruses: In the May 1993 *American Academy of Child and Adolescent Psychiatry* Richard Livingstone of the University of Arkansas for Medical Sciences in Little Rock and coworkers reported their additional research on the previously studied statistical relationship between babies born on May, June, and July and those born during the rest of the year. Late spring and early summer babies are in their second trimester of fetal development in the late winter, when various viral diseases usually grouped as "the flu," as well as true influenza, abound. Previous studies had linked exposure to such viruses to a host of mental problems, including schizophrenia, autism, mental retardation, and hyperactivity. Livingstone's research adds dyslexia (inability to read, thought to be caused by brain damage) to the list; babies born in the late spring or early summer are twice as likely to have dyslexia as those born in other months of the year. As a result, children born in May, June, and July accounted for 40 percent of all the children with dyslexia in the study group of 585 boys, all of whom had been referred to a clinic for psychiatric evaluation. This figure is even more surprising since births in the U.S. are lowest in April and May and rise to a peak in September.

Exercise: In the May 15, 1993 *American Journal of Epidemiology* Maureen Hatch and coworkers at Columbia University reported that studies of recreational exercise in pregnant women showed that babies born to women who burn up to 1000 calories a week in recreational exercise were five percent heavier than those born to women who are more sedentary during pregnancy. Mothers who work out more, burning between 1000 and 2000 calories a week in their exercise routines, have babies that weigh ten percent more than babies born to mothers who do not exercise.

Tobacco: In July 1993, Peter A. Fried of Carleton University in Ottawa, Canada, reported to the Neurobehavioral Teratology Society that smoking during pregnancy results in hearing loss in newborns which continues into early childhood, possibly interfering with speech acquisition. The study did not attempt to trace such hearing problems into adulthood, and it is not known how long the problems persist.

An earlier study showed that children whose fathers smoke are somewhat more likely to develop brain cancer or leukemia, suggesting possible damage to sperm. Other studies have indicated that a father's exposure to environmentally risky chemicals or radiation may also cause cancers in their offspring.

Vitamin and mineral supplements: The August 19, 1993 *New England Journal of Medicine* carried a report of a study by Greta Bunin of the Children's Hospital in Philadelphia and coworkers which showed that use of iron, calcium, and vitamin C supplements reduced the risk of a relatively common form of brain cancer in children.

(Periodical References and Additional Reading: *New York Times* 12-11-90; *New York Times* 8-19-92, p A19; *New York Times* 10-12-92, p A1; *New York Times* 11-18-92, p C18; *New York Times* 12-4-92, p A29; *New York Times* 12-15-92, p C3; *Science News* 5-1-93, p 278; *Science News* 7-10-93, p 23; *Science* 7-11-93, p 1592; *Science News* 7-17-93, p 36; *New York Times* 7-20-93, p C3; *New York Times* 8-19-93, p A20; *New York Times* 11-3-93, p C8; *Science News* 11-6-93, p 302; *New York Times* 11-17-93, p C17)

FETAL DIAGNOSIS

The time is long past when the only method of determining information about a fetus was through external clues of shape and sound and reports from the prospective mother on what she was feeling.

What's Going On In There?

At one time, the only clues to development were what could be observed by looking at or feeling the pregnant mother. Today ultrasound examinations are almost routine, though viewed with mild caution by a few doctors. In cases of suspected future trouble, more invasive tests can sample fetal cells. But the most popular of these, amniocentesis, poses some risk, so new approaches are continually sought. Among the new diagnostic tools is a blood test.

A pregnant woman and the fetus are partly fused creatures. It has been known for over a hundred years that more than nutrition passes through the placenta—a mother's antibodies pass on to the fetus, for example. At the same time, there is some traffic in the other direction. A few fetal cells find their way into the mother's bloodstream. Researchers have demonstrated that they can sometimes locate a single fetal cell amid 100 million maternal cells in a blood sample. Studies by Diana Bianchi of the Tufts University School of Medicine in Boston, Massachusetts, show that the number of fetal cells can vary widely, from as low as 0.2 percent of blood cells during the 11th week of pregnancy to as high as 8.5 percent. Abnormal pregnancies are more likely to leak a high percentage of cells into the bloodstream, making such pregnancies easier to diagnose. This ability to diagnose abnormalities in the fetus by examining the mother's blood is expected to find clinical application in the near future, with earlier and safer blood tests for hereditary disorders to augment or replace the more established amniocentesis and chorionic villus tests.

The best successes so far are with erythrocytes (red blood cells), although some researchers are investigating other cells that leak into the mother's bloodstream. Although mature erythrocytes are not full-fledged cells because of the lack of a DNA-containing nucleus, immature cells of the type produced mostly by the fetus still contain nuclei. This is a double benefit in fetal diagnosis, since (1) any erythrocytes in the mother's blood that have a nucleus are almost certainly fetal and not maternal, making fetal cells identifiable; and (2) it is the DNA in the nucleus that is needed for identification of genetic diseases or for sex determination (important for X-linked diseases).

In one experimental study, Sherman Elias and Joe Lee Simpson of the University of Tennessee were able to use erythrocytes found in the mother's blood to identify chromosomal abnormalities, including Down's syndrome fetuses from women with a high risk for such problems. They were also able in nearly all cases to determine the sex of the fetus. Their method combined monoclonal antibodies with a laser based fluorescence-activated cell sorter.

A German group, including Dorothee Ganshirt-Ahlert of the University of Münster, conducted similar experiments that also were successful. They used a magnetic sorting device instead of the laser, however; the magnetic sorter is both cheaper to use and faster.

The next step in this technology will be to use chain reactions of DNA to develop tests for individual genes and not just for extra chromosomes.

In the meantime, another kind of maternal blood test has been developed, one that offers a simpler and safer way to predict which fetuses have Down's syndrome. Called Bart's Triple Test because it was developed at St. Bartholomew's Hospital in London,

United Kingdom, and screens for three different blood chemicals, the measurements it provides are intended to predict which women should then resort to amniocentesis for a definitive conclusion. According to its proponents, universal use of Bart's Triple Test would have two complementary effects: younger women would be less tempted to unnecessarily risk the fetus by undergoing amniocentesis and younger women who might need amniocentesis would be nevertheless identified. The benefits of the blood test to women older than 37 are somewhat less clear.

Does Chorionic Villus Testing Cause Birth Defects?

Chorionic villus testing for genetic or chromosomal abnormalities started in the U.S. in 1983 and is probably administered to more than 30,000 pregnant American women each year. The main virtue of the test is that it is performed in the first trimester of pregnancy and thus allows women who choose to have an abortion on the basis of the analysis to have one sooner and therefore more safely. Until 1991, there was little reason to think that the test posed any harm to mother or child.

In 1991, however, a group from Oxford University in England suggested that chorionic villus testing caused birth defects. The procedure requires the removal of a small portion of the placenta because the villi involved are hairlike projections on the placenta; in doing so physicians may also be cutting off the blood supply to parts of the fetus. The parts of the fetus most likely to be affected are the extremities, resulting in babies with stubby or missing fingers or toes. The facial area may also be affected, resulting in a shortened tongue and an underdeveloped lower jaw. The Oxford group thought that such defects had occurred in five out of 289 women they studied.

The Oxford report led others to look at their own records of children born to women who had chorionic villus testing. An Italian study found almost as many children per birth with the rare defects as did the Oxford study. In Chicago a similar analysis showed somewhat less incidence than the Oxford or Italian studies, but still a high incidence for such rare defects. All three studies involved small populations of fewer than 400 births.

When larger studies were conducted in 1992, however, such birth defects in chorionic villus sampling were found to occur at the expected rate for all births, and not just births in which chorionic villus sampling had been used. Thus, there is at present no definite evidence that chorionic villus sampling can cause birth defects.

FETAL DIAGNOSIS

Name of Test	Test Procedure	What Can Be Learned
Amniocentesis	Fluid is removed from sac surrounding a fetus via a thin needle inserted through the mother's abdomen.	Chromosomes and genes are studied for genetic defects and for sex determination; primarily used when mother is older or when there is some reason to expect hereditary disease; there is some risk to the fetus and the test is not completely accurate.

Name of Test	Test Procedure	What Can Be Learned
Chorionic villus biopsy	A sample of villus tissue is snipped from the outer sac surrounding the fetus.	Cells in the villus can be studied for genetic defects and sex determination; the advantage of this test over amniocentesis is that it can be performed earlier in pregnancy; a disadvantage is a slightly higher risk of miscarriage than amniocentesis; introduced to U.S. in 1983 after successful trials in Europe.
Ultrasound (also known by the name of the image produced—sonogram)	A small device is placed on the mother's abdomen, which produces ultrasound pictures viewed on a monitor.	The basic shape of the baby can be observed, so that the physician can observe abnormalities (if any) in body parts or position and monitor state of development; a bonus usually available is the opportunity to discern the sex of the fetus; although ultrasound methods now in use produce two-dimensional images, by 1993 several teams of researchers had developed equipment to produce three-dimensional versions.

(Periodical References and Additional Reading: *New York Times* 7-15-92, p C13; *New York Times* 8-19-92, p C12; *Science* 11-19-93, p 1207; *Sciences* 3/4-94, *Focus* p 48c)

BIRTH

BIRTH, NATURAL AND OTHERWISE

The concept of natural childbirth, while older in one sense than any other form—though the common name was only introduced in 1933—seemed to have gained new life in the U.S. during the politically conscious 1960s and environmentally conscious 1970s. Today it is almost routine for educated, middle- or upper-class Americans to have classes in natural (or any) childbirth, birthing coaches, and an exercise program for muscles that might be used in birth. At the same time, starting in 1975, the least natural form of childbirth, known as the caesarean section, began a strong rise.

Surgery and Birth

By 1975 the rate of caesarean births in the U.S. had climbed to 10.4 percent of all births, and the upward trend was continuing. The high point in the ratio of caesareans to all births was in 1988, when the rate reached almost one in four (24.7 percent). Similar rises were occurring in a few other Western nations, notably Brazil, for which caesareans were performed in 32 percent of all births. After 1988, the U.S. rate dropped slightly, remaining at 23.5 percent in both 1990 and 1991, the last years for which there are available U.S. records.

Both the U.S. Centers for Disease Control and Prevention (CDC) and the American College of Obstetricians and Gynecologists agree that too many caesarean deliveries take place in the U.S. The CDC is more specific. On April 22, 1993 they released figures they said showed that of the 966,000 caesareans in 1991, about 349,000 were unnecessary. According to the CDC, the rate of necessary and appropriate caesareans is 15 percent, and they base their categorization of unnecessary caesareans on that. Lower rates than 15 percent may even be appropriate: one hospital established a peer-review system for all caesareans and a second-opinion for non-emergency situations which resulted in the rate of caesareans being cut in half from 22 percent to 11 percent. Among the industrialized nations with a very low rate of caesarean deliveries, Japan has only a seven percent rate of babies delivered by caesarean section.

A less drastic way to aid childbirth surgically also came under fire in the early 1990s. Many doctors attending birth almost routinely make a small cut, called an episiotomy, in the vagina, with the intention of making birth easier and preventing accidental tearing. After birth the cut is sewn up. In the U.S. and Canada, an episiotomy is performed in an estimated 70 to 80 percent of all births that are not caesareans. This makes the episiotomy one of the most common surgical procedures in medicine. But a Canadian study released on July 2, 1992 found that nearly all episiotomies failed to accomplish any of the presumed goals of the operation: babies born in the experimental group who received no episiotomies unless there was a clear medical need were just as healthy; the time of labor was statistically the same—nine minutes longer for first-time mothers without the episiotomies—and there was no evidence that the neat cutting and sewing of the surgeon resulted in enhanced sexual functioning after the birth, an argument sometimes advanced in favor of the operation. Thus, the Canadian doctors argued that an episiotomy ought to be an exception rather than nearly the rule and should be used only when there is a clear-cut need to protect the baby or mother.

Premature Birth

Any baby born before it has fully developed in its mother's uterus has the more difficult task of completing development on its own or with whatever help modern medicine provides. Careful measurements show that the normal development process is completed in 38 weeks after conception. Uncertainty about the actual date of conception means that physicians usually figure 40 weeks from the last menstrual period. So with a margin for error, birth before 37 weeks is "premature."

Since the exact date of conception is seldom known, one measure traditionally used to label early babies as *premature*—meaning too undeveloped for good health—has been birth weight. Physicians somewhat arbitrarily have called any babies weighing less than five-and-a-half pounds premature, even though birth weight depends on many factors, not just the amount of development time between conception and birth. Approximately 250,000 U.S. infants weighing less than five-and-a-half pounds are born annually.

In November 1993 Marilee Allen, Pamela Donahue, and Amy Dusman at the Johns Hopkins University School of Medicine developed an evaluation of premature survival risks that was based on estimated length of development in weeks since conception. They found that for birth at 25 weeks since conception, 79 percent of the infants in their study survived with modern medical help; at that number of weeks, about eight percent have severe birth handicaps. In that time of development, each week makes a significant difference. A week earlier and 34 percent (instead of eight percent) will be born with severe handicaps, a figure that rises to 50 percent at 23 weeks. None of the children believed to be 22 weeks along at the time of birth survived.

At the same time, another study showed that the use of the common drug

---

Background

Tradition has it that the operation of surgically removing a child from the mother was named for Julius Caesar, who, it is sometimes claimed, was born that way (although it was Macduff who was "from his mother's womb untimely ripp'd" in Shakespeare's familiar line). But some scholars have argued the other way, that the name Caesar came from the operation—in Latin *caesus ab utero matris*—although this seems to be merely a coincidence. Indeed, the operation was mentioned in the laws supposedly proclaimed by Numa, the second King of Rome in traditional Roman legend (circa eighth century B.C.). In all those early cases, however, the operation was performed only after the death of the mother during labor. Various attempts to perform a caesarean (or "caesarean section," as it is more formally called) on a living woman invariably resulted in the death of the mother until quite modern times. Even in the 1950s the operation was considered quite risky, and most doctors avoided it unless circumstances indicated that birth could not possibly be accomplished naturally.

indomethacin to delay birth before 30 weeks of development could harm the fetus, causing the number of infants with bowel-tissue disease or bleeding in the brain to triple. A larger study was called for to determine the exact relationship between the benefits of delaying birth and the harm caused by the drug used to cause the delay. Indomethacin is actually an FDA Category D drug, meaning that it should only be used in pregnancy if there is no safer choice to preserve life or in serious disease. Indomethacin, which goes by more than a half-dozen trade names, is a mild analgesic and anti-inflammatory, similar in effect to aspirin and acetaminophen.

Other drugs often used to delay birth are ritodine and terbutaline. Terbutaline is actually approved only as an asthma medication, but physicians are known to prescribe it, as well as the chemically similar ritodine, to relax the uterus and stave off labor.

Since 1980, ritodine has been the only chemical approved by the FDA for suppression of premature labor, which was originally done by administering the drug both intravenously and orally. A Canadian study published in the July 20, 1992 *New England Journal of Medicine* showed that ritodine could cause maternal heart arrythmias and even, in a few cases, death; but as then used, it was no more effective than a placebo in delaying labor. An FDA panel later reexamined the Canadian findings and recommended that the drug be used only as an injection before the 33rd week of pregnancy, being too dangerous to use late in pregnancy. Oral use was found to be ineffective.

Much of the development of the fetal brain takes place in the last trimester. For example, nearly all the docosahexaenoic acid, which accounts for more than a third of the brain's fatty acids, is accumulated during that time. As a result, premature babies often have visual problems resulting from too low an amount of docosahexaenoic acid in the brain and in the retina, which is closely associated with the brain. In October 1992 Eileen R. Birch and coworkers from the University of Texas Southwestern Medical Center in Dallas, and then in July 1993 Susan E. Carson and coworkers at the University of Tennessee in Memphis both reported that adding fish oil supplements to a premature baby's formula improves visual acuity. Because a baby organizes the universe through its eyesight, it is considered especially important to encourage good eyesight in the few months right after birth.

(Periodical References and Additional Reading: *New York Times* 9-2-91, p 9; *New York Times* 7-2-92, p A12; *New York Times* 7-30-92, p A1; *New York Times* 2-14-93, p III-1; *New York Times* 4-23-93, p A16; *Science News* 7-17-93, p 38; *New York Times* 11-28-93, p I-36)

NON-GENETIC BIRTH DEFECTS

While many of the disorders people class as birth defects result from hereditary conditions, many others have different causes. Some problems, such as Down's syndrome, are not present in the body cells of either parent, but happen sometimes on the way to conception or even after conception. Others develop as a result of disease or trauma to the fetus, including diseases caused by inadequate nutrition or drugs. About 250,000 babies are born each year in the U.S. with a birth defect that is apparently physical, such as a deformed body part. In 60 to 80 percent of such cases, we do not know the original cause of a birth defect. Animal studies suggest that one of the causes of nonhereditary birth defects is damage to sperm from environmental chemicals. Many defects that are classed as nonhereditary, such as defects of the nervous system (often called neural tube defects), tend to run in families, suggesting some sort of hereditary disposition toward them.

Although ova are formed before a prospective mother is even born herself, sperm are made daily throughout a man's life. Thus, a chemical can more easily interfere selectively with the development of a sperm than with an ovum. Also, sperm have been known to carry environmental chemicals along with them on their journey to the ovum.

One notable 1991 study, discussed in several places in the *Handbook of Current Health and Medicine*, is that folic acid (also known as folacin) helps protect against spina bifida, a common defect of the neural tube in which the vertebrae enclosing the spinal cord fail to close properly, and against anencephaly, another neural-tube defect in which most of the brain fails to develop at all. Folic acid had been suspected since the early 1960s of preventing neural tube defects, but convincing evidence was lacking until a study reported in the July 20, 1991 *Lancet*. Conducted by a team led by Nicholas Wald of St. Bartholomew's Hospital in London, United Kingdom, the study of more than 1800 mothers showed that neural tube defects were more than four times as likely for the children of mothers who did not take folic acid supplements. It should be noted, however, that six children whose mothers were taking the supplements were born with neural tube defects anyway.

Older Mothers

Many mothers in the present cultural situation of industrialized countries put off having children until they are older. Until recently, it was thought that a major risk of this strategy was that birth defects seem to rise with age, but with this in mind no one had ever done a careful study of birth defects other than Down's syndrome. Down's syndrome has been extensively studied and definitely does rise in incidence with the age of the mother.

Patricia A. Baird of the University of British Columbia and coworkers published a study in the March 2, 1991 *Lancet* for which 26,859 cases involving 43 different types of birth defects in British Columbia (from 1966 through 1981) were analyzed. The defects did not include any known hereditary problems; diabetes, which is thought to be partly hereditary; or defects caused by such environmental factors as alcohol consumption and use of medicines known to cause birth defects. Because the focus of the analysis was on the age of the mother at birth, Down's syndrome, known to increase with the age of the mother, was also excluded. Even with all of these birth problems eliminated, the 43 disorders that remained affected five percent of all the births in British Columbia over this period. It is worth noting that the province keeps very good birth records, so there was little ambiguous data.

Included among the 43 types tracked were spina bifida, cleft palate, harelip, congenital heart defects, limb defects (such as clubfoot), and hypertrophic pyloric stenosis (narrow stomach). Not only did none of these rise with age, but it appears from the analysis that two of them, hypertrophic pyloric stenosis and the heart defect patent ductus arteriosis, decline steadily with age. Furthermore, although the defect called a congenitally dislocatable hip does rise with age up to the age of thirty, thereafter it decreases. Although this study is statistically strong, the results for these three defects are unexpected; most doctors would like to see more focused research on the relation of those defects to age before ruling the results conclusive.

Cerebral Palsy

About half a million Americans are classified as having the cluster of birth defects known collectively as cerebral palsy, and half of those have severe forms. Symptoms include loss of motor muscle control often coupled with hearing or visual impairment and a delay in growth and development. In some cases this condition may be linked to such learning disabilities as dyslexia or even to mental retardation. It is the most frequent birth defect that is observable in young children and is especially common in premature babies.

In the December 1992 *Pediatrics* Karin Nelson of the National Institute of Neurological Disorders and Stroke and Judith K. Grether of the California Department of Health reported their study of cerebral palsy in 155,000 children born in northern California. They discovered that the rate of the birth defect increased dramatically for children who were one of twins, especially if the other twin had died before birth. The rate for children that developed alone in the mother's uterus was only 1.1 per thousand, but it rose to 12 per thousand among twins and to 118.8 per thousand among babies whose twin died before birth. Although twins often have low birth weights—a known factor in cerebral palsy—even when surviving members of twin pairs were over the five-and-a-half-pound weight (the borderline for prematurity), the members of the twin pairs had three times as many occurrences of cerebral palsy as the single-birth infants.

Since the discovery of chemicals that increase fertility and *in vitro* fertilization, the number of multiple births has risen. The percentage of twins, for example, increased somewhere around two to three percentage points during the 1980s. Thus the number of children born with cerebral palsy could also be expected to rise in view of the findings of this study.

(Periodical References and Additional Reading: *New York Times* 1-1-91, p A1; *New York Times* 3-2-91; *Science News* 7-10-93, p 30; *New York Times* 7-19-91)

INFANT MORTALITY

According to the United Nations Population Fund, the 1993 rate for infant mortality worldwide was 69 deaths per 1000 live births (the U.S. Bureau of Census *World Population Profile* had 65 per 1000 in 1991 as its latest figures). The rate for industrial nations taken as a whole was only 12 per 1000 in 1993 (13 per 1000 in the 1991 *World Population Profile*). The *World Population Profile* reported the highest rate as 177 per 1000 in Western Sahara and the lowest as four per 1000 in Japan.

In the United States

Infant mortality has greatly improved over the rates of earlier years in the U.S. and has been at the lowest level in history since the early 1990s. But mortality is still from one to five more deaths per 1000 live births than in Japan or any of the nations of Western Europe. Furthermore, goals set by the U.S. Public Health Service are not being met.

In addition to Japan and Western Europe, the *World Population Profile* puts the U.S. behind Taiwan (six per 1000), Canada (seven per 1000), Australia and Singapore (eight per 1000), and Israel (nine per 1000). The same summary lists the U.S. rate as ten per 1000 in 1991, instead of 8.9 per 1000 as given by the U.S. National Center for Health Statistics, whose figures are the basis of the table below.

INFANT MORTALITY RATES IN THE U.S.
(Rate per 1000 life births)

Year	All births	African Americans	European Descent
1992	8.5	*	*
1991	8.9	17.6	7.3
1990	9.2	18.0	7.6
1989	9.8	18.6	8.1
1980	12.6	21.4	11.0
1970	20.0	32.6	17.8
1960	26.0	44.3	22.9
1950	29.2	43.9	26.8
1940	47.0	72.9	43.2
1915	99.9		

*Exact rates not available early in 1994, but the U.S. Department of Health and Human Services reports that rates among African Americans in 1992 were about double those of European descent, suggesting that the rates are approximately 14 percent and 7 percent respectively.

(Periodical References and Additional Reading: *New York Times* 4-6-91, p 1; *New York Times* 8-1-93, p A13; *New York Times* 4-3-94, p I-11)

Childhood and Growth

THE STATE OF PEDIATRICS

The state of children's health worldwide was a major topic of the 1990 World Summit for Children, held at the United Nations. Among the goals that participants voluntarily set were immunizing 90 percent of their country's children by the end of the century and reducing overall mortality rates in children under five by a third or reducing mortality rates to below 70 per thousand, whichever would be lower.

The health of children is certainly no small matter. At the time of the conference it was estimated that 142 million children were born each year. The World Health Organization estimated that in 1990 about 13.1 million children under the age of five had died, of whom about 3.7 million were over a year old. Different countries' death rates for children under five varied widely; most of the developing countries averaged about 140 deaths per thousand, but the rate reached nearly 300 per thousand in Mozambique and as low as 12 per thousand in the U.S. at that time.

The United Nations Children's Fund (UNICEF) projected that when a country's rate reached somewhere around a level of 100 deaths per thousand children under five, birth rates would begin to drop in that developing country. Parents would see that they no longer needed to produce extra children to ensure a certain number survived. UNICEF posited that in nations with high death rates for children, birth rates would drop more than the gain in the number of children that survived. This would lower the overall rate of population growth at least from the birth end of growth; actual experience in the 1990s has shown that a lowering of death rates is a major factor in rising population worldwide.

Major causes of death for children under five in 1990 were, in order, acute respiratory disease (nearly all pneumonia), dehydration from diarrhea, failure to breath at birth (birth asphyxia), malaria, neonatal tetanus (most often from infection of the severed umbilical cord), and measles.

By the end of 1993, UNICEF could report that considerable progress was being made. Among the death rates for children that fell dramatically over a ten-year period and not just since the World Summit were those from pneumonia, diarrhea, measles, neonatal tetanus, whooping cough, and malnutrition. One striking case was measles, for which the worldwide death rates between 1983 and 1992 had fallen from 2.5 million a year to one million a year. In the same period, deaths from dehydration caused by diarrhea in children fell from over four million a year to less than three million annually. Deaths from neonatal tetanus were cut in half from just over a million in 1983.

Some Concerns in the U.S.

The health of children in the U.S. is far from perfect, but the problems are somewhat different than in developing countries, though concern about adequate vaccination exists worldwide.

Changes in the U.S. economy and in social attitudes have combined to put more mothers to work even when children are very young. By 1976 these trends had progressed to the extent that the U.S. Census began to include surveys of working mothers. That year they found that 31 percent of mothers with a child under a year old were also counted as in the labor force. By 1990, the figure had risen to 53 percent. Although some studies starting in 1986 suggested that children of working mothers suffered problems in socialization and development, the most recent and most careful research has found that having a working mother is not hard on a child. This is especially true when compared to socioeconomic factors: that is, a child in a family with a livable income is better off for the most part even if mother works away from home than is a child in a poverty-stricken family with a mother who is home. One study published in the August 1992 *Pediatrics* looked closely at nutrition and found no significant difference in diet between children of working mothers and those of non-working mothers. Unfortunately both the study group and the control group had too much fat in their diet and not enough calcium, iron, zinc, or vitamin E.

In the U.S., the Federal Centers for Disease Control and Prevention consider lead poisoning to be the most common preventable childhood health hazard (*See* "Lead," p 253).

Allergies and Asthma

Although worldwide progress is being made against childhood disease, most success arises from attacking infectious disease or improving nutrition. In the U.S. and other industrial nations where there is a long tradition of vaccination, sanitation, medical treatment, and adequate nutrition—although all of these still need improvement in every country to reach high technological levels—other problems surface. Not all of these health problems are acute causes of death, but they are the cause of a great deal of suffering and often lead to death.

In the U.S., for example, asthma is "the most common chronic disease of childhood" according to William R. Taylor of the U.S. Centers for Disease Control and Prevention. A report in the November 1992 *Pediatrics* calculated that in 1988, the latest year with good statistics, 2.7 million children under the age of 18 had asthma, which is 4.3 percent of the whole population (slightly better than one in twenty). This percentage had increased from 3.2 percent only seven years earlier, a dramatic increase in rate of more than 0.1 percentage points a year. About 200,000 children were hospitalized annually with asthma. Although several thousand Americans die from asthma attacks each year, nearly all deaths occur in older persons, not children.

Asthma is really the name for a type of lung dysfunction and not a disease at all. During an asthma attack, air passages into the lungs, the bronchial tubes, close up and thus reduce the ability to breathe. The cause of this dysfunction is most often an allergy, but essentially the same dysfunction can occur as a result of infection or even psychological stress. The main difference between asthma and other conditions that restrict passage of air through the bronchial tubes is that the asthmatic person will have periodic asthma attacks for years, while other conditions come for a time and are then gone. Often children have fewer and fewer asthma attacks as they grow older, and the rate of asthma among adults is a percentage point or two lower than that of school-age children.

Children with asthma do die, however, although usually death is preventable if proper medical steps are taken. Death is not a direct result of the asthma itself but of a massive reaction to an underlying allergy which is expressed in part as asthma. Children with severe asthma are more likely than other children to have an anaphylactic reaction to an allergen. Such a reaction includes not only an asthma attack but also at least one other symptom, such as nausea or vomiting, hives or swelling, or sudden low blood pressure (shock).

Although many parents associate such reactions with insect bites, experts believe that anaphylactic reactions more commonly result from exposure to food. A particular problem in the 1990s has been that food manufacturers introduce many proteins from peanuts (use of peanut oil), eggs (as an emulsifying agent), milk (for various purposes), or soybeans (for texture or for oil). These, along with nuts and shellfish, are also the protein sources most likely to induce anaphylactic reactions. Combined with the general rise in childhood asthma, the food additives constitute an increasingly serious problem for children.

A "New" Childhood Illness

In recent years people have come to fear the advent of illnesses that were previously unknown—Legionnaire's disease, Lyme disease, AIDS, hantavirus, and others. For the most part, the new or newly identified diseases have stricken adults, but one major disease affecting children became known in the 1990s.

The story actually started in 1986, when six adults in the U.S. and in Jamaica came down with a previously unknown lymph disease. It was discovered by scientists from the National Cancer Institute in Bethesda, Maryland. The culprit was a virus.

Physicians in Japan found that the newly discovered virus, by then named HHV-6 and recognized as a member of the herpes family (which includes the viral causes of chicken pox and "cold" or "fever" sores), caused a common contagious disease of young children. The disease is named roseola, but its cause was previously unknown. Symptoms are a rash and a high fever. Usually the fever comes first, and then the characteristic rash (flat pink spots, especially on the trunk) starts and the fever abates, reversing the course of many other childhood diseases. It tends to strike children in the spring and affects children between the ages of six months and two years, but can also affect those up to the age of four. Roseola is considered one of the relatively harmless childhood diseases, but it often alarms parents and health workers with the sudden appearance of a fever that can reach 106° F with no apparent cause. When the rash appears, allowing the disease to be recognized, everyone breathes a sigh of relief.

The Japanese doctors found the situation to be more complicated than the simple answer that roseola is caused by HHV-6. In testing for HHV-6, they also found some infants who got the fever but not the rash. They even found infants with the virus and no fever.

In the U.S. a team including physicians from the University of Rochester, the U.S. Centers for Disease Control, and Dupont, Merck Pharmaceuticals looked for the virus in children admitted to a hospital emergency room with high fevers in Rochester, New York during the winter and early spring of 1989-90. They were surprised by two findings. First of all, 14 percent of the children who had fevers higher than 100.4° F were infected with HHV-6. Second of all, the rate of children with high fevers who later developed the rash that indicates roseola was only one in five. Most of the HHV-6 infected children had infected eardrums, not roseola.

The main lesson to be learned from this small study is that a better test for HHV-6 would save money. It took about $600 to $700 to diagnose the unexplained high fevers in children reaching the emergency room. If most of them actually have HHV-6 and not some more deadly disease, a lot of time and money would be saved by a quick test; it would also lower the anxiety level of parents. Also, further study is warranted. Not only were the numbers involved in this study small, but children without high fevers were not tested.

New Remedies

Both vaccination (*See* "Vaccine UPDATE," p 325) and antibiotics make the most significant difference in the health of children, but not all infectious diseases can be prevented by vaccination or halted in their tracks by antibiotics. But almost every year physicians and researchers gain new tools that can help deal with childhood diseases.

Although the orally administered polio vaccine proved to be even more successful than injections, sometimes when there is a choice between an injection and oral administration, the injection is the winner. This is the case with drugs used to treat children's ear infections caused by bacteria. When there is doubt that the patient will follow a full course of antibiotics lasting ten days, the injection of a drug usually used for more serious diseases is better than the oral antibiotic, according to a study of 233 children reported in the January 1993 *Pediatrics*.

Taking antibiotics for less than the required time or in less than the required amount is very risky, in part because any bacteria not killed by insufficient amount of administered medication are likely to be resistant to medical treatment. Thus when the disease comes back, it can no longer be easily treated with the same antibiotic. Moreover, because of crossover mechanisms in bacterial reproduction, the bacteria may develop resistance to all antibiotics, not just the one previously tried.

A study by Steven Rothrock of the Orlando Regional Medical Center in Florida, Steven Green of the Loma Linda University School of Medicine, and coworkers found, however, that a single injection of the antibiotic ceftriaxone was just as effective as a ten-day course of the oral antibiotic amoxicillin, though ceftriaxone is more expensive. Other research suggests that only 30 percent of children out of hospital settings actually take the ten days of the oral drug. Another factor, important to many parents, is that insurance plans more often fully cover emergency room injections rather than oral medicine intended to be taken at home. The injection is also appropriate when the child has been vomiting.

An even more dramatic improvement in treatment involves any fever that produces convulsions in infants or young children. Although the long-term harm of most convulsions is slight, they are dramatically terrifying to parents and in some cases may cause continuing epilepsy. Thus physicians have looked for some way to stop such febrile seizures, as they are called. But until recently, the drug of choice has not proven very effective and may even cause more harm than the febrile seizures. The drug, phenobarbital, is a sedative with sometimes dangerous immediate side effects and possibly negative long-term drop in IQ scores. Some physicians prescribe daily doses of phenobarbital for periods as long as a year after febrile seizures have taken place, mainly in hopes of avoiding further episodes. Children who take this drug, which adults often use as a sleeping pill, are at best lethargic or, perhaps surprisingly, hyperactive. Many physicians concluded years ago that the side effects were worse than the convulsions the drug was intended to prevent.

A different idea was tried in a six-year study in Boston that was reported in the *New England Journal of Medicine* in July 1993. Instead of phenobarbital, the study group took Valium (diazepam) while the control group received only placebos. The study revealed that for the most part, if the Valium regime began after the first episode of convulsions, there were fewer recurrences of the seizures and no observable side effects. About a third of children who received no treatment or a placebo did not have recurrences in any case, but there was an 82 percent drop in this figure among those who started Valium promptly.

In adults, Valium has been found to be addictive if taken in large doses for periods of four weeks or more.

(Periodical References and Additional Reading: *New York Times* 12-19-90;*New York Times* 5-29-92, p A15; *New York Times* 8-2-92, p A17; *New York Times* 8-5-92, p C12; *New York Times* 10-6-92, p A1; *New York Times* 11-7-92, p 10; *New York Times* 1-26-93, p C3; *New York Times* 12-21-93, p A15)

TIMETABLE OF CHILD CARE AND PEDIATRICS TO 1990

1730	George Martine performs the first tracheotomy for treatment of diphtheria.
1891	An antitoxin for diphtheria is tested for the first time on humans.
1901	Emil von Behring [born Hansdorf, Germany, March 15, 1854; died Marburg, Germany, March 31, 1917] wins the Nobel Prize for Physiology or Medicine for his discovery of diphtheria antitoxin.
1913	Emil von Behring introduces a toxin-antitoxin mixture for immunizing children against diphtheria.
1923	The French bacteriologist Gaston Ramon introduces a more effective vaccine against diphtheria.
1943	Leo Kanner [born 1894; died 1981] in the U.S. describes the symptoms of autism and, independently, Hans Asperger [born in Austria, 1906] does the

same; both adapt the word "autism" from a word orginally coined to describe loss of contact with reality by adult schizophrenics.

1952   Virginia Apgar [born Westfield, New Jersey, June 7, 1909; died New York, New York, August 7, 1974] introduces the Apgar Score which predicts the health of a newborn baby by measuring the pulse, respiration, muscle tone, color, and reflexes; its use soon becomes universal in the U.S. as well as in much of the rest of the world.

1963   The first vaccine against measles is introduced; it uses a killed virus and is not reliably effective.

1964   R. Guthrie and A. Susi develop a method for screening newborn infants for phenylketonuria (PKU).

1966   Harry M. Meyer, Jr. [born Palestine, Texas, November 25, 1928], and Paul D. Parkman [born Auburn, New York, May 29, 1932] develop a live-virus vaccine for rubella (German measles).

1967   A live-virus vaccine against measles which is more effective than the previous killed-virus version becomes available.

1968   Live attenuated vaccine against mumps is introduced.

1989   On May 10 Thomas H. Shaffer [born 1908] and coworkers show that a premature infant can breathe an oxygen-suffused liquid called perfluorocarbon, thus reducing lung damage that such infants often encounter; in this first test, the infant's lungs had already been damaged beyond repair by conventional treatment, but the fluid treatment was clearly helpful even though it came too late.

TESTING THE SENSES

Physicians, midwives, and nurses give newborns more than a cursory glance before putting them into the mother's arms or a cradle for the first time. While they have always looked for any signs of ill health, since 1952 they have also used a specific set of criteria to score a newborn's health status. In the 1990s, research suggested that even more tests of a newborn's health or health status in the first few months of life might prove useful.

Hearing

In March 1993 a panel of 15 experts assembled by the U.S. National Institutes of Health met to consider issues relating to hearing impairment in children. Hearing impairment needs early detection for two reasons: children who have difficulty hearing are often mistakenly thought to be mentally retarded, and hearing-impaired children often fall behind their abilities in school because of poor language skills. If the hearing difficulty is discovered early, educational steps can prevent the development of poor learning skills. Unless there is some specific reason to suspect deafness however, most hearing problems in children are not detected until the child is about three years old.

The panel recommended that a newly developed hearing test be used for all children before the newborn leaves the hospital. The idea behind the test is to look for inducted otoacoustic emissions in the inner ear. These are small sounds the normal ear produces by itself, which can be heard with a tiny microphone inserted into the ear. Children who fail to produce the sounds have impaired hearing. Although children can have hearing impairments from other causes not detected by this test, most would be expected to be caught. If the test shows a problem, the panel recommended further checking by scanning the brainstem, similar in principle to an electroencephalogram but focused directly on the auditory nerves and parts of the brain involved in hearing.

Sight

Since 1975 researchers from the Massachusetts Institute of Technology (MIT) have been tracking vision in a group of hundreds of children. Although when the study began, physicians believed that myopia (nearsightedness, or the inability to focus on objects unless they are close to the eyes) did not begin until later in life, the MIT study found that many children tested with a retinoscope turned out to be myopic very early in life. As infants grew older, up to about the age of six, myopia diminished. After six the children who had been found with myopia as infants were most likely to redevelop the condition. Based upon their analysis, the MIT researchers recommended in April 1993 that all infants be tested for myopia early, preferably between 6 months and a year.

Another vision problem called amblyopia, or lazy eye, which is double vision that results from one eye looking off in its own direction, can be prevented if detected early. The brain compensates by shutting down the offending eye, contributing to what may even develop into legal blindness. A computerized test can detect amblyopia even in very young children and the condition can usually be prevented by simply wearing a patch over the wandering eye until development of the brain and muscles deal with the problem.

Background

Myopia is at least partly hereditary. If both parents are myopic, 42 percent of their children are as well, but only eight percent of children from parents of whom neither are myopic develop the condition. Thus the potential of myopia can be predicted to a large extent without testing. Furthermore, there is no generally accepted treatment for young children that would prevent myopia from developing. Surgery has been known to cure myopia in adults, although this remains somewhat controversial. Exercises are sometimes prescribed but also are not generally accepted as effective.

(Periodical References and Additional Reading: *New York Times* 3-10-93, p C12; *Science News* 5-1-93, p 277)

MILK, MOTHERS, AND FORMULA

The defining characteristic of a mammal is the production of fluid food for offspring in special glands of the mother, the food we call milk. Although nature clearly intended humans under the age of about two to subsist on the human version of this fluid, that is often not the practice. Instead, both in industrialized and developing nations, a large percentage of all children are fed some alternative fluid. This fluid may be enriched cow's milk, milk from some other nonhuman mammal, milk based on proteins in plants, or even a totally artificial substance. Nearly all such substitutes for breast-feeding in the U.S., however, use either cow's milk or a soybean product called soy milk as a base.

Perhaps because nearly all of the first such substitutes for mother's milk were mixed into water (most today are premixed), the substitutes have come to be called by the generic name *formula*. This perhaps suggests the old advertising slogan "better living though chemistry." On the other hand, many critics in the 1990s have proposed that something may be wrong with this whole picture or at least some parts of it. The critics for the most part call for reductions in the use of formula and increases, for one reason or another, in the use of mother's milk. Among the reasons put forth are properties of mother's milk such as antibodies which are passed on to the children. Of course, formula manufacturers can point to toxins such as alcohol or drugs that may also be passed from mother to infant along with the milk.

Formula manufacturers have been accused of using many underhanded devices to sell their products in the U.S. and in developing nations. For example, it appears that leading formula manufacturers have for years paid one of the leading medical societies large sums of money so that the society would oppose advertising of formula. The motive apparently was that the ties between the manufacturers and individual doctors were considered to be the best way to sell formula, and advertising might allow new companies to enter the field. In 1992 the three leading infant formula manufacturers were charged with illegal overpricing by the U.S. Federal Trade Commission, and two of the three settled out of court immediately.

A more direct example, involving the Mead Johnson subsidiary of Bristol-Myers Squibb Corporation, one of the leaders in the field, is the case of Ricelyte, a supplement to formula used for treating infant diarrhea, which was introduced by Mead Johnson in October 1990. Rice water has long been a folk remedy for infant diarrhea. Ricelyte was promoted as rice based, but a federal court ordered the promotion to be stopped and also the name to be changed. It seems that Ricelyte has nothing to do with rice at all.

Breast-Feeding

In the period before the 1990s, the trend away from breast-feeding and toward use of formula had been up and down in the U.S. Breast-feeding increased from 34 percent of all women a week after leaving the hospital in 1951 to 61 percent of all mothers in 1982, and then declined somewhat to 53 percent in 1992. Surveys showed that breast-feeding was much higher among better educated, higher income, older women: about 70 percent of such women breast-fed while they were still in the hospital, although what happened later is not known. Yet in 1990 sales of infant formula in the U.S. were greater than $1.6 billion.

Breast-feeding not only affects the baby's health, but it also has profound effects on the mother. Commonly, for example, many women stop menstruating while breast-feeding and therefore enjoy natural birth control and spacing of children, but physicians warn that one should not count on breast feeding for true birth control. A study reported in the June 23/30, 1993 *Journal of the American Medical Association* shows that breast-feeding mothers lose some bone mass during the first six months of the process but gain it back during the next six months. If the baby was weaned before the age of nine months, the mother's bone density returned to its original state a year after the baby's birth. There was some concern by the study's investigators that mothers on an inadequate diet—which was not true of any of the women in the study group—might not regain the lost bone and thus be more likely to experience fractures later in life.

Choosing *not* to breast-feed also affects the mother's health in many cases, for the breasts produce milk that has no place to go, resulting in a swelling known as engorgement. Often medicines are prescribed to prevent engorgement. One such medicine, bromocriptine mesylate (trade name Parlodel), was determined to be of no benefit as early as 1989, but it continued to be used. Finally on September 3, 1993 the U.S. Food and Drug Administration announced that it would take steps to remove breast engorgement from the list of conditions that could be treated with bromocriptine.

Colic and Cow's Milk

Physicians have suspected for many years that the condition known as colic—a pattern of irritability in children between two weeks and three or four months old that includes a lot of unpleasant high-pitched crying, some spitting up of food, and often apparent muscle spasms in the abdomen—is caused by something in cow's milk. Despite this suspicion, colic is just as common in nursing children as in those using a cow's milk formula. In April 1991 Patrick S. Cline of St. Louis Children's Hospital in Missouri and Anthony Kulszycki, Jr. of Washington University in St. Louis, Missouri, announced in *Pediatrics* that they had solved the riddle. They found that certain antibodies found in cow's milk make their way into mother's milk when the mother consumes dairy products. Although not everyone agrees this is the final explanation of colic, mothers whose children suffer from the problem might try avoiding dairy products while nursing. If the theory is correct, the colic should go away after ten days or so of the mother's dairy-free diet. Of course, babies on formula, according to the theory, should be switched from cow's milk to a soy-based formula, which is already a common recommendation of pediatricians.

Experts also levelled a more serious charge against cow's milk in 1992—the charge that it could trigger Type I (juvenile, or insulin dependent) diabetes. Although preliminary studies suggest a connection, results of large-scale studies will not be available until the late 1990s. In the meantime, breast milk might be the best choice if there is any suspicion of Type I diabetes in the genetic profile of an infant. So far, breast milk is generally safer than any of the alternatives in any case, although sometimes environmental factors can even pollute mother's milk.

(Periodical References and Additional Reading: *New York Times* 3-30-91; *New York Times* 6-12-92, p A1; *New York Times* 7-30-92, pp A10 or A12; *New York Times* 8-2-92, p D4; SN 6-26-93, p 407; *New York Times* 6-15-93, p D1; *New York Times* 7-14-93, p C12; *New York Times* 9-3-93, p A10; *New York Times* 10-10-93, p IV-6)

SIDS UPDATE

SIDS means Sudden Infant Death Syndrome. Before most parents in the U.S. learned to call it SIDS, a popular name for it was "crib death." SIDS is the name used by physicians when a previously healthy infant only several months old is found dead with no signs of any kind as to the cause of death. Although the cause is still not known, there are some hypotheses and some recommendations that seem to aid in reducing the incidence of the syndrome.

One suspicious circumstance has to do with the material from which the "crib" mattress is built. In Tasmania, infants sleeping on soft, fluffy mattresses filled with substances such as kapok (which has long silky natural fibers) have 20 times the risk of SIDS as those who sleep on harder mattresses. Similarly, in the late 1980s, when bean-bag cushions for infants were introduced in the U.S., there was a rash of SIDS cases in which infants left to sleep on such cushions were found dead. In 1990 the bean-bag cushions were recalled by the U.S. Consumer Product Safety Commission because of the strong suspicion that babies were smothering themselves in the cushions. Studies using rabbits conducted by James F. Kemp and Bradley T. Thatch of Washington University in St. Louis, Missouri, and published in the June 27, 1991 *New England Journal of Medicine* showed that expelled air could be trapped in pockets in the cushions and then rebreathed. As the carbon dioxide levels in the air increased, the rabbits died. Kemp and Thatch concluded that suffocation also caused SIDS. The same may have happened with the fluffy Tasmanian mattresses.

At least 16 separate studies around the world have found that more infants who sleep on their stomachs die from SIDS. Lying on the stomach is called *prone*, while lying on the back is *supine*, although many people fail to make this distinction. As a result, campaigns to change the way parents put their children to bed have taken place in a number of countries in the 1990s. Results are now in for some of these campaigns, and the news is encouraging. In Australia the 1991 campaign lowered the SIDS rate from 3.6 per 1000 in 1981 to 1.7 per 1000 in 1991. A check in one Australian state also showed that the number of babies sleeping prone has declined from 33 percent to eight percent. A one-year campaign in Britain in 1991 halved the number of crib deaths. The American Academy of Pediatrics began to recommend the supine sleeping position in the U.S. in 1992.

Perhaps the latest study of SIDS is one conducted in Tasmania by Anne-Louise Ponsonby and coworkers and reported in the *New England Journal of Medicine* in August 1993. Their results included the risks of various factors when compared with a healthy infant sleeping supine and not wrapped in blankets (*swaddled*). They found that:

Background

If SIDS happened rarely, it would be no surprise; medicine has many unsolved mysteries. But in the U.S., SIDS is the leading cause of death in infants who are born healthy, accounting for one death in five of children carried to maturity and born without birth defects. (When all infants are considered, it strikes about one in a thousand.) Furthermore, there is a pattern to SIDS that suggests that most cases result from the same unknown cause; SIDS strikes more in winter, for example, and it is mysteriously higher in New Zealand and Tasmania. In general, however, it seems more common in places with cold climates, such as Scandinavia as well as Tasmania.

Suspicion that crib death is more than just any infant death with an unknown cause began in Norway in the middle of the nineteenth century. A hundred years later physicians had named it but still did not know the cause.

Changes in sleeping habits of infants have occurred in industrial countries. Early in Western culture, infants slept in the same bed with their mothers. Some authorities today still think that this was an ideal situation. But as people became wealthier and average people began to live in houses with several separate rooms, infants got their own beds and eventually in many households, their own rooms.

It seems most natural that an infant sleeping in the same bed with its mother would sleep on its back. But when the infant was moved to a separate bed, a choice had to be made. It is not clear at this time what that choice was originally. But starting in the 1960s, pediatricians recommended that babies too young to roll over by themselves be put in their cribs face down to sleep. This kind of recommendation occurred in most of the industrial world, but the cause for it has not been discovered. It is thought that the pediatricians had observed that premature babies breathed better on their stomachs and then extended this concept to full-term, healthy infants.

Depending upon the study, 28 to 52 percent of SIDS victims are found lying face down.

- three times as many infants who sleep prone without being swaddled die from SIDS;
- ten times as many of the prone infant victims have some disease, including respiratory distress, fever, vomiting, or diarrhea;
- twelve times as many die if they are both sleeping prone and swaddled;
- fifteen times as many of the prone victims are sleeping in rooms in which the temperature is higher than 57° F;
- twenty times as many died sleeping prone on soft mattresses made from natural materials (which perhaps could induce allergic reactions).

Although these risk factors have been documented, there are still many infants who sleep supine on hard mattresses and die from SIDS anyway. Thus the possible causes of those deaths remain elusive.

(Periodical References and Additional Reading: *Science News* 6-29-91, p 405; *New York Times* 8-10-93, p C3; *Science News* 12-4-93, p 380)

Autism UPDATE

For over fifty years, psychologists have recognized in some children a fairly common cluster of disorders that has come to be known as *autism*. Autism by today's standards occurs to some degree in one or two out of every thousand live births, about the same incidence as Down's syndrome. Its main symptoms were originally recognized as a preference for aloneness; a liking for sameness, including repeating certain elaborate routines; and often some remarkable ability that seems out of keeping with the rest of the autistic child's intellectual development. Today it might be more accurate to say that autism consists of difficulty in communicating, imagining, and socializing. Experts agree that Raymond, the character played by Dustin Hoffman in the movie *Rain Man*, is an excellent example of a person who has carried a typical autistic personality into adulthood.

Cognitive Basis of a Biological Disorder

In October 1991 Uta Firth of the Medical Research Council in London, United Kingdom, and coworkers John Morton and Alan M. Leslie put forth in *Trends in Neurosciences* a model for autism that locates a single underlying problem. Autistic children are unable to imagine what someone other than themselves is thinking.

A simple puppet show demonstrates how different autistic children are from other

Background

A total list of behaviors that have been termed autistic would include: absence of pretending, bizarre behavior, desire for routine, focus on a single topic, inappropriate giggling and laughter, indifference, lack of eye contact, lack of social play with other children, parroting words, spinning or handling objects, and using a adult's hand to show needs. Most children show some or all of such behaviors at one time or another; in autistic children, such behaviors are consistent or incessant and form a cluster.

As with most severe mental disorders in the twentieth century, informed opinion has gradually swung away from experiential explanations of the problem to biological ones. Today the cause of autism is thought to be damage to the brain, especially to the frontal lobes, perhaps as a result of an inherited condition. Twin studies and family studies show that autism has a genetic component: autism occurs in some families about a hundred times as much as in the general public. Although most workers in the field of autism think that there is a definite brain defect, the exact defect is yet to be found.

In addition to a genetic component, autism has been linked to several of the most common causes of birth defects: maternal rubella (German measles), chromosomal abnormalities similar to those that cause Down's syndrome, and physical injury to the brain. Furthermore, autism may also occur along with seizures or convulsions in infants. There is also some evidence linking autism and other mental disorders to viral infections of the mother other than rubella.

children with regard to following another person's train of thought. This test, originally invented by Austrian psychologists Heinz Wimmer and Josef Perner, is called the Sally-Anne task. A puppet, Sally, puts a marble in a basket and leaves the stage. Puppet Anne enters and moves the marble to a box. When Sally returns, she wants to get her marble back. The Sally-Anne task is to predict where Sally will look for the marble. While normal children predict that Sally will look in the basket where she left the marble, in one study, about 80 percent of autistic children will predict that Sally will look in the box. Firth, Morton, and Leslie claim the reason for the poor predictions of autistic children on this task is that they cannot picture in their own minds the state of Sally's mind. They don't see that Sally could believe something that is not true.

Similarly, in play situations, autistic children do not pretend that teddy bears are people or that dolls are babies.

(Periodical References and Additional Reading: *Scientific American* 6-93, p 108)

CHOLESTEROL, FAT, AND CHILDREN

Sometimes it is tempting to look at an overweight adult and to think that weight gain started with the parent's providing or allowing an improper diet when that adult was a child. Not only is this relationship problematic, but even the question of what is a proper diet for a child has not been completely answered. Although it is fairly certain that very young children need a substantial amount of fat, it is far more difficult to determine how young and how much fat. The same is true for cholesterol, which, although often thought of incorrectly as a fat, is actually a steroid.

Cholesterol

At the beginning of the 1990s, the trend toward lowering fat and cholesterol in children's diets was quite strong—perhaps because it seems easier to monitor your child's eating habits than your own. Then on December 19, 1990 Ronald M. Lauer of the University of Iowa published a report in the *Journal of the American Medical Association* in which he demonstrated that high cholesterol levels in children did not correlate with high cholesterol levels in the same individuals after they had become adults. Surprisingly few of even those children who were in the top ten percent of childhood cholesterol readings had high cholesterol as adults: 30 percent of the men and 57 percent of the women did not have high cholesterol levels. In an interview, Lauer noted that there were no studies linking children's cholesterol levels to heart disease, so there was no reason to be concerned about high cholesterol in children.

In 1990 as well a Canadian task force known as the Toronto Working Group determined that screening young adults for high cholesterol was unwarranted, a conclusion that Stephen B. Hulley of the University of California at San Francisco and coworkers also reached. Specifically, the Hulley reanalysis of previous studies showed no justification for cholesterol screening in men under the age of 35 or women younger than 45. Hulley himself told an interviewer that cholesterol reduction should not be a goal until middle age and that virtually no young adult should use drugs to lower cholesterol levels.

A few months after Lauer's original report on cholesterol levels in children, a U.S. government panel of the National Heart, Blood, and Lung Institute encouraged keeping the diet of children and teenagers three years old or older low in cholesterol. The Institute advocated that all members of the family except for infants should consume less than 300 milligrams of cholesterol daily. The chairman of the expert panel was the same Ronald M. Lauer, who at this time—April 8, 1991—said that "we should not miss the opportunity to prevent the disease from beginning in children." However, he called for no cholesterol testing of young children unless there was some indication of hereditary high cholesterol levels, such as a family history of heart disease. If followed, this advice could result in testing as many as 25 percent of all children, since heart disease is so widespread in the U.S. The panel did suggest testing for all young adults over the age of 20, however. Drugs for cholesterol reduction, according to the panel, should be used only in children ten years old or older and then only if diet changes fail to lower cholesterol levels.

Fat for Children

The same federal panel suggested limiting fat intake for children over the age of two in essentially the same proportions recommended for all adults: 30 percent of all calories of which only a third of the fat calories should come from saturated fat (*See* "Fat UPDATE," p 171). In September 1992 the American Academy of Pediatrics endorsed the same levels and also the suggestion that cholesterol intake be kept below 300 milligrams daily. Previously the Academy had recommended 30 to 40 percent fat in children's diets. But the Academy also recommended that fat consumption not fall much below the 30 percent level for children, since children need a certain amount of fat for proper growth and development. In fact, instead of suddenly quitting breast milk (which is 50 percent fat, mostly saturated) and going to the recommended low-fat level, the pediatricians suggested gradually tapering off after the age of two.

According to the Academy, fat consumption in American children during the early 1990s averaged about 35 percent of total calories with 14 to 15 percent coming from saturated fats. Cholesterol intake was normally below the recommended maximum of 300 milligrams daily.

Autopsy studies have shown that by an age of 15 to 20, about 14 percent of Americans already have plaque in their coronary arteries, the first stage of heart disease.

(Periodical References and Additional Reading: *New York Times* 12-19-90; *Science News* 4-13-91, p 229; *New York Times* 9-5-92, p 5; *New York Times* 3-17-93, p B8)

Growth UPDATE

Growth of children has always been of interest to parents, grandparents, and, of course, older children themselves. With the availability of human growth hormone from genetic engineering, the possibility of changing growth patterns has become a controversial issue. Some children thought to be short but not abnormal have been administered human growth hormone in the hopes of increasing their adult heights. The results of these experiments which are more often conducted outside the framework of scientific research are not known as yet. Furthermore there are frequent reports of people using human growth hormone for other purposes, such as to increase muscle mass. The effects of this practice have also yet to be fully studied, although most specialists on growth would oppose it.

Growth Spurts

Parents have long known that older children go through fairly brief periods of significant growth amid long periods of little change. In adolescence, a boy can grow from as little as 5 feet at age 13 to 6 feet 2 inches at age 14, a height that he will then maintain for years. Some parents have also noticed a similar pattern in even shorter time periods and rapid changes of infancy. One day baby's clothes suddenly don't fit. But when the same parents look in a book on infant growth and development or see a graph at their pediatrician's office, they find that growth of infants is described as continuous and illustrated with graphs of smooth curves or even straight lines.

Advice is even offered suggesting that parents should be alarmed if their infant goes through periods of little or no growth. Not to worry. Michelle Lampi of the University of Pennsylvania and Johannes D. Velduis and Michael L. Johnson of the University of Virginia made some careful measurements of infant growth, using 31 different healthy babies, three of whom were measured every day, while 18 were measured twice a week and ten weekly. Not only were periods of no growth as long as 63 days in the most extreme instance, but also growth spurts were commonly only 24 hours in duration. In other words, the babies that were measured every day would not grow at all for a time and then be found to have grown after the next measurement. Results of the study were published in the October 30, 1993 *Science*.

Careful steps were taken to eliminate errors in measurement (although not all the infants cooperated in the project). Daily jumps in the three infants measured every day took place 23 times, while five times there were growth spurts that lasted longer than a day. Total growth in a spurt ranged from half a centimeter (about a fifth of an inch) to 2.5 centimeters (1 inch) in length over periods that may have been as long as a week, although data from the three measured daily suggest that the growth probably occurred in one or two spurts of about half an inch each, which is the average for all the 31 children. In between spurts, the average periods of no growth measured from about 12 days in the infants measured daily to about 25 days in the infants measured once a week, suggesting that if all the infants had been measured daily, periods of no growth might run around 18 to 20 days.

Unpublished data from one of the authors also suggests that the pattern of no growth and spurts continues right through adolescence.

(Periodical References and Additional Reading: *New York Times* 10-30-92, p A12; *Science* 10-30-92, p 801)

Care of the Body

In the second half of the twentieth century, people gradually came to see that health was more than simply not being ill. People merged the concept of preventing illness or injury with the knowledge that it was also possible to feel better physically and mentally, beyond merely continuing existence. The new way of looking at health came to be called "wellness," and it included improvements in diet, physical activity for health, elimination of chemicals that interfere with health (drugs such as nicotine, alcohol, cocaine, and opiates, and so forth), better care of teeth and other parts of the body, etc.

A sign that the age of wellness was at hand in the U.S. came in November 1992 when the famed Centers for Disease Control in Atlanta, Georgia, changed its name, with the official sanction of the U.S. Congress, to the Centers for Disease Control *and Prevention*. Despite the new name, the agency continues to use the familiar acronym CDC.

Wellness is largely a self-help movement. Doctors may aid the movement by encouraging better care of the body; spas, gyms, or rehabilitation centers ("rehabs") may start people on the right track; and researchers may locate and publicize better diets or other practices. Nevertheless, the changes in life that improve wellness are carried out by the individual. The practice of wellness is therefore unlike Western medicine, which relies heavily on external intervention through drugs or surgery.

Although the new wellness awareness is about a quarter of a century old, many of its basic tenets concerning diet, exercise, and cleanliness can be traced back to the earliest thinkers about medicine.

Diet and Nutrition for Wellness

Among the oldest parts of wellness awareness is the need for a proper diet, but the definition of a good diet is constantly changing. In Woody Allen's movie *Sleeper* a health food store operator awakens in the future from a slumber to discover that in the future red meat is considered good for a person, just as it was in the not-so-long-ago past. What seems like a good diet to one age may indeed differ from the desirable diet of another for good reasons. For example, tribal peoples living north of the Arctic Circle may need amounts of fat that would cause heart attacks and contribute to diabetes among sedentary urban dwellers living in a temperate climate.

Despite the focus on reducing fat, sodium, and calories—which is a major part of wellness awareness—Americans continue to gain weight and die from heart disease at an alarming rate. The main reason is that concern about diet, universally expressed, fails to result in action. In 1993 in the U.S. about 25 million children were in school lunch programs, 27 million people used food stamps, and about ten million were in government hospitals or other government care programs. Thus, more than 60 million people could be affected by U.S. official views, including the dietary guidelines issued by the U.S. Department of Agriculture as early as 1980. Yet few of the persons in these programs were fed according to those guidelines.

One of the reasons for the current emphasis on a diet low in fat and high in fruits and vegetables is that many different research studies in the second half of the twentieth century have demonstrated that heart disease, diabetes, strokes, and probably cancer could to some degree be prevented by such diets. Although this information was for the most part obtained by medical doctors, the conclusions have not significantly affected medical education. Only 23 percent of U.S. medical schools require a course in nutrition; some of them do not even offer such a course.

A typical experience in some ways is that of Dean Ornish, a medical doctor who, like Nathan Pritikin did, came to suspect in the 1970s that a diet very low in fats combined with a lifestyle of reduced stress and regular exercise might reverse the course of heart disease. He also found out that the traditional sources of funds for research, including the American Heart Association and the U.S. National Institutes of Health (NIH), were not interested in supporting research based on such a "weird" idea. Ornish therefore found private funding and ran a small controlled study that showed his method reversed the narrowing of coronary arteries for nearly all of the 22 patients who followed his regime for several years. In his control group, however, more than half the people who did not change their lifestyle got worse, as their coronary arteries became narrower. Publication of this study in the *Lancet* and the changing climate of wellness awareness finally prompted the NIH to fund Ornish's research in 1990. The second three-year study, the results of which were announced in November, 1993, confirmed his initial findings.

Indeed, the Ornish results were sufficiently impressive that a half-dozen hospitals signed up with Ornish so that they could also institute the program, which calls for a 12-week training program for patients, including a two-day introduction and ten hours weekly of further instruction and help. For a patient, such a program costs about $5000, but compared with balloon angioplasty at about $18,000 or coronary artery bypass surgery at about $43,000, it is a bargain. Furthermore, at least one major insurer, Mutual of Omaha, agreed on July 27, 1993 to reimburse their subscribers for the Ornish program. Such official and semi-official recognition of a wellness approach could not have taken place before the 1990s, when wellness research finally came to light.

Diet trends are complicated and often overlap, but a simplified account of how attitudes toward the six major nutrients—proteins, carbohydrates, fats, vitamins, minerals, and water—have changed might run as follows: In the 1930s people were excited about the newly synthesized vitamins and knew that they needed more. The 1940s brought World War II and rationing, so nutrition concerns mainly focused on obtaining enough calories. The 1950s were dominated by the discovery that saturated fat was implicated in heart disease and that unsaturated fat (this was before the sophistication of polyunsaturated and monounsaturated) offered protection against clogging of the arteries. During the 1960s, the importance of protein became apparent, particularly in conjunction with the worry about obtaining essential amino acids—by balancing rice with beans, for example. In the 1970s, the idea of reducing carbohydrates became pivotal to various weight-loss schemes, such as the famous Scarsdale Diet. But in the 1980s all the talk was about increasing carbohydrates—not the simple ones marijuana smokers craved in the 1960s but the complex ones found in grains and vegetables. Then in the 1990s, thoughts turned to fat—not to ways to increase the amount, but instead to ways to choose fats carefully.

Regulation of Food in the U.S.

In the U.S. there was considerable official action concerning food during the early 1990s. Regulation of food had begun in earnest in the U.S. in 1906, spurred in large part by concerns about the meat packing industry raised by Upton Sinclair's novel *The Jungle* and particularly by U.S. President Teddy Roosevelt's experience with bad tinned beef during the Spanish-American War. The wave of regulation in the 1990s was a reaction to a combination of factors: a series of deaths from several unrelated food sources; continuing evidence that chemicals in food can prevent or cause certain chronic illnesses; and David A. Kessler, appointed by President Bush, the most aggressive Commissioner of the U.S. Food and Drug Administration (FDA) in many years. The U.S. Department of Agriculture (USDA) under the Clinton Administration also had a new leader in Mike Espy. Here is a brief list of actions; more details are in individual articles.

TIMETABLE OF FOOD REGULATION

December 2, 1992	U.S. announces that starting in May 1994 food labels on packaged foods will use specific definitions of "low-fat," "light," "less," "reduced," and "healthy." Labels also must list calories from fat; amounts of saturated fat, cholesterol, and dietary fiber; and recommended levels for two levels of consumption (with percentage of nutrients in the foods for total consumption of 2000 calories per day).
December 29, 1992	The FDA proposes rules for labeling bottled water and for guaranteeing its safety.
March 22, 1993	David A. Kessler announces that the FDA will develop a new and stricter method for inspecting fish and other seafood.
May 6, 1993	U.S. Department of Agriculture announces that it will require raw meat and poultry to be labeled with safe-cooking instructions; implementation of this plan is slowed by court challenges.
June 10, 1993	The FDA announces that restaurants, starting in February 1994, will be required to provide concrete information backing up any health claims on menus.
October 30, 1993	After food handlers file a lawsuit against initial rules announced in August 1993 and obtain an injunction, the USDA announces that new labels for meat and poultry will go into effect on April 15, 1994.
December 29, 1993	The FDA rules that, beginning in July 1994, sellers of diet supplements

will be required to limit health claims for diet supplements to those proven in scientific studies and vetted by the FDA.

Progress in the U.S.—or Lack Thereof

The best information about American wellness habits as a whole comes from a 1992 telephone survey of 91,428 adults conducted by the U.S. Centers for Disease Control and Prevention, which was not compiled and published in the *Morbidity and Mortality Weekly* until February 1994. The risk factors assessed were chosen because of their negative effects on heart disease. The factors included current cigarette smoking, physical inactivity, and obesity, all largely within the ability of otherwise healthy persons to control—although it is difficult to stop smoking and there is some question about whether or not certain individuals can control their weight with diet and exercise. The survey also included two factors that have a genetic component, but which can be controlled by medication if diet and exercise fail: these are high blood pressure and high blood cholesterol. Finally, the survey included diabetes as a risk factor, although most persons would identify it as a disease. Diabetes is a risk factor for heart disease, and it may in some cases be controlled or forestalled by diet, exercise, or medication. Diabetes is also a risk factor for many other diseases, including kidney failure, eye diseases, and circulatory problems other than heart disease.

When the factors listed above were considered as risks, the survey found that fewer than one in five, or 18 percent, of Americans live lives that are risk-free from a wellness point of view. People aged 50 to 64 were by far the most likely to fall into the higher-risk group, with only 9.4 percent of the men and 1.6 percent of the women having none of the cited risk factors. Above age 65, the wellness quotient rises to 9.2 percent for women and falls to 3.4 percent for men. Mortality may be a factor in these changes, since some of the higher-risk middle-aged people die before reaching age 65.

Geography was found to be a factor as well as age. People in Utah and Colorado, where there are high numbers of nonsmoking, nondrinking Mormons and a widespread outdoor lifestyle, have 26 percent of the survey population without the cited risk factors, which is eight percentage points higher than the national sample. South Dakota has the highest percentage of citizens who have at least one of the risk factors—90.6 percent.

While the incidence of some risk factors appeared to be decreasing over time, notably smoking and to a lesser extent high cholesterol, the number of sedentary Americans, which had been about 25 percent in 1987, was still the same, while the number of overweight Americans actually rose, from 26 percent to 28 percent.

Despite the relative stability of these risk factors, deaths from heart disease have dropped about 50 percent since 1970. The exact cause of this drop is still hotly debated (*see also* "Heart Disease and Strokes UPDATE," p 400).

Risk Reduction Strategies

In addition to changing diet to reduce risk from illness, which has been a major concern since the 1950s, there are many other risk reduction strategies that individuals can use to protect their health. Here are some of the other strategies that will help individuals in the early 1990s to care for their own bodies. Many of these will be dealt with in detail later in this chapter, and some have already been mentioned.

Stop Using Tobacco   Most authorities say that stopping smoking (or chewing or using snuff) is the single most important health step an individual can take, reducing the risks of cancer, heart disease, and various lung ailments all at once.

Start Using Your Body   Exercise in moderation can improve fitness; it is not necessary to run six miles a day. Although we tend to think of exercise primarily with respect to heart disease and weight loss, there is a body of evidence that suggests that other effects are also important. Some studies suggest that a sedentary lifestyle increases the risk for colon cancer by 50 percent, for example; a 1991 study of 17,148 Harvard alumni suggested that as little as 1000 calories per week of exercise would cut the risk of colon cancer in half, provided the exercise is continued year in and year out. Women who were athletes in college were shown to have substantially less cancer of the breast or reproductive system than the non-athletes did. Three large studies in 1992 showed that exercise protects against type II diabetes.

Protect Yourself Against Sunshine   Although people have relied on sunscreen compounds to protect against the cancer-causing rays of the sun for the past quarter century, melanoma, the most dangerous form of skin cancer, is still on the rise. One possibility is that even visible light at higher frequencies (toward the violet, away from the red) may cause melanoma, suggested by a study of specially bred fish reported in the July 15, 1993 *Proceedings of the National Academy of Sciences.* A broad-brimmed hat and loose clothing may be better protection when one has to be in the sun than any available sunscreen; staying in the shade when possible may be even better.

See Your Doctor Regularly   Visiting the doctor is a wellness step, since it is something a person does for himself or herself. Many of the most devastating diseases can be controlled better, or sometimes even prevented, when diagnosed early.

Expectations for the Future

Wellness is a particularly trendy part of health and medical science. Often a single report of a small study that shows a statistical connection between a health problem and a lifestyle practice results in extensive media coverage and changes in the behaviors of thousands of persons. Prediction of the future is therefore fraught with uncertainty. Nevertheless, some things are known now.

The 1994 *Diagnostic and Statistical Manual* of the American Psychiatric Association contains binge eating as a specific eating disorder for the first time. This is expected to result in increased insurance coverage for treatment of the disorder, which will no doubt lead to extensive recruiting by treatment centers wishing to be reimbursed.

A number of long-term studies will release their reports in the next few years. These may provide a much sounder basis for the use of antioxidant chemicals in prevention of disease (notably vitamins C and E, beta carotene, and selenium), although they may also show that earlier results are flawed. Similarly, the relationship between dietary fat and breast cancer should become more clear.

Fats are bound to be in the news one way or another. Since the 1950s doctors have found over and over that different fats have different effects. The fats formed by hydrogenating vegetable oils to make margarine (also used as an ingredient in many baked or packaged foods), called trans fats, appear to be the next ones to be fingered as a villain or hero—in this case, almost certainly in the villain role.

New food labels and changes in labels on diet supplements will come into effect. The new labels on packaged foods will tell a great deal more than the old ones did, labels on meat and poultry with health advice will appear for the first time ever, and unapproved claims in diet supplements will be eliminated. One can therefore expect more wellness-related reading in the next few years.

(Periodical References and Additional Reading: *Harvard Health Letter* 3-92, p 5; *Harvard Health Letter* 11-92, p 6; *New York Times* 11-3-92, p C8; *New York Times* 6-10-93, p A1; *Science News* 7-24-93, p 53; *New York Times* 7-28-93, p A1; *New York Times* 12-23-93, p A17; *New York Times* 12-28-93, p C4 *New York Times* 12-30-93, p A15; *Harvard Health Letter* 1-94, p 1; *New York Times* 2-9-94, p C13)

TIMETABLE OF WELLNESS AWARENESS TO 1990

24,000 BC	Pits dug at sites in the East European plain reveal the first unequivocal evidence of food storage over the winter; the same pits are apparently used during the summer for storage of such nonfood items as fuel and raw materials for manufacture of tools and jewelry.
13,000 BC	At Mezhirich in Ukraine, as at other sites from the same region and time, pits are dug into what was then permafrost and were used to store food, the first known form of cold storage.
8000 BC	Beer is brewed in Mesopotamia.
7000 BC	Sugar cane is being grown in New Guinea.
6000 BC	It is believed that wine-making may have started in northern Mesopotamia (now northern Iran and Iraq) or in the Levant.
3500 BC	Wine is known from around this time, as evidenced by residues found in a jar from Godin Tepe (present-day Iran), an outpost of the ancient city of Uruk (Iraq).
1500 BC	Bone inscriptions in China refer to the brewing of beer.
	Liquor is distilled in parts of Asia.
1000 BC	Several food preservation techniques exist in China: salting, use of spices, drying and smoking, and fermentation in wine (vinegar).
1070	Trotula of Salerno advocates cleanliness, a balanced diet, exercise and avoidance of stress for maintaining health in *Practica brevis* and *De compositione medicamentorum*.
1100	Italians learn to distill wine to make brandy.
1400	Coffee, which grows wild in Ethiopia, is made into a beverage there.
1503	Raw sugar is refined.
1527	Paracelsus's *Archidoxis* (not published until 1570) reports that frozen wine will have a higher proof than liquid left unfrozen.
1747	Andreas Marggraf [born Berlin, March 3, 1709; died Berlin, August 7, 1782] discovers sugar in beets, laying the foundation for Europe's sugar-beet industry.
1753	*Treatise on Scurvy* by James Lind [born Edinburgh, Scotland, October 4, 1716;

died Hampshire, England, July 13, 1794] establishes the curative effect of lemon juice on scurvy.

1765   Lazzaro Spallanzani [born Scandiano, Italy, January 12, 1729; died Pavia, Italy, February 11, 1799] suggests preserving food by sealing it in containers that do not permit air to penetrate.

1795   Napoleon offers a prize for a practical method of preserving foods, which is eventually won by Nicolas Appert, who introduces a sterilization process for food by bottling or canning, heating, and sealing in 1804 and wins the prize in 1809.

Physician Sir Gilbert Blane [born Blanefield, Scotland, August 29, 1749; died London, June 26, 1834] makes the use of lime juice to prevent scurvy mandatory in the British navy as proposed by James Lind; this is the origin of the nickname "limey" for the British sailor.

1796   Christoph W. Hufeland [born Langensalza, Germany, August 12, 1762; died Berlin, August 25, 1836] publishes *Macrobiotics, or The Art to Prolong One's Life*.

1802   The chemist Archard founds the first factory for manufacturing beet sugar.

1804   Nicolas Appert [born Châlons-sur-Marne, France, October 23, 1752; died Massay, France, June 3, 1841] invents canning foods as a means of preparation and opens the world's first canning factory; along the way, he also invents the bouillon cube.

1810   Nicolas Appert's *Le livre de tous les ménages, ou l'art de conserver pendant plusieurs années toutes les substances animales et végétales* (Art of Preserving Animal and Vegetable Substances for Several Years) explains heat sterilization of food.

1810   Pierre Durand patents food preservation in cans made of iron, but mysteriously fails to provide any way to open them.

1822   Anselme Payen [born Paris, January 6, 1795; died Paris, May 12, 1871] discovers that charcoal can be used to remove impurities from sugar.

1865   Karl von Voit shows that the pathways by which food is converted to energy are complicated; food is not merely burned to produce energy, but many intermediate reactions take place as well.

1870   Francesco Selmi claims that ptomaine (food poisoning) comes from spoiled or putrefying food.

1873   The Australian wool merchant T. S. Mort and the French engineer E. Nicolle build the first refrigeration plant for meat in Australia.

1880   The first refrigerated meat from Australia arrives in London aboard ships.

1881   Refrigerated railway cars are used in the United States for transporting meat from the slaughterhouses in Chicago and Kansas City.

1897   Christiaan Eijkman [born Nijkerk, Netherlands, August 11, 1858; died Utrecht, November 5, 1930] shows the relationship between the occurrence of beriberi and the consumption of polished rice. He does not attribute the disease to the absence of a vitamin in polished rice, however; the role of vitamins in preventing diseases will not be discovered until 1906.

C. W. Post introduces his first breakfast cereal, called "Grape Nuts," just as it is today, even though it contains neither grapes nor nuts. (Post erroneously thought that the manufacturing process resulted in grape sugar and that the cereal had a "nutty" taste.)

1898   The bacteria-killing effect of X rays are noted; however, no scientific work on preservation of food with radiation is pursued until the 1940s.

1901   Gerrit Grijns shows that beriberi is caused by the removal of a nutrient from rice during polishing.

Adolf Windaus [born Berlin, December 25, 1876; died Göttingen, July 9, 1959] shows that the molecule of vitamin D can be affected by sunlight.

1903   Ludwig Roselius, searching for a way to decaffeinate coffee, finds that coffee beans accidentally soaked in sea water can be used to produce 97 percent caffeine-free coffee with an acceptable flavor; he names his product "Sanka," for *sans caffeine*.

1904   C. W. Post calls his new brand of corn flakes "Elijah's Manna" at first, but finds that Christian clergymen oppose it under that name, so he renames the cereal "Post Toasties."

1906   Upton Sinclair's novel *The Jungle* reveals the problem of dangerous food contamination in the meat-packing industry, thus contributing to the passage of the U.S. Pure Food and Drug Act.

1912   Polish-American biochemist Casimir Funk [born Warsaw, February 23, 1884; died New York, November 20, 1967] coins the term "vitamin" for a class of substances that Frederick Hopkins had found to be important to health and which had previously been called accessory food factors.

1913   The first home refrigerator goes on sale in Chicago.

1915   Austrian-American physician Joseph Goldberger [born Girált, Austria-Hungary (now Giraltovce, Slovakia], July 16, 1874; died Washington D.C., January 17, 1929] establishes that a vitamin deficiency causes pellagra.

1918   Kelvinator launches a mechanical refrigerator for home use that is the first successful entry into the field.

1923   "Bob" Birdseye launches his first commercial venture in frozen foods in New York City, with the Birdseye Seafood Co., which goes bankrupt but leads the way to further and more successful operations and eventual merger into the newly formed General Foods in 1929.

1929   Christiaan Eijkman of the Netherlands and Sir Frederick G. Hopkins [born Eastbourne, Sussex, June 20, 1861; died Cambridge, May 16, 1947] win the Nobel Prize for Physiology or Medicine for their work with vitamins.

1930   The Postum Company begins marketing frozen foods for the first time.

1934   Freeze-dried coffee is manufactured in Switzerland.

R. Minot, William P. Murphy [born Stoughton, Wisconsin, February 6, 1892], and George H. Whipple [born Ashland, New Hampshire, August 28, 1878; died Rochester, New York, February 1, 1976] of the United States win the Nobel Prize for Physiology or Medicine for the discovery and development of liver treatment for anemia.

1936   Vitamin E is isolated.

1937   Vitamin K is isolated.

1937   Vitamin B_1 is synthesized as the chemical thiamin.

1938 The Food, Drug and Cosmetic Act of 1938 becomes law in the U.S., leading to establishment of the U.S. Food and Drug Administration.

Vitamin E is synthesized.

T. D. Spies, C. Cooper, and M. A. Blankenhorn demonstrate that pellagra is a vitamin-deficiency disease and that it can be successfully treated with nicotinic acid; they recognize, however, that other B-vitamin shortages may also be involved, such as thiamin (vitamin B_1).

1939 The first precooked frozen foods are marketed under the Birds Eye label.

1940 Freeze drying, developed earlier for medicines, is used for food preservation for the first time in the United States.

1941 Freeze-dried orange juice is supplied to the American army.

Folacin, a B vitamin (also known as folic acid), is discovered.

1946 In response to research that showed many children do not obtain enough energy from food, the first national school lunch program is established in the United States.

The chemical structure of folic acid is unraveled, identifying it as a B vitamin.

1948 A group at Merck & Company headed by Karl August Folkers [born Decatur, Illinois, September 1, 1906] discovers that certain bacteria require vitamin B_{12} for growth, enabling them to use the bacteria as indicators so that they can isolate the pure vitamin.

1950 The artificial sweetener cyclamate is introduced.

1953 The first of the numerous reports linking heart disease to saturated fats and prevention of atherosclerosis to unsaturated fats is published.

1955 The chemical structure of vitamin B_{12} is determined.

Deep freezers capable of preserving fresh food go on sale in the United States.

1957 Selenium is found to be necessary for human health.

1961 The nondairy coffee "creamer" is introduced.

1965 The artificial sweetener aspartame, eventually marketed as Nutrasweet in the U.S., is invented at the Searle Laboratory in the U.S.

1967 The National Academy of Sciences reports in June that the practice of adding antibiotics to animal food produces greater yields, but may leave traces in meat and also may increase drug resistance in bacteria.

The U.S. Department of Agriculture starts a test project in irradiating wheat and other foods to kill insects.

1968 The Nuclear Materials Equipment Corporation begins sterilizing bacon and potatoes with radiation from radioactive cobalt-60 as a means of preservation.

In April, James L. Goddard, commissioner of the U.S. Food and Drug Administration, refuses to permit the use of radioactively sterilized canned ham for human consumption in the U.S. Army.

1974 In the U.S., iron is now added to all enriched flours to help prevent iron-deficiency anemia.

1981 Aspartame, an artificial sweetener, is introduced in the United States.

1983 Aspartame is approved for use as an artificial sweetener in soft drinks.

EATING AND HEALTH

WEIGHT AND HEALTH

Many doctors routinely weigh patients, even when the appointment is for a muscle pull or a sore throat. The reason for this practice is that changes in weight are among the best indicators of health. Furthermore, obesity is statistically connected to numerous health disorders, including diabetes and heart disease, while low weight may point to a variety of diseases, ranging from cancer to clinical depression, not to mention AIDS.

A study by Harvard and Stanford Universities found that a stable weight is the most healthy weight. Gains or losses exceeding 1 kilogram (2.2 pounds) in the 11,703 Harvard graduates studied predisposed them to higher death rates. The highest death rates in the study, published in the *Journal of the American Medical Association* in October, 1992, were associated with gains or losses of more than 5 kilograms (11 pounds). Other studies in the past have shown that weights much higher or lower than the norm are both associated with higher death rates.

Earlier studies showed that the consequences of weight-fluctuation could be even more dramatic. On June 27, 1991 Kelly D. Brownell of Yale University in New Haven, Connecticut, used data from the ongoing Framingham Heart Study in Massachusetts to determine the results of frequent weight change. She found that over a 14-year period the risk of heart disease or death from any cause as a result of weight changes in the 3130 men and women studied was 25 to 100 percent higher than for those who maintained a stable weight.

Americans Gain Weight

Working out and aerobic exercise are still in vogue; television and radio advertisements promise significant weight loss; advice in newspapers and magazines tells how to lower the amount of fat in the daily diet; and nonfat yogurt, diet soft drinks, sugar substitutes, reduced fat margarine, and light beer are popular. On the basis of such indicators, one could conclude that in the past few years the average American has slimmed. Certainly one would expect the health-conscious new generation have heeded all the advice and taken the opportunities to achieve both good health through weight loss.

No such thing has happened.

Instead, as separate studies have shown, Americans of all ages, including Generation X (ages 25 to 30 in 1992-93), are gaining weight. Diane Bild of the National Institutes of Health, Cora E. Lewis of the University of Alabama in Birmingham, and coworkers analyzed the Generation X situation, and Lewis reported the results to the American Heart Association on March 17, 1994. According to her findings, the Generation X group studied weighed ten pounds more than a similarly aged group she examined in 1985-86. The earlier average was 161 pounds and the later was 171 pounds. According to guidelines issued in 1990 by the U.S. government, acceptable weights for persons in the age group from 25 to 30 could range from a low of 97 pounds (for the smallest persons 5 feet tall) to a high of 216 pounds (for the heaviest acceptable person 6 feet 6 inches tall). The median in this table, which might be considered by some criteria as an "ideal" weight for the age group, is 149 pounds for a person 5 feet 9 inches tall. Thus, the study found the average young person about 12 pounds (or about eight percent) overweight in the mid 1980s and about 22 pounds (almost 15 percent) overweight in the early 1990s. Most authorities define obesity as beginning at 20 percent over the desirable weight.

A total of 5,115 persons in four cities were included in the group, divided into approximately equal groups by sex and race.

	Black Men	White Men	Black Women	White Women
1985-86	174.2	171.1	158.5	140.6
1992-93	185.8	181.9	166.2	150.8

The gain of approximately ten pounds during this period was effectively the same across all the groups, with black men gaining slightly more and black women somewhat less.

The study also measured cholesterol levels, which dropped 9 points, suggesting that although the study participants were gaining weight, they might also be watching their diet in ways that contributed to a reduction in saturated fat, the main cause of high cholesterol levels in most people. A separate study reported early in 1994 by the Centers for Disease Control and Prevention found that Americans in general are consuming more calories, but smaller amounts of both cholesterol and saturated fat. Cora Lewis thinks that at least some of the weight gain is more the result of poor exercise habits than poor eating habits, however.

Almost All Weight Back after Five Years

In 1992 a panel of the U.S. National Institutes of Health found that 90 to 95 percent of dieters regain all or almost all the weight they lost within five years. The research focused on various commercial or self-help weight-loss programs and materials, including liquid diets and over-the-counter appetite suppressants.

Appetite Suppressants Actually Work

For the most part, specialists have been skeptical of the efficiency of diet drugs for long-term weight loss. Consequently, there was considerable surprise when a federally funded study released in July 1992 in *Clinical Pharmacology and Therapeutics* showed in a blind study of 121 obese patients that a combination of prescription drugs not only reduced weights by an average of 30 pounds, but also maintained the weight loss for as long as the patients kept taking the drugs. On the average, participants using the drug combination lost about 15 percent of their weight. The drugs involved previously had been prescribed as appetite suppressants for short terms only.

The study participants were also given diet counseling, exercise programs, and behavior modification training, as were the control group members, who received a placebo instead of an actual hunger suppressant. Significantly, people in the control group lost only about ten pounds on average. In addition, at the end of 34 weeks, the placebo users were heading back toward their original weight, while the suppressant patients maintained relatively consistent lower weights. Furthermore, when the groups switched, the new suppressant users lost weight and the former suppressant patients began to gain back lost weight. At the end, all patients in the study stopped taking any drugs and almost all of them returned to their original weights. Six participants in the study failed to lose weight even when taking the drug combination for years.

The entire study took several years, instead of the several weeks more common in such studies. Some people in the study took drugs for three and a half years. The research was conducted by Michael Weintraub of the University of Rochester School of Medicine.

Although the two drugs used in combination in the study (fenfluramine and phentermine) are both called appetite suppressors, their mechanisms and side effects are completely different. Fenfluramine works somewhat like the popular antidepressant Prozac, by stimulating production of the neurotransmitter serotonin in the brain. It not only makes people eat less, but also reduces the speed at which they eat. Phentermine, a common ingredient in various prescription appetite suppressants, works somewhat like an amphetamine, making the neurotransmitters dopamine and norepinephrine more available to brain cells. Like amphetamines, sometimes also used for weight loss, phentermine not only reduces the amount people eat, but also causes them to eat (and do everything else) faster. Both drugs are chemically closely related to amphetamines and have been prescribed for years for short-term weight loss. In the study, lower doses of both drugs were given than is usually prescribed when one of them is used alone.

Phentermine is not recommended for people with high blood pressure, one of the conditions necessitating weight reduction. Doctors conducting the study hoped to be able to use the drugs with patients who had high blood pressure, as well as with those who had other diseases that respond positively to weight loss, including various forms of arthritis and diabetes. Both drugs used together can cause dry mouth, diarrhea, or jitteriness, however.

Start Weight Reduction Early

A study directed by Aviva Must of the Human Nutrition Research Center on Aging of Tufts University in Boston, Massachusetts, and published in the November 5, 1992 issue of the *New England Journal of Medicine* showed that heavier teenage boys died before the age of 70 at a twice higher rate boys whose weight was somewhat below the midpoint of desirable weights. For girls, although the death rate did not increase before they reached their 70s, the heavier ones as teenagers had eight times as many problems with simple physical activities, such as walking or lifting.

The men who had been heavier and who died before the age of 70 had experienced fatal heart attacks, strokes, colon cancer, or other health problems. In addition to diminished physical abilities, the women who had been heavier ran a greater risk of arthritis or atherosclerosis.

The population studied was taken from the Third Harvard Growth Study, which began in 1922 with more than 3000 students in first and second grade and then followed their physical growth until 1935. Only participants with at least eight consecutive years of data were used, and after selection and tracing, 508 individuals, 161 of whom died before 1988, were included in the final statistics.

As noted above, people were more active in the 1920s and 1930s than they are today, which resulted in lower weights. The half the participants that were counted in this study as heavy were in the upper 25 percent of relative weights based on today's relative-weight scales. Although only the top 15 percent of the relative-weight scale is considered obese, the study needed to reach farther to get enough participants to make the statistics meaningful.

These heavy participants were paired with a group that was not the slimmest, but that was in the 25 percent just below the middle of the scale. Some studies have shown that lower-than-normal weights can also raise death rates, but people in that category were not included in the study.

Possible Inability to Lose Weight

An honest effort to reduce calories may not accomplish the goal for another reason. National brands are usually honest about labeling the calorie content in packaged foods (although sizes of a "serving" can be unrealistic). According to a study in the December 31, 1992 issue of the *New England Journal of Medicine*, however, regional or local brands average 85 percent more calories per serving than the amount stated on the labels.

But people should know what will make them fat and thus can stay away from that sort of food without ever looking at the labels. Animal studies show that craving for fats or carbohydrates are caused by chemicals in the brain, chemicals whose levels in later life are often determined at very early stages. This is what Sarah F. Leibowitz of Rockefeller University reported to the Society for Neuroscience in November 1993. The rats she worked with were compelled to eat either carbohydrates or fats depending upon preferences that were first expressed as early as the rats were weaned. (Other investigators tend to think the situation is more complicated, even in rats.)

A study by Valerie George and coworkers at Laval University in Quebec, Canada, reported in the February 1991 *American Journal of Clinical Nutrition* compared 40 women who consumed an average of 2400 calories a day with 50 who consumed an average of 1500 calories a day. The group eating less weighed about ten pounds more than the group eating more despite identical amounts of carefully monitored exercise. The additional pounds on the women who ate less were mainly caused by body fat.

(Periodical References and Additional Reading: *Harvard Health Letter* 5-91, p 7; *New York Times* 6-27-91; *New York Times* 7-5-92, p I-12; *Science News* 10-9-93, p 235; *New York Times* 10-21-92, p C12; *New York Times* 11-5-92, p A27; *Science News* 11-13-93, p 310; *New York Times* 3-18-94, p A17;)

DIET SUPPLEMENTS UNDER FIRE

Every day about 60 million people in the U.S. take some form of diet supplement, ranging from vitamins and minerals in pills to herbs and amino acids in one form or another. Most people think that even if these pills and nostrums do not work, they cause no harm. But late in 1989 and early 1990 a food supplement, L-tryptophan (one of the amino acids), was implicated in 38 deaths and about 1500 cases of a painful muscle disorder. After that experience, considerably more attention was paid to the possibility that supplements might need regulation.

Diet supplements escaped regulation by the U.S. Food and Drug Administration (FDA) because most of them consist of extracts of ordinary foods. The FDA does not regulate garlic, so it also does not regulate garlic pills, according to the thinking prevalent at the start of the 1990s. Earlier attempts by the FDA to regulate supplements in the 1960s and 1970s failed.

When the U.S. Congress passed the Nutrition Labeling and Education Act in 1992, it included a requirement for labeling food supplements, which had previously been unregulated as to safety, nutritional content, and health claims. The health food industry reacted against the labeling with dramatic advertisements on television, displays in health food store windows, and what amounted to a national day of mourning. The FDA brought some of this on themselves by a raid on the Tahoma Clinic in Kent, Washington, on May 6, 1992, to confiscate what they said were illegal vitamins and minerals that were being injected into patients. Because a local sheriff involved in the raid drew a gun, there were widespread reports that FDA agents made armed raids. A patient videotaped the raid, and the tape became part of the campaign against the FDA. The FDA has always claimed that the raid concerned the sterility and safety of the products used in the clinic.

Other anti-FDA stories claimed that the FDA planned to outlaw high-potency vitamins if the size of individual pills exceeded recommended daily allowances. Other rumors or accounts suggested that the FDA planned to fine distributors or to prevent vitamin and mineral supplements from entering the U.S. While these reports were not true, they were given widespread publicity, not only by health food distributors, but also by regular news sources.

Despite all the commotion, when FDA regulation of diet supplements began early in 1994, the rules were much milder than what the rhetoric on either side had suggested in 1992, when the FDA supporters in Congress were proposing legislation to empower the agency and the health food industry was claiming that stores would no longer be able to sell any supplements.

Nutritional Need vs. Other Powers

Although nutritionists may emphasize different food choices as science learns more about the relationship between nutrition and disease, they generally agree that whatever is needed to prevent or help cure disease should come from a proper diet. The opposing point of view has been voiced largely by people promoting a particular diet supplement or by people in the health food industry. ("Health food" refers primarily to materials sold by stores that emphasize specific food ingredients and diet supplements.)

Food and diet supplement benefits that have been proven in controlled, double-blind studies concern chemicals that, if missing from the diet, result in conditions such as pellagra, beri-beri, rickets, scurvy, and so forth. No one disputes the need to have these chemicals present in the diet in sufficient amounts and the virtue of providing the chemicals as supplements when for some reason they are or have been lacking in a person's diet. The argument is over adding specific chemicals beyond the amount known to be needed to prevent diet-deficiency diseases in the hopes of (1) preventing diseases not shown to result from diet deficiency or (2) curing such diseases when already present.

On July 29, 1993, David Kessler, Commissioner of the FDA, reported to the U.S. House Commerce Committee that they had identified 500 diet supplements that claimed to treat such diseases as bacterial infection or cancer, or to have unproven effects such as lowering blood pressure or improving the immune system.

The business of making claims has been complicated in the past by manufacturers of diet supplements who correctly believed that any warning labels on a supplement would bring on regulation of the supplement as a drug. Thus, various preparations that claim to increase energy and produce weight loss contain a powerful herb, known in supplement circles by its Chinese name of *ma huang,* but more familiar to botanists as the genus *Ephedra*. *Ephedra* is the original source of the drug ephedrine, used for treating asthma, blocking allergic shock, and restarting a heart that has stopped. In many ways the effects of ephedrine are similar to those of amphetamines, which ephedrine chemically resembles. Diet supplements based on *ma huang* are thus sold for increasing energy or weight reduction, the same powers for which amphetamines were used before their destructive side effects became better known.

One side effect common to both ephedrine and amphetamines is chemically induced psychosis. On May 27, 1993, for example, a bank manager who had been taking a diet supplement for weight loss and increased energy was admitted to an emergency room in Redmond, Washington, with psychotic symptoms. Three days after stopped taking the diet supplement, which contained *Ephedra,* however, he returned to normal. There are many herbal diet supplements on the market that contain *Ephedra,* but none so far have been labeled with any warning stronger than "Keep away from children."

Even a diet supplement believed by the FDA to be useful may need regulation. A report in the August, 1994, issue of *American Journal of Health* on 70 different calcium supplements available in health food stores found that nearly a quarter of them contain harmful amounts of lead.

Health Claims Limited

At the end of 1993 the FDA, after a more than six months of consideration, announced that it would, beginning in July 1994, require sellers to limit health claims for diet supplements to those that the FDA deemed to have been proven. At that time, December 29, 1993, the FDA added folic acid (folacin) to the extremely short list of supplements permitted to make claims, bringing the list to two. (Calcium to ward off osteoporosis had previously been endorsed by the agency.) Some public advocates for better regulation claim that health food stores contain hundreds of products whose manufacturers make claims that cannot be substantiated.

(Periodical References and Additional Reading: *New York Times* 8-9-92, p A1; *Harvard Health Letter* 11-92, p 4; *New York Times* 6-15-93, p A25; *New York Times* 7-30-93, p A17; *New York Times* 12-30-93, p A15)

TEA AND OTHER "MAGIC" FOODS

Since earliest known times humans have looked to foods for magic, to protect against evil spirits, to improve chances for love, and to impart such qualities as courage. Although this impulse has often been overcome by rational and scientific thought, people still look for magic foods. Before biochemistry, the "scientific" magic foods were often supported on a basis of analogies or anecdotes that were not necessarily more scientific than the herbs prescribed by traditional healers and shamans. A typical line of thought might be as follows: Yogurt is good for you because people in the Caucasus Mountains who ate yogurt regularly lived to be hundreds of years old; and in any case, yogurt contains active cultures of good bacteria that will overwhelm bad bacteria in your digestive tract. Similar claims, with rationales different in detail, were made for blackstrap molasses, wheat germ, brown rice, and other magic foods.

In view of modern biochemistry, magic foods are expected to have a magic ingredient—although attention is often first called to the food by population studies, the equivalent of anecdotes in the modern day. In the early 1990s, for example, there was a flurry of interest in tea. Tea is exceptionally high in flavonoids, thought to be "magic" chemicals.

Flavonoids were first brought to most people's attention as a possible explanation for why the population of France, where people eat rich food and drink wine, is not plagued with heart disease to a greater extent. Something in wine, especially red wine, seemed to be at least part of the cause of a relatively low rate of heart disease in France—a June 1992 study compared the population of Toulouse, France, with 89 deaths per 100,000 from heart disease, to that of Stanford, California, which has 230. For a brief period in November, 1992, the Beringer Vineyards even had a "neck hanger" on its red wines, permitted by the U.S. Bureau of Alcohol, Tobacco and Firearms, proclaiming its health benefits, but the U.S. Federal Trade Commission and the Food and Drug Administration then interfered and spoiled the promotion.

The ingredient in red wine that caused whatever benefits there were could not be the alcohol, since any magic protection from wine failed to extend to people drinking vodka or beer. Flavonoids, known to be present in red wine, were perhaps the protective agent. But flavonoids are found in many different foods, and are especially high in tea, apples, and onions. So a look at tea was in order.

In Norway, in 1992, a large study reported that fewer deaths from several causes, and not just fewer heart attacks, were found among the people studied who drank tea.

In the Netherlands, Michael Hertog and coworkers of the National Institute of Public Health surveyed a population of 805 elderly males (reported in the October 23, 1993, *Lancet*). The scientists counted the heart attacks and the amount of flavonoids that the men consumed. The 805 were grouped by the amount of flavonoids presumed to be obtained from apples (13 percent of the flavonoids), onions (10 percent), and tea (63 percent). The group with the highest intake of flavonoids had about half as many heart attacks as the group with the lowest consumption of the chemicals. Other risk factors, such as high blood pressure or cholesterol, smoking, and obesity were balanced out between groups.

The Dutch study involved flavonoids from all sources. An apple has about as many flavonoids as 4 cups of tea, although the particular flavonoids are not the same.

A two-day conference in 1991 on the health effects of tea, which was supported in part by tea manufacturers associations, focused on a different group of chemicals in tea, polyphenols, which are the main ingredient in tea. One group of polyphenols, catechins, seemed to reduce cancer in animal studies. Chinese researchers have shown that tea itself can reduce experimental cancer in rats. Green tea is thought by some to account for low cancer rates in Japan, where it is the favorite drink.

In Britain, which is still the leading Western tea-drinking nation despite a rise in coffee-drinking in recent years, heart disease rates are among the world's highest, and cancer is rampant as well. It is thought that other factors in British life undermine the benefits of tea.

(Periodical References and Additional Reading: *New York Times* 3-14-91; *Science News* 10-30-93, p 278; *New York Times* 11-11-92, p D3; *Discover* 1-93, p 46; *New York Times* 10-26-93, p C6)

NEW FOOD CHART AND LABELS

Some people in the U.S. may remember the seven basic food groups of long ago. These included the following essentials for daily health: (1) dark green and yellow vegetables and fruits (e.g. apricots); (2) citrus fruits and salad vegetables (such as lettuce and tomatoes); (3) vegetables and fruits not previously mentioned; (4) milk and milk products; (5) meat, poultry, fish, dried legumes, and cheese (also in group 4); (6) bread, flour, and cereals; (7) butter or margarine (with butter also in group 4). Popular wisdom once held that to be well nourished, one needed a reasonable amount from each of the seven groups every day. No group was to be omitted. The U.S. Department of Agriculture (USDA) issued a diagram showing the seven groups on a wheel, similar to a pie chart.

Sometime in the 1960s educators realized that the group of seven was too complicated and even contradictory. The next generation had a simpler list to remember— the four basic food groups: (1) fruits and vegetables; (2) milk and milk products; (3) meat and meat substitutes, and (4) bread and cereals. These were shown on a simpler pie chart.

It is easy to see that the gang of four is simply the seven with the first three lumped together and the last one folded into milk or meat. As before, the healthy diet included a reasonable amount from each of the four, preferably at each meal.

The Food Guide Pyramid

In the spring of 1991 the Agriculture Department tried again. In an effort to modify U.S. eating habits, it introduced a new diagram, this time with four different groups that restored, in a modified form, the fats and oils group from the 1950s, but also combined the meat and milk groups from the old gang of four. The change in the groups was less noticeable than the change in format: the new grouping is shown as layers in a triangle, which the Agriculture Department called a pyramid, apparently mimicking the ecologists' use of "pyramid" to describe how the food chain (who eats whom) is broader at the base.

Group 4 from the previous list, breads and cereals, surfaced as the "grains and cereals" layer at the base of the pyramid. "Fruits and vegetables" became the next to the bottom layer. The newly combined "meat and dairy" group was above that in a layer that not only was less broad, but also less deep than either of the layers below it. Finally, the restored "fats and oils" group appeared as the tip of the pyramid. There was a clear aim to suggest that the diet should be based upon a lot of cereals and not include very much in the way of meat or fat.

In 1992, however, the "Eating Right Pyramid," somewhat modified, became the "Food Guide Pyramid" as well as the official USDA diet guideline—although many continue to call the chart the "Eating Right Pyramid." The aim of the pyramid image was to encourage people to eat six to 11 servings a day of grains, four or five of fruits and vegetables, and not very much in the way of meat or dairy products. The dairy and livestock industries, who had been the prime movers behind the development of the previous four-group pie chart, were incensed.

The August 1992 booklet from the USDA, *The Food Guide Pyramid,* broke the four tiers into six groups subdivided into 18 categories. The base, now called the bread, cereal, rice, and pasta group, is suggested for six to 11 servings each day. The second tier contains both a vegetable group (three to five servings) and a fruit group (two to four servings). Tier three is also divided into two groups, the milk, yogurt, and cheese group (two to three servings) and the meat, poultry, fish, dry beans, eggs, and nuts group (two to three servings). The top triangular tier is the fats, oils, and sweets group (use sparingly). The maximum number of servings are intended for persons with high-energy requirements, such as a large teenage boy. The minimum would be for someone with the opposite physical characteristics, such as a small elderly woman.

With the whole diet plan thus laid out, more critics than just the meat and dairy producers appeared. For example, critics pointed out that sweets (simple carbohydrates) and fats are not even in the same nutritional group (the six nutrients, chemically defined, are proteins, carbohydrates, fats, water, vitamins, and mineral). Makers of low-fat milk products, like nonfat yogurt, were unhappily lumped with suppliers of high-fat cheese. For other reasons, fats with possibly some health benefit, such as olive oil or fish oil, do not seem to belong in the apex with butter.

Another point of criticism was the concept of serving, which varied from the illogical (one and a half ounces of natural cheese, but two ounces of processed cheese) to the inadequate (a slice of bread). Meat servings were cut to two to three ounces, but an egg serving was still two eggs. Why was a serving of fruit only half a cup (less than a medium apple or orange when chopped into chunks) but more concentrated fruit juice allowed three quarters of a cup? Perhaps there would have been fewer questions if the USDA had used a neutral word, such as "unit," instead of serving. It might make some sense to say that a cup of cooked dry beans, four tablespoons of peanut butter, and a cup of raw leafy greens are each a unit. Even then, however, there would be problems, as the USDA guide makes no distinction between a cup of whole milk and one of skim milk

Furthermore, it was learned in 1993 that the General Accounting Office, the investigative arm of the U.S. Congress, had discovered that the official USDA guideline for nutrition in food, known as Handbook 8, had not followed the right rules for gathering and accepting data and that therefore the data in the book probably contained serious errors.

With the above caveats in mind, here is what the Pyramid people list as servings:

Grains: 1 slice bread; 1 ounce ready-to-eat cereal; 1/2 cup (4 fluid ounces) cooked cereal, cooked rice, or cooked pasta.

Vegetables: 1 cup raw leafy vegetables; 1/2 cup other vegetables, cooked or raw; 3/4 cup (6 fluid ounces) vegetable juice.

Fruits: 1 medium apple, banana, or orange; 1/2 cup chopped, cooked, or canned fruit; 3/4 cup (6 fluid ounces) of fruit juice.

Dairy: 1 cup milk or yogurt; 1 1/2 ounces of natural cheese; 2 ounces processed cheese.

Meats, dry beans, eggs, and nuts: 2 to 3 ounces of cooked meat, poultry, or fish; 1/2 cup cooked dry beans; 2 eggs; 4 to 6 ounces of peanut butter.

New Labels on Packaged Food

Starting in May 1994, eating according to Pyramid rules can also include some micro-management based upon the labeling requirements that took effect in 1994. Instead of trying to match mysterious servings from the Pyramid book, one can use the new labels to combine specific nutrients (and one non-nutrient) according to numerical guidelines. This is possible because the new labels not only assign a serving size and tell how many such servings are in the package (which earlier labels also did), but the labels also tell:

- the percent of calories derived from fat, widely suggested to be less than 30 percent (but set at less than ten percent in some heart-disease prevention diets);
- the number of grams of saturated fat, cholesterol, and dietary fiber;
- the percent for each nutrient that a serving supplies for a person on a 2000-calorie-a-day diet—for example, a meal listed with a percent value of 25 percent for saturated fat is getting a fourth of all that undesirable fat needed all day; while a listing of 10 percent for vitamin A suggests that only a tenth of the amount of that desirable nutrient is in a serving of the food.

The labels also give the levels by mass (milligrams and grams) suggested for fat, saturated fat, cholesterol, and sodium that would be considered too great a part of either a 2000- or a 2500-calorie diet, as well as the mass of carbohydrates and fiber that would be considered reasonable for such diets.

Finally each label tells how many calories are in a gram of fat, carbohydrates, or protein, numbers that the sort of person likely to read the new labels in detail probably knows already.

For the casual customer, there are some new aids as well. "Low fat," "less," and "reduced" have been defined strictly so that their use on labels will have a definite meaning. The actual definitions are fairly complicated. A "low fat" food cannot contain more than 3 grams of fat per serving and cannot be more than 6 percent fat by weight.

In 1993, the U.S. Department of Agriculture, with a set of new leaders appointed by the Clinton Administration, took further steps to redirect its interest away from the income of farmers to the provision of healthy food for all. Steps were taken to bring school lunches, largely financed through the government, into line with the Eating Right Pyramid. A position of Under Secretary of Food, Nutrition, and Consumer Services was proposed, (requiring Senate confirmation of its appointee); this put nutrition on the same level as other concerns as far as the organization chart shows. The school lunch program would nearly double the amount of fresh fruits and vegetables. Hearings on the new program continued through December of 1993.

(Periodical References and Additional Reading: *New York Times* 12-3-92, p A1; *New York Times* 2-10-93, p C11; *New York Times* 9-8-93, p C1; *New York Times* 11-24-93, p C4; *Natural History* 1-94, p 72)

PRIMATES ARE ADAPTED TO EAT FRUIT AND NUTS

In the late 1980s Katherine Milton of the University of California-Berkeley, and Montague W. Demnent of the University of California-Davis demonstrated that the digestive system of chimpanzees, probably the species closest to humans in every way, is very similar to that of humans. But chimpanzees, and many other primates, do not have a diet similar to modern humans, especially those humans in industrialized counties. The typical primate diet is high on fruit and nuts (technically, a nut is a either a fruit or a seed), supplemented by some young leaves or flowers for additional fiber and protein and some small animals, most often insects but sometimes small vertebrates. In an earlier study, for example, Milton found that a spider monkey's diet is 72 percent fruit, 22 percent leaves, and six percent flowers, with a few insects (some of which are in or on the fruit, leaves, or flowers). Primates that deviate from this kind of pattern generally do so in favor of more leaves. Aside from industrialized humans, no primate has a diet in which most of the calories come from animals and seeds. (Wheat, rice, corn, and so forth are seeds.)

In the early 1990s, a number of studies of diet and health suggested that parts of a typical primate diet would be healthier for most humans. This is not surprising any more and it has become part of the conventional wisdom in the U.S. (*see* "New Food Chart and Labels," p 151). This article and the ones that follow explore some of the reasons for food choices in more detail, beginning with fruit and nuts.

An Apple a Day

The Food Pyramid calls for from two to four servings of fruit every day. As a part of the Harvard School of Public Health's research program called the Health Professionals Follow-Up Study, nearly 31,000 men between the ages of 40 and 75 reported on their eating habits. Although overweight contributed the most risk of heart disease to those in the study, one factor that tumbled out was that the men with a high fruit diet—the equivalent of five apples each day—had significantly lower risk of high blood pressure. Put another way, the low-fruit group had a 46 percent greater risk. Vegetables and cereals did not provide this benefit. Results were published in the November, 1992 *Circulation.*

Similar results for cancer were found by a different study of the same population conducted by the Harvard Medical School, who also looked at women participating in the Nurse's Health Study. In the June 2, 1993 *Journal of the National Cancer Institute,* the researchers endorsed fruits as a way to keep precancerous colorectal cancer from developing or from turning malignant. These studies also found benefits for vegetables and grains.

Nuts to Heart Disease

While the Food Pyramid proposes almost five servings of fruit a day, it puts nuts into the "use sparingly" group. But a 1992 study of Seventh Day Adventists suggests that for protection against heart disease, a serving of nuts almost every day would be helpful. Of the 31,208 Adventists in a survey conducted by Gary Fraser and co-workers at Loma Linda University in California, those who consumed nuts five or more times a week had a 50 percent lower risk of heart attacks. Even one serving of nuts a week reduced heart-attack risk by 25 percent.

The survey, which was mailed to every adult Seventh Day Adventist in California between 1977 and 1982, was predicated on the observation of longer life and fewer heart attacks of Adventists when compared with other Americans. In general, Seventh Day Adventists are less likely to smoke tobacco or drink alcohol or even coffee, while they are much more likely to be vegetarians. Fraser and co-workers wanted to find specific practices of the group that contributed to a heart attack rate that is about 15 percent of the U.S. norm.

Analysis of the questionnaire, published in the July, 1992 issue of the *Archives of Internal Medicine,* showed that after excessive weight, high blood pressure, smoking, and similar factors had been adjusted for, the only heart benefits in the diets of Seventh Day Adventists came from nuts and, to a much small degree, from whole wheat bread.

The Adventists who ate a lot of nuts were most likely to eat peanuts or almonds. A study in 1993, however, suggested that walnuts, consumed at half the rate of peanuts, might well be the magic nuts. The Loma Linda researchers put groups of male students on low-fat diets for four weeks at a time. Although all the diets used were relatively low in fat (kept at 30 percent), some groups of students got much of that fat from walnuts. In the March 4, 1993 issue of the *New England Journal of Medicine* the researchers reported that the group eating the walnuts had blood cholesterol levels that dropped 18 percent, while the group eating other fats saw only a 6 percent drop. The groups were then interchanged, and the result was the same: walnuts produced a greater drop than simply lowering total fat.

Walnuts were chosen for this study because it was financed by the California Walnut Commission. Other nuts might well have the same, or perhaps even greater, effect.

(Periodical References and Additional Reading: *Science News* 7-25-92, p 52; *Harvard Health Letter* 2-93, p 8;*New York Times* 3-4-93, p B8; *Science News* 3-13-93, p 175; *Science News* 6-5-93, p 358; *Scientific American* 8-93, p 86)

VIRTUES AND VICES OF VEGETABLES

"Eat your vegetables" is well-known advice from mothers to children, although often not willingly taken. Vegetables were in the political news in the early 1990s, as President George Bush proclaimed his dislike of broccoli and First Lady Hillary Clinton told children on television that nobody likes peas. Despite these aversions, mom's advice has been borne out by research. And, of course, many people throughout the world eat nothing else, provided all plant food is called "vegetable." In the following, the word *vegetable* refers primarily to those green or yellow fruits, leaves, seeds, and roots that are served in the U.S. alongside or as the main course in a meal. But *vegans* (strict vegetarians) also eat other plant foods, such as the sweet fruits often part of dessert or the nuts that might even follow dessert in a "soup-to-nuts" meal.

In 1990 a National Cancer Institute (NCI) conference reported that soybeans may contain chemicals in high amounts that would tend to prevent cancer and heart disease. The anti-cancer chemicals were thought to work by lowering estrogen levels, which is known to reduce breast cancer, or by slowing down the proliferation of blood vessels that a tumor needs to grow. The heart disease effect is thought to result from different chemicals that may reduce absorption of dietary cholesterol.

Similar results for colon cancer were found by a study of the same population conducted by Edward Giovannucci and coworkers of the Harvard Medical School, who looked at data from men in the Health Professionals Study and women participating in the Nurse's Health Study. In the June 2, 1993 *Journal of the National Cancer Institute* the researchers endorsed fruits and vegetables as a way to keep precancerous colorectal cancer from developing or from turning malignant.

In addition to cancer, vegetables (including fruit and grains) were found to be beneficial in heart disease. Conventional wisdom is that persons who have had one or more heart attacks should be on a diet that reduces fat, especially saturated fat, and cholesterol. An investigation reported in the *British Medical Journal* of April 19, 1992, found, however, that some two hundred heart attack patients fared better on a diet based on high amounts of vegetables, fruit, grains, and fish than they did on the conventional low-fat diet. A like number of patients with similar histories of diet and other factors had almost twice as many fatal heart attacks within the first year after leaving the hospital. One possible reason for the difference may have been that the low-fat diet is more difficult to maintain than the high-vegetable diet, but other possible reasons include the additional fiber and antioxidants in vegetables and fruits.

(Periodical References and Additional Reading: *Harvard Health Letter,* 10-92, p 8; *Science News* 6-5-93, p 358; ; *University of California at Berkeley Wellness Letter* 10-93, p 1)

PROMISES AND PERILS OF MEAT

Although humans need only vitamin B_{12} from animal products, meat in small amounts has been a significant part of the higher primate diet for millions of years. Our closest relatives, the chimpanzees, consume what is now considered a good diet for primates—mostly fruit, nuts, shoots, and tender leaves, with occasional forays into animal products (in their case, termites and once in a while a monkey).

Before the Industrial Revolution, the average European ate about half a pound of meat *a year.* Along with the factories and better transportation, the nineteenth century also saw advances in large-scale farming, presaged a few decades earlier by enclosure of the common fields in England. Although a few vegetarians begged to differ, "the Sunday roast" ("joint" in England) became a tradition, and meat for breakfast, lunch, and dinner became common. Not until the mid-1970s did an anti-meat message, preached by some nonvegetarians as early as the 1950s, begin to make any reduction in the recently acquired habit of meat-eating. In the 1990s, despite warnings of nutritionists that meat in large amounts is unhealthy for humans, meat and poultry continued to form a major part of the U.S. and European diet, although still used in small amounts only in poorer nations and even in some wealthy Asian populations. At the beginning of the 1990s, however, about one man in seven and one woman in eight had heeded the warnings and stopped eating red meat completely, while others had tapered off. But two or three years later, the food news in the U.S. included the return of the "steakhouse" to the restaurant scene.

A new look at meat, however, suggested that in addition to problems connected with the kind of fat it contains (*see* "Fat UPDATE," p 171), meat also poses health problems of a more immediate nature.

Contamination

On January 13, 1993, a gastroenterologist in Washington State called the Department of Health to report an outbreak of bloody diarrhea. Within four days the Department had located the cause: hamburgers from a Jack-in-the-Box fast-food outlet. By then, 37 persons had been diagnosed as victims of the bacterium in the burgers, a strain of the common bacterium *Escherichia coli* called 0157:H7. By the end of February the number of cases of *Escherichia coli* infection from various Jack-in-the-Box franchises had reached 497, and three children, all younger than three years old, had died, the first on January 22, 1993. Only one of the children is known to have eaten the tainted meat, but the bacteria can spread easily from child to child if the children are in close contact, as in a day-care center.

Earlier than this, two people had died in Washington State from *Escherichia coli* contamination in 1986, and six cases of the same bacterial disease, possibly linked to fast-food hamburgers, had appeared in San Diego County, California, with one death, a six-year-old girl. On March 13-14, 1993, nine customers of a Sizzler steakhouse in Seattle and in October 1993 six people from Butte, Montana, also were infected with the bacterium.

The problem in the Northwest had its origin in meat from six slaughterhouses in the U.S. and Canada, but proper cooking would have killed the bacteria. When Jack-in-the Box added 30 seconds to its hamburger cooking time, the epidemic stopped—although the public relations problem may be with the chain for a long time.

Much more disturbing was a report by Ellis Avner and coworkers from the University of Washington's Children's Hospital and Medical Center in Seattle. In November, Avner told a meeting of the American Society of Nephrology in Boston that 35 of the

Background

According to the Federal Centers of Disease Control and Prevention in Atlanta, Georgia, about 15,000 Americans a year develop serious illness from infected meat and poultry. Of these, about 15 persons a year in the U.S. die from the effects.

U.S. Federal meat inspection consists of looking for discoloration or feeling the meat for lumps or other problems. Since the 1980s, equipment has also been used to test for pesticide residues or other unwanted chemicals in meat and poultry. About 7400 inspectors sample 7 billion chickens and turkeys, 89 million pigs, and 30 million cattle each year at 6400 slaughtering houses. *Escherichia coli* has been known since the nineteenth century and is the common bacterium found by the billions in human intestines where it normally causes no difficulty. It is well known, usually by its abbreviated name *E. coli*, as the bacterium for which water is tested to see if it is safe for swimming or drinking. Many experiments in gene engineering use *E. coli* because it is so common and so well known.

The bacterium does not necessarily pose a threat to water supplies and ocean beaches. However, tests are conducted for the presence *E. coli* because of a significant number of bacteria indicates that fecal matter, which may contain dangerous microbes, has gotten into the water.

Consequently, workers were surprised when in 1982 investigation of outbreaks of bloody diarrhea in Oregon and Michigan were traced to a strain of *E. coli* that was infecting people as a result of too-rare hamburgers. The strain, known as 0157:H7, was investigated further. In addition to the bloody diarrhea that was its first known and most common symptom, the bacterium releases a toxin that is picked up from the intestinal wall and transmitted by blood to other parts of the body. This toxin can cause a form of kidney failure called hemolytic uremic syndrome in about ten to 15 percent of infections, especially in young children, and a bleeding disorder in adults known as thrombocytopenic purpura, as well as anemia. Hemolytic uremic syndrome was the cause of the three deaths in Washington. Dozens of people developed kidney failure, however, but were saved by kidney dialysis. The syndrome was first observed in Switzerland in 1955, but not connected to *E. coli* until 1982. Since then it has been known to have killed 21 persons.

children had developed kidney failure, anemia, and low blood platelet counts, a pattern called hemolytic uremic syndrome (HUS). An earlier French study suggests that many patients with HUS who appear to be cured as children go on to have serious kidney problems as adults, a problem that may affect as many as ten to 14 of the HUS victims from the Northwestern epidemic.

After the illnesses in the Northwest, the Clinton Administration, led primarily by Secretary of Agriculture Mike Espy, proposed revising procedures to include scientific testing for bacteria. The Agriculture Department also conducted surprise investigations of slaughterhouses and temporarily closed 30 after discovering violations.

The Clinton proposal also called for the use of ionizing radiation from radioactive sources to kill pathogens (bacteria, fungi, and parasites) in meats and poultry. Scientists are divided on whether or not such treatment chemically alters the food in undesirable ways, but all agree that it does not make food radioactive and that the treatment kills most pathogens.

The U.S. Food and Drug Administration further recommended raising the minimum cooking temperature at restaurants and in institutions from 140° F to 155° F.

In May 1993 the U.S. Department of Agriculture (USDA) agreed to a settlement in a consumer-group court action that led to an August 1993 USDA announcement that they would order new labels on uncooked meats. The labels would recommend protective steps for protection from bacteria. These steps included thawing in the refrigerator or in microwave ovens instead of on the counter; separating raw meat and poultry from other foods; washing surfaces that raw meat or poultry touched; thorough cooking; keeping hot foods hot; and immediate refrigeration of any undiscarded leftovers. Although similar advice is commonly given in cookbooks and periodicals that deal with recipes and food, the National American Wholesale Grocers Association managed to get a federal district court to prevent, in a ruling on October 14, 1993, the label requirement from taking effect. Within a week, two three-year-old boys in the same court district died from food-borne bacteria (probably *E. coli* 0157:H7). The Agriculture Department developed a new order for labels for uncooked meat and poultry that would sidestep court procedural objections and be put in place in grocery stores by April 15, 1994. In the meantime, some stores and food processors voluntarily added similar labels.

COOKING TEMPERATURES FOR SAFETY

U.S. minimum for cooking processed beef (hamburger)	140° F
Jack-in-the Box standards before 1993	about 140° F
Washington State standards since May 1992	155° F
McDonald's Corporation standard for burgers	at least 157° F
U.S. recommended temperature for home-cooked hamburger	160° F

Additional Bad News

Throughout the early 1990s there was little reason to believe that even uncontaminated meat cooked properly could do you any good. Red meat consumption was linked to colon cancer in a report on the Nurses Health Study that was published on December 13, 1990. So if red meat was a problem, many thought they should stick to poultry and fish.

Although the wave of illness caused by *E. coli* was a major news story, nine deaths from tainted shellfish in Florida in 1992 were not much noticed, perhaps because they were spread over nine months. The bacteria in these instances were various species of the genus *Vibrio*, which the U.S. Food and Drug Administration (FDA) estimates contaminated five to ten percent of the clams, oysters, mussels, and scallops that reach the supermarket or fish store in the U.S. The species *Vibrio comma* is well known as the cause of cholera, which suggests the kind of symptoms that its near relatives produce—fever and chills, diarrhea, and nausea and vomiting. *Vibrio* bacteria are killed by proper cooking, but many people enjoy eating raw clams and oysters, while mussels may be undercooked.

Even eating a contaminated raw oyster will not cause illness in most cases because stomach acid kills most of the bacteria (one of its regular jobs). Research in the early 1990s also showed that hot chili sauce also kills bacteria in raw shellfish. For people with damaged or inactive immune systems or various gastrointestinal problems, however, *Vibrio* can multiply enough to sicken or even or kill, warns the March 1993 *FDA Medical Bulletin.*

And Finally, the Good News

There are some things in meat that are healthy for humans. Animal products are needed to obtain vitamin B_{12} from the diet, although food supplements can be used by strict vegans. Also, vitamin B_6 can be better obtained from beef than from any other source, although grains and such fruits as bananas or watermelon have significant amounts. Both iron and zinc are more readily absorbed into the body from red meat than from other sources. Protein, however, which people tend to associate with meat, can easily be obtained from a diet with a variety of vegetables, including legumes and grains.

Fat, the main meat villain, has been reduced in red meat since the 1950s. As a result of the customer revolt against saturated fats, beef producers and marketers have aggressively trimmed the fat off of meat before it is sold. Over a 40-year period, beef has lost 27 percent of the fat and pork about 31 percent fat, nearly all as a result of trimming.

Scott M. Grundy and coworkers at the University of Texas have even found that stearic acid in red meat and poultry may lower cholesterol levels.

(Periodical References and Additional Reading: *Harvard Health Letter* 3-91, p 1; *New York Times* 1-23-93, p 7; *New York Times* 1-27-93, p A10; *New York Times* 2-9-93, p C3; *New York Times* 2-22-93, p A11; *Scientific American* 6-93, p 132; *New York Times* 3-17-93, p A1; *New York Times* 3-28-93, p I:28; *New York Times* 5-6-93, p A18; *Harvard Health Letter* 6-9, p 8; *New York Times* 10-31-93, p I:25; *New York Times* 12-20-93, p A1; *Science News* 12-18/25, p 414; *Discover* 1-94, p 86)

Vitamin UPDATE

When vitamins were first recognized around the turn of the twentieth century, nutritionists began a century-long campaign to persuade people that eating a well-balanced diet would provide all the vitamins a well-working body would ever require. Only people with rare metabolic deficiencies would ever need to take supplemental vitamins.

Despite a constant drumbeat of this essential message, many people who learned about vitamins persisted in the belief that if a little bit of vitamins in food was good for you, then a lot of vitamins in pill form would be even better. This belief was encouraged by maverick doctors who also went against the nutritionists in favor of one form or another of massive vitamin supplement, often to cure some chronic illness. Vitamin manufacturers were also eager to propose that the average person should consume additional vitamins in pill or liquid form, even if only one multiple-purpose vitamin per day. Vitamins for children were promoted in advertisements that suggests to the children that if they took their cartoon-shaped, multi-colored, candy-flavored pills, they would grow tall and quickly become adults.

Because one of the maverick doctors touting a miracle vitamin, Linus Pauling, had previously won a Nobel Prize for medicine, the scientific community began, albeit skeptically, to test his claims for the utility of massive doses of vitamin C. Today, while many nutritionists still cling to the creed that a well-balanced diet contains all the vitamins one will ever need, the evidence is piling up that for some vitamins at least, a megadose a day does keep the doctor and—better yet—the ambulance or hearse away. More specifically, although the nutritionists are probably correct regarding most vitamins, the ones classed as antioxidants have been shown to have effects that go far beyond the nutritional role of vitamins. These are vitamins A, C, and E, although vitamin A is probably more effective and safer in the form of a precursor, beta-carotene. Furthermore, the B vitamin folacin is known to prevent some birth defects in moderately high doses.

One study, published by Ranjit Chandra in the November 7, 1992 *Lancet* showed that elderly people who took vitamin and mineral supplements endured fewer than half as many days of illness from infection as a matched group receiving a placebo. The placebo did contain calcium and magnesium among its ingredients, and thus could have had beneficial effects. The supplements, which included all the important vitamins as well as the minerals calcium, copper, iodine, iron, magnesium, selenium, and zinc, were heavy on beta carotene and vitamin E (three to four times the RDA) and light on vitamin A (half the RDA). The subjects were 96 middle-class New-foundlanders over 65, about a third of whom were found to have vitamin deficiencies before the study began. At the conclusion, after a year, tests also showed that the immune system in the group taking the supplements had improved as well.

A study directed by M. Christina Leske at the State University of New York at Stony Brook and coworkers, published in the February 1993 issue of the *Archives of Ophthalmology,* showed that middle-aged and elderly people (people over 40) who took a multivitamin supplement of the "one-a-day" form had 37 percent fewer cataracts. Antioxidants in the supplements were suspected at the cause of the reduction, but further study is needed to be certain.

The September 15, 1993 issue of the *Journal of the National Cancer Institute* contained two articles about success in using vitamin supplements to reduce cancer rates in rural areas of China. Diets there are normally poor in fresh fruits and vegetables. Cancer of the stomach and esophagus are very high in the region studied, and those rates were reduced by a combination of beta carotene, B vitamins, vitamins C and E, and other nutrients. Vitamin-mineral supplements also reduced rates of a precancerous esophageal condition.

Here are some of other recent results:

Vitamin A (retinol) Because a lack of vitamin A caused a clearly defined visual impairment, this vitamin has since its discovery been primarily associated in the public mind with improving visual acuity. Regrettably, this seems to be beyond its powers. Nevertheless, vitamin A deficiency causes night blindness and flaky skin.

There was also a degree of public awareness that an excess of vitamin A could be lethal; a notorious case involved stranded Arctic explorers who died as a result of vitamin A overdose from consumption of polar-bear liver—a quarter pound of polar-bear liver contains about 450 times the RDA of vitamin A for an adult male.

Vitamin A does aid in slowing the symptoms of the eye diseases grouped under the heading retinitis pigmentosa (RP). RP is the general name for any degeneration of the rod and cone cells of the retina (the actual cells used for detecting light). Worldwide, about one in every 4000 persons has RP. According to a study of 601 patients reported in June 1993 by Eliot L. Berson and coworkers of Harvard Medical School in the *Archives of Ophthalmology,* a daily supplement of 15,000 international units of vitamin A in the form of a palmitate derivative slowed the loss of rod and cone cells in the retina, a loss that is the hallmark of RP. Slowing the degeneration could prolong vision for years. Vitamin A therapy is the first known useful treatment for the diseases.

Cataracts are another eye disease for which vitamin A is useful, according to a study of 50,000 women that was published in the August 8, 1992, issue of the *British Medical Journal.* There was a 20 percent lower rate of need for cataract surgery among the women whose diets were rich in vitamin A.

Also vitamin A, like its precursor beta carotene (see below), may have a preventive effect on breast cancer. David J. Hunter and coworkers reported in the July 26, 1993, *New England Journal of Medicine* that their analysis of a diet study of the 1439 nurses who developed breast cancer from a group of 89,494 studied from 1980 through 1988 showed that small amounts of vitamin A lowered the risk of breast cancer by about 16 percent, although larger amounts made no difference. In other words, nurses who had virtually no vitamin A in their diet had about a 20 percent higher chance of developing breast cancer. The same study revealed no similar protection from vitamins C or E.

Vitamin A can be dangerous, however. Excessive use most commonly leads to itching, hair loss, dry skin and mouth, pain of various kinds, and even nausea and vomiting. But a study at St-Luc University Hospital in Brussels, Belgium, found that nearly 30 of their patients with liver damage, including 17 patients with cirrhosis, had caused their own diseases with excessive use of vitamin A supplements. Research with rats has also shown that vitamin A can magnify liver damage caused by toxic chemicals, such as carbon tetrachloride.

B vitamins   All the water-soluble vitamins except for vitamin C are classed as "B vitamins," but they are really separate chemicals with somewhat different properties and are increasingly called by their own names, e.g., thiamine or pantothenic acid. Several of the B vitamins are essential for the functioning of small bodies in cells called mitochondria, which do the actual work of metabolism—i.e., changing the fats, carbohydrates, and proteins in foods into energy. The nerves are very sensitive to problems in metabolism, so deficiencies in B vitamins are first manifested as symptoms in the nervous system. Most B vitamins are found in larger amounts in meat and dairy products than in vegetables, so B-vitamin deficiency diseases, such as beriberi or Strachan's disease, often appear in people who do not eat a lot of meat. Beriberi can also be prevented by eating whole grains, such a brown rice.

A mysterious disease that first surfaced in 1991 and then swept through Cuba in 1993 is now thought primarily to have been caused by a vitamin B deficiency, though not all evidence from the epidemic was consistent with the vitamin-deficiency hypothesis. The primary symptoms reported were nerve damage and loss of vision, essentially the same symptoms as in Strachan's disease, which is known to result from B-vitamin deficiencies. In mid-June 1993 Cuban authorities claimed there were 43,412 cases of the disease. Earlier in May and into June, U.S. doctors visited Cuba as part of several international programs. The U.S. doctors used various criteria for visual damage to identify patients and claimed that patients that were counted and did not show loss of vision were misdiagnosed and suffered from unrelated conditions. After the U.S. doctors' visits, the Cuban government began distributing multivitamin supplements to the entire population, and the epidemic drew to a close. More than 60 percent recovered within three weeks.

In December 1993 a report from the ongoing Framingham Heart Study showed that low levels of vitamins B_6, B_{12}, and folacin (a B vitamin) in the blood correlated with high levels of the blood chemical homocysteine, which previous studies have shown to be a predictor of heart disease. Further studies are needed, but it seems possible that the B vitamins protect against heart disease by lowering homocysteine. Researchers involved with the study thought that a diet high in fruits and vegetables could bring vitamin B levels high enough to provide protection. They also felt that few people actually ate such a diet. Red meats and organ meats are also good sources of vitamins B_{12} and B_6.

Except for vitamin B_{12}, which has no generally used chemical name but is sometimes called cyanocohbalamin, B vitamins are listed below by their specific names.

Vitamin B_{12}   The main thing to recognize about this vitamin is that it is not found in vegetable sources, so vegans (strict vegetarians) need to use it as a supplement unless they use eat vegetable-based foods that have been fortified with the vitamin. It is needed for red blood-cell development and maintenance of nervous system, so lack of the vitamin can cause pernicious anemia.

Beta carotene   Technically, beta carotene is not a vitamin, but it is converted to vitamin A in the body. Unlike vitamin A, high doses of beta carotene do not produce adverse health effects, although if high enough they can color the skin orange.

A study by Charles Hennekens and coworkers at Brigham and Women's Hospital in Boston demonstrated that beta carotene was effective in preventing recurrence of heart attacks in men, although it was not as useful as aspirin. But the people in the study who took both had no recurrence whatsoever. In another analysis of beta carotene's effect on the elderly, Hennekens also found that high levels of beta carotene cut the death rate from heart attacks nearly in half.

In another study, beta carotene has been shown by Harinder Garewal of the University of Arizona Cancer Center in Tucson, Arizona, to reduce the size of precancerous lesions in the mouth that are often caused by smoking tobacco. In a few cases, it removed them altogether. In 1994 a Finnish study made headlines, however, when its results included higher cancer levels among heavy smokers who took very high doses of beta carotene for several years.

Either beta carotene or its derivative vitamin A helps prevent cataracts. A Finnish study of 1419 persons during the late 1960s and early 1970s, the results of which were published in the *British Medical Journal* in December, 1992, took blood samples and measured beta carotene (and other nutrients, including vitamin E—see below) in the blood. This method is considered to be much more reliable than one based on what people report eating. The same people were watched for cataract problems for a dozen years after the blood samples had been taken. The persons in the lowest third for beta carotene in their blood were 1.7 times as likely to undergo cataract surgery as the persons in the top third for beta carotene in their blood.

Biotin   This is an unnumbered B vitamin that is important in metabolism.

Vitamin C   This is ascorbic acid, a simple chemical. Even before it was recognized as a vitamin in 1927, fruits containing vitamin C were used to prevent scurvy, a disease that begins with fatigue and bleeding gums and progresses to serious illness and death. Since 1970 Nobel Prize winner Linus Pauling has promoted large doses of the vitamin to ward off colds and prevent cancer, although he was not taken seriously for many years. The main reason for doctors today to recommend doses of vitamin C above the amount needed to prevent disease is that it is another antioxidant. As such, it is thought to reduce the risk of some forms of cancer and coronary artery disease and to prevent or delay formation of cataracts on the eyes.

A retrospective study by James Enstrom and coworkers at the University of California—Los Angeles, reported in the May 1992 *Epidemiology,* found that men who got at least 300 milligrams of vitamin C each day (in their diet or with added supplements) lived up to six years longer than those in the study group who averaged just 25 milligrams from diet alone. The current Recommended Daily Allowance of vitamin C is 60 milligrams for adults; Pauling, however, has proposed much higher doses, ranging from a thousand to 18 thousand milligrams, his personal amount. Women in the Enstrom study of 11,000 Americans showed much less of a gain in longevity than men: larger doses of vitamin C added only a year to their already longer average life spans.

Smokers, as well as persons exposed to second-hand smoke, definitely need additional vitamin C. A study by Diane L. Tribble and coworkers at the Lawrence Berkeley Laboratory in California reported in the December *American Journal of Clinical Nutrition* that passive smokers had reduced levels of vitamin C when exposed to tobacco smoke for 20 to 95 hours a week, some of them even lacking the minimal amount of the vitamin needed for good health. Previous research has also indicated that vitamin C may help fight the diseases caused by smoking, making it more essential for those exposed to cigarette, pipe, or cigar smoke to take supplemental vitamin C.

Vitamin D   Technically, vitamin D is not really a vitamin at all, since it is produced by the body in the liver and kidneys from precursors activated by sunlight. Therefore, vitamin D is a hormone. True vitamins can only be obtained from food or vitamin pills, and not from the body. A deficiency in vitamin D causes rickets.

A normal amount of vitamin D is needed for absorption of calcium and hence for growth of bones and teeth. Lack of vitamin D may increase the risk of osteoporosis, but too much vitamin D is toxic. One recent study showed that different alleles of the gene for the vitamin D receptor molecule influence how effectively the vitamin fights osteoporosis, so some people get more benefit from the vitamin than others do. A French study reported in the December 3, 1992 *New England Journal of Medicine* demonstrated that women over 80 can have 30 to 40 percent fewer hip or other fractures if they take daily supplements of vitamin D and calcium.

At the end of the 1980s researchers found that vitamin D in the form of an ointment containing the activated form known as calcitrol is effective for about seven out of ten patients suffering from the skin disease psoriasis. Oral vitamin D, however, does not achieve the same effect.

Vitamin E   In many ways vitamin E has had the most spectacular history of all the vitamins. Vitamin E was discovered in 1922 by H. M. Evans and K. S. Bishop. It achieved great notoriety when it was found necessary for the sex life of male rats; this discovery quickly created a major market for massive doses to enhance the sexual potency of men—however, scientists have not found any evidence to support this claim. Among the other claims for the vitamin E in recent years has been a promise to remove muscle aches and pains, circulatory and lung damage or disorders, and premenstrual syndrome. It is said to slow the development of breast cysts and the progress of macular degeneration of the retina. The most amazing claims included erasure of wrinkles and general reduction of deterioration caused by age. The only reported side effect ever noted from vitamin E has been a possible mild fatigue. As a result, about 15 percent of Americans take vitamin-E supplements.

Some claims, like the purported improvement in male sex performance, have not held up under further study. Perhaps because vitamin E is thought to slow macular degeneration, a condition of the retina, it was also thought to slow retinitis pigmentosa as well. In 1993, however, the same study that found vitamin A useful in treating RP also disclosed that moderately large doses of vitamin E actually speed rather than slow progress of eye diseases.

Other claims have fared better. A U.S. Department of Agriculture Study conducted in 1992 by Mohsen Meydani and Simin Nikbin Meydani of the Human Nutrition Research Center on Aging at Tufts University in Boston confirmed the claim that vitamin E can protect against muscle damage and reduce soreness after exercises. In a double-blind study, volunteers took a placebo or 800 International Units of vitamin E before a treadmill exercise for 45 minutes. Blood chemistry studies showed that the vitamin reduced the byproducts of fat oxidation and of chemical messengers that enhance inflammation.

One definite benefit of the American predilection for vitamin E is that large numbers of people, whether they take the supplementary doses or not, are available to scientists who want to study the effects of the vitamin. In fact, studies have revealed that some of the benefits promised to humans are real: the vitamin protects babies' eyes from excessive oxygen, reduces the leg pains known as claudification, and protects heart muscles during heart surgery.

In 1991 and 1992 various researchers in Austria, Sweden, and Texas found that vitamin E (and the other antioxidants, beta carotene and vitamin C) reduced low-density lipoproteins (LDL, or "bad" cholesterol) in the blood. This led to further studies of the possibility that vitamin E could protect against heart disease.

Two massive studies of the effects of vitamin E were reported in the May 20, 1993, issues of the *New England Journal of Medicine,* following a preliminary report to the American Heart Association in November, 1992. Together, the studies included tens of thousands of medical workers, male and female, over a period of several years. The Nurses' Health Study, for example, used questionnaires to compile data on 87,245 female nurses between the ages of 34 to 59 who were considered free of heart disease when the study began in 1980. The research, directed by Frank Speizer and Meir J. Stampfer of Brigham and Women's Hospital in Boston, covered a period of eight years. The study of male medical workers, directed by Eric B. Rimm of the Harvard School of Public Health, included 51,529 male health professionals between the ages of 40 to 75 and covered a five-year span. After accounting for every known life style factor, both studies showed that people who took additional vitamin E supplements had about a 40 percent lower risk of heart disease than those who got vitamin E from their diet alone (46 percent for women and 37 percent for men). These results were independent of the general quality of the respondents' diet. The people taking supplements took from ten to a hundred times the recommended daily amounts; while it did not matter whether the supplements were high or low, the best results came from respondents using over 100 units of vitamin E daily for longer periods of time. The doctors who conducted the studies espoused the standard nutritionist theory and did not expect this kind of a result. Despite their results, they refused to recommend vitamin E supplements and said that they themselves did not take the supplements.

Since statistical evidence is always viewed skeptically, extensive controlled studies with placebos will be needed to established results to everyone's satisfaction. Yet in this case there is another approach that has shown chemical evidence that vitamin E has effects that reduce plaque formation in the arteries, the primary cause of heart disease. Various studies have demonstrated that antioxidants prevent low-density lipoprotein (LDL) cholesterol from forming plaque. Among the more dramatic studies was one by Scott Grundy, director of the Center for Human Nutrition at the University of Texas Southwestern Medical Center in Dallas, in which volunteers were fed doses about ten times the daily requirements of vitamins E and C and beta carotene. He showed that all three, but especially vitamin E, blocked the transformation of LDL cholesterol by oxidation. Other studies had established that oxidation was necessary for plaque formation.

The Finnish study that showed beta carotene helped prevent cataracts (see above) also indicated that those in the bottom third for the chemical equivalent of vitamin E were 1.9 times as likely to develop cataracts as the persons in the top third. Since beta carotene and vitamin E are often found in the same food sources, e.g., in dark-green vegetables, it is not clear which of the two substances actually prevents cataracts. Moreover, it is conceivable that some other substance found in foods rich in beta carotene and vitamin E could be the preventive agent.

Folacin (folic acid; folate): Like biotin, folacin is an unnumbered vitamin B vitamin that is involved in some metabolism of proteins. As a vitamin, it is called "folacin" to match the "-in" suffix familiar from vitamin, biotin, niacin, riboflavin, and thiamine. The "in" suffix, however, has many chemical meanings. In reference to the form used by the body, the preferred name is usually "folate." In either case, the chemical in foods is folic acid. Its name comes from the Latin *folium,* for "leaf," suggesting correctly that one of its principal sources is leafy vegetables, such as spinach.

In the 1990s a major discovery about folacin was that it belongs to the group of vitamins that prevent spina bifida, a common birth defect. Its role in preventing spina bifida, anencephaly, and other neural tube birth defects was recognized by British researchers as early as 1991, and may have something to do with its effect on DNA synthesis. There is also some evidence that folacin might reduce the risk of cervical cancer. Following a recommendation of the U.S. Public Health Service on September 14, 1992, the U.S. Food and Drug Administration (FDA) announced on December 29, 1993 that it accepted as valid the particular claims according to which folic acid prevented neural-tube birth defects when taken during the first weeks of pregnancy.

Most people do not get enough folacin. Some experts recommend that pregnant women get at least 800 micrograms a day, which is four times the normal amount needed by men, as well as more than four time the amount most Americans get in their diet. Therefore, women of childbearing age are encouraged by many doctors to take folacin supplements.

Folacin has also been found to have unexpected effects on the health of adults. Although it was originally discovered in conjunction with a form of anemia which occurs when folate absorption is blocked by either alcohol consumption or digestive problems, folacin is now recognized for its ability to correct a metabolic defect which, if uncorrected, may triple the risk of heart attacks in males. In this case, it works as part of the enzyme that breaks down the amino acid homocysteine, which contributes to heart attack risk if reaches high levels in the blood.

Lately it has seemed that every dietary or lifestyle change to lower heart attack risk also lowers cancer risk, and increased intake of folacin is no exception. In June, 1993, a study directed by Edward Giovannucci of Brigham and Women's Hospital in Boston showed a connection between low levels of folacin intake and adenomas, or precancerous growths, of the colon or rectum. Animal studies also demonstrate that a lack of folacin increases the risk of colon cancer. Other studies show similar increases in risks of cancers of the lung, esophagus, and breast when folacin intake is low. For once the mechanism involved is suspected, if not proved: folacin is a component of the enzymes used in DNA repair; without such repair, more cancers, all of which are known to result from DNA damage of one sort or another, are likely.

In October, 1993, the FDA put forth a proposal, unresolved as of early 1994, to enrich white flour and cornmeal grits so that each serving would contain 100 micrograms of folic acid. Various special interest groups who commented on the proposal either felt that the proposed amount was too small or worried that the folic acid might mask a vitamin B_{12} deficiency, especially in older persons.

Vitamin K   This vitamin is essential for normal blood clotting and perhaps has a role in maintaining strong bones, thus possibly helping to prevent osteoporosis. A good diet supplies enough of this vitamin for most purposes.

Niacin (B_3)   A deficiency in niacin causes pellagra. Long known to be involved in metabolism and in maintaining skin, nerves, and the digestive system, niacin is now thought to also lower elevated blood cholesterol. Although it is not as effective in lowering cholesterol as drugs developed with cholesterol in mind, some prefer it as a natural "medicine." Unlike many water-soluble vitamins, it is possible to get too much niacin, which can cause liver damage or irregular heart beat. Active alcoholics need more niacin than people who do not drink.

Pantothenic acid (B_5)   Needed in metabolism and in production of essential chemicals used by cells, it may cause diarrhea if taken as a supplement.

Pyroxidine (B_6)   Perhaps pyroxidine is better known as vitamin B_6. It is needed in various chemical reactions involving amino acids and proteins, helping to maintain the nervous system and to form red blood cells. There is a possibility that it can boost the immune system of older people, although it may cause numbness and other neurological disorders when taken as a supplement.

Riboflavin (B$_2$)   Riboflavin is yet another B vitamin that is important for metabolism, growth, production of red blood cells, and the health of the skin and eyes.

Thiamine (B$_1$)   Thiamine, like other B vitamins, helps to convert carbohydrates into energy (metabolism) and is needed for healthy nerve and brain function. A deficiency causes the disease beriberi or other nervous disorders. It is also involved in regulating the heart.

(Periodical References and Further Reading: *Harvard Health Letter* 4-90, p 2; *New York Times* 11-28-90, p C3; *New York Times* 2-20-91; *Harvard Health Letter* 12-91, p 7; *Science News* 8-1-92, p 86; *Harvard Health Letter* 9-92, p 8; *New York Times* 9-15-92, p C2; *New York Times* 9-22-92, p C1; *New York Times* 10-21-92, p C12; *New York Times* 11-6-92, p A16; *New York Times* 11-19-92, p A19; *New York Times* 11-25-92, p A16; *New York Times* 12-8-92, p C8; *Discover* 1-93, p 54; *Science News* 5-22-93, p 327; *Harvard Health Letter* 5-93, p 4; *New York Times* 5-20-93, p A1; *Science News* 5-1-93, p 277; *Science News* 5-22-93, p 327; *New York Times* 5-25-93, p C3; *New York Times* 5-26-93, p C11; *New York Times* 5-30-93, p I-17; *New York Times* 6-15-93, pp A4, C3; *Science News* 6-19-93, p 390; *New York Times* 7-27-93, p C3; *Science News* 9-18-93, p 183; *Science News* 12-18/25-93, p 414; *Discover* 1-94, p 87; *University of California at Berkeley Wellness Letter* 1-94, p 4; *New York Times* 1-5-94, p C4; *New York Times* 3-1-94, p C1; *Harvard Health Letter* 3-94, p 3; *Harvard Health Letter* 5-94, p 1)

Mineral UPDATE

Among the six major nutrients, minerals are the least well understood. Although nutritionists call this group of nutrients *minerals,* chemists know that they are elements—mostly metals. A few elements, notably calcium and phosphorus, are used in large amounts in hard tissues, such as bone and teeth. Others, such as sodium and potassium, have known importance in maintaining the chemical composition of blood. Some, like iron and molybdenum, are important in specific biochemical molecules. But all of these apparently have many other roles, probably in other specific molecules that occur in key reactions.

Here is the latest information and new results considering the elements that are also known as nutritional minerals.

Calcium   Calcium is one of the two food supplements that the U.S. Food and Drug Administration (FDA) has approved for health claims. The FDA allows sellers of products containing calcium to publicize the claim that calcium is useful in preventing osteoporosis, the loss of bone mass, which often occurs with aging. Indeed, a French study reported in the December 3, 1992, issue of the *New England Journal of Medicine* found that even women over 80 who took daily calcium supplements and vitamin D needed to incorporate calcium into bones and teeth had 30 to 40 percent fewer fractures of hips and other bones.

Although the practice is still controversial, a number of drinks consumed by children are now fortified with calcium, especially orange juice. In August, 1993, Proctor & Gamble introduced Hawaiian Punch fortified with both calcium and vitamin C. A year earlier, Proctor & Gamble had joined the U.S. National Institute on Aging in funding a study that showed that preadolescent children who consume almost twice as much calcium as in the recommended daily allowance (RDA) develop denser bones, presumably putting them at less risk for fractures later in life. In July, 1992, Conrad Johnson and coworkers from the Indiana School of Medicine reported in the *New England Journal of Medicine* on their controlled study of 71 pairs of twins which was financed in part by Proctor & Gamble. The twins in their study who took calcium pills developed five percent more bone mass than the twins taking a placebo. Johnson suggested that five servings of calcium-rich foods would be better for children than the three such servings previously recommended. An August 18, 1993, report in the *Journal of the American Medical Association* also showed that 12-year-old girls gained bone mass after taking calcium supplements for 18 months.

A problem that surfaced in August, 1993, is that many calcium supplements contain dangerous amounts of lead, a mineral that is definitely not good for anyone, and especially harmful to children. Supplements labeled as approved by the USP (United States Pharmacopeia) are less likely to contain harmful amounts of lead.

Chromium   Chromium is involved in metabolism of sugar and regulation of fat.

Cobalt   This mineral is needed because it is a part of vitamin B_{12}, but no other use is known.

Copper   Although copper in large amounts is toxic—which is why copper cooking pots are lined with tin or stainless steel—in small amounts it is needed to help formation of red blood cells, maintain communications in the nervous system, and produce normal hair. In appropriate amounts, copper also lowers cholesterol levels. The genetic disease Menkes' syndrome results in low copper levels resulting from interferences with normal transport of the metal across cell membranes. Injections of copper compounds at birth can prevent some of the worst symptoms of the disease.

Fluorine   As a part of the mineral that forms the hardest bones and layers of teeth, fluorine is essential in strengthening bones and preventing tooth decay. The U.S. Environmental Protection Agency approves of water systems where natural fluorides are low, i.e. having up to 4 parts per million of fluorides in total as a result of adding fluorides, a process known as fluoridation. Fluoridation has been in use in the U.S. since the 1940s, although there have always been some persons who oppose the practice.

On August 17, 1993, a committee of the U.S. National Research Council of the National Academy of Sciences reported that there was no evidence that fluoridation of drinking water causes cancer, kidney disease, stomach or digestive problems, infertility, or birth defects, all of which had previously been proposed as ill effects by opponents of fluoridation. The only effect besides strengthening teeth and bones is mottling or staining of teeth in about ten percent of the exposed population.

Iodine   A key ingredient in thyroid hormone, iodine regulates energy and promotes growth.

Iron   The key mineral in hemoglobin is iron. Lack of iron results in fewer effective red blood cells (anemia). Too much iron, however, can occur in persons with a hereditary disorder that causes them to store iron in their organs, where it interferes with functioning. Also, in 1991 the deaths of 16 children were attributed to accidental poisoning from iron supplements.

A Finnish study published in the American Heart Association's journal *Circulation* in September, 1992, showed that too much iron may have other ill effects even at levels that are considered normal for men, but high for women. Jukka T. Salonen and coworkers from the University of Kuopio followed 1900 middle-aged men for five years, concluding the study in 1989. During that time 51 of the men had heart attacks, resulting in the death of 9 from these attacks. All the men in the study were tested periodically for iron in their blood. A higher iron level was associated with the risk of heart attack, doubling the relative risk at high levels. In this study, high iron levels in blood ranked second behind cigarette smoking as a heart-attack risk. (There were some odd results to the study that need further explanation. This was one of the few groups in which high levels of low-density lipoprotein cholesterol, or LDL, did not show up as a heart attack risk.)

The relationship between iron and heart attacks was predicted as early as 1981 by Jerome L. Sullivan of the Veterans Medical Center in Charleston, North Carolina. Animal studies and population studies also suggest iron as a factor. Premenopausal women, who normally have much lower iron levels in their blood than men, also have much less risk of heart disease. One possible mechanism is that iron promotes oxidation of LDL and aids it in forming obstructions in the arteries.

One way to lower iron levels is bleeding or—even better—donating blood. Three donations a year would reduce most men's iron levels to those of a premenopausal woman.

Magnesium   Magnesium is believed to relax blood vessels and thus improve blood flow, but it may also have a role in regulating the heart beat. Studies in Great Britain (published in June 1992) and in Baltimore, Maryland (published in the November 4, 1992, *Journal of the American Medical Association*) showed that injecting a magnesium solution immediately after a heart attack reduced problems with heart rhythms and speeded recovery. Two earlier British studies, both published in the March 30, 1991 *Lancet*, demonstrated that magnesium helped relieve symptoms of chronic fatigue syndrome and that patients with the syndrome have slightly depressed levels of magnesium in their red blood cells when compared to patients without symptoms of the syndrome.

Manganese   Manganese is believed to be necessary for bone formation and health of the nervous system.

Molybdenum   The atom of molybdenum is needed for some enzymes to assume a working configuration.

Selenium   Recently selenium has been added to the antioxidant vitamin supplements, not because it is itself an antioxidant, as vitamins C or E are, but because it is thought to promote the action of antioxidant vitamins. Thus, it reduces cell damage that can result in cancer or heart disease. Regions where there is not enough selenium in the soil have been shown to have populations that are more likely to have heart disease. Selenium is also thought to promote growth.

Zinc   Once thought to be unimportant, zinc is now known to be a part of various enzyme molecules, including some which play an important role in sex development and sperm growth. In addition, zinc appears to be involved in healing wounds and in the sense of taste. A severe zinc deficiency can lead to dwarfism and skin disorders as well.

At least one study has suggested that zinc in appropriate doses can halt the progression of the eye disease macular degeneration. Yet physicians are cautious about zinc. An overdose can cause nausea, vomiting, and abdominal pains and interfere with the immune system.

(Periodical references and additional reading: *New York Times* 4-20-91; *Harvard Health Letter* 2-92, p 5; *New York Times* 6-9-92, p C6; *New York Times* 7-14-92, p C3; *New York Times* 8-5-92, p C4; *New York Times* 8-9-92, p A1; *New York Times* 9-8-92, p A1; *New York Times* 11-6-92, p A16; *Tufts University Diet and Nutrition Letter* 1-93, p 3; *Science News* 1-9-93, p 30; *New York Times* 8-25-93, p C4; *Science News* 9-4-93, p 150; *New York Times* 12-30-93, p A15; *Harvard Health Letter* 3-94, p 3)

Fat UPDATE

Probably no health issue is as much on the minds of Americans as fat, although some of the emphasis is related to appearance and self-perceived sexual attractiveness rather than health. Not only do Americans and many, though not all, peoples throughout the world attempt to change their eating habits in an effort to reduce fat intake, but they also try through exercise to remove excess fat from the body. People who try to keep up with the latest on fat information from medical studies now know to grade foods by fat in several ways, ranging from the actual amount as a percentage of the diet to types of fat such as saturated, unsaturated, polyunsaturated, monounsaturated, and omega-3, to mention the main varieties.

Food manufacturers are aware of this interest in fat, so they advertise lunch meats—a notorious source of fat in diets—as "97% FAT FREE." Health columnists in newspapers and magazines counter that "97% FAT FREE" means three percent fat, which also means that a one-ounce slice of ham contains about two grams of fat, or 20 calories worth of fat. If the slice has a total of 60 calories of energy (a typical amount), then the ham gets about 33 percent of its calories from fat. Although 33 percent fat calories is not really that high (most authorities recommend 30 percent as the maximum amount of fat calories in overall diet), "97% FAT FREE" clearly sounds more attractive than "33% FAT CALORIES" or the equivalent, "One third of the energy in this meat comes from fat!"

How has this concern for fat affected the American diet? The best available information only reaches 1990, but it does show that people in the U.S. eat less fat than they once did. The U.S. National Center for Health Statistics reported in 1994 on the results of the Third National Health and Nutrition Examination Survey, which showed a slight but perceptible drop in the percentage of fat calories:

Year	Percentage of calories from fat	Percentage of calories from saturated fat
mid-1960s	42 percent	16 percent
1978	36 percent	13 percent
1990	34 percent	12 percent

Various health authorities endorse the goals of ten percent saturated fat calories and 30 percent total fat calories; these goals are certainly in sight. Some feel that the goals are far too high, however, and would prefer 25 percent fat calories or even 10 percent.

Despite the reduction in fat calories, the survey revealed an overall increase in calories of about 231 per day, resulting in a substantial increase in the number of overweight Americans.

What's Wrong with Fat

In the 1950s the original charge against fats was that the saturated versions cause heart disease. This remains valid, but by the 1990s other reasons for reducing fat were being found.

Breast cancer: There are many well-known reasons why excessive fat is bad for a person's health. Besides a greater risk of heart disease, diabetes, and a shorter life in general, researchers in the early 1990s found links between fat and breast cancer. Other studies, however, showed no connection.

As is often the case in trying to relate diet and health, the most suggestive information comes from comparing populations from different nations. Ethnic groups that eat less fatty food throughout their lives have fewer cases of breast cancer. People in Japan, for example, eat much less fat than Americans do and the breast cancer rate in Japan is about a fourth of what it is in the U.S. Significantly, women from Japanese backgrounds who are born and grow up in the U.S. have the same high breast cancer rates as other Americans.

However, detailed studies of diet and breast cancer in the U.S. do not seem support the hypothesis linking breast cancer with fat intake. A study of 5,485 women showed no link. A larger study of 35,000 women in Iowa also failed to corroborate a correlation of fat intake and breast cancer incidence. Research by Walter C. Willitt of Brigham and Women's Hospital in Boston, published on October 21, 1992 in the *Journal of the American Medical Association,* apparently confirmed the absence of a relation between fat and breast cancer. Among 89,494 nurses studied for eight years, the lowest 20 percent as rated by fat consumption had the same rate of breast cancer as the highest 20 percent, even though the ones in the low group received only 25 percent of their calories from fat. (The high group got 49 percent of their calories from fat.) Other recognized risk factors for breast cancer, such as a late pregnancy or an early first menstrual period, did produce an increase in cancer rates. Fat, however, did not.

A May 1993 study by Stephanie J. London and coworkers from the Massachusetts General Hospital and the School of Public Health at Harvard University compared nearly 400 women with breast cancer to about the same number of women with no tumors and nearly half as many with benign breast tumors. They found that the body fat in the three populations had about the same chemical composition—that is, there were no significant differences in the amounts of saturated fats, polyunsaturated fats, monounsaturated fats, trans fatty acids, and omega 3 fatty acids. The researchers also found no difference in levels of such antioxidants as beta carotene and vitamin E. Total amount of fat and distribution of fat, both of which have also been suggested as part of the problem, were not studied.

Prostate cancer: A study reported in the October 6, 1993 *Journal of the National Cancer Institute* showed a link between fat and prostate cancer. The prostate cancer study by Edward Giovannucci of the Harvard Medical School in Boston and coworkers found that a high consumption of monounsaturated fats increase the risk that prostate cancer would progress to a deadly stage. It did not find a connection between increased fat consumption and the onset of prostate cancer.

Lung cancer: Two studies in 1993 reported that men and women who eat a low-fat diet have fewer cases of lung cancer, even when consumption of vegetables and fruits is average. One study looked at women nonsmokers between the ages of 30 and 84 in Missouri; it found that women whose diet produced more than 40 percent of calories from fat were highest in risk for lung cancer.

Fat Surprises

Margarine   Millions of Americans tolerated margarine during World War II, when butter was in short supply. Margarine or oleomargarine or "oleo" is a nineteenth-century invention intended as a substitute for butter. Although the first margarine in 1868 used butter as one ingredient, later versions were based on vegetable oils such as soybean oil, corn oil, cottonseed oil, or even sunflower or rapeseed oils. Most Americans returned to butter after the war.

A decade after the war, however, many went back to margarine when the role of cholesterol in heart disease was made clear. Animal fats and some vegetable fats that were high in hydrogen (saturated) had been shown to raise levels of blood cholesterol. The less saturated fats in margarine were preferable, although observant nutritionists realized from the beginning that the partial saturation needed to achieve a semi-solid butter substitute was less desirable than the "polyunsaturation" of liquid vegetable oils.

Between 1990 and 1992, however, beginning with a Dutch study in 1990, scientists found that the partial saturation in margarine was more harmful than anyone had suspected. The process of converting liquid vegetable oils to semi-solid form produces a group of fats that are known as *trans fatty acids.* The Dutch study showed that the trans fatty acids actually raise the blood level of the "bad" low-density lipoprotein (LDL) cholesterol that clogs arteries, while lowering the level of the "good" high-density lipoproteins (HDL) that tend to scour out arteries. Alarmed, the U.S. Institute of Shortening and Vegetable Oils asked the U.S. Department of Agriculture (USDA) to review and extend the Dutch study, presumably in hopes of showing that it was false. But the USDA confirmed Dutch results.

These conclusions apply only to solidified fats as they are used at home, but there are implications for fast-food chains as well. In an effort to get away from saturated fats such as beef tallow, fast-food chains since 1990, some chains even earlier, have used vegetable oils for deep frying foods like french fries. But because saturated fats stay fresh longer, some chains substituted solid margarine for tallow. Consequently, nutritionists now regard the new fast-food french fries as no improvement over the pre-1990 variety from the point of view of heart disease risk.

The Morning After   When you drink too much alcohol in the evening, you are not surprised if you have a hangover the next morning. When you eat a high-fat meal in the evening, however, you do not expect to wake up with a heart attack. Yet, according to statistics, that can happen. In January 1993 George J. Miller of the Medical Research Council in London, England, told the American Heart Association's conference of science writers that the reason most heart attacks occur in the morning is very likely that most high-fat meals occur in the evening. His studies of middle-aged men in London showed that levels of the blood-clotting chemical factor VII are raised by a high-fat meal. Higher levels of factor VII could theoretically cause heart attacks in those with already clogged arteries.

It's Good for You   It fits with common sense that fat, evident in gross overweight, might be a factor in heart disease, as was first established in the 1950s. Fat people therefore have shorter lives than thin people, according to common wisdom. You are never too thin, as a popular saying goes. A telephone survey conducted for the American Dietetic Association found that 29 percent of its 1000 respondents agreed with the statement: "It's important to totally eliminate fat from the diet."

Consequently, when careful studies showed that people who were too thin actually led shorter lives than those who might by some standards be viewed as too large, people were surprised. Parents were also surprised to learn that young children should not be on fat-reduced diets, though obesity in children should also be avoided. One obesity expert, Wayne Calloway of George Washington University, reports that low-fat diets below the age of 17 to 20 can retard growth.

Furthermore, in an animal study reported in the November 1993 *American Journal of Clinical Nutrition,* fish oil (high in omega-3 fats) was found to ward off sudden-death heart attacks. Earlier research has also suggested beneficial effects from omega-3 fats in fish oil.

Some Fat Helps Weight Loss   A study of fat in mice, reported in *Nature* in December 1993, showed that mice bred to have reduced amounts of one kind of fat, known as brown fat or brown adipose tissue, became obese. In other words, brown fat prevents the development of high body weight.

The reduced-brown-fat mice studied by Bradford Lowell and coworkers at Harvard Medical School were bred in two varieties. One strain had about 70 percent as much brown fat as normal mice, and grew to be massively obese. The other type had even less brown fat, but after they started out as obese young mice, the brown fat returned and they became normal adults. Brown fat has long been suspected to have a role in maintaining normal weight since it burns more calories than it needs just to sustain normal cellular operations.

(Periodical References and Additional Reading: *New York Times* 10-7-92, p A1; *New York Times* 10-11-92, p IV-2; *New York Times* 10-21-92, p C12; *Science News* 1-9-93, p 23; *New York Times* 1-21-93, p A18; *New York Times* 5-19-93, p A13; *Science News* 10-9-93, p 228; *New York Times* 12-28-93, p C5; *Science News* 12-4-93, pp 373, 380; *Harvard Health Letter* 1-94, p 8; *New York Times* 1-12-94, p C10; *New York Times* 3-8-94, p C6)

Cholesterol UPDATE

The Third National Health and Nutrition Examination Survey conducted by the National Center for Health Statistics released early in 1994, and previewed in June 1993 revealed average cholesterol readings for the U.S. population in 1978 and 1990.

The average in the earlier year was 213 milligrams of cholesterol in 100 milliliters of blood serum, but it had dropped eight milligrams to 205 milligrams by 1990. The reduction is consistent with figures showing a slight drop from 13 to 12 percent in the amount of saturated fat in the American diet between those years.

The average figures and the effect of diet on cholesterol are not the whole story, however. Exact figures are difficult to come by, but it is believed that blood cholesterol levels were higher than 240 milligrams per 100 milliliters of blood serum—a level considered too high for good health—in perhaps as many as 26 percent of all U.S. adults in the late 1970s. By the early 1990s, that percentage had dropped to about 20 percent, largely as a result of diet changes but also in some cases because of the use of cholesterol-lowering drugs. A decline in alcohol consumption also has affected total cholesterol levels, although evidence suggests that lower use of alcohol primarily results in lower levels of high-density lipoproteins (HDL), the "good" cholesterol.

This latest drop in cholesterol levels is part of a 30-year trend that accelerated through the 1980s and early 1990s. At the same time both cigarette smoking and the incidence of hypertension decreased. The consequence of these changes is a 54 percent decline in heart disease in the U.S.

At the same time the U.S. National Cholesterol Education Program, chaired by Scott M. Grundy of the University of Texas's Southwestern Medical Center at Dallas issued new guidelines, suggesting cholesterol reduction through low fat diet and exercise, and not through cholesterol lowering drugs. The report also urged more frequent measurement of HDL levels, with both HDL and total cholesterol to be measured at least once every five years in adults.

A Look at Low Cholesterol

Too little cholesterol is also connected with higher death rates, but the reason for this is poorly understood. Several studies in the early 1990s which were primarily intended to examine the effects of high cholesterol also found as a sort of bonus that cholesterol levels below 160 milligrams per 100 milliliters of blood are associated with increased mortality. But there are multiple causes of death for people with low cholesterol, in contrast to the increased risks of heart attacks and stroke for people with high cholesterol. For example, the deaths that seem to increase with low cholesterol are due to a variety of conditions including liver cancer, noncancerous lung disease, intracranial hemorrhage, suicides, and homicides. One possibility is that some conditions that lead to higher death rates also produce low cholesterol levels, although the exact connection is not known. For example, the list of causes of death is suspiciously similar to common causes of death linked to alcoholism, and alcohol is known to affect cholesterol levels, usually by increasing the ratio of HDL cholesterol to LDL.

In an interview on this subject, Dean Ornish of the University of California—San Francisco noted the links between alcohol damage to the liver and low cholesterol, and added that depression (often linked to alcoholism, though not by Ornish in this interview) typically led to poor diets that might contribute to low cholesterol as well as to high rates of suicide. The situation with regard to intracranial hemorrhaging, an uncommon kind of stroke, is different from the others listed. Ornish speculated that lower blood cholesterol might reduce blood's clotting ability and thus be involved in that risk, which would be a trade-off with the much more prevalent type of stroke, for which the risk is increased by high blood cholesterol levels.

The idea that low cholesterol levels and higher death rates are connected to alcohol abuse tended to be confirmed by the Honolulu Heart Program, a study of men of Japanese ancestry in Hawaii. An analysis by Carol Iribarren of the University of Southern California reported in March 1993 that of the 8000 men in the study, only low-cholesterol men who were heavy drinkers, heavy smokers, or afflicted with gastrointestinal diseases had higher death rates. Healthy moderate drinkers or smokers or abstainers from alcohol and tobacco who had low cholesterol levels did not have elevated death rates.

Cholesterol Briefs

- In March 1993 a researcher reported in the *American Journal of Clinical Nutrition* that nibbling produces less serum cholesterol than eating three large meals a day, even when calorie intake remains unchanged. Nine meals a day was the standard set for the nibblers.
- In August 1993 Richard R. Love's study in the *Journal of the National Cancer Institute* showed that the cancer drug tamoxifen drastically reduced levels of serum cholesterol.
- In November 1993 Richard B. Weinberg reported that a mutant gene allows some people escape danger from high cholesterol. (*See* "The State of Genetic Medicine," p 19.)

(Periodical References and Further Reading: *New York Times* 8-16-92, p IV-2; *New York Times* 8-19-92, p C4; *New York Times* 3-21-93, p I-25; *New York Times* 6-16-93, p A18; *Science News* 6-19-93, p 390; *Science News* 9-25-93, p 207; *Science News* 11-20-93, p 325; *New York Times* 2-9-94, p C13; *New York Times* 3-8-94, p C6)

FOOD PRESERVATION AND PROTECTION

At least since World War II, food scientists have been experimenting with using radiation to preserve food. The idea is not that dissimilar to canning, in which high temperatures kill bacteria and render enzymes inactive (active enzymes cause chemical changes in food that contribute to the rotting process). A significant difference between irradiation and canning is that radioactivity, and not heat, kills the bacteria and inactivates the enzymes. In addition, although canning has been accepted for nearly 200 years, legions of critics continue to attack food irradiation as unsafe.

The argument against food preservation by irradiation is as follows: Gamma rays, the penetrating component of radiation, not only kill bacteria and parasites and inactivate enzymes, but they also they knock electrons out of molecules, producing free radicals. In some cases, these are the same free radicals we try to eliminate with vitamins C and E and beta carotene. Free radicals also contribute to new and sometimes unknown chemical combinations, called *radiolytic products,* in irradiated

Background

The word *radiation* has a broad meaning, and can refer to any part of the electromagnetic spectrum from radio waves through light and X rays and beyond. The same word is often used for other phenomenon that transmit energy through empty space. Since physicists have shown that all short waves act like particles and all small particles act like waves, it is reasonable to use the same word for both forms of transfer of energy. Light, for example, can be treated as the small particles called *photons,* while electrons are used as waves in an electron microscope. In the context of food preservation, radiation is high-energy wave/particles produced by radioactive substances. Such radiation is often referred to as *ionizing radiation,* meaning that it has enough energy to move large numbers of electrons from their normal places in atoms. In quantum theory, even low-energy radiation, such as light, can ionize some atoms some of the time, but with a very low probability. The probability becomes higher with increasing energy.

The most common radioactive sources of radiation are the artificial isotopes (forms of atoms not found in nature) cobalt-60 or cesium-137, both also used in medicine as a source of radiation. The main radiation from these metallic sources is a high-energy form of electromagnetism known as gamma rays. Cobalt-60 produces gamma rays with about twice the energy of cesium-137. In food irradiation, food is exposed to gamma rays from the source from various directions for about 45 minutes.

Gamma rays are simply higher-energy X rays. In a crude analogy to the light spectrum, gamma rays are to X rays what violet is to blue, while radio waves are like red, while visible light is like green. The only difference is the frequency. A higher frequency brings along more energy with it. When thought of as photons, gamma rays are just maximum energy photons.

Cobalt-60 and cesium-137 also emit beta rays, which are electrons. Beta rays do not penetrate very far into matter and are usually not considered when thinking about radioactive preservation of food because the energy of the beta rays from cobalt-60 or cesium-137 is hundreds of times less than that of the energy from gamma rays. Electrons also create free radicals, however, when they attach themselves to stray molecules or knock other electrons out of atoms. Beta rays of the same energy as gamma rays are considered to have the same degree of biological damage when considering radiation as a hazard, while alpha rays (energetic helium nuclei produced in some radioactive decay, but not involved in radioactive food preservation) are 20 times as dangerous.

Some forms of radiation can induce radioactivity in other materials, but gamma rays and beta rays cannot. The most likely way to induce radiation is by radiation of neutral particles called neutrons.

food. Some of the known radiolytic products have been identified as carcinogens, e.g. benzene and formaldehyde.

Using radioactive sources is most common in medicine, where strong radiation is a common way to treat cancer. Other uses of radiation include sterilization of bandages and medical equipment and also tampons and condoms.

The U.S. Food and Drug Administration (FDA) finally decided to permit irradiated food to come to market. Permission was given to use a measure equivalent to a hundred thousand rads of radiation on fruits, vegetables, fresh pork, and cereal products. The explanation given by the FDA for permitting this form of food preservation is based on the view that irradiation causes fewer chemical changes, or free radicals, than canning or cooking. An FDA spokesperson puts the amount of radiolytic products in food preserved by radiation as 30 parts per million. Animal experiments have not shown any harm from consumption of irradiated food. Gamma rays do not render irradiated food, or other materials, radioactive.

Irradiation, like other methods of food preservation, reduces the amount of some nutrients. Vitamins A, C, and E—just the ones that would combat the free radicals produced by radiation—lose as much as a quarter of their effectiveness.

Strawberries were apparently the first irradiated food to reach the market. They were sold in January 1992 in Florida. (Herbs and spices used in sausages and preserved meats had been quietly sterilized through irradiation for some time.) Nonsprouting potatoes are not far behind.

Vegetables are not the only target. Two strains of bacteria prevalent in poultry and meat—*Salmonella* and *Escherichia coli* 0157:H7 (the cause of the Jack-in-the-Box epidemic; *see* "Promises and Perils of Meat," p 156) can be killed by radiation. An article by the U.S. Department of Agriculture's Food Safety Research Unit in the April 1993 *Journal of Applied Environmental Microbiology* reports that radiation effectively kills *E. coli* in meat. The American Meat Institute endorses radiation as a means of sterilization for safety—it is more like pasteurization than like canning.

(Periodical References and Additional Reading: *Harvard Health Letter* 8-92, p 1; *Scientific American* 6-93, p 132; *Discover* 1-93, p 44)

OTHER WELLNESS ISSUES

EXERCISE AND HEALTH

Although surveys still show that most people in the U.S. are "couch potatoes" to a certain degree, or simply seem unwilling to exercise, these findings sometimes appear incredible. Urban, suburban, and even some rural roadways are clogged with joggers and walkers for health, a few lifting small weights as they move along. In the winter, cross-country skiing, which is almost pure exercise, has suddenly become popular. Sales of home exercise devices—many unheard of a quarter of a century ago—keep many manufacturers in profits. Health clubs, where swimming, strenuous games, and fancier equipment can be found, are in nearly every community.

However, when, in October 1993, the President's Council for Fitness asked 1018 Americans who were among the estimated 66 percent who do not exercise, what their future exercise plans were, a different picture emerged. Sixty-four percent of respondents, 84 percent of whom watch three or more hours of television each week, said that they knew they should exercise more, but did not have the time. Two out of five of the sedentary people surveyed showed little inclination to exercise in any case, reporting that they were unlikely to start or that they would not exercise even if they had a fitness center at their workplace.

Part of the reason that the "sweaty minority" is working out regularly is cosmetic; people have learned that a firm body is attractive. But the basic reason for exercise activity in the early 1990s is health. Since the 1950s, when running first started competing with golf as a suitable outdoor activity, virtually every popular health writer and family doctor has urged exercise as a way to maintain cardiovascular fitness and reduce the risk of heart disease. Furthermore, because exercise contributes to weight reduction, it is helpful in preventing type II diabetes and its complications, which range from impotence to eye disorders. Given the awareness that fat has something to do with certain forms of cancer, some experts have suggested that fat-reducing exercise may prevent cancer. Indeed, exercise is generally believed to ward off most ills.

A study published in the February 25, 1993, issue of the *New England Journal of Medicine* found that middle-aged or older men could add months to their life by taking up vigorous exercise. (The months could be extended to years by giving up tobacco at the same time.) The main benefit for the elderly is a reduced incidence of heart attacks. Which is, of course, why people are so surprised when noted runners or athletes suddenly die young, often while exercising. But this happens seldom, while some authorities attribute about 250,000 deaths in the U.S. annually to lack of exercise.

On July 29, 1993, the U.S. Federal Centers for Disease Control and Prevention and the American College of Sports medicine announced at a press briefing that they thought only 22 percent of Americans exercised enough—but also that it was not necessary to work very hard at exercise. The main point of the gathering, however, was to say that they were changing their recommendation for exercise: instead of three to five periods of vigorous, continued activity each week, the new goal for every

American was milder exercise—the equivalent of walking briskly for a half hour—at least five days a week. It would not be necessary, however, to perform all the activity in 30-minute periods. A few moments of climbing stairs or light gardening here and there would suffice. Comments at the press conference indicated that although the spokespersons for CDC and the College of Sports medicine still preferred the continuous periods of active exercise, they were willing to compromise, since Americans had refused to take their initial advice.

Blood Pressure

Although various factors are thought to be involved in the recent declines in heart disease in the U.S. and other industrialized countries, reduction of blood pressure is high on the list and, in the view of some, actually accounts by itself for all of the decline. (This argument is based on the idea that not enough people have changed their diets or taken up exercise to account for the observed declines.) While blood pressure can be reduced by losing weight and quitting smoking, the primary reason for reduced blood pressure in the U.S. is the use of various drugs that lower blood pressure.

A study reported in the October 1993 *Circulation* not only reports on blood pressure lowering as a result of regular exercise, but also provides an explanation for

HARDENING OF THE ARTERIES?

Fifty years ago the expression "hardening of the arteries" was used to describe the cause of many of the problems of the elderly, including symptoms that would now be attributed to Alzheimer's disease. When the link between dietary cholesterol, saturated fat, and artery disease was made in the 1950s, many people, including much of the popular press, assumed that the artery disease in question was "hardening of the arteries," but as knowledge of the situation increased, writers began carefully to distinguish between *atherosclerosis,* the build-up of plaque inside arteries caused in part by some forms of cholesterol, and *arteriosclerosis,* which was identified as hardening of the arteries.

Probably the main symptom of arteriosclerosis observable to the afflicted person is pain in the lower legs during exercise, which abates almost as soon as the exercise stops. Sometimes there is also pain in the toes while resting, e.g., in bed; the pain can be relieved by dangling the feet over the end of the bed. More damaging, but less noticeable, is increased blood pressure. Arteriosclerosis is considered the main reason blood pressure tends to increase with age.

The reason arteries become stiffer and lose elasticity with age is the loss of the protein elastin, whose name says it all. Elastin gets replaced with other proteins in the walls of the blood vessels as people become older. Stiffening of the arteries would be a more accurate description than "hardening," an expression that incorrectly suggests that arteries become stonelike in old age.

how it works. One reason the blood pressure rises with increasing age is that arteries lose flexibility.

Edward G. Lakatta of the U.S. National Institute on Aging (NIA) and coworkers used two different approaches to find the effect of exercise on arteries. In one study, they took 146 healthy nonexercisers and put them on treadmills. The more flexible the arteries were, the longer it took the person to become exhausted on the treadmill. The second approach was to look at people who exercised hard on a regular basis — the subjects were 15 men from age 54 to 75 who jogged at least 30 miles every week. Those exercisers were found to have 30 percent less stiff arteries than nonexercisers matched for age and other health habits.

The interpretation of the NIA study is that exercise slows down the rise in blood pressure associated with age. This was not demonstrated directly, however. Further research is planned to find if there is any direct effect of moderate exercise on blood pressure resulting from arteriosclerosis. A small earlier study, by James A. Blumenthal at Duke University and coworkers in 1991, had found that no form of exercise lowered blood pressure in sedentary people with moderately elevated pressure. (All participants experienced a slight lowering caused by "the Hawthorne effect," a result that comes simply from participating in a study, whether they exercised or not.)

Other Health Benefits

Since 1985 the American Cancer Society has listed exercise among the ten steps a person should take to possibly avoid cancer. The rationale for this may not be obvious, since cancer is caused by changes in genes, and exercise does not have a clear or direct effect on DNA. But studies show that people, especially women, who exercise, engage in formal athletics, or do well on a treadmill test have lower death rates from cancer. Estrogen seems to be involved. Women who are athletes have lower rates of breast cancer and cancer of the reproductive organs, possibly because they have less fat which in turn results in less estrogen in the blood.

Changes in the incidence of colon cancer reflect the beneficial effects of exercise. According to the hypothesis linking exercise with lower colon cancer rates, exercise moves wastes through the body faster, thus diminishing the colon's exposure to toxins. One study looked at 17,000 Harvard alumni and found that the exercisers among them had considerably fewer cases of colon cancer than those who were sedentary.

There is also a number of theories that suggesting exercise may strengthen the immune system, which would not only aid in reducing cancer of all kinds, but would also lead to less infectious disease. Moderate exercise has been shown to raise levels of immune cells and their products for a limited time after exercise. And the body temperature rise that accompanies exercise is like a little fever, perhaps aiding the immune system as illness-induced fever seems to do.

(Periodical References and Additional Reading: *New York Times* 10-16-91, p A22; *New York Times* 2-25-93, p B7; *New York Times* 7-7-93, p C11; *New York Times* 7-30-93, p A1; *Science News* 10-16-93, p 246; *New York Times* 11-7-93, p 28)

TO SLEEP

As the 1990s progressed, there were some hints that another health movement might join or replace diet and exercise as the mainstays of wellness—i.e., sleep. Even Jane Brody of health column and healthy cookbook fame admitted in 1994 that she was "sleep deprived." Since people spend considerable time sleeping, although perhaps not the "half your life" or even "a third of your life" that is often mentioned, sleep is an important aspect of wellness.

Since 1980 it has been known that cycles of light and darkness affect various body functions in humans. Indeed, prominent health topics in the early 1990s included considerable thought and experimentation on using light to "reset the internal clock" of shift workers or international travelers. The concept of Seasonal Affective Disorder (SAD), winter depression thought to be caused by deprivation of daylight, gained new respectability. In 1992 researchers at the Oregon Health Sciences University in Portland also identified melatonin as a second biological messenger, along with light, that sets or resets the body's rhythm, known as the body's "clock." Melatonin pills can also be used to reset that clock even in the blind.

But the newly emerging story was not on how light affects sleep, but on how sleep may be related to bodily functioning.

Why Sleep?

The short answer to the question "why sleep?" is that you will die if you do not, although evidence for humans is anecdotal. For animals—at least for rats—there has been no doubt of this truth since experiments in 1983. Rats deprived of sleep for about three weeks die, although there is no apparent symptom of ill health. In 1993, however, Carol Everson of the U.S. National Institute of Mental Health conducted a thorough study of bacteria in the blood of rats that had been killed by sleep deprivation. She concluded that bacteria that normally have no ill effects on health somehow multiply in late stages of sleep deprivation and kill the rats. The apparent reason is that sleep deprivation weakens the immune system.

There are other reasons to suspect that sleep has some relation to the immune system in humans. One clue is found in a possible genetic basis for narcolepsy, which is the inability to prevent falling asleep, or the compulsion to fall asleep whatever the circumstances. Actually, people with narcolepsy (narcoleptics) may fall asleep when they don't want to, but they often fail to sleep properly when they want to; a person can thus be both a narcoleptic and an insomniac. As early as 1983, Japanese researchers found possible links between narcolepsy and a specific immune condition in about 90 percent of narcoleptics. In the April 15, 1991, *Proceedings of the National Academy of Sciences,* Emmanuel Mignot and coworkers from Stanford University School of Medicine reported on their genetic study of narcoleptic dogs. Some inbred lines of Dobermans and Labradors have high percentages of dogs that behave like narcoleptic humans. The Stanford team found that the gene in the affected dogs is similar to the gene that in humans controls production of antibodies. Thus a defect in the immune system might be a cause of narcolepsy, although narcolepsy has probably more than one cause.

Another clue to the link between sleep and the immune system is that people with AIDS are tired and sleepy during the day to a greater extent than what their symptoms would indicate. Since AIDS is fundamentally a virus-caused defect of the immune system, drowsiness in AIDS patients could also be connected to the immune system. Indeed, researcher Dennis Darko found that one component of the immune system—a chemical called tumor necrosis factor—increases and decreases in synchrony with sleep waves in most people but fails to follow this pattern in people with AIDS.

Tumor necrosis factor is one of the immune system messenger chemicals called cytokines. Another well-known cytokine is interleukin-1. Both of these chemicals were investigated by James Krueger of the University of Tennessee—Memphis as possible causes of sleep. When injected into animal brains, he discovered, these cytokines induced sleep, as he reported in 1993 at the annual meeting of the Society for Sleep Research. Other speakers at the same convention also linked the immune system to sleep. For example, David Dinges of the University of Pennsylvania found that healthy sleep-deprived people had increased amounts of several of the immune-system cells, notably the monocytes, granulocytes, and macrophages, as well as higher levels of cytokines.

Interestingly, this all ties into a theory, first propounded by Krueger in 1980, stating that macrophages operating in the small intestine during the day produce chemicals, including cytokines and protein fragments, which build up gradually and eventually cause sleepiness. Darko notes that the cytokine he has been investigating (tumor necrosis factor) is related to movements of the small intestine that push food wastes into the colon. The pattern of pushing is synchronized with sleep patterns, as recorded in studies of sleepers' brain waves.

Failure to Fall Asleep

Some people feel sleep deprived because they cannot fall asleep as quickly or when they want to or because they wake up too soon. Insomnia is one of the major symptoms of clinical depression, but it also strikes the healthy at times. As many as one in four people over 65, for example, reports insomnia as a problem in their lives.

One research effort to correct insomnia used an instrument that creates a low-energy electrical field in the vicinity of the brain. Insomniac volunteers held such a device or a look-alike placebo in their mouths for 20 minutes three times a week. Although neither the doctor nor the insomniac knew which was which, when the records were checked at the end of a month, those who used an actual emitter fell asleep 52 minutes earlier and slept 1.5 hours longer on average than the controls. The study using the device was directed by Milton K. Erman of the Scripps Clinic and Research Foundation in La Jolla, California, and reported at the 1991 annual meeting of the Bioelectromagnetic Society.

Another study of insomnia, directed by Charles M. Morin of the Virginia Commonwealth University in Richmond, showed that cognitive-behavior therapy—which involves much more than simply telling people to stop fretting and go to sleep—was effective in more than half of the 23 older insomniacs who received the training. The idea that education about sleep may contribute to an insomnia cure could become more popular than holding an electrical device in one's mouth for an hour a week.

(Periodical References and Additional Reading: *Science News* 4-27-91, p 271; *Science News* 7-6-91, p 15; *New York Times* 11-3-92, p C1; *Science News* 3-6-93, p 156; *New York Times* 8-3-93, p C1; *Science* 11-19-93, p 1207)

Dental Health UPDATE

Dental health is partly the business of professionals and partly the responsibility of the individual. In *Handbook of Current Health and Medicine*, however, the subject is addressed in articles with an emphasis on individual responsibility. It is largely up to the individual not only to take care of his or her own teeth, but also to regularly visit to a dentist, and also a periodontist, for professional care of teeth and gums.

The widespread use of fluorides, as well as other healthy practices, has apparently resulted in less need for some aspects of professional dental care. In the United States, children in the early 1990s developed fewer than half as many cavities as children did in the 1970s. Opponents of fluorides point out, however, that in several studies in the late 1980s fluorides were shown to cause cancer. The U.S. Environmental Protection Agency (EPA) announced on January 3, 1991, that it would take another look at the fluoride issue. More than two years later the U.S. National Research Council, assigned to the task by the EPA, gave fluorides the seal of approval (*See* "Minerals UPDATE," p 168).

Gum Disease and Losing Teeth

Gums are a different story from cavities, however. A 1992 survey by the Harvard School of Dental Medicine and the New England Research Institute found that gum disease in the elderly had increased over the amount found in previous studies. About 86 percent of the persons over the age of 70 had at least some amount of gum disease. Gum disease is even more the responsibility of the individual than is tooth decay, but treatment is increasingly high-tech work performed by periodontists. Proper cleaning of teeth, which usually involves more than brushing, prevents or greatly reduces plaque build-up that has been identified as the first step toward bone-destroying (and therefore tooth-destroying) gum disease. After disease has developed, new surgical methods using freeze-dried bone or synthetic materials can build up lost bone or redirect blood flow to favor beneficial changes in the gums. Experimental techniques also include new ways to deliver antibiotics to places where they are needed to fight gum disease.

Despite all efforts, advanced periodontal disease can lead to tooth loss in individuals who—although it happens seldom—have not lost their teeth for some other reason. The last available survey, from 1986, showed that 42 percent of Americans 65 or older had lost *all* of their teeth; often loose and troublesome teeth are deliberately removed, but even healthy teeth are sometimes taken out to allow a better set of bridgework. It is widely believed that a similar survey taken today would show many fewer missing teeth.

Increasingly, missing teeth are replaced by individual artificial teeth directly implanted into the bone of the jaw—an *implant*, for short. The implant was invented in

Sweden in 1977 and ten years later over a hundred thousand had been installed in the U.S.. The number is still rising: in 1990 there were 435,700 implants in the U.S., and hundreds of thousands more around the world. The rise would probably even be swifter if the cost of an implant were not much higher than the next best artificial alternatives. The exact price ratios are difficult to establish, since each implant costs about the same no matter how many are installed, while the cost of a bridge, or a set of dentures, does not rise according to the number of teeth being replaced.

In another alternative for those who still have some jawbone, a natural tooth already implanted in bone can be saved from removal by killing it in place and filling the nerve cavity with a neutral material (often the rubberlike gutta percha). That process, known familiarly as a root canal, was used about 13 million times in the U.S. in 1991, so it is almost 30 times as common as using an implant. Animal research suggests that the number of root canal operations, which are painful and costly, can be reduced by use of a human protein that causes bone growth, known as OP-1 (for "osteogenic protein 1"). Although drilling into the tooth would still be needed for insertion of the OP-1 into the tooth's interior, there would be less drilling than necessitated by a traditional root canal. Provided it works in humans, once in the tooth, OP-1 would cause dentin, the main part of the interior of the tooth, to grow and harden, protecting the living pulp. The tooth would be left alive, a clear gain, since a root canal procedure effectively kills the tooth. As far as cost is concerned—the OP-1 procedure might even be more expensive than a root canal, reaching the price of an implant—but many people would surely choose less pain and a living tooth over more pain and a dead tooth. Human trials with OP-1, approved by the U.S. Food and Drug Administration in July 1993, are expected to continue into 1994.

A Mouth Full of Metal

In December 1990 the popular television show *60 Minutes* ran a segment on how dental fillings made from amalgam leak toxic mercury into the body. (*See* "Danger from Mercury," p 250.) Amalgam, the most popular form of tooth filler, is half mercury and half other metals. The inspiration for the segment was research demonstrating that sheep who had teeth filled with amalgam absorbed mercury into their tissues. Studies conducted by Fritz J. Lorscheider and Murray J. Vimy of the University of Calgary Medical School in Alberta, and published in August 1990 and in November 1990, showed that monkeys and sheep with amalgam dental fillings accumulated enough mercury in body tissues to cause an observable decline in kidney function. The actual evidence that this occurred was slight and much disputed by dentists.

Earlier in 1990 the Swedish Health Administration recommended that dentists cease using fillings made from amalgam as soon as possible. The Health Administration called amalgam "unsuitable and toxic." Furthermore, the Swedish government banned outright the use of amalgam fillings in pregnant women, starting in 1991. Researchers in Sweden and at the University of California Dental School had tested cadavers that had several amalgam fillings for mercury. The tests showed the cadavers to contain as much as three times the mercury in the brain and nine times the amount in the kidneys as controls with no fillings.

These findings (and *60 Minutes*) prompted the first review of amalgam by the U.S.

Food and Drug Administration (FDA) since the 1970s. In the 1970s the FDA approved the amalgam filling, explaining that the alloy is widely employed and not known to have caused problems other than rare allergic reactions. The allergic reactions are more often due to the copper or silver in the amalgam than to the mercury. Amalgam has been used in dental fillings for at least 150 years; more than one American in ten has amalgam fillings.

The FDA reported in 1991 that its review showed that amalgam is still safe and could continue to be used in dental fillings. Alternative materials—gold, ceramics, and plastics—are generally more expensive and harder for dentists to install. Furthermore, plastic, the least expensive of the group, causes more allergic reactions than amalgam does.

Chewing Gum for Dental Health

For generations, some chewing gum manufacturers have implied or openly stated that chewing their brand of gum would somehow improve dental health. But dentists have doubted such claims because the bacteria that produce dental caries (decay) thrive on sugar, a traditional gum-sweetener. Brands containing artificial sweeteners, however, have received a half-hearted endorsement from some dentists.

Dentists may be more enthusiastic about gums containing the sweetener xylitol, used in some sugarless gums. Xylitol is not a low-calorie substitute for sugar, but a natural sweetener found in small amounts in fruits and vegetables. Commercial xylitol is made from cornstalks. In March 1993 Kauko K. Makinen, a University of Michigan biochemist, told a meeting of the International Association for Dental Research that, according to his study of children between the ages of nine and 11 who chewed either xylitol gum or sugar-sweetened (with sucrose) gum for several months, a dental health test based on cavities and other tooth problems showed a two-to-one score advantage in favor of the group using xylitol gum. Makinen thinks that xylitol actually promotes the sealing of small cavities as they develop. Also, bacteria do not break down xylitol as easily as they do sugar.

Another natural sweetener, sorbitol, was also tested in the study, and average dental health scores for children using sorbitol gum were halfway between the sugar scores and the xylitol scores.

Going Under

Although modern high-speed dental drills make minor tooth repair tasks completely pain free, many patients do not believe this. Indeed, there are other, more invasive, dental procedures that still cause considerable pain. When effective anesthesia was developed in the nineteenth century, dentists were the first to discard whisky and biting bullets in favor of ether, chloroform, and nitrous oxide ("laughing gas") . The tradition of general anesthesia in dentistry is longer than in any other branch of medicine. This tradition does not make dentists into anesthetists, however, and, according to various estimates, about one in 350,000 to one in 860,000 dental visits ends in death from the effects of general anesthesia.

Many patients undergo complex root canals and dental surgery with only local

anesthetics, but some persons are so terrified of dental pain, even in minor procedures, that they refuse to settle for local anesthesia. Many dentists offer them conscious sedation. This method provides the patient enough of an oral drug such as
valium or chloral hydrate (the traditional "Mickey Finn"), or perhaps a small amount
of laughing gas, to alleviate fears and provide relaxation. Meanwhile, the normal
amount of local anesthetic, injected directly into the gums, acts as a pain block.
Neither local anesthetics nor conscious sedation poses a significant risk to patients,
though any medication can trigger an allergic reaction.

General anesthesia, however, can slow down heart function, and may even
suffocate a person whose breathing passages are blocked. Consequently, the American Dental Association in 1992 issued guidelines for dental anesthesia and in the early
1990s a number of U.S. states issued new laws regulating the practice. Most of the
new requirements involve education for the dentists, require the proper equipment
for monitoring patient health while under anesthesia, and recommend drugs for
correcting problems that arise. These rules may not be enough and the ADA is now
considering recommending two years of regular schooling in anesthesia for dentists
who wish to practice it.

(Periodical References and Additional Reading: *New York Times* 2-20-91; *Harvard Health Letter*
9-91, p 4; *Harvard Health Letter* 6-92, p 3; *Harvard Health Letter* 4-93, p 6; *Science News*
4-3-93, p 220; *New York Times* 6-16-93, p C13; *Scientific American* 11-93, p 106)

TIMETABLE OF DENTISTRY TO 1990

3000 BC	Tooth filling occurs in Sumer.
2250 BC	A Sumerian dialogue known as "The Worm and the Toothache," inscribed on a clay tablet about this time, in which a priest talks to the "tooth worm," is perhaps the earliest record of any form of dentistry.
1000 BC	Etruscan goldworkers are the earliest known makers of dental bridgework, mostly for cosmetic purposes.
1450	Gold is used for filling teeth.
1490	About this time, the Chinese invent the modern form of the toothbrush, with pig bristles at a right angle to the handle.
1530	The first book on dentistry is published in Leipzig.
1728	The post crown, an artificial top portion of a tooth mounted on a post inserted into the root canal, is introduced.
1756	Philipp Pfaff [born 1715; died 1767] publishes *Abhandlung von den Zähnen*, giving the first description of casting models to make false teeth.
1771	*The Natural History of the Human Teeth* by John Hunter [born East Kilbride, Scotland, February 13, 1728; died London, October 16, 1793] lays the foundations of dental anatomy and pathology.
1790	Around this time, porcelain begins to serve as a baseplate material for dentures, thereby replacing ivory, bone, and gold, all of which were hard to fit.
	American dentist Josiah Flagg [born circa 1763; died 1816] invents the dentist's chair.

1790	George Washington's dentist, John Greenwood [born Boston, May 17, 1760; died New York, November 16, 1819], invents the dental drill.
1828	Amalgam, a mercury alloy, is introduced to dentistry, but does not replace gold until about 1910, following experimental work by G. V. Black in 1895 that shows that mercury in amalgam is safe.
1832	The reclining dentist's chair is constructed, but manufactured versions do not become available until late in the 1860s.
1844	About this time, plaster of Paris begins to replace beeswax for making impressions of teeth.
1855	Robert Arthur introduces the technique of filling teeth with cohesive gold foil: he heats the foil to rid the surface of impurities and then cold-welds it in the cavity with pressure from instruments.
1857	Around this time, a special mixture of resins and soapstone known as impression compound begins to replace plaster of Paris for making impressions of teeth.
1858	The first practical powered dental drill, driven by a foot pedal, is constructed.
1860	Vulcanized rubber begins about this time to be used as a baseplate material for dentures, thereby replacing porcelain.
1864	S. C. Barnum invents the rubber dam for controlling saliva while working on teeth.
1872	The first electrically powered dental drill is constructed.
1874	The role of fluorides in preventing dental decay is discovered.
1882	The modern form of the saliva ejector for draining a patient's mouth during dental work is introduced.
1885	An American dentist, Dr. Scott, patents an electric toothbrush 75 years before the device would become common; it does not become a commercial success because the tool is too noisy and too expensive.
1889	Baked porcelain inlays for lost teeth are introduced.
1890	Cocaine is used as a local anesthetic in dentistry.
	The porcelain jacket crown to cover lost portions of teeth is introduced by C. H. Land; in the procedure, the dentist removes the enamel from the tooth and mounts a porcelain shell baked onto a platinum matrix over what is left of the tooth.
1904	Procaine, a local anesthetic, is discovered.
1906	Procaine is introduced as a local anesthetic in dentistry.
1907	W. V. Taggart introduces a practical method of casting gold inlays for teeth using wax impressions and lost-wax casting of molten gold, which is cemented in place after the inlay cools.
1918	Tooth implants, driven directly into a patient's jaw instead of being surgically implanted, as is done today, are introduced.
1945	Fluoridation of a water supply to prevent dental decay is introduced in the United States.
1952	Per-Ingvar Brånemark observes that a titanium microscope he is using to study

bone tissue has bonded to the bone; following up on this discovery, he learns by 1965 to make dental implants that bond to the jawbone.

1957   The high-speed dental drill is introduced, making it possible to work on teeth painlessly without anesthetics for simple fillings; it is driven by a tiny turbine powered by pressurized air.

1965   Harald Löe and co-workers demonstrate that lack of dental care, particularly brushing, allows plaque to build up, resulting in gingivitis—red, swollen, and bleeding gums—in a few days or weeks.

1967   Bonding using composite resins is developed as an alternative to filling teeth with metal alloys.

A 20-year study of fluoridation in Evanston, Illinois, shows that dental cavities have been reduced by 58 percent as a result of adding fluorides to the water supply.

1977   Per-Ingvar Brånemark in Sweden publishes convincing evidence that living bone tissue can be induced to grow in the jaw around the base of an implanted tooth, thereby producing a bond that usually lasts for many years.

ULTRAVIOLET RAYS FROM THE SUN

It has long been recognized that most skin cancer occurs in parts of the body exposed to the sun and that people who spend a lot of time in direct sunlight are more susceptible to skin cancer. Furthermore, there is considerable evidence that exposure to sunlight causes other changes in the skin, most notably the cluster of changes associated with aging. Although a "healthy tan" has been viewed as desirable since the 1920s—before that time the ideal, for European women at least, was milk-white skin—people are beginning to realize that sunlight does more harm than good. It may be better to get vitamin D from fortified milk or even pills than by too much solar exposure.

Because ultraviolet light (UV radiation) has more energy than visible light, it has long been suspected of being harmful. Higher-energy UV radiation causes the chemical changes in a suntan. Experiments have showed that the higher energy UV, which came to be called UV-B, not only caused tanning, but also possibly affected DNA. DNA damage is one of the chief causes of cancer. Furthermore, people with an ineffective allele of one of the genes for DNA repair are especially susceptible to melanoma, the most dangerous form of skin cancer.

More new cases of skin cancer are diagnosed each year than all other cancers combined. Skin cancer usually consists of easily treated squamous cell or basal cell cancer, with about 900,000 to about 1.2 million new U.S. cases each year; melanoma, a less common and more malignant form, of skin cancer, affecting about 32,000 Americans annually, is often fatal even with treatment. Melanoma has been rising in the U.S. as a fairly constant rate since the 1930s, and is now twelve times as likely to strike as then. The rise has been particularly concentrated in women under the age of 40, particularly those who spend time developing a tan. Sunburns, which result from UV-B radiation, are also thought to considerably increase the risk of melanoma.

Because of the accepted view ascribing the truly dangerous effects to UV-B radiation, scientists were startled when Richard B. Setlow and coworkers at Brookhaven National Laboratory in Upton, New York, showed that research on fish indicated that while UV radiation caused melanoma, cancer was induced in the fish by the lower-energy UV-A, not the DNA-damaging UV-B. This result, published in the July 15, 1994, *Proceedings of the National Academy of Sciences,* was alarming to people who work outside or spend a lot of time at the beach, because the commonly used sun screens only block out UV-B. It had been thought that there was no need to stop UV-A from reaching the skin.

Several studies also connect UV radiation to cataracts of the eyes. Fishers who spend a long time in direct and reflected sunlight have an 160 percent increase in the incidence of certain cataracts, while residents of sunny Tucson, Arizona, develop cataracts at a 58 percent higher than people living in cloudier Albany, New York. Sunglasses or special coatings on prescription glasses can block UV radiation and help reduce the risk. As usual, it is thought that UV-B radiation does most of the damage, although UV-B is mostly trapped in the outer structures of the eye.

SUNGLASSES ARE NOW RATED FOR PROTECTION

Cosmetic lenses:	Absorb 70% UV-B and 20% UV-A
General-purpose lenses:	Absorb 95% UV-B and 60% UV-A
Special-purpose lenses:	Absorb 99% UV-B and 60% UV-A

Some coatings are labeled as capable of absorbing "UV up to 400 mm," which means that they absorb 100% of all UV radiation, both A and B.

UV Radiation and Ozone

Since 1974, when it was first predicted that chlorofluorocarbons then used in aerosols and refrigeration were thinning the high ozone layer in the stratosphere, the main concern has been the effect such thinning has on UV radiation. Not only does UV-radiation cause skin cancer and cataracts in humans, it also damages other animals and plants.

Since 1988 UV radiation at ground level has been monitored on the southern tip of Argentina. In the summers of 1990 and 1992 the radiation suddenly shot up to 45 percent above expected levels, probably due to the expansion of the ozone "hole" at the South Pole. Similar but not so dramatic rises are occurring in the more densely populated northern hemisphere. James B. Kerr and C. Thomas McElroy of Environment Canada in Downsview, Ontario, measured UV radiation in Toronto once or twice an hour every day for four and a half years and then reported their findings in *Science* on November 12, 1993. The ozone layer above Toronto was shown to be at its thinnest in winter, ground level UV-B increasing as much as 35 percent on some winter days. The wavelengths that showed the rise in radiation consisted mainly of rays at the correct frequency for absorption by ozone, demonstrating that the increase in UV radiation resulted directly from ozone thinning. Satellite observations in 1992 had shown that atmospheric chemicals that destroy ozone had increased. Direct

Background

Like oxygen, ozone is a gas. In fact, ozone is oxygen—but oxygen with a difference. Ordinary oxygen consists of molecules containing two atoms. This is the oxygen we breathe. With a slight energy boost, however, three atoms of oxygen can combine to form an ozone molecule.

Ozone has different properties from oxygen. For example, oxygen is odorless, but ozone has a distinct odor, which can often be noticed near electric sparks or powerful ultraviolet lights. Oxygen is transparent, but ozone is blue.

Ozone is to oxygen rather like hydrogen peroxide is to water. Ozone is much more reactive than oxygen. Also, just as hydrogen peroxide gradually turns into water, ozone gradually turns into ordinary oxygen. The action of light speeds up these processes.

Although ozone is damaging when it interacts with life directly, ozone high in the atmosphere is important in protecting life. In the upper atmosphere, ozone is both formed by ultraviolet light and broken down by ultraviolet light. When ozone is broken down by light, one atom of oxygen quickly replaces the ozone molecule that was broken. In the process, the energy of the ultraviolet light is trapped as energy by the electrons in the ozone. As a result, the ozone keeps some ultraviolet light from reaching the earth's surface, especially the light with higher energy levels known as UV-B. The amount of ultraviolet light that does reach the surface is blamed for most skin cancers. Furthermore, high-energy ultraviolet light kills microorganisms.

Scientists believe that if more ultraviolet light reached the surface, the number of skin cancers, some of them fatal, would drastically increase. It is also thought that small ocean algae, which produce much of the oxygen in the air and break down much of the carbon dioxide, as well as bacteria important to crop production, would be greatly reduced.

Chlorofluorocarbons—freon is the most familiar type—are gases that have been used as spray propellants, in refrigeration, as cleaning agents, and in plastic foams, such as styrofoam. Since 1974 scientists have known that chlorine may be produced when chlorofluorocarbons break down in the upper atmosphere. The chlorine then can destroy ozone, turning it into ordinary oxygen. Each chlorine molecule destroys only one ozone molecule, but it does so in a process that leaves the original chlorine molecule intact, so it can then proceed to destroy another ozone molecule. Consequently, each chlorine molecule destroys many, many ozone molecules.

Since the discovery that chlorofluorocarbons can destroy high-atmosphere ozone, growing evidence has indicated that the amount of ozone in the upper atmosphere is decreasing. This process is especially noticeable in the Antarctic, where tiny ice particles increase the rate of breakdown, producing an ozone "hole" during the Antarctic summer, when there is nearly continuous sunlight. Increasing evidence shows that the same forces are also at work in the Arctic, where the "hole" is more dangerous because the region is more populated by living beings than the Antarctic.

Steps are being taken to protect the ozone in the upper atmosphere. Chlorofluorocarbons have not been used as spray propellants in the U.S. for years, although they continue to be used in other ways. An international treaty in 1987, signed by the U.S., calls for limiting production of chlorofluorocarbons and related gases, but in 1989 the European Economic Community agreed to eliminate chlorofluorocarbon production in its 12 nations completely by the turn of the century. It called on other nations to join in sharper reductions more immediately than the 1987 treaty requires and to work toward a complete ban, a call that the U.S. joined the following day. Steps to find acceptable substitutes for chlorofluorocarbons have been undertaken in the U.S. and the United Kingdom. Substitutes found so far are less effective in use and more expensive to manufacture than chlorofluorocarbons, but nearly everyone agrees that anything is better than permanent ecological damage.

measurements of the ozone layer by satellite showed a 10 percent drop over the winter of 1991.

Despite international efforts to control ozone-thinning gases, scientists expect that thinning will continue until around the turn of the century, after which the ozone layer will gradually return to its normal state.

Sunscreen Protection

Sunscreens provide protection against skin cancer, but there is solid evidence only for protection against squamous or basal cell cancer. A report in the October 14, 1993, issue of the *New England Journal of Medicine* by Sandra C. Thompson and co-workers from the Anti-Cancer Council of Victoria and the University of Melbourne in Australia described a double-blind study in which 588 men and women spent a summer wearing either SPF (Sun Protection Factor) 17 sunscreen or a look-and-feel-alike lotion with no built-in sunscreen. The people using the real sunscreen developed fewer pre-cancerous spots than the controls. However, the kind of spots, small wart-like growths called keratoses, are not precursors of melanoma. Keratoses are forerunners of squamous-cell skin cancers.

Sunscreens and tanning lotions that are not really sunscreens are all rated for sun protection. Until the early 1990s, the highest levels most people used were labeled SPF 15, but increasingly SPF 30 and even more protective sunscreens have become popular. SPF numbers are based upon exposing real human skin to controlled doses of UV radiation and measuring how red the skin becomes in a given amount of time.

(Periodical References and Additional Reading: *Harvard Health Letter* 6-90, p 1; *Harvard Health Letter* 7-90, p 1; *Science News* 10-5-91, p 214; *Harvard Health Letter* 4-93, p 1; *New York Times* 4-15-93, p B7; *Science News* 7-3-93, p 15; *Science News* 7-24-93, p 53; *New York Times* 10-14-93, p B9; *Science* 11-12-93, pp 990, 1032; *New York Times* 11-16-93, p C11; *New York Times* 5-3-94, p C3)

Smoking UPDATE

Around the world, various populations have discovered plants which produce psychoactive chemicals. The plants probably developed the chemicals in their tissues to repel insects or prevent fungal disease, but these chemicals happen to fit into receptors for various neurological functions in humans (*see* "The Ubiquity of NO in

Life," p 305). One of the most effective of such plants, tobacco, was discovered in the Americas in pre-Columbian times and has been used by shamans to induce trances, as well as for other ceremonial purposes. The main psychoactive chemical in tobacco is nicotine. Early European explorers took the practice of using tobacco back to Europe, where it soon became popular as a mildly relaxing and mind-altering drug, most often burnt in pipes so that its smoke could be tasted or inhaled.

In 1860 in the U.S. the first crude machines that could mass-produce small paper tubes containing dried tobacco leaves were exhibited, but production of such tubes—cigarettes—did not begin in earnest until 1880, when better machines became available. Unlike pipes or handmade cigars, cigarettes produced small amounts of fairly cool smoke that could be easily inhaled deep into the lungs.

By 1895 there were four billion cigarettes made in the U.S. and probably most of them were smoked with much of the smoke inhaled. There were still more handmade cigars puffed in the U.S. than cigarettes until the 1920s, when cigarettes took the lead. By 1950, 75 percent of all tobacco consumption in the U.S. was in the form of cigarettes.

About that time there was also widespread recognition that inhaling cigarette smoke contributes to the development of lung cancer, which by then was rising rapidly in the U.S. The increase has continued since the 1950s. In 1990, according to an analysis by the U.S. Centers for Disease Control and Prevention (CDC) in an August 1993 *Morbidity and Mortality Weekly Report,* cigarette smoking in the U.S. accounted for 418,690 deaths. The report also stated that each cigarette stole seven minutes from a person's life.

In 1993, although 44 million Americans had given up smoking, there were 46 to 54 million people still smoking cigarettes (estimates vary). Increasingly, however, it was difficult for the smokers to find a place to smoke, as a wave of bans swept the U.S. in the early 1990s, starting with the 1990 ban on smoking on shorter domestic airplane flights. All indications were that the restrictions on smoking would be even stricter in 1994, possibly even including a national ban on smoking in all public places.

Decline of Smoking Continues Slowly

As a result of the realization of the connection between smoking and health, smoking in the U.S. has significantly declined for almost a quarter of a century. The practice should decline even further if threatened new restrictions and taxes are imposed. As a goal for the year 2000, the CDC is aiming to lower the rate of smokers to 15 percent of the U.S. population. But news in 1993 suggested that change would not come that fast; a projection of 19 percent for the beginning of the new millennium seems more realistic.

In 1965, according to the CDC, somewhat more than 40 percent of all adults smoked cigarettes. By 1991 that figure had fallen to 25.7 percent. But some studies showed that despite new taxes, restrictions, warnings, and media coverage of bad news about health effects, the 25-year decline in smoking was coming to an end. In statistical terms, the 1991 rate showed no improvement over the previous year; in fact, it rose by two tenths of a percentage point. Furthermore, a survey conducted by the Princeton Survey Research Associates for *Prevention* showed a dramatic *rise* in smoking in 1993 to the highest levels since the magazine began its own regular survey in 1983. Indeed the actual survey of 1250 people over the telephone showed a rise to 30 percent with a margin of error of three percentage points. Thus, the previous year's survey, with the same margin of error, showed a range of 22 to 28 percent smokers and the 1993 survey showed a range from 27 to 33 percent. The probability that smoking has actually stayed at the same level (either 27 or 28 percent, the overlap in range) is 17 percent, while the probability of an actual increase is 83 percent.

The largest increase in smokers in the *Prevention* survey came from African American smokers, who were targeted by tobacco promotion efforts in the early 1990s. Both the *Prevention* survey and the CDC report found that more men smoke than women; more than half of all smokers are between the ages of 25 and 64; a greater percentage of African-Americans smoke than European-Americans; better education is generally related to lower rates of smokers; and low income is positively related to high rates of smoking.

In 1965, taking into account CDC calculations that more than 40 percent of all people smoked, it is believed that 188,000 deaths in the U.S. were caused by the habit. But smoking takes years to destroy the body with lung cancer, heart disease, emphysema, and cancers other than lung cancer. In the 1990s the death rate directly attributable to high rates of smoking in the past soared higher than 400,000 a year, more than twice the number in 1965. More than ten percent of the current deaths are thought to be the result of someone else's smoking—known as second-hand smoke—which is discussed below.

Nonsmokers Affected

Second-hand smoke or environmental smoke is tobacco smoke produced by a smoker that is later breathed by a nonsmoker; what is imposed on the nonsmoker has been termed passive smoking. Environmental smoke has been branded as a health hazard since the U.S. Surgeon General's 1986 report on smoking and health. Partly for that reason, most airlines, and an increasing number of businesses, have banned smoking.

Starting in 1989, the U.S. Environmental Protection Agency (EPA), which had long studied second-hand smoke as an indoor air pollutant, asked a professional advisory board to prepare a report on the health effects of passive smoking. Preliminary results started appearing late in 1990, and the report made headlines every year until it was finally issued on January 7, 1993, as "Respiratory Health Effects of Passive Smoking: Lung Cancer and Other Disorders." The report was not based on new research, but re-examined previous studies. It concluded that 3000 persons a year died from lung cancer solely because of second-hand smoke. (Other sources suggest that perhaps ten times that number are killed annually by heart attacks caused by changes produced by environmental smoke.) EPA Administrator William K. Reilly commented that second-hand smoke was a higher risk than virtually all of the chemicals regulated by the agency. The report classed environmental smoke as a Group A carcinogen, the same group that includes such known hazards as benzene and asbestos.

A second part of the report dealt with the effects of passive smoking on children, which included a higher incidence of asthma and between 150,000 and 300,000 cases of other respiratory disorders in infants. On July 21, 1993, the EPA followed up its report with a set of voluntary guidelines to use in restricting smoking in the workplace or providing ventilation.

In a separate effort, the EPA conducted original research on the presence of nicotine by-products in the blood of both smokers and nonsmokers. Two weeks after releasing the study on respiratory diseases, the EPA said they found a nicotine by-product in the blood of the first 800 people—smokers and nonsmokers—they tested. The blood studies were scheduled to be completed sometime in 1994. In the mean-time, another study (reported in the December 1993 *American Journal of Clinical Nutrition*) found that people exposed to environmental smoke were deficient in vitamin C.

The EPA report on second-hand smoke met with strong resistance, including legal action, from the tobacco companies, but it seems likely that the EPA position will prevail in court.

What Happens If You Quit?

Most studies of people who successfully stop smoking tobacco find that the health risks associated with smoking disappear within five to ten years. However, a study of 900,000 people, consisting of 25 percent ex-smokers, 25 percent smokers, and 50 percent nonsmokers, showed that the risk of lung cancer is the lowest for those who have never smoked. Furthermore, according to research by Michael T. Halpern, Kenneth E. Warner, and coworkers at the University of Michigan, the younger a smoker was when he or she quit, the lower the likelihood of developing lung cancer. Their study appeared in the March 1993 issue of the *Journal of the National Cancer Institute*.

The statistics of the University of Michigan study are difficult to follow because so many groups are being compared: people who never smoked; people still smoking (until they die); and people who stopped smoking in their thirties, their forties, their early fifties, their late fifties, or even their sixties. Furthermore, there are separate data for men and for women. Half the people studied were 57 or over in 1982, and the death rates are based on the period between 1982 and 1988. Despite the fragmentary data, researchers were able to conclude that at age 75 male smokers were 14 times as likely to die from lung cancer as men who quit in their thirties. But there was still a bit more than twice the risk for the quitters as for lifetime nonsmokers. Nevertheless there is a definite lowering of risk that results from quitting. As the age of quitting increased, however, the benefits of quitting decreased.

It is hard to quit smoking. Many studies rate nicotine as more addictive than heroin, cocaine, or alcohol. A study by John P. Pierce from the University of California—San Diego, presented to the American Society of Addiction Medicine in November 1993, found that successful quitting is usually a gradual process. Tapering off smoking and delaying the first cigarette of the day are practices that work better in the long run for most people than trying to cease instantly. The increasing restrictions on smoking at work or in public places have therefore made it easier to quit by forcing some smokers to cut down on the number of smokes a day. The study of 4624 Californians, interviewed twice, with an 18-month gap between interviews, also showed that it often takes more than one attempt before quitting successfully.

Since 1991 a popular device to aid smokers wishing to quit has been the nicotine patch, which delivers nicotine through the skin. The idea is that to satisfy the addiction itself, thus enabling the smoker to break the oral and nervous attachment to smoking. This approach proved so popular that there was more demand than supply for patches at some periods in the early 1990s. The patch also created a new health problem: some smokers responded well to the patch "treatment" but remained addicted to nicotine. Smoking while wearing the patch produced an overdose of nicotine that, according to inconclusive evidence, caused heart attacks.

It's Not Just Lung Cancer

The statistical connection between smoking and lung cancer has been recognized for at least fifty years and remains strong. The adverse changes in the heart and blood vessels that come from smoking are also well documented. For example, heart flow through the small blood vessels called arterioles is about 30 percent less than normal in smokers, and drops by up to 38 percent in the coronary arteries after each cigarette. A person who smokes two packs a day is likely to have a heart attack 11 years earlier than a nonsmoker, according to a March 5, 1991, report by Arnold Moss of the University of Rochester. If lung cancer and heart disease are not enough to motivate a person to quit smoking, here are a few other discoveries about the health effects of tobacco from the early 1990s.

Low-weight infants: The CDC reported in August 1992 that mothers who smoke have babies under the weight of 5 1/2 pounds at a rate of 11.6 percent, which more than doubles the 5.6 percent rate for nonsmoking mothers. A birth weight of 5 1/2 pounds is the dividing line for the common physician's classification of premature birth. Such low-weight babies are more prone to respiratory problems or to sudden infant death syndrome.

Cataracts: Two studies, both published in the August 26, 1992, issue of the Journal of the American Medical Association, showed that smoking is associated with cataracts in the eyes of smokers, doubling the rate of cataract formation for people who smoke a pack or more of cigarettes daily. Data for the statistical study came from tens of thousands of doctors and nurses. An editorial in the journal attributed one of five cataract cases in the U.S. to smoking.

Disrupted thought: A controversial report in the September 1992 *British Journal of Addiction* claimed that smoking makes it more difficult to collect one's thoughts in order to perform complex tasks. One reason this study is controversial is that people who quit smoking usually lose the ability to concentrate for several months until their brain adjusts to life without nicotine. Indeed, another study in the September 1992 *Psychopharmacology* found that small amounts of nicotine improve concentration.

Thyroid disorder: Smoking is one of the contributing factors to an overactive thyroid, causing the condition known as Grave's disease that often results in bulging eyes and blurred vision. Nearly twice as many smokers as nonsmokers were found to have thyroid overproduction in a Dutch study published early in 1993, but there were 7.7 times as many smokers as nonsmokers with vision problems caused by thyroid hyperactivity.

Asthma: Asthmatic children exposed to high levels of second-hand smoke have 80 percent more attacks than those not exposed, according to a study published in the *New England Journal of Medicine* in June 1993.

Strokes: A ten-year study of 22,000 originally healthy male doctors showed that smokers were twice as likely to have strokes as nonsmokers, as reported by JoAnn Manson of the Harvard Medical School to the American Heart Association on November 8, 1993.

(Periodical References and Additional Reading: *New York Times* 2-1-91; *New York Times* 3-7-91; *New York Times* 7-7-92, p D4; *New York Times* 8-5-92, p C12; *New York Times* 8-26-92, p C12; *New York Times* 11-22-92, p I-39; *New York Times* 1-6-93, p A10; *New York Times* 1-7-93, p B10; *New York Times* 1-8-93, p A14; *Science News* 1-16-93, p 46; *New York Times* 1-21-93, p A10; *New York Times* 2-2-93, p C2; *New York Times* 3-21-93, p I-31; *New York Times* 4-2-93, p A21; *New York Times* 6-15-93, p C9; *New York Times* 6-23-93, p A1; *New York Times* 7-22-93, p A14; *New York Times* 8-27-93, p A19; *New York Times* 11-14-93, p I-34; *Science News* 12-18/25-93, p 414; *New York Times* 12-19-93, p I-24; *New York Times* 2-9-94, p C13)

Drug Addiction and Alcoholism UPDATE

There are many different chemicals that affect the human mind. Some of these are considered harmless, or nearly so, such as caffeine. Nicotine is known to be addictive and dangerous, but is legal (*see* "Smoking UPDATE," p 192). So is alcohol. Some substances, such as morphine, amphetamines, and various antidepressants or tranquilizers, are legal but controlled: their medical use is recognized along with their dangers. The active ingredient in marijuana is controlled, but marijuana itself is illegal in most places. A large number of chemicals, often simply called *drugs,* including heroin, various forms of cocaine, and various artificial psychoactive chemicals, are illegal, except when used for research purposes.

A study conducted by researchers from Brandeis University in Waltham, Massachusetts, and released in October 1993 — "Substance Abuse: The Nation's No. 1 Health Problem" — tried to quantify the effects of nicotine, alcohol, and controlled and illegal drugs on U.S. society. Using figures from the U.S. National Center for Health Statistics for 1989 or 1990, the researchers estimated that substance abuse causes 520,000 deaths annually in the U.S., and that most of these deaths, by far, result from smoking tobacco. Alcohol and other drugs account for about 100,000 of those deaths, resulting mostly from alcohol abuse. In addition, about 25 to 40 percent of all hospital admissions have been attributed to alcohol abuse. Other research shows that about 24,000 persons each year are killed by drunk drivers, and another half million are injured.

The U.S. National Institutes of Mental Health surveyed a population of 20,291 individuals in five communities between 1980 and 1985 on the mental problems reported by people living in urban areas of the U.S. The survey found 7.4 percent of the population willing to admit to alcohol abuse or dependence and 3.1 who would admit to dependence on drugs other than alcohol. Since many people who are addicted to alcohol or drugs deny or minimize their problem, the survey figures probably represent the most conservative statistical snapshot of drug abuse in the urban U.S. Results of the survey were reported in the February 1993 *Archives of General Psychiatry.* A 1991 report from the National Institute of Alcohol Abuse and Alcoholism claimed that 15.3 million Americans show symptoms of alcohol abuse, which would be 6 percent of the total population that year.

Alcoholic Lives

Alcoholism and the designation of a chronic alcohol abuser as an alcoholic have been widely used terms mostly since the founding of Alcoholics Anonymous (AA) in 1935. Widespread accounts of the success of the AA program in helping people stop drinking and get on with their lives also included the information, new to many people, that alcoholism is a disease, not a sign of moral turpitude, or a failure of will power.

A few years after AA was founded, two groups of young men were recruited to participate in a long-term study which eventually spanned a period of 50 years. Both groups were located in the Boston, Massachusetts, area between 1940 and 1943, and included 456 teenagers from the poorest part of Boston and 268 sophomores at Harvard University. Starting in 1977, George E. Vaillant of Brigham and Women's Hospital in Boston used data from other researchers as well as his own findings to examine alcohol dependence in both groups. Vaillant reported on his study at a meeting of the American Psychiatric Association in June 1993.

For this research, alcohol abuse was defined as heavy and uncontrolled use of alcohol on a daily basis. About a third of the men in the impoverished group became alcohol abusers in their twenties, suffering the devastating effects of alcohol. Only a fifth of the Harvard students abused alcohol, starting later in life, typically in their 40s or 50s. Characteristically, the respondents from the student group were able to maintain jobs and families better than those who grew up in the inner city.

AA members, and many others, believe that no one ever recovers from alcoholism, except by death. Nevertheless some alcoholics in the study were able to stop drinking. About two out of five of the alcoholics ended up in AA. Most of those who managed to stay sober for five years, whether in or out of AA, continued to be sober thereafter. Those who could not stay sober for five years typically resumed alcohol abuse. "Moderate" drinking seldom lasted more than a year before the drinker returned to old patterns of abuse, or worse. All in all, about one in five of the alcoholics was still abusing alcohol at the age of 60. Active alcoholics had a three times higher death rate than those who managed to stop drinking.

Drinking generally starts early in life. The U.S. Centers for Disease Control and Prevention reported on September 16, 1991, that, according to their findings, 46 percent of high school students admitted to having an alcoholic beverage in the past 30 days. A survey of small colleges found that 86 percent of the students drank sometimes, 45 percent weekly, and 42 percent had consumed at least five or more drinks on one occasion in the past two weeks. Data was compiled by researchers for Southern Illinois University and from the College of William and Mary and released in September 1993.

Other types of drug abuse also start early in many cases. A smaller amount, 11 percent of high school students, told the CDC they had used marijuana in the past month. The small-college survey found that 27 percent had smoked marijuana and that 6.1 percent had used cocaine in the past year.

Alcohol and Heart Disease

A number of studies, inspired by lower rates of heart disease in France, have suggested that drinking—especially red wine—in moderation helps prevent heart disease. The cause of this effect is that consumption of two or three drinks a day improves the ratio of high-density lipoprotein (HDL), or "good" cholesterol, to low density lipoprotein (LDL), or "bad" cholesterol. Indeed, moderate drinking raises the amount of HDL cholesterol, as reported by J. Michael Gaziano of Brigham and Women's Hospital in Boston and others in the December 16, 1993, issue of the *New England Journal of Medicine*. Other research, however, shows that the same amount of alcohol that raises HDL cholesterol also increases liver fat, which can lead to cirrhosis of the liver, a serious and often fatal disease. Thus, although no careful study has directly compared the two effects of moderate drinking, the moderate drinker may be gaining a safer cholesterol level while endangering his or her liver. Also, although alcohol in small amounts may be good for coronary arteries, it is not healthy for the heart itself, since alcohol is one of the leading causes of heart arrhythmias.

Chemical Remedies for Chemical Dependence

If tests support its claims and if federal regulators agree, in the year 1998 or thereabouts the public will have access to a prescription drug that enhances the body functions that normally metabolize ethyl alcohol. The new drug, reportedly developed at a major university with the aid of federal funding, is already being promoted by the medical-equipment manufacturer Compumed Inc. of Manhattan Beach, California, which has bought an option on it from the unnamed university. The drug, named Detoxahol, is said by Robert Stuckelman, president of Compumed, to reduce the time it takes a person to eliminate alcohol from the system from as much as eight hours to a few minutes. As a prescription drug, it would be intended for use by ambulance staff and emergency-room doctors, who often deal with alcohol overdoses. Treatment of accident victims is also frequently complicated by alcohol intoxication. Compumed also hopes that there will eventually be an over-the-counter (or over-the-bar) version for self-medication as needed.

The drug primarily increases the ability of the small intestine and liver to remove alcohol from the blood, prompting them to overperform those natural functions. No side effects are predicted for accelerating this natural process, but the benefits might be dubious, since alcohol may already have damaged a person's brain before the drug takes effect.

While the prospects for Detoxahol are far from certain, the stock of the small company rose over 18 percent on the announcement of the new drug. In the meantime, in China, doctors at the Shanghai hospital claimed to have found a herbal medicine that would accomplish about the same results as Detoxahol.

Another Chinese herbal drug for alcohol abuse was also touted in the early 1990s, but it reportedly prevented drinking rather than helped recovery from drinking. The drug in question is kudzu, an herb which drapes itself over entire hillsides, and is a familiar import in the U.S. South. Wing-Ming Keung and Bert L. Vallee of Harvard Medical School in Boston tried kudzu, which is used to treat alcoholism in China, on a strain of hamsters known to drink large quantities of alcoholic beverages whenever allowed. The hamsters cut their imbibing in half, however, when given injections of two chemicals—daidzin and daidzein—extracted from kudzu root. The report of these experiments appeared in the November 1, 1993, *Proceedings of the National Academy of Sciences.* In China, physicians claim to cure about 80 percent of the alcoholics that they treat with kudzu extract or closely related potions. Research in 1992 had shown that the opiate blocker naltrexone also blocks desire for alcohol by filling the same receptors in the brain that alcohol uses.

However, the Chinese have no monopoly on herbs with dramatic effects. In West Africa the herb ibogaine is used to induce trance states during puberty rites. In 1962, a heroin addict and his friend in quest of a new high tried ibogaine. One result of the experiment was that five of the seven heroin addicts who tried it lost their desire for heroin for a period of time. In the 1980s, the initiator of the experiment, now a former addict, began to treat heroin addicts with ibogaine, mostly in the Netherlands. Some success has led to animal trials, with varying results, and late in 1993 it prompted a small-scale test on humans in the U.S. If the first phase convinces scientists that the drug is safe, it may be tested further in the U.S. in 1994. In addition to heroin, proponents claim that ibogaine can reduce craving for other drugs, including cocaine and alcohol.

In a different chemical strategy against drugs, an enzyme has been designed to attack and destroy cocaine molecules while they are still in the bloodstream, knocking them out before they reach the receptors in the brain. The scientists developing this enzyme hope that people undergoing treatment for cocaine addiction would tolerate the otherwise harmless enzyme which would circulate in their blood at all times, ready to attack any cocaine molecules. So far, this experiment has only been tried in the test tube, and clinical trials may be years away.

(Periodical References and Additional Reading: *New York Times* 9-20-92, p I-33; *Science News* 11-21-92, p 341; *Science News* 2-27-93, p 134; *New York Times* 3-26-93, p A18; *Science News* 3-27-93, p 199; *New York Times* 5-3-93, p A16; *New York Times* 5-11-93, p A20; *Science News* 6-5-93, p 356; *New York Times* 10-24-93, p I-20; *New York Times* 10-27-93, p C11; *New York Times* 11-2-93, p C6; *Science News* 11-13-93, p 319; *New York Times* 12-8-93, p D5; *New York Times* 12-16-93, p B16)

WELLNESS TABLES

REVISED RECOMMENDED DAILY ALLOWANCES

Amounts:

IU	International Unit—varies with vitamin
mcg	microgram—millionth of a gram; thousandth of a mg (microgram abbreviated µg by scientists)
mg	milligram—thousandth of a gram
RE	retinol (a form of vitamin A) equivalents
tbs	tablespoon
tsp	teaspoon
oz	ounce (28.350 grams)

Nutrient	*Women*	*Men*	*No RDA*	*Typical Source*
Vitamin A	800 RE (8000 IU)	1000 RE (10,000 IU)		1 cup milk = 140 RE
Beta carotene			5–6 mg	1 med. carrot = 12 mg 1 sweet potato = 15 mg
Vitamin B$_{12}$	2 mcg	2 mcg		1 cup milk = 0.9 mcg
Biotin			30–100 mg	
Vitamin C	60 mg	60 mg		1 orange = 70 mg 1 cup broccoli = 115 mg
Vitamin D	5 mcg (200 IU) *After age 25:* 10 mcg (400 IU)	5 mcg (200 IU) *After age 25:* 10 mcg (400 IU)		1 cup milk = 2.5 mg (100 IU)
Vitamin E	8 mg (12 IU)	10 mg (15 IU)		1 tbs canola oil = 9 mg 1 tbs margarine = 2mg 1 cup kale = 6mg
Folacin (folic acid)	180 mcg	200 mcg		1 cup raw spinach = 110 mcg 1 cup asparagus = 180 mcg
Vitamin K	60–65 mcg	70–80 mcg		1 cup broccoli = 175 mcg 1 cup milk = 10 mcg
Niacin (B$_3$)	13–19 mg	13–19 mg		3 oz chicken = 12 mg 1 slice enriched bread = 1 mg
Pantothenic acid (B$_5$)			4–7 mg	
Pyroxidine (B$_6$)	1.6 mg	2 mg		1 cup lima beans = 0.3 mg
Riboflavin (B$_2$)	1.2–1.3 mg	1.4–1.7 mg		1 cup milk = 0.4 mg 3 oz chicken = 0.2 mg
Thiamin (B$_1$)	1–1.1 mg	1.2–1.5 mg		1 cup oatmeal = 0.5 mg

(Periodical References and Additional Reading: *University of California at Berkeley Wellness Letter* 1-94, p 4)

SOME BIOLOGICALLY ACTIVE FOOD COMPOUNDS

Dieticians traditionally recognize six categories of nutrients (proteins, carbohydrates, fats, vitamins, minerals, and water), along with two important classes of non-nutrient — soluble and insoluble fiber. Evolution has produced in plants, animals, and fungi a vast array of chemical compounds that serve various purposes in the living organism. When an organism, or its remains, is consumed by animals, many of these compounds are destroyed during digestion. Others, however, survive and enter the consuming animal's bloodstream, where they may or may not interact with other physiological processes. Some of these biologically active compounds have long been known. Dramatic examples include poisons produced by herbs, amphibians, and mushrooms, or chemicals such as nicotine in tobacco and THC in marijuana. Among the beneficial compounds are those found in medicinal herbs, ranging from quinine to the hormones used in birth control pills. These compounds have long been known, although scientists have not always been able to verify benefits claimed for such plants as garlic or ginseng.

Nutritionists and other scientists have recently observed various biologically active compounds in foods usually eaten to provide the six nutrients and the two fibers. As with poisons, psychoactive drugs, and herbal medicines, some of these appear to be beneficial, and some, dangerous. The newly discovered chemicals may resemble the previously known active ingredients in certain respects. For example, their effects may be harmful or beneficial depending on the circumstances. Thus, digitalis from foxglove is helpful in small doses to people with certain heart conditions, but dangerous in large doses to anyone.

The following table is arranged by compound (or family of compounds) with one or two food sources given as examples of where such a chemical might be found. The table "Sources of Vitamins and Minerals," which begins on page 207, is arranged by food sources and lists vitamins and minerals.

COMPOUNDS

Compound	Biological activity	Found in
Allylic sulfides	May stimulate an enzyme (glutathione-S-transferase) that helps eliminate toxins, including carcinogens	Garlic, onions
Carotenoids	Antioxidants; also involved in cell differentiation; betacarotene is famous member of family	Orange or dark green vegetables and fruits
Catechins	Antioxidants	Green tea, berries
Flavonoids	Block hormone receptor sites; in some cases the hormones promote cancer growth; may protect against heart disease by reducing plaque or by lowering cholesterol or hypertension	Most fruits and vegetables, but especially apples and onions; also in red wine and tea
Genistein	May block growth of new blood vessels, a benefit when cancer is present	Soybeans and the cabbage family

Compound	Biological activity	Found in
Indoles	Induce protective enzymes	Cabbage family
Isoflavones	May protect against cancer by reducing estrogen production	Soy products
Isothiocyanates	Induce protective enzymes	Radishes and mustards
Limonoids	Induce protective enzymes	Citrus fruits
Linolenic acid	Regulates prostaglandin production	Seeds and leafy vegetables
Lycopene	Antioxidant	Tomatoes, red grapefruit
Monoterpenes	Inhibit cholesterol production in tumors; aid protective enzymes; mild antioxidant	Carrot family and cabbage family
Phenolic acids	Inhibit nitrosamine formation and affect enzyme activity; mild antioxidant	Carrot family and cabbage family
Phthalide	Lowers blood pressure	Celery
Phytosterols	May prevent cholesterol from being absorbed	Soy products
Plant sterois	Aid cell differentiation	Cabbage and squash families
Reservatol	Reduces tendency of platelets in blood to clump	Red wine and purple grape juice
Tannins	Antioxidants such as catechins and phenolic acids	Tea
Sulforaphane	Encourages enzyme formation	Cabbage family

(Periodical References and Further Reading: *Discover* 1-93, p 46; *New York Times* 4-13-93, p C1; *New York Times* 10-26-93, p C6; *University of California at Berkeley Wellness Letter* 10-93, p 1)

HEALTH CONCERNS AND COMMON FOODS

The People's Diet Guide

A miscellany of advice on food culled from various sources.

Do not be alarmed by contradictions or take these lists too seriously. They reflect news reports from all sorts of sources of varying quality; detailed explanations of recommendations for diet choices are found in articles on particular topics throughout *Handbook of Current Health and Medicine*.

WHAT YOU *SHOULD* EAT OR DRINK AND WHY

Alcohol (in small amounts)	Prevents heart attacks
Apples	Protects against heart attacks and high blood pressure
Broccoli	Protects against cancer
Celery	Lowers blood pressure

Fiber	Reduces risk of colon cancer and type II diabetes
Fruits and vegetables	Reduces risk of many forms of cancer, heart attack, stroke, and type II diabetes
Honey	Prevents intestinal polyps from progressing to colon cancer
Magnesium (in foods)	Prevents chronic fatigue
Milk	Nature's perfect food
Nuts	Reduces risk of heart attack
Onions	Protects against heart attacks
Protein (in foods)	Needed for growth and development
Soybeans	Slows growth of cancers, especially prostate cancer
Tea (any kind)	Protects against heart attacks
Tea (green)	Reduces risk of stomach cancer

WHAT YOU *SHOULD NOT* EAT OR DRINK AND WHY

Alcohol (in large amounts)	Causes liver and pancreatic disorders as well as throat cancer and brain damage (irreversible)
Alcohol (in small amounts)	Increases susceptibility to colds and flu
Caffeine	May cause miscarriages
Calcium oxalate (in foods)	Causes vulvodynia (inflammation of the vulva)
Fat	May increase risk of lung, breast, and colon cancer, heart attack, or type II diabetes
Fish (large, ocean)	May contain ciguatera toxins, causing food poisoning
Margarine	Contains trans fatty acids that act like saturated fats
Milk	Physicians Committee on Responsible Medicine claims that cow's milk has too much fat, not enough iron, and causes children to develop diabetes, colic, allergies, and digestive problems
Protein (in foods)	Some say too much causes liver cancer or stresses the kidneys
Rare meat	May contain E. coli 0157:H7
Red meat	Risk factor for prostate cancer according to study of 86,000 male health professionals
Salt and sodium in foods	Raises blood pressure in sensitive people
Salted or pickled foods	May contribute to stomach or liver cancer and stroke
Water (chlorinated)	Related to small increases in the risk of rectal or bladder cancer

Classifications of Foods

For the most part, common foods can be grouped into plant families or other large categories for which all members are sufficiently alike that any one will have the same benefits or cause the same problems as any other member of the group. Where possible, such large groupings are used below, although sometimes there is a singular member of a family that merits special notice. Foods from one group that can also appear in another are listed in the alternate group in square brackets, such as "[asparagus]." The groups used below are the following.

Beet family: beets, (Swiss) chard, [quinoa], spinach

Cabbage family (Brassica, crucifers): bok choy, broccoli, brussels sprouts, cabbage, cauliflower, Chinese cabbage, collards, kale, kohlrabi, mustards, rape, rutabagas, sauerkraut (preserved cabbage), turnips

Carrot family: carrots, celery, parsley, parsnips

Citrus fruits: grapefruit, kumquat, lemon, lime, orange, shaddock (pummelo)

Cranberry family: blueberries, cranberries, huckleberries

Currant family: currants (black, red, and white), gooseberries

Dairy products: cheese, creme fraiche, ice cream, milk (from cows, goats, horses, reindeer, sheep, yaks), sour cream, whey, yogurt

Eggs: eggs from chickens, ducks, geese, guinea fowl, gulls (black-headed), moorhen, ostrich, partridge, penguins, pigeon, plover, quail, turkeys, turtles; fish eggs are called roe or caviar

Fish: nutritionally, fish are either oily or non-oily. *Oily fish* include eel, herring, mackerel, salmon, sardines, shad, swordfish, tuna. *Non-oily fish* include bass, brill, catfish, cod and scrod, dab, flounder, hake, halibut, lemon sole, mullet, perch, pike, plaice, sole, turbot, walleye, witch, whitefish. *Ocean fish* include brill, dab, flounder, grouper, haddock (dried, it is finnan haddie), hake, halibut, herring, lemon sole, mackerel, mullet, plaice, red snapper, salmon*, sardines, shad*, sole, sturgeon*, swordfish, tilefish, turbot, witch. *Freshwater fish* include catfish, eel, perch, pike, trout, walleye, whitefish. *Sharks (not classed by biologists as fish):* rays, sharks, skates.

Flowers: artichokes—also called "globe artichokes," [broccoli and cauliflower], figs, okra (pods, not really flowers)

Fruit (miscellaneous) (*see also* citrus fruits, cranberry family, currant family, rose family): ackee, avocado, banana, breadfruit, cactus fruit, dates, durian, figs, grapes and raisins (dried grapes), jackfruit, jujube, kiwi (Chinese gooseberry), loquat, lychee, mango, mulberry, olive, papaw, papaya, passionfruit, persimmon, plantain, pineapple, pomegranate, sapodilla, tomatillo (usually treated as a vegetable)

Fungi: chiefly what we know as mushrooms, including cêpes, champignons (ordinary cultivated mushrooms), huitlacoche, morels, portobellos, puffballs, shiitake, truffles; but also yeasts such as brewer's yeast

Grains (Cereals and cereal products): [amaranth], barley, [buckwheat], bread, corn (maize), farina, flour (of various types), grits (ground dried corn), groats (cracked wheat), hominy (hulled corn), macaroni, masa harina (ground hominy), millet, noodles, oats, oatmeal, pasta, popcorn, quinoa, rice, rye, sorghum, spaghetti, wheat, wild rice. *Whole grains,* such as whole wheat or brown rice, have not had any edible parts of the grain removed during processing.

Greens: amaranth, asparagus, [beet greens and chard], [cabbages], chicory, [collards and kale], dandelions, endive, fennel, fern shoots (fiddleheads), grape leaves

* These fish live most of their lives in the ocean, but are usually caught in freshwater while spawning.

(vine leaves), lamb's-quarters, lettuce, nasturtium, nettle, rocket, salsify (a lettuce relative grown for its roots)

Legumes: beans, black-eyed peas (cowpeas), broad (fava) beans, chickpeas (garbanzos), flageolets, green beans, lentils, lima beans (butter beans), mung beans, [peanuts], peas, runner beans, snap peas (sugar snaps), snow peas (edible-pod peas), soybeans (including tempeh and tofu), tamarinds

Oils: almond; avocado (20% unsaturated, 50% monounsaturated, 15% polyunsaturated); candle-nut, canola or rapeseed (5% saturated, 15% monounsaturated, 15% polyunsaturated); coconut (75% saturated); colza (combined rapeseed and mustardseed); corn (10% saturated, 35% monounsaturated, and 50% polyunsaturated); cottonseed (25% saturated, 20% monounsaturated, 50% polyunsaturated); fish (varies: herring oil, for example, is 20% saturated, 25% monounsaturated, 50% polyunsaturated); olive (15% saturated, 70% monounsaturated, 10% polyunsaturated); palm (45% saturated, 40% monounsaturated, 10% polyunsaturated); peanut (15% saturated, 50% monounsaturated, 30% polyunsaturated); safflower (5% saturated, 70% polyunsaturated); sesame, soybean (10% saturated, 25% monounsaturated, 55% polyunsaturated); sunflower (5% saturated, 25% monounsaturated, 65% polyunsaturated); walnut.

Onion family: [asparagus], chives, garlic, leeks, onions, scallions, shallots

Organ meats: foie gras (goose liver), kidneys, heart, liver, sweetbreads, tripe

Nuts: almonds, brazil nuts, butternuts, candle nuts, cashews, chestnuts, coconuts, hazelnuts, hickories, filberts, macadamias, marzipan (almonds and sugar), peanuts (actually legumes), pecans, pine nuts (pignolos), pistachios, walnuts, water chestnuts

Poultry: chicken, duck, frog*, goose, grouse, guinea fowl, ostrich, partridge, pheasant, pigeon, quail, rabbit*, squab, turkey, turtle*

Potato family: eggplant, sweet and hot chiles (red, green, or bell peppers), potatoes, tomatoes

Red meats: bacon, beef, corned beef, goat, ham, hare (but not rabbit), horse, kid, lamb, mutton, veal, venison

Roots and tubers (*see also* the beet, carrot, and cabbage families): Jerusalem artichoke (sunchoke), radish, [salsify], sweet potatoes, tapioca (cassava), yams

Rose family: apples, [almonds], apricots, blackberries, cherries, damsons, medlars, peaches, pears, plums and prunes (dried plums), quinces, raspberries, strawberries

Seeds: poppy seeds, [pumpkin seeds], sesame seeds and tahini, sunflower seeds

Shellfish: Abalone, calamari** (squid**), clams, crabs, crayfish, cuttlefish**, langouste (spiny lobster), lobster, mussels, octopus**, oysters, prawns, scallops, scampi, shrimp, snails (not usually called shellfish, despite the shells), squid**, whelks.

Squash and melon families (green): chayote, cucumbers, honeydews, marrows, pattypan squashes, zucchini

Squash and melon families (yellow): acorn squashes, butternut squashes, cantaloupes, casabas, crookneck squashes, hubbard squashes, muskmelons, pumpkins, vegetable spaghetti, watermelon

---

* Not poultry, but treated like poultry in cooking.

** Shell not evident, but these are in same biological group as clams and oysters.

Yellow fruits and vegetables (also included above by family):   apricots, carrots, mangoes, peaches, pink or red grapefruit, red capsicum peppers, sweet potatoes, tomatoes, yellow squash or melons

Sources of Vitamins and Minerals

Vitamin A: Dairy products, organ meats, oily fish, carrot family, sweet potatoes, squash and melon family, greens, and any yellow or red fruits or vegetables.
Beta carotene: Carrot family, greens, sweet potatoes, squash and melon family, greens, and any yellow or red fruits or vegetables.
Vitamin B$_{12}$:   Organ meats, red meats, poultry, eggs, dairy products, shellfish.
Biotin: Eggs, dairy products, organ meets, fungi, fruit, tomatoes, whole grains.
Vitamin C: Citrus fruits, the currant family, the rose family, the potato family, the cabbage family, squash and melons.
Calcium: Dairy products, sardines or other whole fish (including the bones), dark-green leafy vegetables (greens).
Chromium: Brewer's yeast, wine, oysters, potatoes, meat, liver, egg yolk, seafood, whole grains, cheese.
Cobalt: Meats.
Copper: Oysters, nuts, organ meats, oils and fats, legumes, greens, raisins, chocolate, meats.
Vitamin D: Dairy products and oily fish.
Vitamin E: Oils, nuts, wheat germ, greens, and seeds.
Fluorine: Tea, seafood, legumes.
Folacin (folic acid):   Greens, wheat germ, organ meats, legumes, whole grains, cabbage family, citrus fruits, and liver.
Iodine: Seafood, algae, cod-liver oil, iodized salt.
Iron: Red meats, organ meats, legumes, dried fruit, tomato juice, poultry, nuts, eggs.
Vitamin K: Greens, the cabbage family, dairy products, legumes, and eggs.
Manganese: Nuts, whole grains, tea, coffee, greens.
Molybdenum: Legumes, cereals, coffee, tea, greens, meats.
Niacin (B$_3$):   Nuts, red meat, fish (oily and non-oily), poultry, organ meats, dairy products, fungi.
Pantothenic acid (B$_5$):   Whole grains, legumes, dairy products, eggs, organ meats, red meat (especially beef), bananas, watermelon.
Pyroxidine (B$_6$):   Whole grains, fruits, red meats, legumes, nuts, wheat germ, fungi, poultry, fish (oily and non-oily), organ meats.
Riboflavin (B$_2$):   Dairy products, organ meats, red meats, poultry, fish (oily and non-oily), greens, legumes, nuts, and eggs.
Selenium: Seafood, meats, organ meats, cabbage family, onion family, tomatoes, tuna, milk, egg yolk, whole grains.
Thiamine (B$_1$):   Whole grains, legumes, red meats, organ meats, wheat germ, nuts, fish (oily and non-oily), fungi.
Zinc: Oysters (but not other shellfish), meat, liver, eggs, brewer's yeast, pumpkin seeds.

(Periodical References and Additional Reading: *New York Times* 1-31-91; *Harvard Health Letter* 3-91, p 1; *New York Times* 7-1-92, p A18; *New York Times* 6-9-92, p C3; *Science News* 9-25-93, p 207; *New York Times* 9-30-92, p C2; *New York Times* 10-7-92, p A1; *Science News* 3-13-93, p 175; *Harvard Health Letter* 4-93, p 8; *New York Times* 10-26-93, p C6; *University of California at Berkeley Wellness Letter* 1-94, p 4; *New York Times* 1-5-94, p C4)

OLD AND NEW WEIGHT TABLES

On November 5, 1990, the U.S. Departments of Agriculture and of Health and Human Services issued new guidelines for weight. These were intended to replace the Metropolitan Life weight table that had been a standard for over 30 years. The newer guidelines, given below, are both different in content and format. For one thing, heavier people, especially older heavier people, can find themselves within the guideline limits for their height—the table is separated into a young-person section and an over-35 section. Also, unlike previous guidelines, there are no separate figures for males and females. The authors of the new chart think that a healthy weight is the same for either sex. Also, the old MetLife tables allowed a person to rate himself or herself by "frame," wherein those with larger frames were allowed extra pounds. There was no widely accepted definition of frame.

It should also be noted that the 1990 tables are not the only attempts to replace the 1959 MetLife tables. In 1983 MetLife itself issued a new table, with weights averaging 13 pounds heavier for men and 10 pounds for women, with no allowance for different frames. The basis for this revision was the weights of people who had lived the longest. These tables were criticized by medical groups and not accepted by the public. In 1985 a set of tables was issued by the National Institute of Aging that was organized by age instead of by gender, and frame.

The 1990 tables combine some features of the 1983 MetLife tables (heavier weights) and the National Institute of Aging table (some adjustments for age, none for gender). Here are some cross-table comparisons:

	Man, age 40, 5'8", medium frame	Woman, age 40, 5'6", medium frame
1959 MetLife	143 to 155, midpt: 149	130 to 144, midpt: 137
1983 MetLife	137 to 171, midpt: 154	120 to 160, midpt: 140
1985 Aging Ins.	137 to 174, midpt: 155.5	129 to 164, midpt: 146.5
1990 U.S. Gov't	138 to 178, midpt: 156	130 to 167, midpt: 148.5

It is apparent from both the high weights allowed and the midpoints that each subsequent table has allowed heavier weights. Some have called this is a departure from standards, while others claim that the new tables simply reflect a better understanding of health. In the meantime, mannequins used to display clothing to prospective buyers in department stores have slimmed significantly since 1959, losing inches about their waists, derrieres, and thighs. Thus Americans, especially women, have received mixed signals about a desirable weight.

	1990 U.S. Departments of Agriculture and Health and Human Services Guidelines		1959 MetLife Guidelines (range from sm. to lg. frame)	
Height	Ages 19 to 34	Ages 35 and up	Men	Women
5'0"	97-128	108-138	123-145	103-137
5'1"	101-132	111-143	125-148	105-140
5'2"	104-137	115-148	127-151	108-144
5'3"	107-141	119-152	129-155	111-148
5'4"	111-146	122-157	131-159	114-152
5'5"	114-150	126-162	133-163	117-156
5'6"	118-155	130-167	135-167	120-160
5'7"	121-160	134-172	137-171	123-164
5'8"	125-164	138-178	139-175	126-167
5'9"	129-169	142-183	141-179	129-170
5'10"	132-174	146-188	144-183	132-173
5'11"	136-179	151-194	147-187	135-176
6'0"	140-184	155-199	150-192	
6'1"	144-189	159-205	153-197	
6'2"	148-195	164-210	157-202	
6'3"	152-200	168-216		
6'4"	156-205	173-222		
6'5"	160-211	177-228		
6'6"	164-216	182-234		

Health by Gender

THE STATE OF
HEALTH BY GENDER

While the feminist movement began with a search for simple political and social equality between women and men, it has evolved to include many of the other issues that divide the human sexes. Although it was always clear that some diseases, such as breast or prostate cancer, were closely related to sexual characteristics of humans, only recently has this recognition become a major issue, especially for women. Furthermore, one of the major concerns of the women's movement since the 1960s has been the treatment of women by male doctors.

La Différence

One significant reason women are concerned about health issues—a reason that transcends the examining room—is that women (and many men) have come to the realization that research on diseases that affect both men and women has been largely conducted on male subjects. Thus if women's bodies react differently than men's, researchers have had little knowledge of it. And in the early 1990s evidence began to accumulate that women do react differently than men: oral contraceptives taken by women interfere with some drugs; almost all drugs are absorbed at different rates by women's bodies; and some drugs produce unexpected reactions in women that do not occur in men for reasons that have not been determined. Heart disease especially differs between men and women in several ways, as is discussed below.

Furthermore, research on animals has demonstrated that reactions can be different in quite subtle ways. Experiments with mice in 1993 showed that the nerve pathways female mice use to deal with pain after severe stress are different than those used by males. In this case, the difference can be attributed to some mysterious effect of estrogen, for the females use the same pain-reaction pathways as males when deprived of the hormone.

Official steps are being taken or suggested to remedy the lack of information about women's reactions to drugs in the U.S. The U.S. National Institutes of Health (NIH) established an Office of Women's Health Research in the early 1990s, for example. A report by the U.S. Congress's General Accounting Office (GAO) in October 1992 proposed that the U.S. Food and Drug Administration (FDA) should require that manufacturers test all new products on appropriate numbers of women. The GAO had discovered that for three drugs out of five the proportion of women in manufacturer's tests was less than the proportion expected to use the drugs, even though then-existing FDA guidelines called for appropriate sex ratios in drug testing. The FDA responded on March 24, 1993 by doing what the GAO had suggested and more. First of all, it lifted a 16-year-old ban on women in the Phase I safety trials of drugs—a ban originally instituted to protect fetuses. Now women taking contraceptive measures or otherwise certain of not becoming pregnant will be recruited. Furthermore, it made the previous guidelines mandatory, as suggested by the GAO, and even strengthened them. Thus future research on drugs and medical devices will have to include women.

Another official reaction to the increasing concern about adequate research on women came from the U.S. National Institutes of Health (NIH) a few days after the FDA announcement. The NIH on March 30, 1993 announced a 14-year, $625 million study of the health problems of women between the ages of 50 and 79. The study would deal with heart disease, cancer, and osteoporosis, with the main focus on diet, hormonal therapy, and lifestyle changes that would help prevent these diseases. The complex research program would be called the Woman's Health Initiative. Eight months later, on November 1, 1993, the independent advisory board the Institute of Medicine, an arm of the U.S. National Academy of Sciences, criticized the NIH plan as too expensive and too complicated. The Institute of Medicine had been asked for its opinion by the House Appropriations Committee, which was alarmed by the amount of money involved.

One suggested way to deal better with women's separate and often unequal health problems would be to develop a new medical specialty that would deal with all aspects of a woman's health. At present, a woman may have at least two separate doctors: one for reproductive functions, which are possibly viewed by males as more important than other parts of a woman's being, and then the same internists and specialists as a man has for everything else. In practice, women often skip the internist and just see the gynecologist. Some have said that women now get poorer treatment because they typically have to see two or three physicians for regular health, whereas a man sees a single internist or family practitioner. These critics would like a new specialty to combine gynecology along with internal medicine.

Such new women's specialists might be women doctors as well; a study published in the August 12, 1993 *New England Journal of Medicine* found that women physicians were twice as likely as male doctors to give their female patients Pap smears and also were more likely to prescribe mammograms. Younger male doctors were more responsive to women's needs than older ones, however.

Women's Problems

Some feminists accuse the medical establishment of more than just neglect. The two most common forms of surgery in the U.S. are performed on women—the caesarean section (*see* "Birth, Natural and Otherwise," p 112) and removal of the uterus (womb), or hysterectomy. In the early 1980s about three quarters of a million hysterectomies were being performed each year. Feminists and some male doctors claim that the popularity of the hysterectomy is largely a result of economics. The surgeon makes a lot of money in short order and the treatment quickly solves such problems as fibroid tumors, endometriosis, sagging of the uterus or other nearby organs, and pelvic pain of unknown origin—all of which are difficult, but not impossible, to treat without surgery. As a result of criticism or of the availability of different treatments, the number of hysterectomies dropped throughout the 1980s and reached 590,000 by 1990, the last year for which figures were available in 1993. Even so, a study published in May 1993 in the *Journal of the American Medical Association* proclaimed that careful examination of hysterectomies randomly selected from several health maintenance organizations found that only 58 percent of the operations should have been performed.

Despite the excess hysterectomies, a frequent complaint is that problems of women's reproductive organs often fail to be taken seriously, especially by male doctors. One such problem is a condition called vulvodynia, or painful itching and inflammation of the vulva, the opening to the vagina. It may affect as many as 200,000 women in the U.S. Until the late 1980s, no one knew what caused vulvodynia. At that time, it was finally connected to calcium oxalate from dietary sources in one patient. Since then other studies have shown that calcium oxalate metabolism is involved in many cases of the disease, but not in all of them. When the problem is calcium oxalate, it can be solved or mitigated by avoiding foods high in oxalate, such as dark leafy vegetables, legumes, and berries.

Women and the Heart

Heart disease has been the leading cause of death for women since 1908, but because men tend to have heart attacks younger than women, heart disease has long been thought of primarily as a male phenomenon. One way to look at the difference between the sexes in this instance is that men really do have more heart attacks than similarly aged women up to about the age of 65. After that, the rates for both sexes are about the same. Because heart disease is by far the leading cause of death in the U.S. (*see* "Heart Disease and Strokes UPDATE," p 400), this is true for both sexes.

But heart disease and its treatment are different for each sex. First of all, there is that age difference. Women seldom have heart disease before menopause. The reason is thought to be that estrogen influences the ratio of "good" high-density lipoprotein (HDL) to "bad" low-density lipoprotein (LDL) cholesterol. A high HDL/LDL ratio is a known protector against heart disease. Estrogen replacement therapy after menopause is thought to reduce the rate of heart disease (or stroke) by 50 percent.

Women frequently suffer from the pain of angina, caused by insufficient oxygen reaching the heart muscle. But angina often seems to be pain in some other part of the body, not necessarily the heart. Physicians may think women's angina pain has some other cause, especially if the doctors are not expecting heart disease. Also, women, like female mice, may use different pain pathways than men (*see* above). Some women fail to exercise when they are older, and angina is masked most of the time, failing to warn of heart disease.

Standard tests often fail to detect heart disease in women for reasons that are poorly understood. The treadmill test is especially prone to unreliable results. Chest images can be harder to obtain because of women's breasts.

Women with heart disease have a worse prognosis than men with similar problems. Women are twice as likely as men to die after a heart attack. According to a study of 4532 heart attacks by Jaime Caro of Medical Research International in Burlington, Massachusetts, reported in March 1993 to the American College of Cardiology, women may survive heart attacks less often because women fail to be treated as aggressively for heart attacks as men do. If women survive, they have more damage to their hearts and are more likely to have a second attack within a year of the first.

Women are also less likely to survive surgical treatments, such as bypasses or angioplasty. Usually women with heart disease are both smaller, with smaller blood vessels, and older than men who undergo corrective surgery or procedures. Another reason for differences in response to heart attacks or surgery may be that women's blood vessels react differently to medications.

What About Him?

Health issues that primarily apply to men are much simpler and most are treated in separate articles (see "Prostate Problems," p 230 and "Impotence Reconsidered," p 233). Despite claims from both sexes, the reason is not only that women are complicated and men are simple. In contrast to women, men have no complaints about being treated primarily by male physicians, and there are no specialists in specifically male problems. Such difficulties as impotence and prostate cancer, for example, are treated by the same urologists who aid women with urinary tract illnesses.

One example of a male health difficulty is chlamydia, one of the most common sexually transmitted diseases, but it normally has been found largely in women. This is not because men fail to contract and spread the disease; it is because until 1993 the only test for the disease was to insert a swab into the suspected infected region of the body and culture the material on the swab for the microorganism *Chlamydia trachomatis*. For women, this is not a big problem as the regions likely to infected are easily reached with the swab. For men the swab has to be inserted into the urethra through the opening of the penis. This is quite painful and men avoid being tested unless they themselves have unpleasant symptoms. But in 1993 a urine test was developed that, combined with follow up, is less costly and more accurate than the standard urethral swab culture. Not to mention a lot less painful.

(Periodical References and Additional Reading: *New York Times* 8-6-91, p C1; *New York Times* 7-1-92, p C12; *New York Times* 10-30-92, p A14; *New York Times* 11-7-92, p A1; *New York Times* 3-18-93, p A18; *New York Times* 3-25-93, p B8; *New York Times* 3-31-93, p A21; *New York Times* 6-30-93, p C14; *New York Times* 10-13-93, p A1; *New York Times* 10-27-93, p C11; *New York Times* 11-3-93, p C16; *New York Times* 11-10-93, p C17; *Discover* 1-94, p 71)

TIMETABLE OF WOMEN'S HEALTH TO 1990

138   Soranus of Ephesus [born 98; died 138], the first great Greek writer on obstetrics and gynecology, dies.

779   St. Walpurga dies in this year; an English princess who studied medicine, Walpurga is often depicted holding a flask of urine in one hand and bandages in the other.

1070   Trotula of Salerno writes *Passionibus mulierum curandorum* (The Diseases of Women), which deals with the medical needs of women.

1179	Hildegarde of Bingen [born 1098; died 1179] (Germany), author of *The Book of Simple Medicine* and *The Book of Compound Medicine*, which treat not only medicine but also sexuality, dies.
1322	Female physician Jocaba Felicie (Italy) is charged by the Dean and Faculty of Medicine of the University of Paris with illegally visiting the sick of both sexes, examining them, prescribing drugs, collecting fees, and curing patients; she defends herself in part on the grounds that male physicians do not understand the "secret nature" of female infirmities, but loses the case anyway.
1513	*Garden of Roses for Pregnant Wives and Midwives* by Eucharius Rosslin is the earliest printed guide for midwives.
1636	Louise Bourgeois [born 1563; died 1636], midwife to the French Court, dies after writing extensively about her profession after her retirement.
1671	Jane Sharp's (England) *The Compleat Midwive's Companion* argues that only women should deal with birth and that male physicians are not sanctioned by the Bible.
1687	Midwife Elizabeth Cellier petitions the Court of James II of England for a Royal Hospital for women to be managed by midwives, but the English College of Physicians scuttles the idea.
1721	Lady Mary Wortley Montagu (England) [born 1689?; died 1762] introduces the practice of inoculating children with smallpox, which she had learned in Turkey.
1853	John Snow administers chloroform to Queen Victoria of England during the birth of her eighth child; prior to this many had believed that it was immoral to give anesthesia to women in childbirth.
1953	Alfred C. Kinsey (United States) [born 1894; died 1953] and coworkers produce a landmark study of sexual practices of U.S. women. Among the conclusions: almost half have sexual relations before marriage; a quarter are unfaithful afterward; and of those unmarried, a quarter have had a homosexual relationship.
1960	About this time some women enlarge or reshape their breasts with a semi-liquid plastic (silicone gel) in a bag that is implanted in the skin. About two million women will use the implants in the next 30 years.
1965	Morris E. Davis reports that estrogen therapy prevents atherosclerosis and osteoporosis in postmenopausal women.
1988	Scientists from Johns Hopkins show that the drug Taxol, made from yew bark, is helpful in fighting ovarian cancer.

WOMEN'S HEALTH

BREAST CANCER

Throughout the early 1990s there was considerable concern, much real and some manufactured, about breast cancer as a major killer. Advocates wanted the amount of money spent on research on the disease, about $158 million in fiscal 1992, to come closer to the amount spent on AIDS research, roughly calculated as $1.1 billion, nearly eight times as much as on breast cancer. Many felt strongly that the discrepancy was in part discrimination against women by the male-dominated medical establishment. The lobbying was effective. In fiscal 1993, while AIDS research only went up to $1.2 billion, planned spending on breast-cancer research was increased to $400 million, more than double the previous year, although $200 million of that was in the Defense Department budget. Regular research spending by the end of the year was still up, however, to $197 million. The next year, regular spending for fiscal 1994 on breast cancer research was estimated at $262.9 million. Although still far below the AIDS level, it was considerably higher than the $90.3 million for lung cancer, which actually causes more deaths among women than breast cancer does. While incidence of breast cancer is by far the highest form of cancer among women, treatment of breast cancer saves more lives. About a quarter of the women diagnosed with breast cancer die from it, but four-fifths of the women with lung cancer are killed by the disease. Furthermore, the greatest fatality risk to women is not cancer in any case — cancer risks are far lower than from heart disease or type II diabetes and even less than that of dying from complications of a hip fracture.

More Statistics

Mark Twain is credited with a low view of statistics. If he had followed the breast cancer controversies of the early 1990s, he would have found little to change his opinion. Headlines that tell the tale include "RISE IN RISK OF BREAST CANCER: One in Nine Women Likely to Get Disease" and "Risk of Breast Cancer Jumps to 1 in 9, Study Says" at the start of 1991; "Chance of Breast Cancer is Figured at 1 in 8" in the fall of 1992; and "Rethinking the Statistics of 'Epidemic' Breast Cancer" early in 1993.

The first headline referred to a change from a 10 percent risk of breast cancer over a woman's lifetime (to 85 years old) to an 11 percent risk. The rise of one percentage point means a change from one in ten (used from 1987 to 1990 by the American Cancer Society) to one in nine, since the fraction 1/9 is equivalent to 11 percent. The American Cancer Society accompanied its press release with a graph showing the chance of breast cancer as 4.9 percent in 1940, 6.6 percent in 1950, 7.0 percent in 1960, 7.6 percent in 1980, and 11.2 percent in 1987. Despite the dramatic-appearing graph and the headlines, the Cancer Society attributed most of the change to improved diagnosis, not to an actual increase in incidence.

On September 26, 1992, the National Cancer Institute (NCI) changed its prediction of the chances for breast cancer in a woman's lifetime to one in eight (actually 12.57 percent), up from one in nine (actually the somewhat higher 11.5 percent). The NCI admitted, however, that the new figure did not come from a rise in the incidence of breast cancer. Instead it was an artifact resulting from a change in their rules so that "lifetime" no longer stopped at age 85. Most breast cancers, according to NCI statistics, develop after the age of 50, so—using their own figures—the chances of getting breast cancer before the age of 50 are only one in 40 instead of one in eight. About 30 percent of those who develop breast cancer, all ages considered, die from the disease. If that death rate were spread equally among women, the chances of dying from breast cancer before the age of 50 would be about one in 130. Looked at another way, the risk of a 40-year-old woman of developing breast cancer before she is 50 is one in 63; for a 60-year-old, the risk of developing the disease before age 70 is one in 28. Nevertheless, campaigns for more money for breast cancer research stressed the one in eight figure.

By the end of February 1993 enough thought had been given to the statistical manipulation to lead to the "rethinking the statistics" article. Much of the information had been released with the original statistics in the previous two years, but had not gotten the attention that the scarier sounding figures had. For example, an apparent rise in breast cancer among women in their twenties and thirties was always noted in responsible publications as being an artifact of there being a larger proportion of young women in the population as a result of past changes in the birth rates. In fact, the underlying incidence of breast cancer has remained the same for decades, with any apparent rise the result of better detection. The basic mortality rates have also stayed about the same for decades.

When examined in five-year intervals, the greatest number of breast cancer cases occur in women from 65 to 69, while the second greatest number are women from 70 to 74, with the early sixties and late seventies about tied for third place. When all women are considered, almost 75 percent of the breast cancer incidence is in women over the age of 60. Looked at another way, however, the same statistic can be stated as more than one out of four breast cancer cases are in women under the age of 60.

Causes, Avoidable and Not

Since statistics have sometimes been misinterpreted to mean that the incidence or severity of breast cancer is on the rise, various theories have been put forth to account for the supposed increase.

Heredity: For breast cancer, as for many diseases including most common forms of cancer, the best prevention had been thought to be to choose your parents wisely. But a study published on July 21, 1993 in the *Journal of the American Medical Association* and revised a few months later showed that in 2389 women with breast cancer, the percentage of cases that could be linked to family history was only six percent. Although that meant that hereditary connections were looser than previously believed, a woman with a mother or sister who has been diagnosed with breast cancer still has twice the risk of breast cancer as a woman without that cancer in her immediate family.

Diet: Starting with the first concern about dietary cholesterol in the 1950s, diseases of all kinds have increasingly been thought to be encouraged, if not actually caused, by diet. Breast cancer is no exception. At the beginning of 1991, a writer on the relationship between food and health could confidently state that "a low-fat diet (that is, one that includes fewer than 25 grams of fat for every 1000 calories consumed) is rated highly effective in protecting against cancers of the breast...." The main evidence for this point of view is that in Japan, where most people have eaten a low-fat diet for most of their lives, the breast-cancer rate is less than a fourth of what it is in the U.S. Similarly, women in one region of Italy who derive fewer than 30 percent of their calories from fat have half the rate of breast cancer of other women from that region.

Similarly, a high-fiber diet was rated as somewhat effective in preventing breast cancer. Fiber's protective power had first been recognized among Finnish women, who ate a lot of fat but also a lot of fiber. Experiments with rats supported the high-fiber diet. Rats who eat a lot of fiber along with a lot of fat have almost half rate of breast cancer as those who take the fat without the fiber. Even low-fat diet rats get breast cancer at reduced rates if they have a high-fiber diet.

Although low fat and high fiber works for rats and for Japanese, Italian, and Finnish women, applying it to Americans has proved difficult. Two studies released in 1992, one of 35,000 American women and one of almost 90,000 American nurses, failed to find any relationship between a low-fat diet and breast cancer. The nurse's study also looked at dietary fiber and found no connection with breast cancer either. There is some reason to suspect that the apparent relationship with diet has less to do with fat than with calories consumed during rapid growth at puberty.

A year later, however, the role of fat in breast cancer was still being debated. Even the directors of both 1992 studies that found no dietary connection still believed that it was possible for a low-fat diet, provided it was low enough, to prevent breast cancer. The studies of women in 1992 used 30 percent of calories from fat as a "low-fat diet." Perhaps if the amount of fat calories was closer to the ten to 20 percent historically common in Japan, the low-fat diet would also work with American women.

At the same time, a plausible reason for relating fat to breast cancer is that fat contains certain chemicals picked up from the environment. This also can be used to explain differences between Japanese and American experience.

Environmental chemicals: The idea is that perhaps environmental chemicals that mimic estrogen are stored in fat, and the chemicals in the environment may be different in different countries. One small Swedish study released in the January 6, 1993 *Journal of the National Cancer Institute* found that some women apparently could prevent a return of previously excised cancer by sticking to a low-fat diet, but only those women with abundant estrogen receptors in their breast cells were so capable.

There is limited evidence that environmental chemicals that act like estrogen, especially some pesticides (DDT, heptachlor, atrazine, and others), polycyclic aromatic hydrocarbons (PAHs), and PCBs (polychlorinated biphenyls), may build up in fatty tissue and increase cancer risk. In the New York University Women's Health Study, Mary S. Wolff of Mount Sinai Medical School in New York City and coworkers found that a DDT by-product that is stored in fat was about 35 percent higher in the women with cancer than in those without.

Estrogen processing: In the December 1, 1993 *Journal of the National Cancer Institute* Michael P. Osborne and coworkers reported that noncancerous tissue of women with breast cancer metabolized estrogen in an uncommon way: that one of the by-products of estrogen metabolism in those women was a chemical implicated in genetic damage and abnormal cell growth.

Drinking: Alcohol consumption has been found in some studies to be a risk factor, especially high alcohol consumption (more than three drinks daily) and alcohol use starting at an early age. As with dietary fat, some studies find an association while others do not.

Electromagnetic fields: A panel of experts from the U.S. Centers for Disease Control and Prevention declared that there was no reason to think that breast cancer rates on Long Island, which have been about 20 percent higher than rest of New York state, were any more than a statistical fluke. Despite this conclusion, the U.S. National Institutes of Health started a major study of breast cancer in Long Island late in 1993. The suspects being examined were pesticides and electromagnetic fields from appliances or overhead wires. Results should be available in 1998 or 1999.

Other factors: In addition to the genetic factor, some other factors beyond a woman's control are statistically associated with increased risk of breast cancer. These include early menstruation and late menopause, both of which also influence hormone levels for long periods of time. Oral contraceptives, for similar reasons, may also result in a slight increase in risk of breast cancer, though in that case the effect of delaying pregnancy might be the important factor. While a postmenopausal woman is taking estrogen, risks are increased, but risks return to lower levels when estrogen therapy is halted. All of these factors were found to increase cancer risk in nearly 90,000 nurses.

Causes and Prevention

Avoiding the avoidable causes may be one form of prevention, provided that eating fat, drinking alcohol, and exposure to pesticides really do promote cancer. Some other approaches have also been proposed.

Vitamins: In the July 22, 1993, *New England Journal of Medicine* Graham A. Colditz, David J. Hunter, Walter C. Willett, and coworkers at the Harvard School of Public Health reported their analysis of data from the 89,494 women in the Nurses Health Study. They found that women who consumed the greatest amount of vitamin A had a 20 percent lower risk of breast cancer.

Tamoxifen: In May 1992 the NCI started a large-scale attempt to chemically lower breast cancer risks in 16,000 healthy women by administering 20 milligrams daily of the chemical tamoxifen. Tamoxifen is a partial analog to estrogen, with important differences. Called Nolvadex in the U.S., tamoxifen is thought to help control cancer by preventing estrogen from being used by tumor cells. Estrogen stimulates breast cells to divide. Tamoxifen has been used for 24 years in the treatment of breast cancer, but in 1991 it was suggested that the drug might also prevent cancer, and trials were begun.

Critics were concerned about possible side effects of giving tamoxifen for reasons other than treatment. Unpublished research in 1993 and a published report in the

March 1993 *Journal of Clinical Oncology* both suggested that women taking tamoxifen were likely to develop a deadly form of uterine cancer. Furthermore, a year into the study, some long-standing research was finally published showing that high doses of tamoxifen cause liver cancer in rats, an event already foreshadowed by a case reported in the April 11, 1992 *Lancet* in which a woman in Nottingham, England, receiving 20 milligrams of tamoxifen daily, succumbed to massive damage to her liver cells. Her doctors asked around and found that several other patients in England had also developed tamoxifen-induced liver damage, including three additional fatalities.

Nevertheless a benefit of tamoxifen that has also been touted is its ability to lower cholesterol levels in the blood by about 12 percent over the course of tamoxifen treatment. This might prevent heart attacks in women recovering from breast cancer. However, an analysis by Trudy L. Bush and Kathy J. Helzsouer of Johns Hopkins University published in September in *Epidemiologic Review* suggests that benefits from heart attacks in the population likely to get breast cancer are much less than had been thought.

All in all, Bush and Helzsouer evaluated several benefits and risks from giving tamoxifen to healthy women. Their conclusion was that there were not enough heart attacks and breast cancers prevented to justify the increased risk of uterine cancer, blood clots, and toxicity to eyes.

Other factors: Other factors have shown a statistical reduction in the risk of breast cancer. Of these, the most reliable seems to be the age of first pregnancy. A lower age means less chance of breast cancer, possibly because of some unknown effect of hormones.

Detection

Both diagnosis and treatment of breast cancer were at least as controversial as the statistics and the risk factors in the early 1990s. Various authoritative medical groups took sides on the need for mammography at different age levels, while the research methods of large-scale treatment studies were shown to be severely flawed.

Mammography is a method for making X-ray studies of women's breasts to detect abnormal tissue. Because it uses X rays, a form of ionizing radiation known to cause cancer under high, repeated, or prolonged doses, the procedure can negatively influence the very condition it is designed to detect. Furthermore, the procedure is expensive enough that attempts to control medical costs that focus on unnecessary diagnostic tests—a common concern of cost accountants—become a large part of the overall controversy. Near the end of 1993 the U.S. Food and Drug Administration set up standards that the 12,000 mammography clinics will have to maintain to stay in business, standards widely viewed as not being met at that time.

Dangers, if any: A Swedish study (published in the October 20, 1993 *Journal of the National Cancer Institute*) reported that high-dose breast radiation used to treat benign cysts in 1216 women in the 1920s through the 1950s showed a statistically significant increase in breast cancer. Of course, mammography uses low-dose radiation, so the situation is not actually comparable. Moreover, there is some reason to suspect that having benign cysts is also a risk factor for breast cancer, which complicates a complex relationship even more. There is some older evidence from the 1980s that suggests that mammograms early in life may increase risks for breast cancer, but no such evidence exists for women who have frequent mammograms (annually, for example) after the age of 40.

Usefulness, and at what age: There is general agreement that women under the age of 40 have too slight a risk of breast cancer to warrant screening and that women over the age of 50 have been shown to benefit from screening. The ten-year gap in between is in dispute. From 1987 until 1993, however, the most authoritative voices in cancer treatment agreed that screening should begin at 40. In 1993, however, opinions began to change.

Suzanne W. Fletcher of the American College of Physicians in Philadelphia and others participated in a workshop review of available research on the effectiveness of mammography in screening for breast cancer, the conclusions of which were published in the October 20, 1993 *Journal of the National Cancer Institute*. The workshop participants concluded that there was no benefit from screening in the 40 to 49 age range, but there was a reduction in the risk of death from breast cancer for women who were regularly screened in the 50 to 69 age range. Their conclusions were immediately rejected in an editorial in the same issue, which claimed that there was too little good data to be sure.

Nevertheless, on December 3, 1993 the NCI ceased recommending screening for women aged 40 through 49. This left the NCI siding with the American College of Physicians and the American College of Family Practice on this issue, but differing with the American Cancer Society and the American College of Radiologists (whose members are paid to do mammography). A few weeks earlier an advisory board to the NCI had suggested that it make no recommendations, but the advice was not followed.

An alternative?   A study reported in November 1993 of more than a thousand cases of breast cancer showed that high-resolution, digital ultrasound scanning could reduce the need for biopsies. It was not reported if ultrasound might also be used in place of mammograms.

Treatment

After screening, the most common treatment involves removal of at least the cancer (lumpectomy), or the breast (mastectomy), or the breast and associated tissue including lymph nodes in the shoulder and pectoral muscles (radical mastectomy). A subcutaneous mastectomy is removal of the breast except for the skin and superficial tissues and replacement of the breast by an implant (more on implants below). In most cases, removal is followed by radiation treatments, chemotherapy, hormonal therapy with tamoxifen, or some combination. On November 29, 1993, Carl Mansfield of Thomas Jefferson University Hospital in Philadelphia, Pennsylvania, told the Radiological Society of North America that breast implants of radioactive substances (not to be confused with the implants discussed below) are as effective as lumpectomy for many cases of cancer if detected early enough.

Breast cancer treatment has caused more public controversy than other forms of cancer treatment. Women with cancer are frequently torn between a desire to keep the affected breast and a fear of the cancer spreading. Well-publicized problems in the major study of the effectiveness of various forms of treatment further contributed to confusion. In 1990 the NCI recommended lumpectomy followed by radiation for the most common kind of breast cancer, which is a small tumor that has not advanced in any obvious way to the lymph nodes. About two-thirds of all cases of breast cancer fit this pattern. But many U.S. physicians were unhappy with this recommendation because they felt there was not enough research to prove lumpectomy as effective as mastectomy. Research continued, resulting in one of a group of notorious studies conducted under the direction of Bernard Fisher of the University of Pittsburgh in Pennsylvania. It was a study of 319 women treated with lumpectomy and radiation who had only ten percent recurrence of breast cancer, of which only three percent was serious; it was published in the *New England Journal of Medicine* on June 3, 1993.

Breast Implants

While not exactly part of the treatment for breast cancer, many women who have had mastectomies have also replaced the breast tissue with a silicone or saline implant so that the shape of the torso would not be changed by breast removal. Throughout the early 1990s such implants—which are used for purely cosmetic purposes 80 percent of the time and to replace breast tissue lost to cancer in the remaining 20 percent— were implicated in various diseases. Since 1988 implant manufacturers have been on warning from the U.S. Food and Drug Administration (FDA). At the start of the 1990s, about one to three million Americans (not all of them women) had such implants installed. The estimates of the number of installed implants have varied wildly, with later estimates often lower than earlier ones. Much of the controversy over the side effects of implants has occupied the courts.

In March 1991, a woman won a court case on the grounds that her implant— actually the polyurethane foam covering of the implant—had caused breast cancer, leading to the removal of one of her breasts. At that time about a tenth of all installed implants had been coated with this kind of foam, about 100,000 to 200,000 implants. In April 1991 the FDA declared that its scientists could establish a definite cause and effect relationship between the foam coats and breast cancer. The manufacturer of implants that used the polyurethane coating, Bristol-Myers Squibb, then stopped selling implants of this type and asked physicians to cease using them. But a month later Bristol-Myers Squibb said that animal tests showed that the actual risk of cancer from the implants was small; the FDA also notified physicians that risks ranged from as high as one in ten thousand to as low as one in a million, depending on which studies were used. Critics, including anonymous sources at the FDA, cited their own choices of animal studies that showed that implanted polyurethane causes cancer in one in seven, one in fifty, or one in five hundred instances in rats and mice. No studies have ever shown cancers caused by polyurethane implants in mammals other than rodents. The chemical formed in the breakdown of polyurethane that is suspected of causing human cancers, 2-toulene-diamene (TDA), has been found in the blood (by the FDA) and urine (by Bristol-Myers Squibb) of women using the coated implants. There was also an earlier report of TDA in the breast milk of a nursing mother who had received a coated implant.

Other concerns besides breast cancer caused the FDA to ask manufacturers (primarily Dow Corning) to stop selling silicone breast implants of any kind on January 6, 1992. A year later the FDA also notified the makers of saline-filled implants (silicone bags filled with salt water) that the safety of those devices was also in doubt. Silicone, either in all-silicone implants or as the envelope in saline-filled implants, has not been associated with breast cancer but has been connected to a host of other diseases caused by immune system malfunctions. (*See* "Implants and the Immune System," below.)

(Periodical References and Additional Reading: *New York Times* 11-28-90, p A19; *New York Times* 1-25-91; *New York Times* 3-24-91; *New York Times* 3-30-91; *New York Times* 4-14-91, p I-18; *New York Times* 6-2-91; *New York Times* 4-18-92, p B13; *Science News* 4-27-91, p 260; *Harvard Health Letter* 5-91, p 3; *New York Times* 7-21-91, p A1; *Science News* 5-9-92, p 309; *New York Times* 5-16-92; *New York Times* 5-17-92, p A14; *Science News* 7-4-92, p 12; *New York Times* 7-28-92, p D2; *New York Times* 8-28-92, p A17; *Harvard Health Letter* 8-92, p 4; *New York Times* 9-27-92, p A30; *New York Times* 10-19-92, p A15; *New York Times* 11-3-92, p D3; *New York Times* 1-7-93, p A16; *Science News* 1-9-93, p 23; *New York Times* 2-28-93, p IV-16; *New York Times* 3-20-93, p 8; *Science News* 4-24-93, p 262; *New York Times* 6-3-93, p A18; *Science News* 7-3-93, p 10; *Science News* 7-24-93, p 52; *Science News* 7-31-93, p 76; *New York Times* 9-8-93, p C4; *New York Times* 9-10-93, p A16; *New York Times* 9-11-93, p 7; *Science News* 9-18-93, p 181; *New York Times* 9-25-93, p 10; *Science News* 9-25-93, p 207; *New York Times* 10-20-93, p C14; *New York Times* 10-21-93, p C12; *Science News* 10-23-93, p 262; *New York Times* 11-25-93, p B1; *New York Times* 11-30-93, p C6; *New York Times* 12-1-93, pp A20 & C15; *New York Times* 12-2-93, p A24; *New York Times* 12-5-93, p I-30; *New York Times* 12-14-93, p C1; *New York Times* 12-21-93, p C13; *New York Times* 12-28-93, p C3)

IMPLANTS AND THE IMMUNE SYSTEM

Four out of five breast implants in the U.S. during the 1960s, 1970s, and 1980s were for cosmetic purposes. Early in the 1990s the U.S. Food and Drug Administration (FDA) effectively halted the use of cosmetic implants. The principal reason for banning new implants was a concern that silicone, used in virtually all breast implants, could activate the immune system to attack the implant wearer's body, causing such diseases as systemic lupus erythematosus (SLE), rheumatoid arthritis, or scleroderma (a disease in which skin hardens). About ten percent of all implants were also suspected of causing cancer because of a polyurethane coating (*See* "Breast Cancer," p 216). Many women were also unhappy with their implants for other reasons. Some silicone sacks broke apart or leaked, causing odd-shaped lumps. FDA Commissioner David A. Kessler estimated that 15 to 20 percent of all implants fail in one of these ways. A few silicone implants hardened, which could be painful. Fairly often, women who had undergone one operation to have cosmetic implants inserted then paid for a second expensive operation to have the implants removed.

One additional risk of cosmetic breast implants, discussed among physicians since at least 1988, is that the implant or changes in the breast caused by the implant can mask cancer, preventing detection by mammography. A before-and-after study released in the October 14, 1992 *Journal of the American Medical Association* confirmed that implants make mammography more difficult and probably could hide cancer.

Scientific data was often difficult to come by during the peak of the implant controversy. The August 29 *Lancet* reported that two children with silicone implants to treat birth defects had developed antibodies against silicone itself. The November 28, 1992 *Lancet* published a study of 28 women who had developed an autoimmune disease, such as SLE, after receiving breast implants. For some of these women, the implants had leaked or even broken apart. The study, led by Eng M. Tan of the Scripps Research Institute in La Jolla, California, found that the women possessed the kind of antibodies that are linked with autoimmune disease. Disease symptoms were more severe in the patients whose implants had permitted silicone to spread, suggesting that the silicone itself was at the root of the symptoms.

Dow Corning had been the biggest manufacturer of silicone implants (approximately 75 percent of the market) and became, along with other manufacturers, a target for lawsuits by women who blamed the implants for their diseases. Dow Corning was vulnerable because as early as 1971 internal company memos, which became public in the early 1990s, showed that Dow Corning scientists knew that silicone leaked from the implants into other parts of the body. Dow scientists were also caught altering some records related to implant safety testing. By the second quarter of 1992 Dow Corning profits had fallen as a result of heavy costs of getting out of the implant business, including estimated legal fees and costs for additional research. A year after Dow Corning stopped making implants and began conducting research they reported that their own animal studies showed that silicone irritates the immune system. On September 9, 1993, Dow Corning proposed that a fund of $4.75 billion be set aside by the implant manufacturers to pay claims against the devices.

The fund, which came into being in 1994, paid claims not only for women who developed SLE or scleroderma, but also those with mixed connective tissue disease or primary Sjogren's syndrome, which also includes dry eyes and mouth, and those with polymyositis or dermatomyositis (inflammation of skeletal muscles and skin). In some cases neurological disease or rheumatic arthritis might also qualify for payments. Individual payments were expected to be as high as $2 million.

One potential solution to several implant problems was a type called a saline-filled implant, which consists of a silicone bag filled with salt water. More transparent to mammograms than silicone implants, the saline-filled implants do not contain semi-liquid silicone in the bag. If they leak, they leak salt water, tolerated by human tissues in reasonable amounts. The silicone bags themselves could provoke immune responses, but research on this possibility is incomplete.

It should be noted that the implant problem is not limited to women or transsexuals. One treatment for impotence involves silicone implants in the penis.

Despite all the problems outlined above, the American Medical Association on November 30, 1993 declared silicone implants to be safe and urged changes in FDA policy so that people who want to use such implants would have the devices available.

(Periodical References and Additional Reading: *New York Times* 7-8-92, p D2; *New York Times* 8-28-92, p A17; *Science News* 10-17-92, p 262; *New York Times* 11-3-92, p D3; *Science News*

12-12-92, p 414; *New York Times* 1-7-93, p A16; *New York Times* 3-20-93, p 8; *New York Times* 9-10-93, p A16; *New York Times* 9-11-93, p 7; *New York Times* 12-1-93, p A20; *New York Times* 12-28-93, p C3)

WOMEN AND OTHER CANCERS

Breast cancer is far from the whole story. As noted in the breast cancer article, lung cancer kills more women. And a variety of cancers of the female reproductive system are major health problems.

Ovarian Cancer

At the end of 1992, Alice S. Whittemore of the Stanford School of Medicine and a large team of researchers from 14 different schools reviewed recent studies of ovarian cancer risks and reported the analysis in five articles published in the November 15, 1992, *American Journal of Epidemiology* and the January 20, 1993, *Journal of the National Cancer Institute.* They found the following:

Childbearing reduces the risk of ovarian cancer by about 14 percent for each successive child. Failed pregnancies, such as miscarriages and abortions, offer some protection, depending on how long the fetus is carried.

Drugs taken to enhance fertility, however, raise the chances of ovarian cancer, apparently by 27 times, although the sample size was very small and therefore the size of the increase could be exaggerated. The suggestion here, as in some previous studies, is that ovulation itself is a risk factor, since fertility drugs increase ovulation (and pregnancy decreases it).

Birth control pills, of which most presently used forms do not affect ovulation, do lower the risk of ovarian cancer, especially in older women. Thus ovulation is not the whole story. Furthermore, infertility by itself does not raise the risk, nor does a woman's age at menopause.

One woman in 70 in the U.S. will over her lifetime develop ovarian cancer and three out of five who have the cancer will die from it.

Cervical Cancer

For a long time now physicians have been aware of a danger from sexually transmitted genital warts in women; they may lead to cancer of the cervix. Test tube studies conducted by Mary M. Pater, Alan Pater, and coworkers at the Memorial University of Newfoundland in St. John's and reported in the January 1994 *Obstetrics & Gynecology* shed light on the mechanisms involved. The natural hormone progesterone and the synthetic hormone dexamethasone cause the RNA of the virus that transmits genital warts, known as a human papillomavirus (HPV), to increase dramatically. It is thought that the HPV messenger RNA codes for proteins that shut off some tumor-suppressing genes, thus paving the way for cancer to start. If the test-tube studies reflect what actually happens with humans infected by genital warts, that would explain the results of previous studies that have linked birth control pills, which contain progesterone, to cervical cancer. Women known to have genital warts caused by HPV might want to switch to some other form of birth control.

The drug RU 486, which blocks the action of progesterone, also prevents the increase of HPV messenger RNA in the test tube. Thus RU-486 might also be tried as a way to block cancer initiation in women thought to be at high risk because of genital warts or other factors.

Cervical cancer kills about 4400 American women annually.

Lung Cancer Controversy

Because women in large numbers started smoking cigarettes some twenty to thirty years after men took up the habit, lung cancer rates for women have until recently lagged far behind those for men. Lung cancer rates among women are now even climbing for passive smoke, however. The death rate among female nonsmokers from lung cancer was higher in the early 1990s than the total death rate from lung cancer among women in the 1960s or earlier.

For unknown reasons, it appears that the lung cancer risk, cigarette for cigarette, is twice as high for women as it is for men. An analysis presented in the *American Journal of Epidemiology* in September 1993 by Harvey Risch of the Yale School of Medicine compared the "pack-years" of men and women smokers and nonsmokers, some with lung cancer and some without. A pack-year is a pack a day for a year, or 7305 cigarettes in a year of 365.25 days. Women smokers with fewer than 30 pack-years of smoking have seven times the risk of female nonsmokers. The study found that this was higher than for men with fewer than 30 pack-years, who only had five times the risk of male nonsmokers. But the most mysterious aspect of this study was that the increased risk for women soared in comparison to increased risk for men as greater and greater numbers of pack-years were considered. By 60 pack-years, the women smokers had 82 times the risk of nonsmokers and the men smokers had only 23 times the risk of nonsmokers. Small numbers of people were used in each group, with the total number in the study only 1617 persons, so some of the differences could be accidental statistical artifacts. Nevertheless two other studies published in the *International Journal of Epidemiology* that same month also supported the notion that women smokers have higher lung-cancer risks. The other research, by Randall Harris and Judy Anderson at Ohio State University and by Edith Zang and Ernst Wynder of the American Health Foundation, furthermore used larger populations.

But two even larger studies, one by the American Cancer Society and one by the U.S. National Cancer Institute, both of which use different statistical means for comparison than the ones reported in the epidemiology journals, still show that when all other factors are taken into account men and women have the same level of risk of lung cancer from smoking. It is difficult to resolve the differences, and cancer researchers have taken sides on the issue.

(Periodical References and Additional Reading: *Science News* 1-16-93, p 38; *Science News* 1-23-93, p 54; *Science* 11-26-93, p 1375; *New York Times* 1-4-94, p C3)

MEANINGS OF MENSTRUATION AND MENOPAUSE

While men's bodies change as they grow older, nothing that happens to men is quite as dramatic as menstruation for women, which typically starts fairly suddenly when a girl is in her teens. This shedding of blood and other tissue through the vagina then starts and repeats, usually quite regularly, unless interrupted by pregnancy.

Not so dramatically, approximately forty years later, menstruation stops. The second change, and associated other changes, are called menopause.

Both sets of changes have seemed sufficiently mysterious that various myths and practices have arisen about them in primitive societies. Often a girl's first menstruation is a major event of great significance to society as well as to the girl herself; the event is greeted with ritual, and the girl is often isolated for a time.

Even in this scientific age, it is not entirely clear why either menstruation or menopause happens, though it is apparent that the bleeding in menstruation is a way of discarding an unfertilized egg and a uterine lining (endometrium) that had been prepared by hormones for implantation of a fertilized egg. But there are other theories for why menstruation and menopause occur.

A Protective Role for Menstruation

Margie Profet of the University of California at Berkeley has studied menstruation in humans and also in the few other mammals known to menstruate (some higher primates, and a few species of monkey, tree shrew, bat, and marsupial). Profet has a new theory on the subject, which was presented in the September 1993 issue of the *Quarterly Review of Biology*. In short, however, Profet thinks that menstruation is an adaptation that evolved as a drastic method for protecting the uterus and Fallopian tubes against infectious disease. (*See* "A Better Pregnancy," p 105, for another theory from Profet, who was given a MacArthur "genius" grant for her original contributions.)

Profet reasons that sperm cells nearly always carry bacteria along with them. Although cervical mucus protects against bacterial infection reaching the uterus, the mucus thins when an egg is ready to be fertilized. The endometrium is shed, instead of simply thinning until the next fertile period, to get rid of any bacteria or other pathogens (germs) that might infect it. Furthermore, large amounts of blood that flow easily instead of clotting not only wash out any germs that are lurking but also provide the special cells of the body's immune system, which tend to accumulate in the blood, where they would be needed to attack the pathogens.

Since menstruation is therefore an important part of reproduction, other mammals could be expected to menstruate as well—and Profet thinks that all of them do, to one degree or another. Scientists, in her view, have simply not looked for the phenomenon and therefore have missed it in most mammals. It is impossible to miss in humans, however, because humans need it more than the other mammals: human females are sexually receptive for more of the year, and menstruation is necessary. Why this happens is not part of Profet's theory.

Supporting the theory is the undisputed fact that human women are provided with special arteries and low-clotting blood, circumstances that would not be the case unless there was an evolutionary need for them. A study of blood samples from the Framingham heart group shows that premenopausal women have more of an inhibitor of a clot-busting substance than postmenopausal women do.

Not everyone agrees with Profet, but her theory does suggest some health-related ideas. First, she thinks that women need to bleed, so that oral contraceptives that prevent this should not be used. But physicians should also search carefully for infection when bleeding occurs at unusual times or in unusual amounts.

Menopause

As the life expectancy for women in industrialized nations hovers around 80, and the average age of menopause in the U.S. is 51, most women will be postmenopausal for about a third of their lives. For many women, the postmenopausal period will be as long as or longer than the number of years they spend menstruating. Thus, postmenopausal becomes the norm and menstruation the exception, reversing the pattern of ages past when many women died before menopause.

Freed from the necessity of ovulating every month, probably because the ova have aged to the point where the body no longer finds it worthwhile to try to protect, fertilize, and use them (see "Encouraging Conception and Pregnancy," p 90 for older women having babies with eggs donated by young women), the evolutionary reasons Profet sees for menstruation are gone. Therefore, neither is there need for the careful orchestration of hormones that prepares ova for fertilization. Production of estrogen declines and for practical purposes shuts down.

But women are less protected after menopause. With little or no estrogen, the ratio of testosterone to other hormones increases, and some postmenopausal women begin to grow face hair or lose scalp hair as men do. Worse, the protection against heart attacks that estrogen gave women is also gone. Before menopause, estrogen helped keep high the ratio of high-density lipoprotein (HDL) cholesterol to low-density lipoprotein (LDL) cholesterol. A high HDL/LDL ratio helps keep arteries clear. Thus for women over 55, heart attacks become as common as they are for men of the same age.

Virtually all of the changes in women's lives caused by menopause also result from the lower levels of circulating estrogen. However, the women whose blood was sampled as part of the Framingham heart study, alluded to above, had less of the substance plasminogen activator inhibitor (PAI) when premenopausal than when postmenopausal. This means that the chemical tissue plasminogen activator (TPA) is better inhibited after menopause. Uninhibited TPA would tend to prevent heart attacks, which is the effect observed in premenopausal women. The analysis of the Framingham blood samples was performed by Otavio C. E. Gebara of Harvard Medical School in Boston, Massachusetts, and reported to the American Heart Association in November 1993.

Estrogen and Health

Estrogen is a mixed blessing at any time of a woman's life, but the difference after menopause is that the postmenopausal woman can easily obtain estrogen by replacement hormone therapy. Hormones become a choice, not a given, as in earlier years. But with this choice come a great many factors to be taken into account.

- As noted above, a low estrogen supply may result in heart attacks. A study of 48,470 healthy postmenopausal women showed that those that took estrogen had about half as many heart attacks over a ten year period as those who did not use estrogen hormone replacement therapy (reported as part of the ongoing Nurses Health Study in the September 12, 1991 *New England Journal of Medicine*).
- Higher levels of estrogen are thought to contribute to the development of endometrial cancer or breast cancer.
- Hormone replacement often sets off bleeding similar to menstrual bleeding as a result of cyclical changes in hormone administration from estrogen to progesterone (or progestin) to protect against uterine cancer. It may also cause breast tenderness.
- Adding progesterone to hormone replacement in order to lower risks of cancer may cause unwelcome bloating or depression.
- Cycling estrogen and progestin (progesterone) not only helps protect against endometrial cancer, but also, according to a study in the April 15, 1993, *New England Journal of Medicine* by a team from the University of Minnesota School of Public Health in Minneapolis, it gives postmenopausal women a better heart-disease profile: less LDL, lower triglycerides (thought to be a risk factor for heart disease), and lower clotting Factor VII, meaning that blood clots more slowly.
- Low levels of estrogen result in thinning bones, or osteoporosis. This is an increasing problem, for unknown reasons. Hip fractures, the worst result of osteoporosis and a leading cause of death for older women, are rising even when adjusted for age. One reason seems to be that women of the past got more exercise through housework or work in trades when they were younger than young women do today. Exercise builds bone as well as muscle.
- Estrogen patches as well as oral estrogen have been shown to increase the thickness of bones, which typically have lost about a third of their mass through osteoporosis. But the patches do not increase HDL cholesterol the way oral estrogen does, and the patches can cause skin irritation (reported in the July 1, 1992 *Annals of Internal Medicine* by researchers from the Mayo Clinic).
- The postmenopausal women with osteoporosis are more likely to get strokes than those with thicker bones, suggesting that decreased estrogen or some similar factor causes both.

To get through this thicket of conflicts, a better guide than currently exists is needed. In September 1993 the U.S. National Institutes of Health began a study expected to include 25,000 women which will attempt to find the proper path though a controlled experiment. The study is planned to last for 12 years. In the meantime, there are already critics who say that the women in the study's estrogen-alone group are too much at risk of endometrial cancer.

(Periodical References and Additional Reading: *Harvard Health Letter* 3-92, p 1; *Harvard Health Letter* 10-92, p 8; *New York Times* 3-16-93, p C3; *Science News* 4-17-93, p 246; *Science News* 7-24-93, p 61; *New York Times* 9-17-93, p A29; *New York Times* 9-21-93, p C1; *Science News* 11-20-93, p 332; *New York Times* 12-1-93, p C15; *New York Times* 12-8-93, p C16)

MEN'S HEALTH

PROSTATE PROBLEMS

The prostate is a walnut-sized cluster of glands in men, found at the base of the penis, just below the bladder where urine is stored. The prostate surrounds the lower part of the urethra, the tube that leads from the bladder through the penis and through which at different times urine and semen pass. The prostate is involved in semen manufacturing, but knowledge of its exact function is surprisingly limited.

Indeed, most of what physicians know about the prostate is bad news. As men age the gland almost invariably causes trouble, providing a man lives long enough. Half the men over 80 develop prostate cancer, for example. With an increased lifespan, prostate problems have multiplied to become one of the major health problems in the industrial world, running behind only cardiovascular disease. Although some prostate problems are not life-threatening, cancer of the prostate is the most commonly diagnosed cancer in the U.S. (165,000 cases in 1993 and 200,000 expected in 1994, accounting for some 27 percent of all cancer cases). Furthermore it is the second leading cause of death from cancer, after lung cancer. In the U.S. in 1993 deaths from prostate cancer or secondary bone cancer that began as prostate cancer reached 35,000 in 1993 and are expected to go to 38,000 in 1994.

There is some reason to think that *incidence* of prostate cancer is higher because of better detection. On April 11, 1991 a study of 1633 men over the age of 50 by William J. Catalona, reported in *New England Journal of Medicine,* found that use of a blood test for the protein prostate-specific antigen (PSA) combined with a rectal examination found 50 percent more cases of cancer than would have been found by the rectal examination alone. Although the PSA tests missed about 20 percent of the instances of prostate cancer that were found and also gave false positive in 16 percent of the men, Catalona said that his results made it conceivable that instead of nearly seven out of ten cases of prostate cancer being caught at an advanced stage, perhaps as many as seven out of ten could be found at an early stage, greatly improving prospects for treatment.

Another possible explanation for the increase in incidence is the rise in performance of vasectomies for birth control, a trend that started a few decades ago. Two separate retrospective studies of health-related professionals and of husbands of nurses showed from 56 to 66 percent greater risk of prostate cancer in men who had undergone vasectomies, with the highest risk in those who had the operation some 20 years earlier. The results are somewhat suspect because instead of indicating a possible cause of prostate cancer, similar statistics might be produced by an increase in incidence from other causes or might be a statistical artifact of the type of people in the study.

The Cancer Dilemma

Advanced prostate cancer is a terrible disease, spreading to the bones and causing muscle loss, inability to walk, and pain that is difficult to control. But many people with prostate cancer do not live long enough to experience advanced prostate can-cer—not because they die from their cancer but because their cancer grows and spreads so slowly that the men die from some other cause (often euphemistically called "death from old age") long before the prostate cancer causes difficulty. A 1992 Swedish study reported in the *Journal of the American Medical Association* found that of 233 older men who chose not to have their prostate cancer treated, 45 percent died within ten years from causes other than prostate cancer; only 8.5 percent were victims of their untreated cancer.

An analysis of this and other studies by the Prostate Patient Outcomes Research Team concludes that: few patients benefit by early treatment; life expectancy is improved only slightly in the best circumstances; and more harm than good is usually the result of invasive treatment in patients over the age of 70. The Prostate Patients Outcome Research Team study reported in the May 26, 1993 *Journal of the American Medical Association* found that for men 70 years old or older, the risks of surgery or radiation to treat prostate cancer are not worth it, since surgery and radiation only increase the potential lifespan by six months. For younger patients with tumors of the type most likely to spread, invasive treatment gains somewhat less than four additional years of life—and there is considerable risk of impotence or incontinence or both.

Effective treatment for localized prostate cancer is surgery or radiation therapy. Many individuals respond to prostate surgery or radiation by developing side effects that are difficult to live with, side effects that can include inability to control urination (25 percent for surgery; six percent for radiation) or, less commonly, bowel damage. Impotence or other damage to sexual function—which 85 percent of men who have undergone surgery claim, as well as 40 percent after radiation treatments without surgery—can also lead to serious depression. About one percent of the time, surgery itself at any age results in death. A second study in the May 26, 1993 *Journal of the American Medical Association* found that two percent of the patients over the age of 74 die, and eight percent suffer major complications. Despite such problems, the rate of surgery in 1990 for complete removal of the prostate was six times the rate of 1984.

Furthermore, it is established that once the cancer has spread beyond the prostate, neither surgery nor radiation is effective. Treatments aimed at neutralizing male hormones, which can include castration, slow the course of the disease but do not cure it.

Thus the choices facing patients and their physicians are extremely difficult. The Hippocratic injunction to do no harm is involved. The peace of mind of a man who is terrified of cancer is also a factor.

Recently the motto for many physicians has been "watchful waiting," which consists of doing nothing until changes in the size of the prostate observed manually or with ultrasound or other scanning suggest further treatment. A suddenly elevated PSA may also prompt additional scanning and warn of developing problems. The difficulty with watchful waiting, of course, is making sure that action is taken while the cancer is confined to the prostate, for after the disease spreads, death is thought to be inevitable, usually occurring within two years.

Avoiding Complications

Clearly, it would be better all around to avoid getting prostate cancer in the first place than to have to deal with watchful waiting. Edward Giovanucci of Harvard Medical School in Boston, Massachusetts, and coworkers, who have investigated environmental effects for several cancers using data from a study of 48,000 health care workers, reported in the May 19, 1993 *Annals of Internal Medicine* that they could find no evidence that diet had any effect on incidence of prostate cancer in their sample.

However, diet was related to prostate cancer's progression to an active and dangerous stage. Diets high in red meat, butter, chicken fat, and other foods containing alpha-linolenic acid led to a risk of prostate cancer advancing that was 3.5 times as great as those diets low in those foods. Skinless chicken and many other dairy products do not contain alpha-linolenic acid and also do not correlate with cancer progression. Another essential fatty acid, linolenic acid (without the "alpha"), seemed to reduce the chance of the cancer advancing.

Prostate cancer most often spreads to the backbone, where it soon causes pain and death. In the July 1, 1992 *Proceedings of the National Academy of Sciences*, Marcella Chackal Rossi of the Massachusetts Institute of Technology and Bruce R. Setter of Children's Hospital in Boston, Massachusetts reported that the reason the backbone is a target is because it is rich in the iron transporter and suspected growth factor transferrin. For unknown reasons, transferrin greatly promotes the growth of prostate cancer, at least in the test tube. Thus, supposedly when a prostate cancer cell that has been carried by the bloodstream to the backbone lodges there, it quickly multiplies under the influence of the transferrin, which is plentiful there. The researchers hope this discovery may eventually lead to development of a way to prevent prostate cancer from advancing to a dangerous stage.

Another approach, which scientists hope will actually prevent prostate cancer from developing, is use of a drug called finasteride, which is a successful treatment for benign prostate hyperthropy (*see below*). In October 1993, the National Cancer Institute began a seven-year study of the drug in which 18,000 men over 55 will be enrolled in a double-blind study in which half the men will take placebos. Results from this trial might be expected around the year 2005.

Prostate Problems Involving No Cancer

Although considerably less dangerous than cancer, other prostate difficulties are common in older men and require treatment. The most common difficulty is that the prostate grows too large, blocking the urethra. Most commonly the result is that it becomes difficult or almost impossible to urinate. In serious blockage, urine builds up in the bladder, which then has a tendency to push through at odd times; thus, urination happens whether one wishes it or not, a condition oddly named *incontinence.* (The word *continence,* of course, means "able to control sexual impulses" as a primary meaning, but *incontinence* means "unable to control excretory functions" first and only in older usage refers to sex.) Neither the inability to urinate nor incontinence is pleasant, and a blocked urethra can result in poisoning by one's own waste products or infection of the bladder as a result of stagnant urine.

Medical workers call an enlarged but not cancerous prostate condition benign prostatic hypertrophy (BPH). Medication sometimes helps, but usually surgery is needed. The standard surgical approach for BPH that interferes with the urethra also has a formidable name: transurethral resection of the prostate (TURP). TURP consists of inserting an electrical device through the opening of the urethra in the penis and using the device to burn away the inner part of the prostate. In younger men a device that mechanically snips into the interior of the prostate is sometimes used instead of the electrical cauterizer. Neither method can be used if the prostate is very much enlarged; in such cases, surgery through the abdominal wall and cutting away part of the prostate from the outside is required. Both TURP and other forms of surgery can have serious side effects.

The newer alternative to TURP is laser surgery of various kinds. Although quicker than TURP and somewhat less invasive (a laser is usually inserted into the urethra), the rate of complications is comparable to TURP. However, laser surgery is still new and improvements in technique are being made rapidly, especially in the use of ultrasound or fiber optics to insure that the laser is pointing in the right direction when fired. Authorities expect laser prostate surgery to become the norm by the end of the 1990s.

There are other alternatives to lasers. Microwave devices can be inserted either through the urethra or the rectum, but preliminary evidence suggests that this technique is not as effective as laser surgery. A short-term solution, used most often with elderly men, is to insert a balloon to open up the interior of the urethra (which is effective usually for a few months) or to put plastic reinforcement inside the urethra to keep it open (which is effective until prostate tissue grows through the mesh used as reinforcement).

(Periodical References and Additional Reading: *New York Times* 4-25-91; *New York Times* 7-1-92, p A18; *Science News* 2-30-93, p 116; *New York Times* 5-26-93, p C11; *Science News* 6-5-93, p 367; *New York Times* 10-17-93, p I-23; *Harvard Health Letter* 12-93, p 6; *Harvard Health Letter* 2-94, p 1; *Scientific American* 4-94, p 72)

IMPOTENCE RECONSIDERED

Male impotence is the inability to achieve or to maintain a penile erection. Until quite recently many physicians were willing to say that as many as nine out of ten instances of impotence were psychological in origin. The tide of opinion on this matter has now turned. Eight out of ten instances of impotence, doctors today believe, have physical causes, although psychological elements soon enter into the picture because of the impotent male's reactions to his state. At a conference called by the U.S. National Institutes of Health in December 1992 to discuss ways to treat impotence, the assembled experts called for dropping the term *impotence* altogether and replacing it with *erectile dysfunction,* which they felt would emphasize that the condition is a medical and not a psychological problem.

At that same conference the committee members estimated that erectile dysfunction (complete failure of erection) occurred in about ten to 15 million American men (perhaps as much as 12 percent of the male population) with about another ten

Background

Despite common nicknames suggesting the penis might encase a part of the skeleton, it is made entirely from soft and spongy tissue. A large artery carries blood into the penis and veins carry the blood back out. Most of the time, when the penis is flaccid, there is very little blood in the penis. When sexually aroused or during the dreaming sleep known as REM sleep—REM stands for the Rapid Eye Movements that can be detected during this sleep stage even when eyes are closed—nerves in the penis release the nerve transmitter nitric oxide. (*See* "The Ubiquity of NO in Life," p 305.) Nitric oxide causes the muscles in the arteries to relax. Now more blood can flow into the penis than is flowing out, and the penis fills with blood which is confined mainly to thin spiral arteries that branch off the main one and to the veins—it is not "loose" in the tissue. This stiffens the penis just as any somewhat flexible container is stiffened when filled with an incompressible fluid. The result is called an erection.

One theory of impotence holds that the amount of oxygen in the flaccid penis is normally less than that in a similar volume of most organs because little oxygen-carrying blood is present. This deficit is overcome by an erection, when the penis is for a time filled with oxygen-rich blood. A lack of erections on a regular basis makes erectile dysfunction worse by letting the muscles of the arteries stiffen so that they no longer expand when stimulated by nitric oxide from the nerves. In most men, however, erections on a nightly basis, usually for about three hours a night, keep muscle stiffening from occurring.

The main causes of impotence are thought to include nerve damage from diabetes, diseases of the circulatory system including high blood pressure, and various neurological disorders. About a quarter of all impotence results from use of prescribed medicines or illicit drugs. While pills used for controlling high blood pressure are well known for causing erectile dysfunction, other medications, including various forms of cortisone, are also frequently involved in the problem. Half of all coronary-bypass patients become impotent, either because of underlying circulatory problems or insufficient blood flow. More than half of the men whose prostate has been removed also experience erectile dysfunction. Some impotence is indeed psychological, with clinical depression probably the main recognized cause. Alcoholism can also be a factor. A January 1994 *Journal of Urology* study found a high correlation between impotence and smoking tobacco, which was even higher among men who also had heart disease and continued to smoke.

Treatment options vary from those that attack the stimulation of the muscles in the arteries to purely mechanical solutions.

Hormones: In a few cases, a man for one reason or another has a low supply of the hormone testosterone. The hormone can be replaced with regular injections every two or three weeks. According to one source, such a deficiency occurs in one percent of men between the ages of 20 and 40, five percent of those between 40 and 65, and more than 20 percent for men over 65. Other estimates are usually lower than that, however. An accurate test for testosterone involves collecting all the urine for a 24-hour period and is expensive, so the test is not commonly performed. Low testosterone usually results in lack of sexual desire, unlike other conditions that can cause impotence.

The survey of Massachusetts men in the *Journal of Urology* study originated as an assay of levels of male hormones, and only later was the data converted for use in studying impotence. The data compiled from the study of Massachusetts men suggest that lack of testosterone is not a major factor in impotence, although many physicians start investigations of causes of impotence with a testosterone test.

Injections: Unlike testosterone injections, administered to veins by a nurse or physician, these injections consist of an impotent man just before coitus injecting very small amounts of such chemicals as prostaglandin E-1, papaverine, phentolamine or a combination into spongy tissue at the side of his penis. The chemicals cause artery muscles to relax and more blood to flow, filling the penis as in an unassisted erection. This method works for most men. Problems include injecting too much, which produces an erection that fails to end appropriately causing possible tissue damage, and development of scars from the injections. In some cases the injections can cause normal function to return and can be discontinued.

Vacuum pumps: Applying a sleeve to the penis and pumping the air out of the sleeve causes more blood to flow into the penile arteries. A rubber band at the base of the penis keeps the blood in the penis for a time. The erection is not as rigid as a natural one in a fully functional penis, but the method is simple and otherwise effective.

Penile implants: Some men have had semi-rigid rods or hydraulic devices permanently implanted in the penis. The semi-rigid rods sustain the penis in a state somewhat similar to an erection all the time. They may abet a partial natural erection. Hydraulic devices work somewhat like arteries, except that the fluid must be pumped in from outside the body and they do not branch throughout the penis. Neither of these implants is very satisfactory. Problems include surgical complications, mechanical failure of the hydraulic system, and concern that silicone, which is used for the implants, can cause cancer or affect the immune system. (*See* "Implants and the Immune System," p 223.)

Vascular surgery: Arteries or veins can be surgically rerouted in the hope of improving blood flow. This method has not been very successful. After a time blood can leak into the wrong part of the system and impotence returns.

The "patch": Two different kinds of transdermal patches can be applied to the thin skin of the scrotum or the penis. (A transdermal patch delivers a chemical to the body through the skin.) One patch, patented in 1992, can deliver testosterone to the blood, removing the need for injections every few weeks in men for whom low testosterone is a problem. It is attached to the scrotum because large hormone molecules can only get through the thinnest skin. The other patch is the familiar nitroglycerine patch used by many persons with heart disease. The theory is that the nitroglycerine patch will deliver nitric oxide directly to where it is needed to relax arteries, just as the nitroglycerine patch aids heart patients by providing nitric oxide to the circulatory system. On the skin of the penis, however, a nitroglycerine patch often delivers too much of the chemical, causing such side effects as fainting or splitting headaches at a time when these effects are particularly undesirable.

Oral drugs: None have yet been developed. One drug has been found to work in experiments with a few men, but it is delivered into the end of the urethra. This concept is only moderately more appealing to most men than injecting a drug into the side of the penis.

million experiencing partial impotence of one kind or another. More than a million men have sought treatment for the condition.

The panel concluded that most cases of erectile dysfunction could be successfully treated by such methods as injections of chemicals or use of a vacuum pump to increase blood flow to the penis. Surgery or a penile implant were considered to be fall-back options.

At present, nearly all the million men who are being treated medically for erectile dysfunction use self-injection into the penis of one of several available drugs. About 30,000 men use a vacuum pump and another 20,000 have chosen penile implants. Surgery to rebuild or reroute arteries or veins has proven to be fraught with difficulties and is seldom done anymore.

Latest Survey Results

Much of the available data about impotence is simply an informed guess, as figures such as "ten to 15 million" might suggest. The January 1994 *Journal of Urology* contains results of the largest actual study of the incidence of the condition in almost 50 years, when the Kinsey Report documented male sexuality in 1948. Even so, the *Journal of Urology* study only included 1709 men (1290 answered the questions about impotence), all of whom lived in Massachusetts, and a period of six months. If the Massachusetts figures can be extrapolated to the whole population, erectile dysfunction is even more common than suspected: 19 million Americans between the ages of 40 and 65 (a total population of 37 million) have some erectile problems during a given six-month period. While this is more than half the population, it should be noted that it includes episodes of impotence as well as longer periods of impotence.

In general, the survey found that impotence increases with age, as might be expected, but increases start earlier than had been previously believed. Survey answers suggest that at the age of 40 as many as five percent of men are completely impotent (or were so, at least, for a six-month period). By the age of 70, however, that figure has only risen to 15 percent, which is not a completely surprising ratio. If one assumed that 15 percent of the 37 million American men between 40 and 70 were impotent, the number would be less than six million, not the 19 million with occasional problems. A more realistic estimate would be that between two million and five million men are completely impotent during a six-month period.

(Periodical References and Additional Reading: *New York Times* 11-2-92, p D2; *New York Times* 12-10-92, p D10; *New York Times* 6-2-93, p C12; *New York Times* 12-22-93, p C13)

MEN AND WOMEN AND SEX

SEXUAL SURVEYS

After the Kinsey Reports on sexual behavior in men (1948) and women (1953) caused considerable uproar in the U.S., the serious scientific quest for information about sex appeared to vanish. The advent of AIDS in the early 1980s, however, caused scientists investigating the progress of this sexually transmitted disease to recognize that Kinsey's data was very old and flawed in significant ways. New surveys that examined a wider range of people were needed if AIDS was to be tracked properly.

In the U.S., conservative Republican administrations at least for a time succeeded in blocking attempts by scientists and social scientists to conduct large-scale surveys about sex. Margaret Thatcher's government in Great Britain also refused to finance such surveys. As a result, the most recent large-scale surveys of sexual behavior were taken in Norway, Denmark, Scotland, France, and, surprisingly, Great Britain (where the private Wellcome Trust paid the $1.7 million for the survey). The first studies to be completed were in France and Great Britain.

Sex in France and Great Britain

The titles of the articles in the December 3, 1992 *Nature* clearly show what the French and British researchers had in mind: "AIDS and Sexual Behavior in France" and "Sexual Lifestyles and HIV Risk." News stories, however, tended to focus on frequency of heterosexual sex and number of homosexuals found.

In France in the winter of 1991–92 a total of 20,055 persons answered a basic list of questions about their sex lives, a part of the survey that took 15 minutes to conduct per respondent. All questions were asked over the telephone to randomly selected individuals who had previously been notified that they would be surveyed. People surveyed were told truthfully that all identifying information about the responder would disappear as soon as the reply to the first question was entered into the computer. Despite this assurance, more than one household in nine refused to participate and, after telephone contact had been made, another one in nine dropped out, although often for reasons that had nothing to do with the nature of the survey. The total refusal rate in France came nearly to one in four. Most people were willing to answer all the questions, although one in 20 balked at discussing anal sex and almost one in 16 women would not answer items about lesbian practices.

If answers to the first part of the French survey revealed a risk factor for AIDS in the respondent, a longer series of questions was asked, looking for more details concerning sexual activity. A number about equal to those with risk factors, but chosen at random from those without, also took the second part of the survey as a sort of control.

In contrast the British survey was conducted by interviewers who visited households and questioned more than 18,000 persons. The refusal rate was only slightly more than in the French telephone survey; 28 percent, mostly older or single men, refused to participate in Britain. Questions thought to be especially sensitive were written on cards and only a number or letter need be given to indicate a response. After the face-to-face interview, the respondent was asked to complete a written survey with additional items.

Investigators for the two studies made a conscious effort to keep the French and British data comparable. Despite this, there were some distinctive national touches to the reports. British results show that the higher the social standing of the respondent, the more sexual contacts he or she had. One in ten French men had his first sex experience with a prostitute 20 years ago, but only one in 50 of the ones who began sexual activity within the past few years began with a prostitute. The sex lives of people in Paris and London were more complex than those in the provinces.

Condom usage was fairly high. In France, more than 65 percent of the men and 43.7 percent of the women claimed to have used a condom during the year preceding the survey, with young people reporting higher rates than that. In Great Britain, results showed that more than one in five persons with high rates of sexual activity also arranged to be tested for the HIV virus that causes AIDS.

How Many Are Gay?

Kinsey reported that one out of ten male Americans was homosexual, which astonished everyone at the time. With almost no surveys that covered the questions of sexual identity in the next 40 years, the ten percent figure from Kinsey was widely quoted, especially by male homosexuals defending their own situation.

As the first new surveys began to appear in the early 1990s, it became apparent that Kinsey's figure was at best suspect. In 1992 the French result was that 4.1 percent of the men questioned had a homosexual experience at one time or another, but only 1.1 percent of the men had sex with another male during the five years before the survey was taken. The British reported that their data showed only slightly higher ratios: 6.1 percent of men ever and 1.4 percent of men in the preceding five years had sex with another man.

In April 1993 new results from the U.S. appeared, revealing that Americans in the early 1990s are a lot like the French and British in sexual practices and quite different from what Kinsey reported 40-some years earlier. Although the new American study, *The Sexual Behavior of U.S. Men,* was based on a smaller sample and only surveyed young men (3321 men aged 20 to 39), the results for homosexual behavior were about the same as in France and England. About one percent of the men asked were willing to call themselves homosexual.

Why More Men Have Sex Than Women Do

Every survey of sex practices that includes data on the number of sexual partners for both men and women shows that men report a great many more partners than women do. On the face of it there is something wrong with these numbers, and this consistent bias has been something of a black cloud over sexual surveys. The discrepancies can be quite large: surveys in the 1960s found that men reported six times as many sexual partners as women. In the French study discussed above, the men report that over their lifetime they had sex with an average of 11.0 partners, while the women report only 3.3 partners over a lifetime. The numbers are somewhat less divergent for the British men and women: 9.9 heterosexual partners for the men as opposed to 3.4 for the women. When only the past year is included, the number of heterosexual partners of British men is only slightly greater than that of British women, 1.2 for men and 1.0 for women.

Although the reported lifetime differential is commonly attributed to bragging by men and modesty in women, there seems to be another factor involved. British men in the oldest age group report 13.6 lifetime heterosexual partners, while women in that group report only 2.6 heterosexual partners. But the variance, a measure of how different the numbers are for different individuals, is enormous for the men: 22,093. This implies that some very few individuals are skewing the data upwards by reporting extremely large numbers of sexual events. This might be called "the Wilt effect," after basketball star Wilt Chamberlain who in his autobiography reported that he had thousands of sex acts with different individuals each year.

The number used in reporting large amounts of data is generally the mean, i.e., the average found by adding up all the data and dividing by the number of addends. Suppose for example that there are 100 men, each claiming three partners in the past year. The mean is three. Now think of 99 of those men and one Wilt, who claims 2000 partners in the past year. The mean is nearly 23.

Looking at the other British data shows the Wilt effect is to some degree operating for every age group: the variance for men is always much larger than for women, although that is in part a result of the higher averages.

Another way of looking at data shows that the Wilt effect is a principal contributor to the discrepancy. When you eliminate all persons who report more than 20 sexual partners from the data in recent surveys, the ratio reported by men to that reported by women drops from 3.2 to 1, to 1.2 to 1. This is the same ratio as was found in the British data for reports of sexual partners in the past year.

Thus, instead of most men exaggerating by a factor of three or more, most men may exaggerate just a little when telling about their sexual adventures. But a few men make enormous claims that are difficult to reconcile with reports from women.

(Periodical References and Additional Reading: *Nature* 12-3-92, p 407, 410; *New York Times* 12-8-92, p C3; *New York Times* 4-18-93, p IV-3; *Nature* 9-30-93, p 437)

Environmental Hazards

THE STATE OF THE ENVIRONMENT AND HEALTH

Although it may seem that concern for the effects of the environment on health is a development of the past quarter century, the truth is quite different. People from early times suspected, often incorrectly but with a grain of truth, that some unknown effect of place or air caused illness—think of *mal aria*, the fever that was thought to be caused by the air from marshes and swamps, which we now know to be the mosquito-borne disease malaria. Ancient Egyptians believed that many other diseases were caused by winds or by changes in weather, and folk beliefs today still include the idea, possibly correct, that weather changes seem to affect various chronic aches and pains. Early records of the first civilizations as well oral tradition in many nonscientific societies right up to the present day attribute poor health to demons, although whether or not you consider demons a part of the environment depends on your general belief structure. The School of Hippocrates in ancient Greece thought that disease was a state in which the body experienced difficulty in mastering its environment.

But the environmental situation has changed since early times, often with serious effects on health. In the past, the effect of the environment on health may have been mostly superstition, but today the link between the environment and health is seen to be true and important. For example, some elements either by themselves—e.g. lead and cadmium—or in various compounds—e.g. mercury—are concentrated by human activities. In their natural state, these elements are dispersed throughout minerals, which are most often buried by soil. Before mining and processing began, people encountered these poisons so seldom that the chemical elements posed little hazard. But today, human activities have put the concentrations of these elements in exactly the same places as people.

Chemists in the nineteenth century tried to combine chemicals to produce improved versions of useful natural substances. But they soon realized that some of their artificial chemicals were different from any that existed in nature. When life encounters such a synthetic chemical, it sometimes ignores it; thus there are nearly inert artificial materials such as teflon. More often, however, life almost recognizes the artificial chemical and tries to use it in place of a natural one that the artificial chemical resembles, which is often the occasion for disaster. Silicone seemed sufficiently inert to use in various kinds of implants, but the human immune system seems to confuse silicone with some body chemicals; as a result, the immune system, failing to attack the silicone itself, instead attacks some tissues in the body. The body confuses some of the synthetic pesticides with estrogen, thereby possibly promoting the growth of cancer. Another example is synthetic "designer drugs," which were originally chemicals that the body mistook for neurotransmitters, thus producing overwhelming emotional reactions craved by some people. But in some cases these drugs caused permanent neurological damage. Today the term "designer drug" is often used for synthetics specifically crafted to fool the body into using the drug instead of natural chemicals, so that cancer or other illnesses can be checked (*see* "Right Keyhole, Wrong Key," p 537).

If the problems of toxic substance concentration and development of modern synthetics were not enough, people have learned in recent years to change the environment all over the globe in ways that could affect health (*see* "Ultraviolet Rays from the Sun," p 189). Environmental priorities, therefore, have shifted from local ones, such as preservation of a lake or pollution of a specific site, to such problems as global warming and loss of the ozone layer. Of course, many local problems remain, but they seem less serious vis-à-vis a new perception of planet-wide change as a result of human activity. Even if people stop short of changing the entire environment, some toxic products, such as acid in the clouds, rain, and snow, spread in space far from their point of origin, while others, such as long-lived synthetic compounds, spread through the years without degrading into safer chemicals.

Coal and Soot

Lead or mercury are poisonous in and of themselves. But even an innocuous element, such as carbon, can become a hazard. Coal, which is mainly carbon, becomes soot when burned. As early as the fifteenth century, people had concluded that soot from burning coal was unhealthy, and by the eighteenth century it was recognized that exposure to a great deal of soot caused chimney sweeps to develop cancer. It is not the carbon itself that is the problem; instead, hydrocarbons formed during burning and some contaminants in coal make soot dangerous.

As early as 1307, burning of coal was outlawed in London because of its noxious smoke. Coal burning was reinstated after better furnaces and chimneys were developed a couple of hundred years later. Soon London was famous for its soot and cloudy skies. Finally in 1952 a smog largely composed of smoke from coal fires kept near the ground by a temperature inversion killed about 4000 mostly elderly or infirm people in London. A few other "killer smogs" also struck around that time in the U.S. and on the European continent.

Today, soot from burning fossil fuels, including petroleum as well as coal, is a major worldwide health problem. In the former Communist countries of Eastern Europe the problem is especially bad because the most common fuel is a high-soot lignite, or brown coal. Health conditions in some places, such as the industrialized Karelian peninsula of Russia, in which Murmansk is located, are as bad as in developing countries, with short average lifespans and much respiratory illness. The same is true of parts of Poland or Slovakia. In the U.S., calculations of the Environmental Protection Agency and the Harvard School of Public Health are that exposure to airborne soot kills as many as 60,000 persons a year—mainly people of all ages with respiratory problems, including asthma, emphysema, and pneumonia.

Coal is also one of the workplace killers (see below), with black lung disease among coal miners a recognized hazard of coal dust. There are still 134,000 coal miners in the U.S. alone, as well as many more around the world. According to the U.S. Department of Labor in April 1991 more than 600 mining companies had altered filters in the 1980s in order to record less coal dust in mines than was actually present. The Labor Department fined the companies six million dollars for the tampering, but the problem is also being fought in the federal courts, where the cases continue—except for a handful in which mining companies pleaded guilty.

Work Can Be Sickening

The part of the environment that often causes the most trouble is the workplace, and with good reason. First of all for many workers, a workplace environment is much the same every day. Outside of work, where would a person be exposed to coal dust at least five days a week? or to dry-cleaning fluid every workday? or to possible radiation from regular proximity to a computer monitor? or to small particles in the air that are too large to travel far, but too small to fall quickly to the ground? or to dozens of separate X-ray exposures daily? In these and thousands of other instances, the regularity of the job environment turns what might be a minor annoyance if encountered infrequently into a serious danger.

A typical example of a workplace problem is coal mining, discussed above. But for coal mining, the cause of black lung disease has been obvious for centuries. Other dusts also produce similar diseases, including silica dust, asbestos particles, cotton dust, sugar-cane dust, and so forth.

In 1989 the U.S. Occupational Safety and Health Administration issued standards for a total of 428 substances that could pollute workplace air, including fumes as well as dusts. But in July 1992 a U.S. circuit court of appeals threw out the standards for lack of evidence that the substances were hazardous in the amounts that the regulations declared unacceptable.

Can We Really Tell What Will Make Us Ill?

The first methods for determining which chemicals in the environment might affect humans adversely began with our pre-human ancestors, who developed taste buds that recognized some foods as dangerous. Fruit that was bitter or sour was likely to cause a stomachache. Fruit that was sweet was likely to be good to eat. Although such simple rules sometimes failed, they provided a good start.

The next step in detecting danger was experience. Higher primates have been shown to learn from their mother's choices what to eat and what to avoid. Thus if the mother has had a bad experience with a food and lived anyway, she can pass that information on to her children. When primates developed into speaking humans, oral traditions carried the message more easily through the generations. Writing provided a further means of communicating.

With a large array of information of this sort, the first crude epidemiology could begin. Some substances that did not kill right away might in large enough quantities or in small exposures over a long period of time cause illness. One of the earliest examples we known of this is the recognition from at least as early as 650 A.D. that exposure to lead could lead to illness. Paracelsus [1493-1541] pointed out that miners and smelters of metals developed a number of diseases from the vapors and dust of mining. A hundred years later Bernardino Ramazzini [1633-1714] discussed how specific diseases were connected to specific occupations, noting that only the lowest class of doctors used mercury because better physicians knew that they could cause illness in themselves from exposure to mercury. Another early example of this epidemiological approach was the recognition alluded to above: in 1775 Sir Percival Potts observed that chimney sweeps were more likely to develop cancer of the scrotum than other people. He correctly reasoned that something in soot was a cause of cancer.

People began to recognize that prolonged exposure to other substances could lead to cancer, and a new word entered the language: carcinogen. After soot, perhaps the next recognition of carcinogens was not until well into the twentieth century, when people learned that exposure to radioactive elements also induces cancer. By the 1950s there was clear-cut evidence that asbestos could be added to the list and evidence enough for most people that prolonged exposure to tobacco smoke leads to lung cancer at least some of the time.

The problem with the epidemiological approach to carcinogens was that the known examples—soot, radioactivity, asbestos, tobacco smoke—all required repeated exposure over many years to cause disease. This was a very different situation from exposure to a poison by eating a toxic fruit that caused a stomachache within hours of a single exposure. Also, not every person exposed to carcinogens develops cancer. Another past difficulty has been that the mechanism by which substances cause cancer was not known until fairly recently, when it was learned that damage to DNA was the actual cause in most instances. Substances that damage DNA in certain genes initiate cancer. Another group of substances are suspected not of damage to DNA but of encouraging cancer that has been started by another substance to grow or spread faster. Synthetics that imitate estrogens are in this latter class (see "Breast Cancer," p 216).

Because epidemiology is slow and uncertain, scientists looked for other ways to determine which parts of the environment might initiate cancer. Animal studies were an obvious answer, but even animals do not develop cancer from small exposures until many generations have passed. Although mice or guinea pigs breed and grow far faster than humans, many years might be needed and the cost of caring for all the animals during the study would be far too high. Thus a "quick-and-dirty" method was developed.

A given animal would be fed or otherwise exposed to as high a dose of a chemical as possible. Nearly every substance when provided in large enough amounts will cause death. From this preliminary work, a "maximum tolerated dose," or MTD, was determined. Then several generations of the animal were exposed to the MTD to find if they developed cancer. Often they did. If so, U.S. policy became, as a result of a succession of laws or regulations in the 1960s through the 1980s, to ban the substance for humans. This concept became one of the key ideas of the "war on cancer" that officially began in the U.S. in 1971.

In the last 30 years, the U.S. government has conducted 450 lengthy studies of possible carcinogens using animals, primarily rodents. There have also been uncounted corporate studies. Some of the best-known results of such research concerned the pesticide DDT, the pesticide and industrial contaminant dioxin, and the artificial sweeteners saccharin and cyclamates. Although all four of these chemicals were found to some degree to cause cancer in animals, their status today is still problematic. Dioxin (see "Dioxin UPDATE," p 260) has turned out to be a much more potent carcinogen in rodents than in humans. Saccharin is such a weak carcinogen in humans that it is not banned in the U.S. Cyclamates, banned for a time, probably do not cause cancer in humans at all. DDT does not seem to cause cancer either, although it has other harmful effects and may promote the growth of cancer initiated by other substances. Part of the problem is that using the MTD test is not realistic; another part of the problem is that the differences between rodents and humans are sufficiently great, so it is often difficult to translate rodent results into human illnesses.

Another problem with rodent tests is time and expense. About 85,000 mice had to be used to find out that saccharin is not very carcinogenic. Biologist Bruce Ames developed a quicker test to screen for chemicals that *might* cause cancer; the Ames test uses exposure of microorganisms to the carcinogen. Although even more unlike humans than rodents are, microorganisms reproduce very quickly (on the order of minutes or hours) and are very cheap to maintain. Ames himself is now well-known as an advocate for less fear of synthetic chemical contamination of the environment. His main point is that natural chemicals in foods are more carcinogenic than many feared pesticides or other synthetics.

Some of the scientists involved in testing chemicals with rodents also think that the animal model is not providing good answers. Better epidemiology might be the answer. For example, rat and mouse studies show that an industrial solvent, 1,2,3-trichloropropane, is a powerful carcinogen. In some industries, humans use the same solvent to wash their hands and also regularly breath fumes. A good epidemiological study, which is yet to be done, might show whether or not the solvent is truly a problem for humans. For example, a few years ago when a rodent study showed that fluorides cause cancer, the epidemiological study that followed determined that this was not the case in humans.

In summary, although the main concern about chemicals in the environment has recently been that some may cause cancer, it is far from certain—except for a very few, such as tobacco smoke—that they actually do. Much more information is needed.

Population and Health

There is some evidence that human beings were generally healthier before the Agricultural Revolution. Confirmed meat eaters claim that health of early humans was harmed by switching to a plant-based diet that provided less concentrated nutrients.

But it seems more likely that the increased population, caused in part by a more regular food supply, was a bigger factor. As people began to live closer together and as there were many more people on the planet, infectious diseases had a reservoir in which to develop. Furthermore, as the number of people living in one region grew, resources were outstripped and wastes began to build up. Population growth by itself became a cause of environmental disease.

In the late 1960s and early 1970s many people became aware for the first time that the earth's growing population is a problem, although Thomas Malthus had proclaimed the evil consequences of growth as early as 1798. Best-sellers in the United States during the first awakening of environmental concern included Paul Ehrlich's *The Population Bomb* (1968) and the Club of Rome's *The Limits of Growth* (1973), while many other prophets of gloom were heard around the world as well. The message was that there would not be enough food for everyone, nor enough energy in any form; such shortages would have unpleasant results for many people. It would be just as Thomas Malthus had predicted around the turn of the nineteenth century, only worse.

The message of the gloom-and-doom books went largely unheeded. Population continued to increase in most of the world at a rapid rate, although much more slowly in developed nations than in the countries that were already poor and overcrowded. Over the course of the 1970s and 1980s, about 1.3 billion people were added to the total world population.

But the Malthusian famines did not come. It appeared that, as had been the case in the nineteenth and twentieth centuries, technological advances would continue to stay ahead of population growth. Throughout the 1980s this was explained by the concept that more people would produce more ideas that would solve any problems caused by population growth. Furthermore, it seemed that all the additional consumers in a higher population group would generate prosperity. Because prices go down with mass production, similar economies of scale could emerge in any situation caused by high population. In this view, the larger the population, the better.

So why did people start fretting about population growth again in the 1990s?

Global warming was one reason. On the one hand, people realized that reduction of carbon dioxide from smokestacks might not make much difference if all the people in China and India got the cars, refrigerators, and perhaps even air conditioners that people in the developed world enjoy. On the other hand, since more industrialized nations produce more carbon dioxide per person than less developed nations with population problems, reductions in population leading to international industrial development might result in more global warming, not less.

According to the United Nations Population Fund, the current world population is about 5.7 billion today. Population is expected to rise to somewhere between 7.8 billion to 12.5 billion by about 2050. Most experts would like to see it stop rising at the lower figure and stay there for the foreseeable future. For some time, various calculations have suggested that the "sustainable yield" for humans in the earthly environment is about eight billion. Some economists think that many regions have already reached a point of complete population saturation. For those regions there is already no more room, energy, or food for further growth, even though population growth continues.

(Periodical References and Additional Reading: *New York Times* 4-2-92, p A15; *New York Times* 3-23-93, p A1; *New York Times* 7-19-93, p A1; *New York Times* 4-3-94, p I-11)

TIMETABLE OF ENVIRONMENTAL HEALTH TO 1990

600 BC   The Chinese develop the art of fumigating houses to rid them of pests.

77   Pliny the Elder writes that the element mercury is poisonous.

100   The Chinese discover about this time that dried, powdered chrysanthemum flowers can be used to kill insects, which is believed to be the first insecticide; the active ingredient, pyrethrum, is widely used today, especially on vegetables, since it is biodegradable and virtually harmless to mammals.

304   An agricultural text by Xi Han mentions the use of carnivorous ants to control insects attacking vegetable gardens.

1763   There are indications that ground tobacco leaves are used in France to control aphids.

1775   Sir Percival Potts suggests that chimney sweeps in London develop cancers of the scrotum and of the nasal cavity as a result of exposure to soot, the first indication that environmental factors can cause cancer.

1800   Copper sulfate, hydrogen cyanide, lead arsenide, nicotine, petroleum, and turpentine are used in fighting plant diseases.

1872   Robert Angus Smith [Scottish: 1817-1884] describes acid rain.

1878   Physiologist Paul Bert [born Auxerre, France, October 17, 1833; died Hanoi, Indochina (Vietnam), November 11, 1886] announces that dissolved nitrogen in the blood of people working under pressurized air causes the disease commonly known as the "bends" or caisson disease; he proposes that if air pressure is lowered by stages the disease will be prevented, which is correct.

1884   A new law in California prohibits using water to extract ores because the wastewater from the process causes pollution of agricultural land.

1885   Bordeaux mixture (a combination of copper sulfate and hydrated lime dissolved in water) is discovered by horticulturist P. M. A. Millardet [French: 1838-1902] to control a serious fungus disease of grapes; invented by wheat farmers to prevent a fungus disease of seed, Bordeaux mixture is blue-green from the copper sulfate and had been applied to the grapes in Bordeaux to discourage grape thieves. Bordeaux mixture is quickly discovered to control other fungal diseases, such as late potato blight (cause of the Irish famine of 1845-46), and it is still used today.

1889   An air lock, called a hospital lock, is introduced to eliminate caisson disease (nicknamed "the bends") as part of an abortive attempt to build a tunnel under the Hudson River at New York City; by providing a place for slow decompression for workers from the pressurized, underwater caissons, the hospital lock completely eliminates the disease, which previously had affected as many as one worker in four.

1896   Selective weed killers are used in France.

1900   Asbestos is linked to a type of lung disease called asbestosis.

1906   The U.S. Congress passes the Pure Food and Drug Act.

Upton Sinclair [U.S.: 1878-1968] writes the novel *The Jungle,* which alerts Americans to contamination of food by the meat-packing industry.

1907   John Scott Haldane [born England, May 3, 1860; died Bhubaneswar, India, December 1, 1964] develops a method for deep-sea divers to rise to the surface safely.

1939   Paul Müller [born Olten, Switzerland, January 12, 1899; died Basel, Switzerland, October 13, 1965] discovers that DDT is a potent insecticide.

1945   Herbicide 2,4-D, the first modern plant poison, is introduced.

1948   Smog lasting five days kills 20 people in Donora, Pennsylvania, and injures 14,000.

1952   The Great London smog is believed to kill 4000 people, mostly the elderly or infirm.

1953   Smog in New York City, New York, is believed to be responsible for 200 deaths.

1955   The link between exposure to asbestos fibers and development of lung cancer, suspected since 1935, is definitely established.

1957   Nuclear waste stored by the Soviet Union in a remote mountain region of the Urals explodes, contaminating thousands of square miles with radioactivity and causing a number of villages to be permanently evacuated.

1959   An illness that has affected people living around the shores of Minimata Bay in Japan is traced to contamination of the bay by industrial wastes laced with mercury.

1961   Acid rain and its consequences are rediscovered in Sweden by Svante Odén; subsequent investigations in Scandinavia and the U.S. Adirondacks confirm that acid rain causes lakes to lose all animal species living in them.

1962   *Silent Spring* by Rachel Carson [U.S.: 1907-1964] attacks pesticide use and stimulates a U.S. wave of environmentalism.

1965   The U.S. Congress passes the Water Quality Act, giving the federal government the power to set water standards in the absence of state standards.

The U.S. Congress passes the Solid Waste Disposal Act, its first major legislation on solid wastes.

1968   Fishing in Minimata Bay in Japan is banned after a second wave of mercury poisonings.

1970   On April 22, the first Earth Day is celebrated around the globe.

The U.S. Environmental Protection Agency is created.

1971   A shipment of seed wheat and barley treated with methylmercury as a fungicide is used for food by people in Iraq; 6530 are hospitalized and 459 die.

1972   In the United States, the use of DDT is restricted to protect the environment, especially eagles, hawks, and other predatory birds, whose eggshells are dangerously thinned, thereby lowering the birds' reproductive rate.

The U.S. Congress passes the Clean Air Act designed to reduce air pollution.

The U.S. Congress passes the Clean Water Act, forbidding discharge of pollutants into navigable waters.

1974   F. Sherwood Rowland [born Delaware, Ohio, June 28, 1927] and Mario Molina [born Mexico City, March 19, 1943] warn that chlorofluorocarbons are destroying the upper-atmosphere ozone layer, which protects lower levels from excess ultraviolet radiation.

1976   The FDA bans the use of chloroform in drugs and cosmetics because it is suspected of being a carcinogenic substance.

The U.S. Congress passes the Toxic Substances Control Act to control hazardous industrial chemicals.

1978   The community of Love Canal, New York, is evacuated because of hazardous wastes dumped in local landfills in the 1940s and covered over in 1953.

1979   A nuclear reactor at Three Mile Island, near Harrisburg, Pennsylvania, suffers a partial meltdown of its core, but nearly all radiation is confined.

1980   The U.S. Congress passes the Comprehensive Environmental Response, Compensation, and Liability Act (known as the "Superfund") to clean up hazardous waste sites.

In Argentina, between seven and ten thousand infants are exposed to phenylmercury, used as a fungicide in cloth diapers; about a dozen become ill.

1984   More than 2000 die and thousands of others are injured by toxic gas from an industrial accident in Bhopal, India.

1985   British scientists discover that a "hole" in the ozone layer of the upper atmosphere develops over Antarctica each year.

1986   In the Soviet Union (Ukraine), Chernobyl nuclear reactor number four explodes and burns, causing 31 deaths locally in the short run; the accident is suspected of causing a rise in cancer incidence throughout a large region.

1987   An international treaty to halve the production of chlorofluorocarbons is signed in an effort to protect the ozone layer of the upper atmosphere.

1988   The U.S. Congress passes the Ocean Dumping Ban Act, which mandates an end to ocean dumping of industrial waste and sewage sludge.

1989   Thirteen major industrial nations, including the U.S., agree to halt chlorofluorocarbon production by the year 2000 to protect the ozone layer.

CHEMICALS IN THE ENVIRONMENT

DANGER FROM MERCURY

In the early 1990s, mercury, one of the first elements to be recognized as toxic, continued to be a problem to humans. But one suspected application, that is, mercury in the alloy known as amalgam which is used in dental fillings, may be harmless (*see* "Dental Health UPDATE," p 184).

A major concern of the early 1990s was mercury in lakes and oceans. Like many other elements, mercury that has been consumed in small amounts remains in the tissues of the consumer. When the consumer is later consumed, as when a big fish eats a large number of smaller fish, the mercury is concentrated at a higher level in the tissues of the larger fish. Unlike the short food chains on land, aquatic and marine food chains often stretch through several levels, so mercury in fish tissues can become quite concentrated.

Loose Mercury

Mercury, the only common metal to be liquid at room temperature, has always seemed somewhat mysterious. Droplets of mercury seem to move around as if they have a life of their own, which gives mercury its other name, "quicksilver." "Quick" in this context means "living," not "speedy." People could mistake tiny drops of mercury that seem almost alive as infused with spirits, not knowing that this "behavior" is caused by surface tension.

On October 18, 1990, *Nature* published a study by Arnold P. Wendroff of Columbia University that showed that 86 percent of 115 *botanicas* (shops selling potions and ritual objects, mostly to Spanish-speaking immigrants to the United States from the Caribbean or from Latin America) sold capsules containing elemental mercury. The capsules were to be used by breaking them open and sprinkling the liquid mercury around the floor of a room to disperse evil spirits.

Because such a practice would release toxic mercury vapor into the air, it is dangerous. Two children in Columbus, Ohio, became ill from mercury vapor when they moved into an apartment where the previous tenant had spilled a jar of mercury. Also, small children might ingest globules of liquid mercury loosed from spirit-removing capsules. So far, no action has been taken by the EPA or other agencies to halt the practice.

Mercury in Fish

In September 1990, Greg Mierle of the Dorset Research Center in Ontario, Canada, reported that his study of a lake in Ontario showed that rain was depositing much more mercury in the lake than previously expected. He believes that most of the mercury in rainwater comes from air pollution caused by combustion of materials containing mercury. Much of this is released by cement and phosphate plants, while most of the rest comes from incinerators.

Because it falls from the sky, mercury can pollute even remote lakes, far from industrial sources. One example is Crane Lake in Minnesota, where almost every fish tested comes close to or exceeds the FDA standard of one thousandth of a gram of mercury per kilogram (one part per million). The Minnesota standard is the strictest in the United States, about a sixth of the FDA standard. Consequently, the state has advised restrictions on consumption of Crane Lake fish, though these are merely warnings, not prohibitions.

Mercury can contaminate the ocean as well as lakes. The most famous instance is Minimata Bay in Japan. Since 1959 it has been known that this arm of the sea has been contaminated by mercury, poisoning the people who eat fish from the bay. About 2000 people living on the bay in 1990 still officially claimed in court to be victims of mercury poisoning. Another 8000 or so who have so far not pressed their claims in court also say that they have been poisoned.

Mercury in the sea accumulates in the tissues of larger fish, which include tuna, sharks, and swordfish. Lakes and rivers contain sturgeon with similar accumulations, and large salmon can become contaminated. Although there is not very much mercury in any one helping of such fish, experts suggest that pregnant women or women of childbearing age should avoid eating a lot of any one of the larger fish. Particularly worrisome is tuna, which some people eat for lunch day after day. The suggestion for expectant mothers is that a little tuna is all right, but it should not be eaten more than a time or two each week. Most salmon available in stores today in the U.S. comes from small, farm-raised fish, which pose less of a hazard.

Where does the mercury in the ocean that causes this problem come from? No one is quite certain, though one ingenious idea holds that it was put there by Spanish silver-smelting operations in the New World in the sixteenth and seventeenth centuries. Others have argued that mercury from that time would have mostly settled since then. A lot of mercury in the sea is probably of natural origin, since it is believed that two to four times as much mercury is produced by volcanoes and other natural sources as comes from human interference with nature. The approximately 13,000 tons of mercury that humans add to the atmosphere each year comes primarily from burning fossil fuels that contain mercury.

Mercury in Paint

A four-year-old boy in Detroit, Michigan, called attention to a widespread problem when he developed mercury poisoning from fumes given off by a latex-based interior paint. The paint was loaded with phenylmercuric acetate, used as a preservative. The amount of mercury detected in the air inside the house was two and a half times the amount permitted by standards of the U.S. Environmental Protection Agency (EPA).

The U.S. Centers for Disease Control and Prevention (CDC) in Atlanta, Georgia, also became involved. Its investigators, Mary M. Agnocs and Ruth A. Etzel, along with John L. Hesse of the Michigan Department of Public Health, studied the effects of using high-mercury paint in interior rooms, a practice common in the Detroit, Michigan, region. Air samples from the 19 homes the investigators monitored revealed high concentrations of mercury vapor in the air at an average level about 600 times greater than that of outdoor air. Most of the samples were taken about a month after paint had been applied. Urine samples from people living in the newly painted homes also

Background

Depending on how hydrogen and arsenic are classified, 87 to 89 of the 109 known elements are metals. Several metals in fairly large amounts are essential for life—notably sodium, potassium, and calcium. Others, such as iron, zinc, and cobalt, are needed in small amounts, but become toxic in large quantities. A third group, which includes lead, cadmium, antimony, tin, and mercury, is toxic even in small quantities. Since the metals in the last group all have atomic numbers greater than 47, they are often grouped as the "heavy metals." For example, it is frequently noted that incinerator ash may be contaminated with heavy metals (principally cadmium and lead). In terms of actual density, not all of the heavy metals are especially heavy, with tin and antimony being especially light, but all are far heavier than sodium, potassium, and calcium.

None of the heavy metals is particularly common. Mercury is only about a sixth as common as lead or cadmium, the two that are most abundant in the earth's crust. But geologic processes easily concentrate mercury into rich deposits. As a result mercury has been known since ancient times and was the first of the heavy metals to be recognized as toxic; its dangers were mentioned by Pliny the Elder in the first century.

Mercury is dangerous in all forms, as an element and in all compounds, but it is also extremely useful in industrial processes, so it continues to be used. The exact process of mercury poisoning is not clear, but it seems likely that mercury removes sulfur from key enzymes, making them useless. It also destroys kidney cells.

Mercury can cross the blood-brain barrier; once in the brain, it causes dementia. Since the sixteenth century, fur used to make felt for hats has been treated with nitrate of mercury. Before the dangers of this procedure became known, hatters often succumbed to mercury dementia; thus, the phrase "as mad as a hatter" entered the language and became the basis of Lewis Carroll's Mad Hatter in *Alice in Wonderland.* Even earlier, mercury was used by alchemists because gold and silver dissolve in it. Mercury fumes are thought to have caused dementia in alchemists who used it, perhaps even in Isaac Newton, who experimented extensively with alchemy and who became noticeably deranged in his later years. The ability to act as a solvent for other metals has led to the extensive use of mercury in mining, as well as to the development of an alloy of mercury used in dental work.

Mercury in water is often converted by bacteria to the compound methylmercury, in which a carbon atom and three hydrogen atoms are chemically bound to each mercury atom. Methylmercury is much more easily absorbed by living organisms than elemental mercury. In water, it moves up the food chain, where it is concentrated in predator fish. Older, and therefore larger, predator fish are especially prized by humans for food. Also, methylmercury tends to accumulate in the parts of fish that people eat, the muscles. Fish are not especially affected by methylmercury poisoning, but humans, especially young ones, can be harmed. At least 21 U.S. states, two Canadian provinces, and Sweden have had to blacklist lakes in which fish have high levels of methylmercury. Typically, pregnant or nursing women and young children are advised not to eat fish from such lakes, while others are told to limit their consumption. The worst lakes for methylmercury contamination are small, shallow ones, or lakes newly created by impounding water. In the smaller lakes it is warmer water and in the younger lakes organic debris that produces conditions suitable for bacterial action. Another factor is acidity; acid lakes develop more methylmercury.

Methylmercury has also been used widely as a fungicide on crop seeds. Usually such seed are also dyed strange colors (lavender corn, for example) to show that treated seeds should not be used for food. In 1971, however, people in Iraq who did not know that grain intended for seed had been treated, cooked and ate the wheat and barley seed. As a result, 6530 became ill and 459 died.

Mercury gets into air not only from industrial processes, but also from incineration of batteries, paints, and switches containing mercury.

Perhaps the most recent case of widespread mercury poisoning occurred in and around the town of Minimata, Japan, on Kyushu Island. In the early 1950s fishers and other villagers in the region began to go mad and develop many neurological problems. There were many stillbirths and children born with serious defects. About a thousand people in all are thought to have died from what came to be known as Minimata disease. The "disease" was recognized in 1959 as mercury poisoning caused by industrial wastes that the Chisso Corporation dumped in Minimata Bay, polluting the fishing grounds of a people whose main source of protein is fish. Fish caught in Minimata Bay had mercury levels 11 times as great as would be permitted by the U.S. Food and Drug Administration (FDA). As recently as the early 1990s about 2000 people living around Minimata Bay continued to suffer from the effects of mercury poisoning.

Because mercury is toxic to all forms of life, it has frequently been used as an additive to prevent growth of fungi or other organisms, especially in paper manufacture and in paint.

revealed in three individuals mercury concentrations high enough to cause illness, though health problems were not investigated in the study. This study was reported in the October 18, 1990 *New England Journal of Medicine.*

On August 20, 1990, the EPA completely banned the use of mercury-based preservatives in interior paints. No recall was initiated, however, so mercury-laden interior paints continued to be sold even though no more were being manufactured. Mercury compounds are still used in exterior paints.

(Periodical References and Additional Reading: *Science* 1-19-90, p 276; *Science News* 10-20-90, p 244; *New York Times* 12-13-90; *Harvard Health Letter* 11-90, p 7; *New York Times* 1-16-91, p A3; *Science News* 3-9-91, p 152; *New York Times* 8-26-91, p A1; *Tufts University Diet & Nutrition Letter,* 4-92, p 7; *Nature* 6-17-93, p 589; *Nature* 9-23-93, p 302; *Nature* 11-11-93, p 118)

LEAD

People have made the environment more dangerous by creating materials that were previously unknown and by accumulating existing substances that are rare in nature. Perhaps the earliest material to be made dangerous primarily by accumulation was elemental lead in large quantities. (Native lead—naturally occurring metal instead of ore—exists, but it is quite rare.) Archaeological evidence for smelted lead exists from 6000 B.C. It is not known when people first recognized that lead is dangerous, although warnings against it exist among early Greek medical writings.

High levels of lead cause symptoms of poisoning, but it has long been argued that even low levels of lead in children reduce intelligence. Sometimes it has been argued that other factors in the environment or even genetics result in a somewhat lower intelligence in the same population that is, for various reasons, exposed to environmental lead. But evidence increasingly indicts lead as the cause of lower intelligence. For example, an Australian study, published in the *New England Journal of Medicine* on October 29, 1992 found that middle-class white children with low levels of lead in their blood—between ten and 35 micrograms—can experience a drop in scores on IQ tests, with a drop of five percent in ten-year-olds at the 35-microgram level. A similar study in Boston, Massachusetts, directed by David C. Bellinger of Boston's Children's Hospital, also found a small but significant drop in IQ scores.

As a result of these and other studies, the U.S. Centers for Disease Control and Prevention (CDC) has declared lead poisoning to be the most common preventable childhood disease. Before 1991 the CDC had said there was no cause for alarm until lead levels reached 25 micrograms per deciliter. Since a re-evaluation in 1991, levels higher than ten micrograms per deciliter were considered dangerous by the CDC. The CDC has called for testing all children in the U.S. between the ages of six months and six years for lead in their blood. The CDC estimates, in the absence of national tests, that four to six million American children exceed its standard of ten micrograms per deciliter.

By 1993 the CDC call for testing had been heeded in New York state, which began to mandate such testing at age one and again at two as part of what may be the toughest set of regulations against lead in the nation. A few days after the New York law went into effect, a study published in the April 7, 1993 *Journal of the American Medical Association* demonstrated that aggressive treatment of lead poisoning in children results in increased scores on IQ tests at a rate of about one point for each three micrograms per deciliter of lead reduction. The most successful treatments reduced lead levels in children with high exposures by 30 micrograms per deciliter.

Later in life, lead may also cause similar damage in adults, usually pregnant or lactating mothers and older adults with osteoporosis. Lead often travels with calcium, and so 90 percent of retained lead accumulates in the bones of the body. In pregnancy, lactation, or osteoporosis, the harmless calcium is leached from the bones, but at the same time the tag-along and very dangerous lead moves into the blood. From there, it can affect various organs, impairing the mind and the operation of the body. Also, the milk of lactating mothers, who are taking calcium from the bones for milk creation, can contain lead in amounts harmful to the nursing baby.

Adults exposed to lead at work often develop lead poisoning as well. It was from work-related lead poisoning that the symptoms of lead poisoning, which can affect not only the nerves, but also the stomach, testes, kidneys, and bone marrow, were first noticed. Inhaled lead dust can also adversely affect the lungs. Among the occupations hazardous for lead today are work with storage batteries, pottery, plumbing and heating, machine maintenance and repair, home renovation, and ship or office construction.

Throughout the early 1990s, despite this long history, battles over lead in water and tableware persisted, although ice cores from Greenland demonstrate that the main lead input into the environment has ceased with the change away from leaded gasoline.

Water Faucets

On December 15, 1992, the Natural Resources Defense Council and the Environmental Law Foundation used California's Proposition 65, a law designed to protect consumers from toxins and carcinogens, to sue manufacturers of water faucets. The two environmental groups had arranged to have faucet output measured for lead in water, which can leach from brass used in the faucets. Although measurements varied from faucet to faucet, the total lead in some samples of a liter of water drawn through the faucet reached levels as high as 25 times the amount California law sets for maximum daily intake. The laboratory that did the testing estimated that about 25 percent of faucets used nationally leach dangerous levels of lead. Such leaching may diminish as faucets age.

In 1992 and again on May 11, 1993, the U.S. Environmental Protection Agency (EPA) issued reports on lead in water systems in the U.S. The second report used a new, tighter standard of 15 parts per billion for the most contaminated households and tested every U.S. water system with more than 3300 customers. Of the water systems surveyed, which together with the previous survey cover about 180 million people in the U.S., a total of 819 failed to meet the new standard. Because some of these were very large systems (New York City, New York; Chicago, Illinois; both Minneapolis and St. Paul, Minnesota; Cleveland and Columbus, Ohio; Portland, Oregon; among others) the total number of persons served by such systems was high—30 million. But because of the way the households were identified, many fewer people actually were being exposed to heavily leaded water. Some samples were over 300 parts per million for individual houses, but that did not mean that the system as a whole was really that contaminated by lead. Lead pipes into a house or lead in faucets could make a big difference.

Lead from faucets and pipes can be minimized be letting water run for a few seconds before using it in most cities, although if lead is leaching from pipes it may take a minute or two to discharge all the lead-tainted water when the water system has not been used for several hours. If, as in Chicago, lead pipes are used to connect the house to the mains, however, running the water for a short period of time does not really help.

Dishes

In another California development, ten leading manufacturers of dishes, including Lenox, Royal Doulton, and Wedgwood, agreed to change their practices with regard to lead as part of a two million dollar settlement in a lawsuit, the largest to that time under Proposition 65. The money will be used for enforcement of lead standards and consumer education concerning lead hazards.

Although dishes have come a long way from the lead jars of the Romans and the pewter plates of the American colonists, some forms of ceramics have continued to use lead glazes and decorative paints or dyes based on lead. Primarily the ceramics in question are the shiny forms often grouped as porcelains or enamels. The less shiny stoneware, unless painted or decorated, has a negligible lead level. Glasses of all sorts, including those used for manufacture of plates and bowls, are nearly lead-free as well. Many manufacturers also certify that their porcelains are low-lead or lead-free. Despite this range of choices, tableware is considered the largest source of dietary lead.

Under the settlement, the manufacturers since June 1, 1993 have put a warning label on dishes with lead levels higher than that permitted in California. The label is actually a sort of insignia, a yellow triangle with a black border; unlike the tobacco warning, there is no text. Instead, stores selling the dishes are to post signs with the legend explaining that the yellow triangle means that use of dishes carrying it expose the consumer to lead, "a chemical known to the State of California to cause birth defects and other reproductive harm." Although this warning seems to bypass the known effects on children after they are born, the Environmental Defense Fund, the other party to the suit, thinks that the warning about birth defects will cause manufacturers to change their use of lead and that other manufacturers, not parties to the agreement, will also abide by it.

Calcium Supplements

Calcium supplements are offered as pills or added to some products, especially drinks likely to be consumed by children (*see* "Minerals UPDATE," p 168). Antacid tablets that are chewed are also promoted as calcium supplements. Some of the sources of calcium are chemicals concocted in laboratories, but ground bone and calcium-rich earths (dolomite) or minerals (calcium carbonate, also known as limestone) are also used. As observed above, lead often travels with calcium. The FDA found lead in calcium supplements, especially in bonemeal, in the 1980s. Bernard P. Bourgoin of the National Water Research Institute in Burlington, Ontario, Alfredo J. Quattrone with the California Department of Health Services in Sacramento, and coworkers looked for lead in 70 calcium supplements sold in Canada and the U.S. They reported in the August 1993 *American Journal of Public Health* that more than 50 of the supplements also contained lead, 17 of them in amounts higher than the six micrograms a day which is the FDA limit for children under six years old. Bonemeal-based supplements were the worst offenders.

If calcium is pure, however, there is some evidence that taking extra calcium along with food will lower rates of lead absorption by the body. Cells prefer calcium to lead, and accept lead only where calcium is not available.

TIMETABLE OF LEAD POISONING

6000 BC	About this time lead beads are produced at Catal Huyuk in what is now Turkey.
400 BC	Hippocrates of Cos [Greek: circa 460 BC-circa 370 BC], about this time, documents illness caused by lead mining.
650	Greek physician Paul of Aegina lists the symptoms of lead poisoning.

1621	Lead mining in the United States starts in Virginia.
1723	Drinkers from North Carolina complain that rum from Massachusetts causes stomach problems and partial paralysis; after Boston physicians attribute the problem to lead parts used in the stills that produce the rum, the Massachusetts legislature outlaws that use of lead.
1767	Physician George Baker [born Devonshire, England, 1722; died 1809] is knighted for having proved that lead-lined cider presses causes paralysis, stomachaches, and other symptoms.
1768	Benjamin Franklin points out to George Baker that in Massachusetts lead still-heads had been banned because of the belief that lead in the rum causes "dry belly ache and the loss of the use of . . . limbs."
1890	About this time physicians in Australia discover that children were being poisoned by ingesting old paint that had turned to powder.
1917	Physicians in the U.S. learn that children develop lead poisoning by eating paint chips that have peeled off of interior walls, especially in poorer neighborhoods (where paint is more likely to be allowed to peel).
1930	Leaded gasoline is introduced about this time.
1955	U.S. paint manufacturers limit lead in paints to one percent or less.
1971	The U.S. government passes the Lead Paint Poisoning Prevention Act, which requires that interior paint applied before 1955 must be stripped from buildings; the Act is never fully implemented, however.
1977	The U.S. government in this year and over the next three years imposes more and more restrictive rules on use of lead shot for hunting migratory birds (mostly ducks and geese) because the shot causes lead poisoning in wounded birds; by 1980 the ban is complete.
1978	The U.S. Occupational Safety and Health Administration sets its first standards for on-the-job lead: if blood-lead levels rise to 50 micrograms per deciliter, the worker must be laid off with full pay until levels drop below 40 micrograms per deciliter.
1979	In March, Herbert Needleman releases an influential study that shows that low levels of lead in children's blood and teeth correlate with lower IQ test scores, suggesting the low-level lead poisoning can reduce intelligence.
1980	The U.S. government bans paints containing lead.
1983	A panel of experts from the EPA at first object to the way the 1979 Needleman study was conducted; however, its final report states that the study's methodology was essentially correct.
1984	The U.S. government takes steps toward a complete ban on leaded gasoline in order to reduce lead concentrations in the lower atmosphere.
1986	The U.S. government lowers its standards for the permissible amount of lead in air and bans the use of solder containing lead.
1989	U.S. government mandates tests for lead in children from low-income families.
1990	A report from the U.S. Department of Housing and Urban Development states that 75 percent of all U.S. homes built before 1980 contain lead paint, amounting to three million tons of lead.
	For the first time since the mid-1970s, a child who has eaten paint chips dies

from lead poisoning.

1991   On May 7, the U.S. mandates tests for lead in tap water; it will take about 20 years for tests to be completed and problems corrected.

In June, Clifford Weisel and coworkers at the University of Medicine and Dentistry in New Jersey–Robert Wood Johnson Medical School report that lead ink used on bread wrappers could be a hazard; lead ink also contributes about 0.8 metric ton (0.9 short ton) of lead each day to the U.S. waste stream.

Donald Smith of the University of California–Santa Cruz finds that California sea otters have up to 40 times the lead in their teeth compared with fossil sea otters of 1000 to 2000 years ago.

On October 7, the U.S. Centers for Disease Control and Prevention in Atlanta lowers the definition of lead poisoning in children from 25 micrograms of lead per deciliter of blood to ten micrograms.

On October 11, the California government settles a lawsuit out of court by agreeing to provide tests federally mandated in 1989 for lead poisoning in poor children.

In October, Claude F. Boutron of the Laboratoire de Glaciologie et Geophysique de l'Environemènt in St. Martin-d'Hères, France, and coworkers report that lead concentrations in Greenland ice had dropped to levels not seen since the early 1900s; between 1967 and 1985, lead levels in the ice dropped by more than 85 percent. This is largely attributed to a decline in the use of leaded gasoline. (The study also reports declines of 60 percent since the 1960s in cadmium and zinc.)

In November, the U.S. government recommends new guidelines limiting leaching of lead from dishes to 3.0 micrograms of lead per milliliter of a four percent solution of vinegar over a 24-hour period and from cups and mugs to 0.5 microgram per milliliter; although not binding, the guidelines are set at about half the previously recommended limits.

On November 12, California sues ten manufacturers of tableware for violating its limits for lead in dishes and mugs, which call for about one-fiftieth the amount of leaching permitted under federal guidelines; the California law does not ban tableware violating its permissible levels, but calls for clear labeling.

On December 7, California obtains an agreement from major wine makers in the state to stop using lead caps over the corks on wine bottles. The U.S. Office of Scientific Integrity asks the University of Pittsburgh to investigate charges that Herbert Needleman's 1979 study violates rules against scientific misconduct.

1993   A French study shows that high levels of lead in the Greenland Ice Cap that accumulated during the 1960s and 1970s were almost entirely the result of leaded gasoline burned in the U.S. during that time; levels began to decline for ice deposited in the 1980s. Other studies showed a similar decline in lead levels in soils in the northeastern U.S. during the 1980s.

1995   Lead is scheduled to be eliminated from all U.S. gasoline.

(Periodical References and Additional Reading: *Science News* 4-28-90, p 261; *New York Times* 12-20-90, p A1; *New York Times* 12-22-90; *New York Times* 2-21-91, p B8; *New York Times* 3-29-91; *New York Times* 5-8-91, p A1; *Science News* 5-18-91, p 308; *International Wildlife* 5/

6-91, p 28; *Science News* 6-8-91, p 367; *Science* 8-23-91, p 842; *New York Times* 9-3-91, p
C10; *New York Times* 8-24-91; *Science News* 9-14-91, p 166; *New York Times* 10-7-91, p C3;
New York Times 10-12-91, p 7; *New York Times* 10-15-91, p C4; *Science* 10-25-91, p 500;
New York Times 11-13-91, p A18; *New York Times* 12-8-91, p L39; *Science* 12-13-91, p 1575;
Harvard Health Letter 5-92, p 6; *New York Times* 10-29-92, p A20; *New York Times* 11-18-
92, p C18; *New York Times* 12-16-92, p A22; *New York Times* 1-17-93, p I-25; *New York
Times* 4-5-93, p B4; *New York Times* 4-8-93, p A18; *New York Times* 5-12-93, p A12; *New
York Times* 8-17-93, p C6; *Science News* 9-4-93, p 150)

CHLORINE

Trend-watchers have observed that chlorine is the fad chemical of the early 1990s.
Despite its long service to sanitation and the popularity of chlorine-based bleaches
since their first introduction in 1783, chlorine has acquired a bad name. Maybe it was
the chlorine in long-lasting chlorinated hydrocarbon pesticides that first got people's
attention; or perhaps it was the chlorine in polychlorinated biphenyls (PCBs); or the
chlorine in the chlorofluorocarbons that erode the ozone layer; or in polyvinyl
chloride plastics. Somehow, however, that "chlor" kept showing up in prefixes,
suffixes, and roots of chemical names. And every time it appeared, the chemical was
bad for people or the environment. Not only that, but white bread, reputedly
unhealthy, is made from bleached flour.

It is not surprising that after a time the element chlorine itself became suspicious.
Nearly everyone in the industrialized world drinks water that has been purified with
chlorine. Could that be good for you? Would it be a good idea to switch to bottled
water?

Chlorination of Water

Chlorine was first used to purify water in England in 1800 by William Cruickshank,
and it has been a common and effective approach to killing pathogens (germs) in
water since about 1900 in the U.S. Chlorine is poisonous to just about every form of
life. Like the other halogens (notably fluorine, bromine, and iodine), it is even more
reactive than oxygen and can easily alter the chemistry of organic molecules. Furthermore, in water, chlorine participates in some chemical reactions that make atomic
oxygen available, which accounts for the bleaching action of chlorine. Atomic oxygen
behaves like those free radicals that people are encouraged to take vitamins to
eliminate.

Research in the early 1990s suggested that chlorine in drinking water, which has
drastically reduced the incidence of typhoid fever and other water-borne diseases, has
as a trade-off the production of an increased risk of cancer. One study in the May/June
1993 *Archives of Environmental Health* suggested that drinking more than 14 cups
of chlorinated water a day raised the risk of bladder cancer in men to double or
quadruple what it otherwise would be. A re-analysis of 22 older studies of chlorinated
water, directed by Robert B. Morris of the Medical College of Wisconsin in Milwaukee,
revealed not only a 21 percent increase in the likelihood of bladder cancer, but also a
38 percent increase in rectal cancer (reported in the July 1992 *American Journal of*

Public Health). If these data are accurate, chlorinated water might cause as many as 4200 extra cases of bladder cancer and 6500 additional cases of rectal cancer in the U.S.

It did not seem likely to the scientists studying chlorine that the element itself would cause cancer. Instead, chlorine might interact with organic molecules to form biologically active compounds. Animal studies, reported in the May 19, 1994 *Journal of the National Cancer Institute* show that this suspicion is true. Rats and mice drinking pure chlorinated water do not have higher levels of cancer (with one minor exception that could be a statistical anomaly). But if chloroform, known to be formed in polluted chlorinated water, or related compounds called trihalomethanes were included, cancer rates soared. By itself this study does not mean that the trihalomethanes are the source of all the cancer, since chlorine interacts with many organics to produce a variety of chemicals, not all of which are even known. It does suggest, however, that removing the organics or the products formed would help prevent cancer.

The truly nervous as well as pregnant women might want to drink bottled water, especially since there are now health standards that apply to it. For most of the rest of us, the safety of sanitation by chlorination is greater than the added risk of cancer.

(Periodical References and Additional Reading: *Science News* 7-11-92, p 23; *Science News* 5-29-93, p 343; *Science News* 7-24-93, p 61)

Dioxin UPDATE

Controversy about dioxins continued into the early 1990s.

In November 1990 a conference at the Banbury Center in Cold Spring Harbor Laboratory, a conference later revealed to have been sponsored by the chemical industry, concluded that the dangers of dioxins to humans have been exaggerated. The only known effect was chloracne, a severe chemically induced skin condition. By February 1991 it appeared that many of the conferees had failed to agree with that reported conclusion and that some felt their names had been used without permission or agreement. However, the main conclusion of the conference—that a low-enough level of dioxins might be harmless—was not disputed at that time.

Despite the defections from the Banbury conference report, the U.S. Environmental Protection Agency (EPA) seemed to take the report seriously and in May called for further study of the significance of dioxin. In August 1991 the EPA touted its incomplete year-long study of the health hazards of dioxins with widely publicized statements suggesting that the hazards of dioxins would turn out to be seriously exaggerated. The main goal of the study was to determine the background level of dioxins to which the public is exposed, and the EPA comments apparently were still based on the Banbury conference.

However, other signs pointed toward a change in attitudes toward dioxins in 1991. On May 28, 1991, Vernon N. Houk, director of Environmental Health and Injury Controls for the CDC, told the twenty-fifth annual Conference on Trace Substances in the Environment that he had, been mistaken in recommending the evacuation of Times Beach, Missouri, in 1982. Shortly before this admission, a federal district judge approved (on January 1, 1991) plans to tear down buildings in Times Beach and to build an incinerator for burning the soil.

In the face of all this optimism, research in 1991 showed for the first time that dioxin does influence cancer in humans. On January 24, 1991, Marilyn A. Fingerhut reported that the largest study ever of the effects of dioxin in the workplace showed a small but significant increase in cancer among workers exposed to high levels of dioxin. The study was interpreted by many, however, as showing that the danger of dioxin to humans was less than previously had been believed, since only high levels of the chemical were involved. Another study, by Alfred Manz of the Center for Chemical Workers' Health in Hamburg, Germany, released on October 19, 1991, also concluded that exposure to dioxins produced during the manufacture of chemicals leads to an increase in the cancer rate in humans, but does not cause any specific cancer. Also, in late September Georg Lucier and Chris Portier of the National Institute of Environmental Health Sciences in North Carolina announced a new study of the effects of dioxin at low doses. The results suggested that low doses also might cause cancer, although further research was needed.

When the EPA panel's preliminary findings became available in September 1992, they failed to settle issues conclusively. Basing a lot of its thinking on Fingerhut's work, the panel declared that only people exposed to high levels of dioxin were at any risk, but that animals throughout the environment were adversely affected by the chemical. Members of the panel interpreted the findings to mean that only chemical workers or people exposed in Seveso-like accidents might be at risk among humans. Panel members also noted that they felt that currently estimated levels of five parts per trillion in fat in humans posed no risk. Much higher levels, however, increase risk

---

Background

Dioxin is the general name for a group of 75 related chemicals. One of the most common of the dioxins and probably the most toxic is 2,3,7,8-TCDD, short for 2,3,7,8 tetrachlorodibenz-*para*-dioxin, a contaminant in the herbicide Agent Orange (2,4,5-T) which was used as a defoliant in Vietnam. Often this dioxin is simply called TCDD. Nearly always the word *dioxin* in medical literature means TCDD.

Dioxins are a class of chemicals formed when compounds containing chlorine are heated to high temperatures or burned. Because chlorine is an important part of many pesticides, dioxins are often found as contaminants in insecticides and herbicides. Chlorine is also used as a bleach in making paper or fibers or other industrial processes, and further processing also produced dioxins, frequently emitted into the environment along with smoke. Incinerators that burn mixed garbage also often produce dioxins in their smoke and in their ashes.

Dioxins are poisonous for many animals, but in humans they have been proven to cause only the skin disease chloracne. There is, however, a great deal of circumstantial evidence and some scientific studies linking dioxins with cancer in animals. Recent studies have shown that the dioxin molecule activates the enzyme cytochrome p450, which disrupts chromosome structure. Such disruption is a likely predecessor to cancer.

from both lung cancer and the cancers classed as soft-tissue sarcomas (*see* "Agent Orange Update" p 263).

Dioxin and Sex

One of the scientific conclusions of the Banbury conference was that the primary effect of dioxin TCDD was to bind to a receptor for steroid hormones called Ah (aryl hydrocarbon). The steroid hormones are best known for those that resemble testosterone, the hormone that promotes masculinity. Such steroids are used to build muscles, although they have dangerous side effects. Estrogen is also a steroid hormone. Once bound to the receptor, TCDD fails to degrade and disappear the way that actual steroid hormones do.

Thus scientists came to suspect that dioxins might influence sex. As is often the case, this suspicion was checked out with experiments on laboratory rats. Dick Peterson, Thomas A. Mably, and coworkers at the University of Wisconsin-Madison, who had previously demonstrated that TCDD reduces concentrations of male sex hormones in adult rats, tested TCDD on pregnant rats to see the effect on developing pups. Even very low doses reduced sperm counts and higher doses produced definite, lifelong feminization of pups, including changes in behavior. Fertility was not reduced, however, although because of differences between rat reproduction and human reproduction, a reduction in sperm count of the amount seen in rats exposed to TCDD in the womb would probably lower fertility in humans.

A study of female rhesus monkeys by Sherry E. Rier of the University of South Florida College of Medicine in Tampa and coworkers that exposed the monkeys to TCDD found that the level of exposure was linked to the disease endometriosis, a painful condition affecting the lining of the uterus. In the condition, cells from the lining form nodules elsewhere in the reproductive system. The more TCDD there is, the more likely the disease will develop, although a third of the monkeys not deliberately fed dioxin also developed a mild form of endometriosis.

Seveso Update

In September 1993 Pier Alberto Bertazzi of the University of Milan and coworkers published in *Epidemiology* a study of the effects of dioxin contamination on the 37,000 persons who were exposed to the chemical as a result of the July 10, 1976 explosion of the ICMESA Factory near Seveso, Italy. This explosion and the widespread deaths of animals near the site brought dioxin to the attention of people around the world. The toxicity of dioxins to some animals, combined with the ability of even small amounts of dioxin to cause cancer and birth defects in laboratory animals, suggested that the Seveso explosion might produce similar results in humans. Immediate destructive effects of the Seveso material on dogs, cats, chickens, other farm animals, and wildlife seemed to confirm those fears.

Bertrazzi's team compared the people in Seveso with an Italian population living in similar circumstances, but circumstances not known to be exposed to dioxins. Overall, the rate of cancer was about the same in both populations, but the frequency of certain types of cancer was much different. An anomaly in the statistics was that the small group (about two percent of the dioxin group) exposed to the highest amount of dioxin in the soil showed nothing either way. The main results occurred in a larger group (about 13 percent) who were exposed to somewhat less dioxin, but had more exposure than the remainder of the 37,000 persons. Group B, the 13 percent with the most striking cancer statistics, had half the expected cases of breast and uterine cancers, but five times the number of cases of gall bladder cancer and multiple myeloma, and a somewhat higher rate of liver cancer. Altogether, however, the rate for Group B of all cancers was close to that of the control group.

It is thought that dioxin interferes with the operation of estrogen in addition to any other effects it may have in humans. Estrogen exacerbates some forms of cancer. Interference with estrogen use by dioxin might explain why the persons who developed chloracne, and therefore are thought to have been the most exposed, were all cancer-free at the time of the study.

Agent Orange Update

Among the measures taken by U.S. troops during the Vietnam War between 1962 and 1971 was defoliation, i.e. poisoning plants in regions where the opposing Viet Cong or North Vietnamese troops might find cover. Defoliation causes leaves to fall off trees, and bushes and shrubs to die. Some 19 million gallons of herbicides were sprayed on forests and fields, mostly from planes or helicopters. Several herbicides were used for defoliation, most notoriously a compound labeled Agent Orange, which was frequently contaminated with dioxins that developed during the manufacturing process. When dioxins became famous as a possible cause of human disease in the 1970s, veterans of the Vietnam War were quick to connect various physical and psychological troubles with their experience with Agent Orange (and, to a lesser extent, other herbicides). Although the U.S. government and chemical manufacturers fought veterans' claims, by the mid-1980s the veterans, or their survivors, had developed a good case. Dioxins or something in the herbicides was a cause of disease. The U.S. Department of Veterans Affairs began compensating members of the armed forces who had been exposed to herbicides and who later developed chloracne or one of two rare cancers: soft-tissue sarcoma (a cancer that sometimes appears in muscle or connective tissue other than bone) or non-Hodgkin's lymphoma (which forms in cells in the lymph nodes, bone marrow, spleen, or liver and affects blood cells). Seven corporations that had manufactured herbicides settled out of court for $180 million.

On July 27, 1993, the Institute of Medicine of the National Academy of Sciences, at the behest of Veterans Affairs, reported that their analysis revealed a statistical association between exposure to herbicides and specific diseases. Specifically the panel found such an association for civilians who use or manufacture similar herbicides. Not only did such an association exist for the three diseases that Veterans Affairs already compensated for, but two additional diseases were added: Hodgkin's disease, a lymphoma with similar symptoms to non-Hodgkin's but a different kind of tumor (and a much higher cure rate), and porphyria cutanea tarda, a rare disease whose symptoms include skin that thins, blisters, or darkens and excessive hair growth. As a result of the report, the Department of Veterans Affairs will add

Hodgkin's disease and porphyria cutanea tarda to the other three diseases for which it compensates veterans.

TIMETABLE OF DIOXIN TO 1990

1949   Monsanto's manufacture of pesticides in its plant at Nitro, West Virginia, exposes its workers to dioxin.

1951   Diamond Shamrock Corporation starts manufacturing Agent Orange at its plant in Newark, New Jersey.

1957   West German workers manufacturing the herbicide 2,4,5-T develop a skin disease later named chloracne; their cases lead to the first recognition that a dioxin frequently contaminates such herbicides.

1962   U.S. troops in Vietnam begin using Agent Orange and other herbicides to defoliate potential hiding places for soldiers of opposing forces.

1971   Used oil contaminated with dioxins is sprayed on the roads in and around the small town of Times Beach, Missouri; birds and animals die and at least one child becomes ill.

            The Vietnam defoliation program is terminated.

1974   The U.S. Centers for Disease Control and Prevention (CDC) in Atlanta, Georgia, investigates the health problems in Times Beach and identifies dioxin-contaminated oil as their cause.

1976   Many around the globe learn of dioxin for the first time when an explosion at the ISMESA Factory near Seveso, Italy, contaminates a large region with about a pound of dioxin, resulting in the death of birds, farm animals, and pets, along with cases of chloracne in humans.

1977   Dutch scientists discover that incinerator wastes are contaminated by dioxins, potentially dangerous chemicals that have been linked to cancer in animal studies.

1978   Dow Chemical releases a study showing that dioxins are produced when garbage is burned.

1979   The U.S. Environmental Protection Agency (EPA) bans the herbicide 2,4,5-T, an ingredient in the Agent Orange herbicide sprayed by U.S. troops in the Vietnam War to defoliate forests, because 2,4,5-T is linked to birth defects; dioxin contaminates 2,4,5-T as a result of the manufacturing process.

1980   A recycling plant in Hempstead, New York, is shut down because of high dioxin levels produced in incineration.

1982   Soil samples collected by the EPA in Times Beach in December reveal high levels of dioxins, resulting in the first large-scale public knowledge of the problem in the United States.

1983   The EPA agrees to buy Times Beach and move the residents out of it; eventually, it spends $37 million on the resettlement through 1991, with another $150 million expected to be needed to clean up the site.

1984   In May, U.S. veterans of the Vietnam War reach an out-of-court settlement with chemical companies that once manufactured Agent Orange; the companies agree to set up a $250-million fund for veterans with health problems from exposure to the chemical.

1988   Italian scientists report that follow-up studies of the people exposed to dioxins
              in the 1976 industrial accident near Seveso, Italy, show no increase in birth
              defects.

(Periodical References and Additional Reading: *New York Times* 9-26-92, p 9; *New York Times*
    10-28-92, p A14; *Science News* 5-30-92, p 359; *Science News* 1-11-92, p 24; *New York Times*
    7-28-93, p A12; *Science News* 9-4-93, p 149; *Science* 9-10-93, p 1383; *New York Times* 10-26-
    93, p C4; *Science News* 11-27-93, p 356; *Scientific American* 1-94, p 25)

Pesticides: Insecticide and Herbicide UPDATE

The continued environmental movement dates itself from the 1962 publication of
Silent Spring by Rachel Carson, a book that indicted insecticides for killing birds and
perhaps affecting humans as well. Although there have since been many other
environmental alarms that took the forefront for a while, the pesticide issue has
remained a significant environmental concern since 1962. Farmers, for example, have
a much higher risk of cancer because of their exposure to pesticides, according to a
U.S. National Cancer Institute report (in the September 1992 *Scandinavian Journal
of Work, Environment, and Health*).

Pesticides and Children

While birds were the concern in *Silent Spring,* human children were seen to be at risk
in two widely publicized studies in the summer of 1993: "Pesticides in the Diets of
Children" by the U.S. National Academy of Sciences and "Pesticides in Children's
Foods" (issued June 28, 1993) by an organization known as the Environmental
Working Group. Both reports claimed that tests to detect pesticide residues in food
are inadequate and that the amounts in children's food, though perhaps not enough to
damage adults, might be harmful to children.

The report of the Environmental Working Group was primarily prepared by
Richard Wiles, who examined unpublished data of 17,000 food samples that had been
tested by the U.S. Food and Drug Administration (FDA) between 1990 and 1992 along
with another 3000 samples from independent laboratories tested during the same
time period. He concluded that a third of a lifetime exposure to pesticides will come
by the age of five because of the kinds of foods children eat. Wiles also thinks that the
FDA underreports the amount of pesticide residues in the food supply. Even Wiles,
however, thinks it is better for children today to eat their fruits and vegetables and
take the pesticide risks as a trade off.

The National Academy of Sciences panel mainly called for more information on
what children eat and what pesticides in that food might or might not do, including
how different pesticides interact with each other. But in the absence of such data, the
panel recommended cutting pesticide residues in food by 90 percent, just to be on the
safe side.

These reports caused the U.S. Environmental Protection Agency (EPA), along with
the FDA and the Agriculture Department, to announce they would reduce the amount
of pesticides in food and create incentives for the development of safer pesticides.

Background

Pesticides can cause harm to humans when they are applied, when they are general residues in the environment, or when they are present in or on food that humans consume. In the U.S., several different government agencies regulate each of these areas.

During application: Responsibility for pesticides at this stage was largely with the Department of Agriculture until 1993, although other agencies could become involved if pesticides were applied beyond the boundaries of farms, either by accident (as in drifting spray) or intentionally (as in the use of an insecticide in homes or specific environments, such as swamps). On August 13, 1992, however, the EPA issued its own set of rules requiring employers to train workers and post notices that would help prevent accidental pesticide poisoning. The new rules would apply to all of the approximately two million farm workers who are not owners or their families by 1995. Starting in April 1993 pesticides had to carry labels saying that they should not be used so that they enable human exposure. When the rules are fully implemented, workers must be trained in the use of protective gear, given a place to clean up after exposure, and be provided with emergency care if needed. Workers would also be barred from the fields for a specified amount of time after spraying.

In the environment or food: The EPA sets officially tolerated amounts of pesticide residues on crops or in food. Mostly the acceptable amounts on food range from 0.2 to 100 parts per million; a tolerance level of one part per million means that less than a molecule out of each 1,000,000 can be a given pesticide. Current EPA guidelines are different for toxic or teratogenic (causing birth defects) pesticides and for carcinogenic pesticides. If cancer is not involved, then the tolerance is set at 1/100 of the dose needed to produce recognizable adverse effects in animal tests. When the pesticide causes cancer in animals, the tolerable amount for humans is set at a level expected to cause about one instance of cancer among a million people who ingest average amounts of the food in question. On the average, the amount for cancer-causing residues is in practice about 1/400 of the amount that causes animal tumors.

On produce: Using EPA guidelines, the U.S. Food and Drug Administration is responsible for testing foods other than meat and poultry. This responsibility includes farm products, such as fresh produce. Somewhat less than two percent of domestic produce is found to be outside the guidelines and four percent is imported into the U.S.

For meat and poultry: The Department of Agriculture is in charge of residues in meat and poultry, although their inspectors rely largely on visual inspection.

Earlier in 1993, however, the EPA had asked Congress to permit 35 pesticides known to cause cancer in animals to bypass the 1958 law that tolerates zero residues in food. The EPA had contended since 1988 that they could maintain pesticide levels that would constitute a "negligible risk" to consumers and had permitted trace amounts of the 35 pesticides in food. In 1992, however, after losing a court case and its appeal, the EPA was ordered to obey the 1958 Delaney Clause of the Federal Food, Drug, and Cosmetic Act, which permits no detectable residues at all. By 1993, however, the change in administrations from Bush to Clinton, plus all the 1993 publicity about pesticides in food, caused the EPA to ask for the authority to ban or restrict more pesticides than ever before, eliminating any that seemed unsafe.

Estrogen Look-Alikes

In 1993 a number of biologists and physicians called attention to the chemical resemblance between a number of pesticides, including DDT, and the human hormone estrogen. Their contention was that the body treats these chemicals as additional sources of estrogen with varying results. One theory is that the clogging of the estrogen receptors with artificial chemicals results in added risk for breast cancer, possibly because with the receptors all in use, the body makes more estrogen, a known risk factor for breast cancer. Mary S. Wolff of Mount Sinai School of Medicine testified at an EPA hearing that DDT itself when present in tissues was associated with increased risk of breast cancer.

Although DDT was effectively banned in the U.S. in 1972, it is so persistent in the environment that most people contain measurable amounts of DDT in their fat. Wolff's work, published in the April 1993 *Journal of the National Cancer Institute,* showed that women in the top ten percent of exposure to DDT had four times the risk of breast cancer when compared with women in the bottom ten percent. Levels of exposure were measured in 229 women, 58 with breast cancer, using a blood test for a chemical formed when DDT is broken down in the body.

In men, estrogen look-alikes may interfere with sperm production. Louis Guillette of the University of Florida has testified before the EPA that the data show that there has been a 50 percent reduction in sperm count worldwide since estrogen look-alikes have been in use (combining studies of 14,947 men between 1940 and 1990). Furthermore, other studies show a 19 percent decline in the volume of semen, which in combination with the lower count suggests that about 40 percent as many sperm are available for fertilization as there were in 1940. Since human fertilization is sensitive to the number of sperm, this effect alone could account for a general decline in fertility.

Herbicides

Often when we think of pesticides we limit our thought to chemicals that kill animals, especially insects. But chemicals that kill plants—herbicides—are used as often or more by farmers. Herbicides laced with dioxin are thought to have caused some cancers among veterans of Vietnam (*see* "Dioxin UPDATE," p 260).

SELECTED PESTICIDES AND THEIR STATUS

Chemical	Intended use	Comments
Atrazine	Kills weeds in corn and soybeans	Nation's largest selling pesticide. It causes cancer in lab animals and would be banned under proposed new EPA guidelines.
Benlate	Halts fungal disease	Accidental contamination with a potent weedkiller caused it to kill the crops it was supposed to protect in 1991.

Chemical	Intended use	Comments
Bt	Kills caterpillars	A natural toxin produced by bacteria.
DDT	Kills insects	Restricted and effectively banned in the U.S. since 1972 but still used in Third World countries; estrogen look-alike.
Dioxins	Contaminant in many different pesticides	Definitely causes cancer in animals and probably in humans as well; also causes chloracne in humans; clean-up efforts to rid the environment of dioxins have been a major activity of EPA.
EDBCs	Kills rot in fruits and vegetables	Proven animal carcinogens used mainly in Florida and the South; would be banned if new EPA guidelines are enacted.
Endosulfan	Kills insects on fruits and vegetables	About two million pounds a year used in the U.S. to kill insects on 45 crops; estrogen look-alike.
Mancozeb	Kills fungal blight on potatoes	Found to cause cancer in animals, it is one of the 35 chemicals the EPA would like to allow in potatoes as long as the risk of cancer in humans is negligible.
Spod-X	Kills beet armyworm	A virus cleared by the EPA for use on tomatoes and other vegetables.

(Periodical References and Additional Reading: *New York Times* 2-2-93, p A1; *New York Times* 8-16-93, p I-23; *New York Times* 2-7-93, p IV-6; *New York Times* 4-22-93, p A16; *New York Times* 5-13-93, p D4; *New York Times* 6-17-93, p A23; *New York Times* 6-27-93, p A1; *Science News* 7-3-93, p 4; *Science News* 7-31-93, p 70; *New York Times* 9-21-93, p A19; *New York Times* 10-24-93, p I-21; *New York Times* 10-10-93, p IV-6; *Harvard Health Letter* 1-94, p 6; *Science News* 1-22-94, p 56)

PROBLEMS FROM THE AIR

RADON AND OTHER DANGER FROM RADIOACTIVITY

In the early 1990s reports reminded people of the danger from cosmic and solar radiation to air travelers and of the danger of excessive use of diagnostic X rays. But the main problems that were extensively discussed involved natural radiation from the earth's crust and nuclear reactors used to produce electricity or weapons.

Radioactivity from Earth

In October 1990, a conference of more than 230 scientists convened in Richland, Washington, to grapple with problems connected with radon.

It has long been clear that miners who work in hard-rock tunnels have an increased risk of lung cancer as a result of radon exposure; it is less clear whether the much lower levels of the gas found in people's homes could also increase risk. A study by Janet B. Schoenberg of the New Jersey Department of Health, reported at the Richland conference and in the October 15, 1990 *Cancer Research,* did establish a link, albeit a weak one because of the small size of the sample, between household radon exposure and lung cancer.

The U.S. Environmental Protection Agency (EPA) was given a congressional mandate in 1988 to reduce exposure to radon, although it was not given regulatory authority. Consequently, efforts of the radon division of the EPA have almost all been educational and voluntary. Indeed, the EPA mounted a campaign against household radon in 1988 that continued into the early 1990s. The EPA claims that radon accounts for 7000 to 30,000 cases of lung cancer in the U.S. annually, which would make it among the leading environmental threats. The EPA bases these estimates largely on studies of miners exposed to radon.

However, a study released on February 1, 1991 by the National Research Council (NRC) of the U.S. National Academy of Sciences suggests that the EPA overestimates the risk of radon by 20 to 30 percent, although that lower level is considered serious by the NRC. Another study, conducted by Naomi H. Harley of New York University Medical Center, demonstrated that people in homes contaminated by radon are less exposed to the gas than previously believed. Another authority, Jan A. Stolwijk of Yale University, said in 1993 that the facts show that the danger from radon is much less than the danger from smoking.

Despite these results and comments, the EPA campaign to eliminate radon from homes continued. On April 6, 1993 the EPA called for protective measures against radon to be installed by builders in new homes in radon-prone regions. About a third of the new homes in the U.S. are built in such areas. At the same time the EPA issued a booklet warning homeowners against the dangers of radon and suggested that all house resales include radon inspection and protection as a condition of sale. Estimates for what all these voluntary measures would cost if implemented ranged from the EPA's guess of less than $100 million to outside experts' opinions that reached as high as $2 billion a year.

RADON

Radon is an elemental gas that seeps into people's homes as a by-product of natural radioactivity of minerals in the earth's crust. Most commonly, radon is released along the way as uranium decays into stable lead. Because radon is a gas at temperatures and pressures that prevail in the upper crust, unlike other common radioactive elements, it leaks out of mineral deposits. If it reaches the outside air, radon disperses and causes little or no damage. But in some places, such as mines or home basements, radon gas can collect. In such situations, humans breathe air laced with radon. Breathing radon-enriched air leaves behind particles of its radioactive daughter products in the lungs. It is these particles that are thought to cause cancer.

Radon is the heaviest of the noble gases (the others are helium, neon, argon, krypton, and xenon). All of these gases are exceptionally inert, meaning they combine with other materials only under unusual circumstances. Thus radon does not present a chemical hazard in the way that sulfuric acid, carbon monoxide, and ozone do. Although it is highly radioactive, radon decays quickly, with a half-life of 3.82 days for the most common isotope and less for other natural isotopes. Thus, radon *per se* is not much of a hazard, but its immediate decay products are several radioactive elements in sequence: polonium-218, lead-214, bismuth-214, polonium-214, lead-210, and so forth (these are also sometimes known as radium A, B, C, C', and D). Collectively, these have a half-life measured in years, not days, and they cause most of the damage associated with radon.

Other Radiation Hazards

Although radon is probably the radioactive element most commonly encountered by the general public, there are some other common radiation hazards. Many of these dangers, like the radon encountered by miners, are work-related. It should be no surprise that people working at nuclear power plants or with nuclear wastes have to deal with dangerous conditions caused by radiation. For example, one study published in the March 1993 *American Journal of Internal Medicine* found that 200 of the 35,000 workers at the U.S. nuclear-bomb facility at Hanford, Washington, had died or were dying as a result of exposure to radioactivity. Medical workers and other workers who use radioactive sources can also have problems, and wastes from these uses, like wastes from nuclear power production or defense efforts, can escape proper disposal and subsequently affect segments of the general public.

Although X rays are not produced by radioactivity, the line between higher-frequency X rays and lower-frequency gamma rays is an artificial border. Scientists think that most people do not have enough exposure to X rays to cause health problems, especially if they take normal precautions. X rays add, however, to an individual's overall exposure to radiation. Thus X rays plus radon or some other radioactive source may be more dangerous than either alone. As early as 1956 it was shown that prenatal exposure to X rays can lead to higher rates of cancer in children.

Background

Hazards of radiation range from skin cancer and aging caused by the relatively low-energy photons of ultraviolet radiation to rapid death caused by large doses of certain subatomic particles. Perhaps because radiation effects were unrecognized until early in the twentieth century, and perhaps because most forms of radiation are undetectable by human senses, many view radiation as scarier than other hazards. Since radiation can result in damage to DNA or other genetic mechanisms, another association in people's minds connects radiation to monstrous births. Much of this concern is exaggerated, but the threat of illness from radiation of one kind or another is real.

Types and sources of radiation vary widely. These include cosmic radiation, which probably originates in violent processes in the Milky Way galaxy; solar radiation, which originates with fusion of hydrogen to helium in the sun; natural radioactivity that is caused by the transmutation of elements in the earth's crust; radiation produced by people, including that from X rays and from radioactivity, both used primarily to observe the interior of material opaque to light or to deliberately destroy tumors or other tissue; incidental artificial radioactivity produced as a result of energy production by nuclear fission or weapons research and development; and other forms of radiation incidental to modern technology. While the incidental forms of artificial radioactivity cause the most concern—largely because of the potential for widespread death and destruction in nuclear accidents—for most people the natural forms of radiation are more damaging to their health.

Radiation that harms living organisms is often called ionizing radiation, because knocking electrons out of atoms to form ions or unpaired electrons is frequently the first step in tissue damage. A compound that has an unpaired electron, which can occur as a result of chemical processes as well as from radiation, is called a free radical. Free radicals have been implicated in tissue damage, in degenerative disease, in cancer, and in aging. Certain isotopes of elements release various forms of ionizing radiation as they change from one isotope or element to another. This kind of radiation is commonly called "radioactivity," and it consists of various types of radiation in different proportions for each isotope.

RADIATION

Common name	Identity	Description	Damage to tissues
Alpha rays	Helium nuclei	Positively charged particles formed from two protons and two neutrons bound together	Because they are slow and massive, they cause the most disruption, but do not penetrate very far into tissues.
Beta rays	Electrons	Negatively charged particles	High-energy beta rays pass through tissues with little harm; lower energy ones cause much ionization and form many free radicals.

Common name	Identity	Description	Damage to tissues
Gamma rays	Photons, or electro-magnetic radiation	Neutral particles of high energy that can often be more easily thought of as waves	Penetrate deeply and are the form of radiation used to treat cancer or to sterilize equipment or food.
Positrons	Antiparticles of electrons	Positively charged particles	Similar in action to beta rays.
Neutrons	Neutrons	Neutral particles easily captured by atomic nuclei	Slow neutrons can transmute one element into another.
Neutrinos	Neutrinos	Neutral particles of little or no mass	Most pass through the body with no interaction.

Radiation is measured in "rads" and radiation-damage-potential in "rems." A rad is based on the amount of energy absorbed per gram of exposed material, while a rem (an acronym for "roentgen equivalent man") is based on the different health effects of the different types of radiation. For example, one rad of slow alpha particles is equivalent to one rem, but so is ten rads of fast electrons. A medical X ray generally produces exposure to about six to seven millirems (a millirem is a thousandth of a rem). A lethal dose of radiation is about 500 rems, but substantial damage occurs at lesser amounts. Repeated exposure to radiation results in additional rems; the average person receives about 360 millirems each year or about 20 rems of radiation over a lifetime.

By 1993, Alice Stewart, who discovered the cancer-causing potential of prenatal X-ray exposure, concluded from studies of her own and others since then that small doses of radiation over long periods of time are more likely to cause cancer than single larger exposures that add up to the same amount of radiation.

Radiation exposure of parents can also produce illness in their children. Men who worked at a nuclear plant in England, for example, were found to have children with higher than expected rates of leukemia and non-Hodgkin's lymphoma.

Of course, an accident at a nuclear facility can lead to exposure of the general public. Regions hundreds of miles away can experience radioactive fallout, as seen after the Chernobyl disaster of April 26, 1986. A letter in the September 3, 1992 *Nature* by Vasily S. Kazakov of the Belarus Ministry of Health in Minsk reported that in regions downwind of Chernobyl, rates of thyroid cancer began to soar starting in 1990. Although Chernobyl is in what is now Ukraine, it is very near the southern border of Belarus; both states were part of the Soviet Union at the time of the accident. Another letter in *Nature,* this one from officials of the World Health Organization, claims that their investigation showed the same rise in thyroid cancer.

About 825,000 people in Belarus, Ukraine, and Russia were exposed to fallout from Chernobyl, while smaller amounts of fallout drifted into Scandinavia. About 80 percent of the fallout from the accident was in the form of radioactive iodine, which is concentrated in humans in their thyroid glands. Children, who are small, growing fast, and drink a lot of milk, are particularly vulnerable, since the iodine that falls on grass is concentrated in cow's milk.

(Periodical References and Additional Reading: *Science News* 10-27-90, p 260; *New York Times* 12-24-90; *New York Times* 12-26-90; *New York Times* 12-30-90; *New York Times* 1-5-91, p 8; *New York Times* 2-21-91; *New York Times* 3-20-91; *New York Times* 3-29-91; *New York Times* 5-22-91; *Science News* 10-26-91, p 264; *New York Times* 10-28-91, p A16; *New York Times* 11-3-91, pp I-1 & I-29; *New York Times* 11-9-91, p 10; *Nature* 9-3-92, p 21; *New York Times* 9-3-92, p A9; *Harvard Health Letter* 10-92, p 5; *New York Times* 12-8-92, p A1; *New York Times* 4-7-93, p A16; *Discover* 12-93, p 26)

Acid Rain UPDATE

Acid rain is often considered more as an enemy of fish and trees than of humans. But since the 1980s there has been a growing body of research that indirectly links acid precipitation with human respiratory illnesses. A study released in the October/ December 1992 *Journal of Exposure Analysis and Environmental Epidemiology* was the first to measure actual acid particles and droplets in air and then relate the amount of acid to the amount of respiratory distress. The study found that on the worst days, admissions to hospitals for asthma increased 23 percent in New York City and 29 percent in Buffalo, New York. Ozone levels were also measured in the study. The investigators believe that the acid particles and the ozone are synergistic, working together to produce bad health (*see* "Ozone at Ground Level (and Related Problems)," p 277).

Trading Dirty Air Rights

On October 29, 1991 the U.S. Environmental Protection Agency (EPA) proposed its first version of regulations under the Clean Air Act of 1990 to go into effect in 1995. These regulations were supposed to cut acid rain in the United States in half; Canada would also benefit. The new rules were expected to cut pollution at 110 electric utility plants in the U.S. East and Midwest beginning in 1995. Then in the year 2000, the coverage is supposed to expand until all plants that burn fossil fuels will be affected. The goal is to cut emissions of sulfur dioxide by 9.1 million metric tons (ten million short tons), which would almost halve total emissions of 1985. The Act also calls for a ten percent reduction in nitrogen oxides, which also contribute to acid rain.

An unusual feature of the new rules is that one company would be able to sell its right to pollute to another company; that is, a company that exceeds the standards can sell that "excess" to another company that would otherwise not be in compliance. The main reason for this provision is to reduce the adverse economic impact of the regulations. The EPA believes that buying and selling pollution rights will reduce the cost of compliance from $3.8 billion to $1 billion.

The first sale of such rights was concluded on May 1, 1992, although it would not go into effect until 1995. The Tennessee Valley Authority (TVA) agreed to pay an amount expected to be $2.5 to $3 million a year to Wisconsin Power and Light for the right to

Background

Acid rain caused by industrial pollution has been known since 1872, when Robert Angus Smith discussed its appearance in England in the wake of the Industrial Revolution, then roughly at its centennial. It was not until 1961, however, that acid rain reached public consciousness. The Swedish scientist Svante Odén rediscovered the phenomenon in Scandinavia and took his findings to the press instead of to obscure scientific journals. In 1976 Odén showed that acid rain is a regional phenomenon. By 1980 acid rain in the United States, Canada, and Western Europe was understood as a major environmental issue, and the U.S. Acid Precipitation Act of that year initiated a ten-year study program. That year also marked the start of negotiations between the United States and Canada on halting acid precipitation that crossed over from one country into the other. More recently still, scientists have recognized that acid rain is found in parts of the world that are not industrialized. Reports in June 1989 showed that acid rain falls almost continuously on the African rain forest and seasonally on the South American rain forest.

"Acid rain" is the commonly used term to denote acidic precipitation of all kinds, as well as acidic dust particles, which may contribute as much as actual wet precipitation in the form of rain, snow, and fog. Although rainwater is normally slightly acidic, precipitation is noticeably higher in acidity in certain regions. One result of the higher acidity is that small lakes become more acidic than they were in the past—technically, they lose the ability to buffer the acidity with alkaline chemicals from the rocks and soil. As these lakes become more acidic, they progressively lose populations of various types of organisms. Many small invertebrates are the first to go. This reduces the food supply for fish, frogs, and other vertebrates. Different species of fish stop breeding at different levels of acidity. Soon there are only a few adult fish left, and little for them to eat. Eventually all forms of animal life are lost. This particular effect was the first to call widespread attention to acid rain. It has affected lakes in Scandinavia, the U.S. Appalachian Mountains, and southeastern Canada. One study in 1988 estimated that more than 25 percent of the lakes in New York's Adirondack Mountains had become too acidic to support life.

More controversial is the effect of acid rain on forests, crops, and human beings. Forests at high altitudes in the United States and at both low and high altitudes in Europe are severely stressed and many trees are dying. Although this would seem to be evidence of acid rain, the situation is more complex. Acid rain may be one of the factors involved, but even that is not clear. Some tests have shown that acid rain injures leaves on some food crops, such as beans, broccoli, and spinach. However, this damage does not seem to be severe; furthermore, few major food crops are grown in regions of highly acid precipitation. As for human beings, it is clear that breathing sulfuric acid, the main component of acid rain, is not a good idea, but it is much less clear how much sulfuric acid from acid rain actually reaches the lungs.

Sulfuric acid is a product of reactions of sulfur dioxide. Sulfur dioxide is released primarily by industrial plants that use coal or oil for fuel. Sulfur is commonly found in both coal and oil, but high grades—the expensive grades—of coal and oil contain much less sulfur than lower grades.

Nitric acid, produced from nitrogen oxides, also contributes to the acidity. Nitrogen oxides are produced largely by reactions at high temperatures of the nigrogen in air with oxygen in air. Thus, nitrogen oxides are found in automobile exhausts as well as in emissions from plants that burn almost any kind of fuel at sufficiently high temperatures. Burning vegetation causes acid rain by a different mechanism, producing formic acid and acetic acid, as well as nitric acid.

A surprising effect of nitric-acid rain is that it can promote plant growth, since availability of nitrogen compounds is one of the factors that limit plant growth. A study released by the Environmental Defense Fund in 1988 revealed that about 25 percent of the excess nitrogen in Chesapeake Bay comes from acid rain. (The remaining 75 percent comes from crop fertilizer runoff and sewage.) This nitrogen is resulting in excessive growth of algae, which is choking out fish and shellfish production in the bay.

Acid rain can travel great distances from its source, with as much as ten to 80 percent increases in acidity noted as far as 4000 km (2500 miles) from the source. In North America, that source is principally the northern part of the United States east of the Mississippi River and the southeastern part of Canada. Because of prevailing winds, however, the eastern Midwest, especially the Ohio valley and Great Lakes region, produces the emissions that cause the most damage. Acid rain from this region is most likely to fall on lakes with little buffering capacity (ability to reduce acidity). Most acid rain in this region is thought to be caused by emissions from electrical power plants, especially those that burn high-sulfur coal or oil.

In Europe, acid rain is produced in various industrial regions, including western Germany, northern England, and parts of Russia. In China, some of the worst acid rain falls on the Xishuangbanna National Nature Reserve in the southwest. The reserve is home to several rare mammals, 35 percent of all of China's bird species, half its butterfly species, and 4000 types of flowering plants. In sub-Saharan Africa, acid rain falls on the tropical rain forest as a result of year-round burning of the savanna to make land suitable for agriculture. The Amazonian rain forest also receives acid rain from land clearing, although burning the rain forest in the Amazon region is seasonal, not year-round.

Reduction in sulfur dioxide can be accomplished in many ways. Among these are switching to low-sulfur coal or oil as a fuel, a switch that does not require capital investment but raises annual expenses. Switching to natural gas as fuel is even more effective, since natural gas contains almost no sulfur, but it requires new furnaces. Devices called scrubbers can be added to smokestacks to remove sulfur dioxide, but these are expensive to install and maintain. Encouraging conservation of electric power is one of the least expensive ways to reduce the need for fuel and therefore reduce emissions. The trick for electric utilities is to reduce power production without reducing profits. Various new technologies, based mainly on getting sulfur out of coal before it is burned, can also be used. Also, alternative energy sources can replace part of the generating capacity.

Reduction in nitrogen oxides is more difficult. Automobile emissions can be partly controlled by various means, including catalytic converters and use of alternate fuels. Converters can also be added to smokestacks.

release 10,000 tons of sulfur dioxide into the air. Wisconsin Power and Light would reduce its own emissions by 10,000 tons below the allowance given it under the law. Although the ability to sell rights is supposed to aid in overall reduction of acid rain and air pollution, Wisconsin Power and Light already had a very low production of sulfur dioxide as a result of tough state laws. Thus the net benefit to air quality might be illusory; in effect, the TVA would simply be paying for the right to pollute higher than its own limit and Wisconsin Power and Light would be getting a windfall.

It was not until October 16, 1992, however, that the EPA, acting under court order, began to make the 1991 rules official. When it did, it was met with lawsuits by New York state and three environmental groups (the Adirondack Council, the National Resources Defense Council, and the Environmental Defense Fund). The main concern was that Wisconsin Power and Light and other companies that had been below emissions standards in 1985 would sell the right to pollute to companies that needed such a right. In November 1993 the EPA responded by changing the rules. Now only air cleaned up in 1991 or later could be used to qualify for the sale of pollution rights.

In the meantime, the estimated sales value of a ton of emitted sulfur dioxide was falling from $1000, when the concept was first explored, to $300, thought to be the amount of the Wisconsin Power and Light deal with the TVA, to $180 at the end of 1993. The reduction came in part because of steadily lowering costs for emission control devices as more moved into production and in part because so many companies saw, as one spokesperson put it, "the writing on the wall" and started clean-up before the 1995 deadline.

Because acid rain had been perceived as a problem in the United States in the late 1970s—but an obstacle that the federal government was reluctant to move against for economic reasons—the government at that time began a ten-year study of the problem, the $600-million National Acid Precipitation Assessment Program (NAPAP). As NAPAP began to wind down in 1989, the U.S. Environmental Protection Agency (EPA) set up an oversight panel to review the assessment. The oversight panel released its report in April 1991, saying that NAPAP was good science but not very useful in terms of its original goal of clarifying what steps, if any, the U.S. government should take to contain acid rain. Although the original NAPAP expired as scheduled in December 1990, a slimmed-down version was created to observe the effects on acid rain of the U.S. Clean Air Act Amendments of 1990.

Progress Anyway

Acid rain was on the decline in North America well before the first trade deal, however. According to the National Acid Precipitation Assessment Program, by the early 1980s U.S. emissions of sulfur dioxide dropped by 30 percent after passage of the Clean Air Act of 1970, even though neither that Act nor amendments to it were intended specifically to attack acid rain.

On May 24, 1991 the major results of the U.S. National Surface Water Survey showed that acid rain is the main source of acidity in 75 percent of the acidified lakes and in 47 percent of acidified streams. The other causes of acidity are tailings from mines (mainly in streams) and natural acidity from decaying plants (mainly in lakes). The survey also showed that while organic sources of acidity dominated lakes in Florida and the upper Midwest and coal mining parts of the Mid-Atlantic Highlands, acid rain accounted for the acidity in the Adirondacks and in non-coal-mining parts of the Mid-Atlantic Highlands. Because of prevailing winds, these data tend to support what most scientists strongly believed before the survey: most of the acid rain in the eastern United States is caused by air pollution from the Midwest. Further analysis of the National Surface Water Survey included a search for the presence of acidity at various times in the past. It had been suggested that regrowth of forests after clear-cutting could produce observed acidic conditions, but the timing of the onset of acidity did not coincide with clear-cutting or regrowth. It did, however, coincide with industrialization. Proponents arguing that organic causes increased acidification of lakes and streams continued, however, to push their case in the face of overwhelming evidence that acid rain causes acidity in many lakes and streams.

A study released in July 1993 by the U.S. Geological Survey found that the sulfur component of acid rain decreased between 1980 and 1991 at 26 out of 33 of its rainwater collection sites analyzed. Furthermore, the acidity of the water was greatly reduced at nine of the stations and slightly reduced at 26 stations. Nitrate concentrations also fell significantly at three stations and slightly at others, showing a sign of reduced nitrogen oxides.

Although acid rain was on the run in North America, a different picture was presented in Eastern Europe. The Communist governments of the past had allowed unbridled air pollution and other toxic wastes. After the fall of Communism, the full extent of this legacy gradually came to the attention of the West. It was found that Poland by itself emits as much sulfur dioxide as the whole 12-nation European Economic Community. Studies in various parts of Eastern Europe show that the industrial regions, where brown lignite is burned, have life expectancies from eight to 11 years lower than in Western European countries.

(Periodical References and Additional Reading: *Science News* 3-3-90, p 143; *Science News* 9-15-90, p 165; *Science* 3-15-91, p 1302; *Science* 4-19-91, p 370; *Science* 5-24-91, pp 1043 & 1151; *Science* 9-20-91, p 1334; *New York Times* 5-12-92, p A1; *New York Times* 5-13-92, p A1; *Science News* 1-23-93, p 52; *Science News* 7-10-93, p 22; *New York Times* 10-27-93, p A16; *New York Times* 12-19-93, p I-57)

OZONE AT GROUND LEVEL (AND RELATED PROBLEMS)

Ozone is unique among environmental health problems in that too little of it high in the atmosphere contributes to a rise in cancer rates (*see* "Ultraviolet Rays from the Sun," p 189), while too much of it in lower levels of the atmosphere adds to respiratory problems. Using data compiled mainly in the late 1980s, the U.S. Environmental Protection Agency (EPA) has set an upper limit of 0.12 parts per million of ozone molecules in air that is breathed. Breathing air with ozone exceeding that level—a situation that occurs often in major cities of industrialized countries—has been shown to cause damage deep in the lungs. This limit had been criticized as too lenient, but on August 3, 1992 the EPA stood by its data and its limit. In March 1993, however, the U.S. federal Clean Air Scientific Advisory Committee informed the EPA that studies conducted before 1989, which they had reviewed, did not provide enough scientific evidence to set toleration levels for ozone.

Soon after the Clean Air advice, new data did become available and they suggest that ozone causes more harm than previously known. Robert M. Aris of the University of North Carolina School of Medicine at Chapel Hill and coworkers reported on a study they had conducted with 18 athletic, healthy young men and women, who exercised periodically for four hours at a time. During some exercise periods the subjects were exposed to ambient air with little or no ozone. In others, the air was charged with 0.20 parts per million of ozone, much higher than EPA maximums but still lower than that found in many major cities. Los Angeles, California, for example, has some 30 to 40 days annually with air containing higher than 0.20 parts per million of ozone.

After the subjects exercised as part of this study, their bronchial tubes were flushed with saline water, and surface tissue from the tubes was sampled. Levels of enzymes in the water used to flush the tubes were higher when ozone was present, which indicated that inflammation was present. The tissue samples confirmed that the bronchial tubes were irritated by the ozone. Previous studies used by the EPA had only found damage to the air sacs deep in the lungs. Ozone makes these sacs stiffen, reducing the ability to breathe.

Hospital admissions for asthma attacks correlate with exposure to ozone (*see also* "Acid Rain UPDATE," p 273), as do deaths from asthma. The rate of asthma fatalities began a sharp rise at the end of the 1970s, increasing by more than 30 percent into the early 1990s. While no one knows for sure what the cause of this problem is, the rise in ground-level ozone certainly has contributed to it.

A study published in the December 9, 1993 *New England Journal of Medicine* claims that air pollution shortens lives by up to two years, although the authors think that particulate matter is more responsible than ozone. The highest pollution levels studied were in Steubenville, Ohio, which had a 26 percent higher death rate from lung cancer, other lung diseases, and heart disease than the least polluted area in the study, Portage, Wisconsin. In this study, smoking, the greatest contributing factor in such deaths, was statistically adjusted to be the same for all regions included.

Automobiles, Fuel, and Ozone

While ground-level ozone is caused in part by the reaction of sunlight with oxygen in the air, it nearly always becomes a problem only when additional ozone is produced by burning fossil fuel at high temperatures, which mainly occurs in the engines of automobiles. Temperature inversions, which keep combustion products near ground levels, can contribute to the build-up of ozone. Ground-level ozone levels tend to be higher in the summer as a result of all these factors, including increased automobile traffic.

A reduction in automobile traffic in central cities and elimination of plants that burn coal or oil for fuel would help but are very difficult to achieve. Ways to reduce ozone by "scrubbing" gases, as catalytic converters and other devices do for automobiles and smokestacks, are not very effective. New gasoline pumps at service stations that prevent vapors from reaching the atmosphere are expected to help. Gasoline manufacturers have also taken steps to reduce the volatility of their product.

Ground-level ozone can be produced by any high temperature combustion, not just that in automobile engines. When satellites observed a vast cloud of low-lying ozone above Africa and the South Atlantic in 1988, few believed it. But enough believed it for a ground-based expedition in 1992, which found that the ozone was really there. In September and October, people burn vast parts of the southern African forest and also the forests of Brazil to create more pasture or crop land. These raging fires produce the ozone. The ozone pool over the South Atlantic, fed mostly by African fires, is large enough to worry scientists about where the ozone might go. Natural wind currents carry ozone from Africa into the Atlantic. In Brazil, the ozone already accumulates near humans and can be presumed to adversely affect health.

Photochemical Smog

Another policy issue that governments are worried about is smog. Although much of the visible smog caused by burning fossil fuels in the United States has been controlled since the end of World War II, photochemical smog has gotten worse during that period. In Los Angeles, California, smog was the butt of hundreds of jokes on nationwide radio programs of the 1940s, but most of the listeners at that time had never seen photochemical smog. Today episodes of photochemical smog are familiar in many major U.S. cities, although the region around Los Angeles continues to lead the United States. International honors for high levels of smog go to Mexico City. Efforts to control photochemical smog have been based on the knowledge that its main cause is the action of sunlight on automobile tail pipe emissions of unburned hydrocarbons and nitrogen oxides. Another source of volatile hydrocarbons has been fumes from stored fuels.

When the Clean Air Act of 1990 was passed, better control of photochemical smog was among the main goals, so the Act required an in-depth study of the problem. The

Background

Burning fuels at high temperatures can result in some unstable molecules that contain oxygen. When exposed to sunlight, these break down and some of their oxygen becomes ozone. Also, some chemicals in auto exhausts can catalyze oxygen in the air to become ozone. Automobile exhaust gases produce ozone, for example. Other sources of ground-level ozone include fumes from gasoline, other volatile liquids such as dry-cleaning fluids, emissions from bakeries, gases released by hazardous wastes, and fires set to clear forests in South America or savannahs in Africa. This ozone, especially if it is trapped near the ground, becomes an important component of air pollution. Because the chemical reactions that produce ozone make the air hazy or even brown, this form of air pollution is called *photochemical smog*, or just *smog*, although it is not the combination of smoke and fog that is the origin of the name *smog*. Increasingly it has become clear that ozone is the most damaging part of smog and the hardest part to control.

Ozone by itself is harmful to plants and animals, so harmful that ozone can be used to sterilize since it kills microorganisms. Ozone at levels found in many cities damages trees. Ozone can damage food crops, especially grains. The EPA estimates that the U.S. loses about $2.5 to $3 billion each year in ozone damage to crops, while the World Resources Institute thinks the losses to crops caused by ozone annually reach $5 billion. When animals breathe ozone, it causes immediate inflammation in the lungs, followed by a long-term abnormal stiffening, reducing the lungs' ability to take in air.

EPA sponsored the review at a cost of $430,000, jointly funded by the Department of Energy, the American Petroleum Institute, and the Motor Vehicle Manufacturers Association. Results leaked by someone from the business community on December 14, 1991 can be presumed to have pleased the sponsors, since the results supported the contention of the oil, automobile, and trucking industries that not enough is known about the cause of photochemical smog to change the way fuels are formulated or engines are built. The report also suggested that efforts to control hydrocarbons have been misplaced because the main contributor to smog is nitrogen oxides. No one really has a good way to control nitrogen oxides at present. Nitrogen oxides are present whenever combustion occurs in air (which is about 80 percent nitrogen and 20 percent oxygen) at a high enough temperature, a condition that seems necessary for the operation of an internal combustion engine. Furthermore, the report states that mismeasurements have led to an overly optimistic estimate of success in reducing volatile hydrocarbons.

In fact, the official EPA listings for ozone claim that emissions have been reduced from 22.7 million metric tons in 1980 to 16.9 million in 1991. Similarly the number of days when selected major metropolitan areas exceeded the EPA air-quality standards, which include other various components of photochemical smog, among them ozone, and particulates (mainly soot), decreased from 610 in total for the 15 metropolitan areas used to 285 in 1991. U.S. air quality continued to improve in 1992. The number of Americans living in counties where air quality fell below the EPA standards, which had already dropped from 100 million in the early 1980s to 86 million in 1991, fell dramatically to only 54 million in 1992.

Near the end of the 1992 lawn-mowing season in the northern U.S., the EPA declared that a gasoline-powered lawn mower produces as much of the hydrocarbon products that produce photochemical smog as an automobile does in the same amount of time. Chain saws, which contribute even more to noise pollution than mowers do, are also worse offenders for air pollution. Outboard motors are worse than either. The announcement heralded an EPA campaign, with cooperation from manufacturers, to reduce pollution from what were dubbed "mobile sources."

Reductions should continue into the mid-1990s in major cities. Stricter emission controls on automobiles were instituted in 1993 in 84 metropolitan areas, with further restrictions and additional regions scheduled to be added throughout the mid-1990s. Another reduction is expected after 1994 in ozone and hydrocarbons in 50 of the largest cities of the U.S. as a result of new requirements for special nozzles and vacuum devices on gasoline pumps to capture fumes. Some localities, however, had already mandated the capture devices a year or two earlier.

(Periodical References and Additional Reading: *Harvard Health Letter*, 5-91, p 5: *New York Times*, 7-14-92, p A1: *New York Times*, 8-6-92, p A1: *New York Times*, 8-14-92, p A9: *New York Times*, 10-12-92, p A1: *New York Times*, 11-3-93,p B14; *Science News* 11-20-93, p 326)

IS EMF A CAUSE OF DISEASE?

For years now there has been a controversy over the relationship between electromagnetic fields (EMF) and health. Most scientists say that EMF in the typical dose most people encounter—even people living near electrical power lines—does not affect health adversely. Many people, especially those trying to keep power lines away from their own backyards, quote statistical evidence that suggests that EMF specifically causes cancer. Some people avoid their microwave ovens, television sets, or computer monitors, in part because of fears of various types of electromagnetic waves or fields. Others have given up their electric blankets.

A typical confrontation between citizens and scientific research occurred in the small town of Guilford, Connecticut, on the shores of Long Island Sound. Residents of one neighborhood came to believe that there was a higher than expected incidence of cancer where they lived, and they attributed it to a nearby Connecticut Light and Power Company facility. A reporter got the story and wrote about the "calamity" along with other tales of EMF-ridden communities in *New Yorker* magazine. The state legislature became involved and asked for a report from the Connecticut Academy of Science and Civil Engineering. The Academy set up a nine-scientist panel that included such well-known epidemiologists as Jan A. J. Stolwijk of the Yale School of Medicine.

On June 4, 1992, the 44-page report from the Academy panel was released; it said that there is no evidence that there are any health effects caused by the low-frequency changes in electromagnetic fields produced as a side effect of the operation of the facility. Typically, newspaper reports discussed "magnetic waves"—which may not exist and certainly would not be produced in a small power station if they did—as a possible cause of the observed illness. The purported effect would be caused either by moving magnetic lines of force (the *field* of EMF) or by long-period electromagnetic waves, such as sub-radio waves. Most research, however, agrees with the Academy in saying that none of these possible forms of electromagnetism is associated with disease or provides a mechanism that even suggests a way of causing harm to human DNA, the only way to initiate cancer.

Theory Argues Against EMF Harm

The power of a magnetic field is measured in units named after the great mathematician Karl Friedrich Gauss, who worked out the mathematics of magnetism in the early nineteenth century. Magnetic fields from power lines are very small at ground level when away from the line itself; they are typically one to two milligauss. A larger exposure to magnetism comes from being in close proximity to a source, such as a microwave oven or house wiring. The magnetic field inside a house from its own wiring and a ground, often through plumbing, can be as much as that found standing outside under the tower of a high-voltage power line, but more than half the homes surveyed show a magnetic field of less than half a milligauss. An inch or less away from the back of a microwave oven might produce a magnetic field of over 1000 milligauss, but at a more typical distance of somewhat over a foot, the field has already dropped to about 30 milligauss—still ten times higher than from the power line.

Most of these artificial sources of magnetic fields pale in comparison to the natural magnetic field in which all life on the earth evolved. While the magnetic field of the earth is different from place to place and both fluctuates daily and changes mysteriously over hundreds of thousands of years, there is not at present any place on earth

Background

Contrary to what many people believe, electromagnetism has always been with us, since EMF includes light. The electromagnetic spectrum ranges from the very long waves of radio (sometimes suspected of adverse health effects) through microwaves, infrared radiation perceived as heat, light, ultraviolet radiation, X rays, and high-energy gamma rays (known to cause death after exposure to high levels). Viewed as radiation, most of the components of the electromagnetic spectrum have health effects.

The controversy, however, primarily concerns electromagnetic *fields* instead of radiation. The relationship between magnetic fields and electromagnetic radiation was first explained by Michael Faraday and James Clerk Maxwell in the nineteenth century. They pictured the field as lines of force, similar to the pattern of curved lines observed when iron filings are affected by a magnet. As these lines move through space, the motion produces electricity, hence the name "electromagnetic." Symmetrically, moving electric charges produce a magnetic field. The interaction between these two effects occurs in waves. The waves are the electromagnetic radiation. In this view, the field and the radiation are intimately connected, although different from each other.

At the end of the nineteenth century the electron was discovered and a new interpretation of the electromagnetic field became possible. Early in the twentieth century that interpretation came to include the idea that the electromagnetic waves also act as particles. The field is seen as a structure that underlies both the wave and the particle, although it is still produced by movement of the particle (or by the wave). In some of the most modern interpretations, the field is the actual entity and the particle/wave is just a manifestation of it.

where the natural magnetic field is as low as that from a high-voltage power line. In the U.S. the typical magnetic field is usually about 450 milligauss, a hundred times greater than that from a power line.

Evolutionary evidence even suggests that the periodic reduction of the earth's magnetic field as the north and south magnetic poles interchange every few hundred thousand years somehow triggers extinctions of species. The earth's magnetic field is a major protection against a rain of radiation in the form of charged particles from the sun.

Thus most scientists think that the small magnetic fields that some think may initiate cancer are swamped by the earth's much larger field. Even if there were some evidence that a magnetic field causes harmful changes in human tissues or cells—a danger which is limited to possible alteration in production of the hormone melatonin, if it exists at all—the fields caused by high-voltage power lines are much less than those for which our bodies are already adapted. Furthermore, the most intense magnetic fields that humans encounter frequently are those used in magnetic resonance imaging (MRI), thought to be the safest diagnostic tool since the stethoscope.

Some point out that it is not stationary EMF, like that from the earth, but changing EMF that they believe causes cancer. They cite alternating current, which in the U.S. has a cycle of 60 times a second (60 hertz). The direction of the field changes 60 times every second in all the household currents and in those high-voltage lines as well. It is the change that is sometimes referred to as "magnetic waves."

Nearly all environmental hazards show up in the workplace before they are found in the general public. About 50 studies have been done of power-station or microwave-relay-station personnel. Most show little or no effects, although a few show odd effects such as the three that unexpectedly found a rise in the rate of men with breast cancer, which is normally close to zero.

Reactions to EMF Concerns

Despite the lack of evidence of harm from EMF, U.S. power companies heeded their public-relations problem and spent about $1 billion annually in the early 1990s in efforts to lower the magnetic fields around power lines. From 1990 to 1992, U.S. power companies conducted a major survey of fields associated with alternating current transmission and use. It found that simple changes in wiring could reduce EMF in houses. Manufacturers have also taken steps to reduce EMF, such as redesigning the wiring inside an electric blanket. Electric blankets made since 1990 have about a tenth the EMF of earlier models.

Six states had by 1993 passed legislation limiting EMF produced by high-voltage lines. Also, the number of lawsuits by people claiming damage to their health from EMF has risen.

Further studies are planned for the mid-1990s on both EMF in the workplace and in proximity to power lines, studies for which considerable funding is already in place. For example the research for the U.S. National Institute of Environmental Health Sciences and Department of Energy is scheduled to cost $65 million and to be completed in 1997.

TIMETABLE OF EMF

1600	William Gilbert [English: 1540-1603] observes that the earth is a great spherical magnet.
1750	John Michell [English: 1724-1793] explains how one magnet induces magnetism in another.
1751	Benjamin Franklin [born Boston, Massachusetts, 1706; died Philadelphia, Pennsylvania, 1790] demonstrates that electricity can magnetize or demagnetize an iron needle.
1819	Hans Christian Oersted [Danish: 1777-1851] accidentally discovers that a magnetized needle is deflected by a nearby electric current.
1845	Michael Faraday [born Newington, Surrey, England, 1791; died Hampton Court, Surrey, England, 1867] introduces the concepts of a magnetic field and lines of force.
1873	In his *Electricity and Magnetism,* James Clerk Maxwell [born Edinburgh, Scotland, 1831; died Cambridge, England, 1879] explains how moving magnetic fields generate electromagnetic waves and moving electromagnetic waves generate magnetic fields, allowing light to radiate through empty space.

1882   Marcel Derprez shows that an electric current can be transmitted over long distances by increasing its voltage.

1884   Nikola Tesla [born Smiljan, Croatia, July 10, 1856; died New York, New York, January 7, 1943] invents an electric generator that produces alternating current, better suited for long-distance transmission than direct current; as a result, alternating current becomes the commonly transmitted electricity.

1979   Nancy Wertheimer and Ed Leeper of the University of Colorado report that children exposed to higher-than-average magnetic fields have two-to-three times the risk of leukemia compared to children not so exposed.

1988   David Savitz of the University of North Carolina finds an increase in childhood cancer from exposure to magnetic fields.

1990   The Electric Power Research Institute in the U.S. institutes a two-year survey of sources of EMF in the U.S.

1991   John Peters of the University of Southern California finds an increase in childhood cancer from exposure to magnetic fields.

1992   Maria Feychting and Anders Ahlbom of the Karolinska Institute in Sweden study half a million Swedes who lived within 1000 feet of a power line between 1960 and 1985; they find that the risk of childhood leukemia in this population is nearly three times as great as among Swedes not living near power lines—although since there are only 70 cases of childhood leukemia in Sweden annually, this risk translates into at most one case that could be attributed to magnetic fields.

Joergen Olsen of the National Cancer Registry of Denmark and coworkers examine all Danish children of the past 20 years who have had either leukemia, a brain tumor, or malignant melanoma; they find that there is no increase in leukemia attributable to magnetic fields, but that a small increase in brain tumors is statistically associated with exposure to high levels of magnetic fields. The association, if true, would mean that one case of childhood brain tumor every five years might be caused by electromagnetic fields.

Richard Doll and coworkers at the British National Radiological Protection Board produce a report for the British government that flatly states that there is no significant evidence for an association between electromagnetic fields and cancer.

The Oak Ridge Associated Universities publishes "Health Effects of Low-Frequency Electric and Magnetic Fields," which concludes that evidence of an association between such fields and leukemia or other childhood or adult cancers is "inconsistent and inconclusive."

(Periodical References and Additional Reading: *Harvard Health Letter* 3-90, p 1; *Science* 9-7-90, p 1096; *New York Times* 6-6-92, p 29; *Science* 12-11-92, p 1725; *New York Times* 6-22-93, p C1; *Harvard Health Letter* 7-93, p 1; *Science News* 8-21-93, p 124)

Mental Health

THE STATE OF
PSYCHOLOGICAL MEDICINE

Over a lifetime, an American has about a 48 percent chance of developing a condition that might be characterized as a mental disorder, provided such conditions as alcoholism and fear of public speaking are included. If the definition of mental disorder is limited to such serious illnesses as various forms of major depression, schizophrenia, or multiple personality disorder, the percentage drops dramatically. The study on which this paragraph and the three following are based was directed by Ronald C. Kessler of the University of Michigan and published in the January 1994 *Archives of General Psychiatry*. It found that the most common mental illness of all is major depression, of which of which there is a 17 percent chance of developing it in a lifetime; major depression is even more common than alcohol dependence (14 percent in a lifetime). Some 13 percent of the persons interviewed for the study claimed phobias in the course of their lives, such as 11 percent with fear of flying. Figures add to more than 100 percent, however, since as many as 14 percent of the interviewees claimed three or more psychiatric problems.

In any given year, however, only 30 percent of Americans claim to have undergone a period of mental disorder, including ten percent with major depression, followed by eight percent with phobias and seven percent admitting alcohol dependence. Some of these figures are no doubt skewed by the people being interviewed—alcoholics and drug users are notorious for refusing to admit their condition. About half the potential subjects refused to take the test when told they would have to promise to answer honestly.

One disorder frequently reported in this survey was what psychiatrists call "post-traumatic stress disorder," the mental stress a person feels after some severe emotional (and often physical) experience. The rate for this problem was 12 percent for women and only six percent for men, a difference fueled by rape or sexual molestation which over a lifetime affected nine percent of the women.

This rate of sexual trauma, which is much higher than the two percent found in previous studies, is thought to be more accurate as well. The interviewers in the study used a printed card with various traumas listed and numbered on it. The respondent did not have to say anything more specific than the number for rape instead of the number for a less emotionally involving trauma, such as an automobile accident. Such printed cards are now common in face-to-face interviews on topics related to sexual practices or anything else that might involve shame or a desire to keep something hidden.

Surveys of mental illness in the past often provided widely varying results, mainly because of different criteria as to what was to be included and what not. More recently, psychiatrists have generally followed the latest edition of their *Diagnostic and Statistical Manual,* and results are therefore comparable. Thus the Epidemiological Catchment Area (ECA) survey of 20,291 individuals in Baltimore, Maryland; Durham, North Carolina; Los Angeles, California; New Haven, Connecticut; and St. Louis, Missouri obtained results that for the same time period are very much like those from the University of Michigan survey discussed above: in a period of one year, the ECA survey found a total of 28 percent of the total people surveyed were affected by mental disorders including drug dependence. Of these, 10.9 percent reported phobias, 10.4 percent reported depression (nearly half of this classed as severe), 7.4 percent alcohol abuse or dependence, 3.1 percent had non-alcohol drug dependence, and 2.1 percent were bothered by obsessive-compulsive disorder (such as a compulsion to wash hands continually or to repeat the same ritual before going to bed).

Of the interviewees, 14.7 percent had obtained help of some official kind for a mental or substance-abuse problem during the year, but only half of these had a current problem. Conversely, of those with current problems in the ECA survey, only 28.5 percent sought treatment. It was thought by the ECA staff that mental-health facilities need to be more available or more attractive to those who might need their services.

Treatment Trends

Although there may have been some herbal remedies, before modern times not much short of confinement was used to treat severe mental disorders. Less severe problems were often ignored, although Biblical accounts tell that King Saul's apparent clinical depression was treated with music. In England in the eighteenth century, facilities and medical attention were instituted for people with "nervous, hypochondriacal, or hysteric diseases" or with "madness" or "feeble-mindedness."

Some early treatments were examples of what today is a sometimes labeled "talking therapy," which would include any treatment that consists primarily of either the patient or the doctor talking to the other one. Among the first such talking therapies was hypnosis, in which the doctor first talks the patient into a receptive state, and then either the doctor makes suggestions, the patient describes feelings, or both. In the late nineteenth, hypnosis evolved into psychoanalysis the most famous talking therapy, in which the patient talks to the doctor about dreams and childhood on a regular basis for long periods of time. Currently the most popular talking therapies focus more on the patient describing immediate problems while the therapist gives small amounts of advice. In numbers, the most popular therapy is group self-help, usually modeled on Alcoholics Anonymous (AA). In group self-help a small number of people who share a specific problem talk mostly about the problem but they also discuss each other their feelings about life in general. As a treatment method, talking therapies of one kind or another have been highly successful with milder neurotic disorders but somewhat less successful with addictions.

Few pure talking therapies assume a physical basis for the mental disorder being treated although AA is an exception to this general rule. Early in the nineteenth century, however, physicians generally assumed that mental illness was the result of a disease of the brain. This concept lost favor when specific evidence—outside of a few known conditions (syphilis, lead poisoning, and so forth)—was found lacking. Moreover, because the talking therapies were showing some success—a success that would be unexpected if there were a physical condition involved—most psychiatrists rejected the idea of a physical basis for mental illness by the mid-twentieth century.

Increasingly since that time, however, modern medicine has found that common mental problems, especially such serious illnesses as bipolar disorder (formerly called manic-depressive disorder) or schizophrenia, can be traced to chemical imbalances in the brain itself, perhaps with a genetic basis in some instances. Most physicians today assume that talking by itself will not change chemistry, so other methods have come to supplant or replace the talking therapies.

Just as tradition has it that a good fright will cure hiccups, some doctors reasoned that disrupting the pathways of the brain might cure incoherent or misdirected thinking. Around 1930 both chemical and electrical shock treatments (ECT, for electroconvulsive therapy) were somewhat successful with both schizophrenia and bipolar disorder. The even more profound shock of removing a part of the brain, called prefrontal lobotomy, was also tried. Except for ECT, which is still used for intractable depression, these violent cures have been almost completely abandoned.

It has long been known that some natural chemicals affect the mind. Shamans used nicotine or chemicals in mushrooms to induce trance states, for example. Modern chemicals that affect the mind were also discovered, starting with the first barbiturates in 1863. While barbiturates were tried as a treatment for mental illness, especially in Swiss clinics, they were not very effective. In the 1950s, the minor tranquilizers such as reserpine, and also the "major" tranquilizers such as Thorazine; were introduced. The minor tranquilizers were used to combat generalized anxiety and specific phobias. By 1989 more than 36.4 million *new* prescriptions were written for these minor tranquilizers, 81 percent of them for such benzodiazepines as alprasolam (Xanax) and diazepam (Valium). In March 1964 a significant study undertaken by the U.S. National Institutes of Health found that major tranquilizers classed as phenothiazines were effective in treating schizophrenia. Lithium salts for the treatment of bipolar disorder as well as for clinical depression gradually became popular in the early 1970s. Other somewhat effective "psychic energizers" or antidepressants also came into use.

The mid-1980s saw the arrival of Prozac, a more effective drug for depression too mild to treat with lithium (which has some alarming side effects) and too much a part of the personality to be effectively treated by talking therapy. Fluoxetine (trade-name Prozac) and similar drugs elevate serotonin, one of the main chemicals used in the brain to signal from one nerve cell to another. For reasons that are poorly understood, higher serotonin levels tend to remove depression and to reduce the impulse toward violence in most people. Furthermore, even obsessive-compulsive disorder, previously thought to have no physical basis, often yields to Prozac or other drugs that raise serotonin levels.

By 1989 the most common drugs used to treat mental disorders were still the oldest in terms of widespread application. They were minor tranquilizers (53.0 percent of psychotherapeutic medications), then antidepressants (29.4 percent), major tranquilizers (12.6 percent), and lithium products (2.4 percent).The remainder consisted of drugs thought to be antidepressant tranquilizers.

The new chemical approach to mental illness has had profound effects on society in general. Fewer people are in mental hospitals and most who are there stay only for a short time. People often leave the hospital in reasonably good mental shape because of the drugs they are taking, but when side effects develop (which happens often, especially for drugs similar to Thorazine or for lithium), they stop taking the drugs and return to their previous state. In many cases, however, the former patients do not go back to the hospital but find themselves homeless as a result of their illness.

In other instances, people became addicted to one of the tranquilizers, adding yet another drug to Western society, which already has considerable drug problems. The common tranquilizer diazepam (Valium), which acts on the same receptors in brain cells as alcohol does, has been the latest habit-forming drug in a long list that perhaps started with meprobamate (Miltown), the first popular tranquilizer in the early 1960s. (Opiates were also first thought in Western society to be relatively harmless; heroin was originally used to break addiction to morphine, just as methadone is used today to interrupt addiction to heroin.)

Some physicians and their patients came to think that Prozac and its relatives were the wonder drug of the ages, solving all the difficulties of life. Others claimed that too many doctors were prescribing Prozac, which is a powerful drug, to ordinary people with normal mental health. Prozac had been introduced in the late 1980s; by 1990 there were critics who felt that Prozac causes some people to become either violent or suicidal or both. After a few more years of experience with the drug, however, most physicians believed that the occasional outbursts of violence or acts of suicide in people taking Prozac were coincidences. Mind-altering drugs, however, have a way of affecting different people in different ways, so it is hard to prove anything about a specific instance. The most famous example of the different effects of a drug is methylphenidate (Ritalin), which is used by some people as a stimulant and is also used to treat hyperactivity in children. But even sleeping pills are known to keep some people awake.

In any case, a new age of drugs is dawning, because for the first time medicine has been able to understand how the mind works well enough to design specific chemicals that can resolve specific problems. For example, the new drug vigabatrin (Sabril—not approved for use in the U.S. in 1993) for the control of epilepsy is the first specifically planned treatment for this condition, which is known to be a direct result of brain damage; vigabatrin has the effect for which it was planned, and works to control the disease. For mental illnesses with a less well-understood physical cause, however, the preferred treatment of the 1990s could be described as a drug therapy combined with one or more talking therapies.

The Relation of Mental States to Illness

As the history outlined above suggests, during the twentieth century there was a strong trend toward believing that the mind is controlled by bodily processes instead of by experiences. Paralleling this has been what might be seen as the opposite change in opinion, i.e., that the body can be controlled by the mind. Just as the belief that the body controls the mind has roots in earlier centuries, the thought that the mind can alter physical processes is quite ancient in some cultures. Perhaps the best known manifestations of this idea are connected to such beliefs as Hinduism or Buddhism.

The modern history of this idea has several beginnings. One is in the conditioning experiments that Ivan Pavlov, B. F. Skinner, and other behaviorists conducted with animals. If saliva production could be controlled by ringing a bell, the behaviorists reasoned, why not control blood pressure by some external or internal stimulus? Another root of this idea was Norman Cousins's (a famous magazine editor) self-cure of a serious disease. He achieved his cure by watching old Marx Brothers movies. The idea was to get well by laughing, which for Norman Cousins at least seemed to have worked, leading him to publicize the connection between cheerfulness and health extensively. A third strand of support for this idea comes from the work of Meyer Friedman and R. H. Roseman whose work with heart disease convinced them that personality (specifically what they labeled Type A behavior) influences who will have heart attacks.

All of these ideas came together in the 1990s with the general idea that stress influences the immune system, which then mediates the outcome of diseases from the common cold to cancer. Previously there had been a general idea that some diseases were specifically caused by stress (notably ulcers, which recent research has shown not to be true, or psoriasis, which may actually be caused by stress). But there had been no clear cut mechanism to explain how the mind could directly influence body processes. Close interaction of the nervous and immune systems appears, however, to be a key that can account for this process. Furthermore, if the body and mind work together through the immune system, the effect of stress or cheerfulness on many diseases with unrelated causes begins to make sense.

(Periodical References and Additional Reading: *Statistical Bulletin* 1/3-91; *Harvard Health Letter* 10-91, p 1; *Science News* 6-19-93, p 399; *New York Times* 11-30-94, p C3; *New York Times* 1-14-94, p A20)

TIMETABLE OF MENTAL HEALTH PROGRESS TO 1990

1751	The first institution to treat mental patients is opened in London.
1764	Robert Whytt [born Edinburgh, September 6, 1714; died April 15, 1766] publishes *Observations on Nervous, Hypochondriacal, or Hysteric Diseases*, one of the first important textbooks on neurology.
1774	Franz Mesmer [born Baden (Germany), May 23, 1734; died Meersburg, Germany, March 5, 1815] uses hypnotism to aid in curing disease.
1829	James Mill [born Fofarshire, Scotland, April 6, 1773; died June 23, 1836] publishes *Analysis of the Phenomena of the Human Mind*, which tries to show that the mind is nothing more than a machine and that it has no creative function.
1840	Johannes Peter Müller [born Koblenz, Rhenish Prussia (Germany), July 14, 1801; died Berlin, April 28, 1858] completes *Handbuch der Physiologie des Menschen* (Handbook of Human Physiology) (volume 1 published in 1834) and is among the first to give a mechanistic explanation of human thinking.

1841   Surgeon James Braid [born Rylawhouse, Scotland, 1795; died Manchester, England, March 25, 1860] renames mesmerism *hypnotism* and gives the practice some medical respectability by correctly explaining why it works.

1843   Emil Heinrich du Bois-Reymond [born Berlin, Prussia (in Germany), November 7, 1818; died 1896] demonstrates that electricity is used by the nervous system to communicate between different parts of the body.

1861   Pierre-Paul Broca [born France, June 28, 1824; died Paris, France, July 9, 1880] is the first to demonstrate that a particular region in the brain (Broca's area) is connected to a particular faculty, in this case the faculty of speech, by discovering a lesion in the brain during an autopsy on a man who could not speak intelligibly.

1863   Johann Friedrich Adolf von Baeyer [born Berlin, October 31, 1835; died Starnberg, Bavaria, August 20, 1917] develops the first barbiturate, which he supposedly names for his girlfriend Barbara.

1868   Sir Francis Galton [born Birmingham, England, February 16, 1922; died Haslemere, Surrey, England, January 17, 1911] shows that mental abilities of human beings form a normal distribution, lying along the familiar bell-shaped curve.

1872   Physician Jean Martin Charcot [born Paris, France, November 29, 1825; died Nievre, France, August 1893] uses hypnosis as part of his treatment for therapy; in 1885, Sigmund Freud is a student of Charcot's and learns this use of hypnotism from him.

1880   Physician Josef Breuer [born Vienna, Austria, January 15, 1842; died Vienna, June 20, 1925] treats a patient suffering from psychological disabilities by having her relate her fantasies, sometimes using hypnosis; this relieves her difficulties. Breuer tells Sigmund Freud of his experience, and Freud soon begins similar treatments for his patients.

1885   Austrian psychiatrist Sigmund Freud [born Freiberg, Germany, May 6, 1856; died London, England, September 23, 1939] studies hypnotism with Jean Martin Charcot, thus beginning his path toward the development of psychoanalysis.

1890   James McKeen Cattell [born Easton, Pennsylvania, May 25, 1860; died January 20, 1944] coins the term *mental test* and develops a test that measures bodily or sensory-motor responses.

1893   Jean Martin Charcot's papers on the use of hypnosis in medicine are published.

        Sigmund Freud's and Josef Breuer's collaboration in studying the psychic mechanism of hysterical phenomena becomes the foundation of psychoanalysis.

1904   British scientist T. R. Elliot correctly proposes that neurons communicate with each other using chemical signals, now called neurotransmitters, instead of with electric currents.

1906   John Newport Langley [born Roxbury, Massachusetts, August 22, 1834; died Aiken, South Carolina, February 22, 1906] correctly proposes that cells contain receptors for curare, nicotine, and other drugs.

1910   Sir John Tuke, John Macpherson, and L. C. Bruce state that "insanity" is a "morbid mental condition produced by a defect or disease of the brain."

1914	The U.S. Congress passes H.R.6282, the Harrison Act; it is the first comprehensive U.S. law against personal drug use, focusing on narcotics.
1921	Canadian-American medical student John Augustus Larson [born Shelbourne, Nova Scotia, Canada, December 11, 1892; died September 21, 1965] invents the polygraph (lie detector).
1929	Manfred J. Sakel [born Nadvorna, Austria, June 6, 1900; died December 2, 1947] introduces insulin shock for the treatment of schizophrenia.
1935	In June, the meeting that leads to the founding of Alcoholics Anonymous occurs in Akron, Ohio.
1937	Italian doctors Ugo Cerletti [born Conegliano, Italy, September 12, 1877; died July 27, 1963] and Lucio Bini [born Rome, Italy, September 18, 1908] develop the first form of electroconvulsive therapy (ECT), often known as "shock treatment," for treating schizophrenia.
1939	The publication of *Alcoholics Anonymous* this year, followed in the next two years by national publicity in newspapers and magazines, leads to the development of what is now a fellowship thought to have several million members in about 135 countries, as well as a large number of similar self-help groups modeled on the same principles that treat other addictions.
1948	Walter Rudolf Hess, Swiss physiologist [born Frauenfeld, Switzerland, March 17, 1881; died Locarno, Switzerland, August 12, 1973] describes in his book *Das Zwischenhirn* (The Diencephalon) his technique of using small electrodes to stimulate specific regions of the brain, which he has used to identify various regions in the brains of dog and cats.
1949	Australian psychiatrist John Cade [born 1912], working from a theory that later was seen to be entirely wrong, accidentally discovers that lithium salts successfully treat a manic patient.
1952	Robert Wallace Wilkins [born Chattanooga, Tennessee, 1906] discovers that reserpine is a tranquilizer, the first one found; he had been using it to treat high blood pressure.
1954	Chlorpromazine (Thorazine) is introduced for the treatment of mental disorders.
1957	The first of the anti-anxiety benzodiazepines, the minor tranquilizer chlordiazepoxide (Librium), is discovered.
1960	Clozapine is synthesized but not yet recognized as a treatment for schizophrenia.
1963	The second anti-anxiety benzodiazepine, the minor tranquilizer diazepam (Valium) is discovered.
1967	Albert M. Cohen [born Boston, Massachusetts, June 15, 1918] and coworkers report that LSD (lysergic acid diethylamide), frequently taken as a drug to induce an altered state of consciousness, produces breaks in chromosomes, creating the possibility of genetic abnormalities in children of LSD users.
	Mogens Schou, who had followed up John Cade's 1949 work with lithium to cure a manic condition, introduces the use of lithium to treat bipolar disorder in Europe, where it gradually becomes popular.
1980	Scientists at the U.S. National Institute of Mental Health discover that light and dark cycles affect human bodily functions.

1985   The minor tranquilizer buspirone (Buspar) begins to be marketed in the U.S.

1987   The antidepressant drug fluoxetine, better known by its trade name of Prozac, is licensed by the U.S. Food and Drug Administration.

Clozapine is found to improve the mental health of about 30 percent of schizophrenics in a study directed by Herbert Y. Meltzer of Case Western Reserve in Cleveland, Ohio, and John M. Kane of Long Island Jewish Medical Center in Glen Oaks, New York. Not only is this a vast improvement over previous drug treatments, but most patients do not develop side effects.

CAUSES AND DEVELOPMENT OF MENTAL ILLNESS

GENES FOR THINKING AND ACTING OUT?

It is sometimes difficult to be certain that a person has a particular physical disease and even more difficult to ascertain whether the disease is hereditary. Mental illness is still harder to diagnose—often it is not clear if certain behaviors are the result of illness or just a different logic. Moreover, the hereditary basis of any purely mental disease is far from proven. Indeed, when a physical basis for a mental disease is determined, as has largely happened with regard to Alzheimer's Disease, the illness is reclassified from mental to physical. Even more elusive are tendencies toward certain habitual types of behavior, such as aggression or addictive patterns (*see also* "Genes for Alcoholism?," p 61).

Despite these difficulties, researchers have long looked for a genetic basis for just about every mental trait from absent-mindedness to zaniness. In many searches for such genes the technique used is the one that has often been successful in locating the gene for a specific physical condition, such as Huntington's disease. The search for genetic markers that might be inherited along with the trait begins by examining the inheritance patterns in large families that seem to display an inherited version of the condition. The patterns allow the family to be separated into one group exhibiting the trait and another group including their relatives that are free of it. When the genes of the two groups are compared, the differences between the genes can sometimes be found. Markers are usually found first. Markers are sections of a particular chromosome that are associated with the trait but that contain hundreds or thousands of genes. Further study is needed to find a specific gene.

Such large-family studies in the 1980s were used to associate clinical depression and schizophrenia with specific parts of chromosomes. By the end of the 1980s, however, those studies had been effectively refuted for one reason or another. Despite this poor track record for mental conditions, however, researchers have continued to use the large-family method along with more traditional studies of adopted children in an effort to better understand the better causes of mental illnesses and such important mental traits as intelligence.

Intelligence

Even when the condition being studied is intelligence and not a disease at all, the same technique can be used. Robert Plomin of Pennsylvania State University has been among the researchers to use the marker technique in an effort to locate genes for intelligence by comparing three groups of children with high, normal, and low intelligence levels. His results so far, presented in January 1993, suggest that there are markers that can be used to identify the three levels of intelligence, but several different genes are involved in complex interactions.

Variations in normal intelligence, like other variations in normal traits, are less likely to be understood through genetics than through very sharp divisions between those with some variety of normal intelligence and those whose thinking has been severely compromised.

Severe lack of intelligence is sometimes known as mental retardation, although this familiar euphemism might better be restricted to low intelligence on the normal curve. Nearly complete failure to develop mentally often has a basis in a single gene. This is because the operation or development of the brain can be damaged by an allele of a gene that fails to make the correct version of a necessary protein. An example is the Miller-Dieker lissencephaly brain disorder, in which the brain is smooth instead of convoluted, which is a result of incorrect migration of neurons in the brain. Although sometimes labeled "mental retardation," children with this defect seldom learn to speak or to behave in normal human ways. In this case, the gene and its causative allele were isolated in 1993 (published in the August 19, 1993 *Nature*).

In such cases, the connection between genetics and intelligence is not in dispute. It is the question of how much or little the genes affect high or low normal intelligence that is undecided. Research through 1993 has not progressed beyond the concept that several different markers may be involved. Ethicists who had discussed such issues are not certain that it would be desirable in any case to know from a person's genes what his or her scores on an intelligence test might be.

Dyslexia

Most often dyslexia, or impairment of the ability to read, refers to a complex of commonly made mental errors in perception that seem to have nothing to do with intelligence. Often individuals identified as dyslexic confuse left and right or up and down as part of their reading difficulty. Dyslexia is generally treated as having a physical basis, often identified as mild brain damage. Most scientists identify about four to five percent of the population as dyslexic, although some psychologists think there are three times as many with the condition. Because boys are more likely to be identified as dyslexic than girls are, it is easy to suspect a typical sex-linked gene, probably on the X chromosome, as the cause of the problems.

In 1991 Shelley D. Smith of Boys Town National Institute for Communication Disorders in Children, Omaha, Nebraska, and David W. Fulker of the University of Colorado found gene markers associated with dyslexia by looking at the members of 19 families that have large numbers of members identified as dyslexic. That same year, Albert Galaburda of the Dyslexia Neuroanatomical Laboratory at Beth Israel Hospital in Boston, Massachusetts observed that part of the visual processing region of the brain was different in autopsies of five persons identified as dyslexic. He observed an average reduction of some 27 percent in the regions associated with the "fast" processes of vision—including seeing motion and locating objects in space. Similarly, Paula Tallal of the Rutgers Center for Molecular and Behavioral Neurosciences has found that dyslexic children have defects in recognizing the fast-components of sound. The exact connection of all these studies is suggestive, but has failed to produce a consistent opinion regarding the cause of dyslexia.

Attention-Deficit Disorder, or Hyperactivity

Like dyslexia, attention-deficit disorder, or hyperactivity—which appears to be one condition with two names—is generally diagnosed by school psychologists. Unlike dyslexia, however, hyperactivity is often treated with a drug such as methylphenidate (Ritalin) or other amphetamines. Some other regimes that have been recommended include changes in diet to avoid certain amino acids or to avoid sweeteners. The often unspoken implication of such treatment measures is that there is a physical basis for attention-deficit disorder, although until recently the basis has been elusive and the new proposals are also controversial. The sweetener hypothesis, for example, gained strength from work by Alan J. Zametkin of the U.S. National Institute of Mental Health (NIMH) that suggests that the cause of the attention-deficit disorder is an inability of certain regions of the brain to utilize glucose properly.

In the April 1993 *New England Journal of Medicine*, Peter Hauser and Bruce D. Weintraub of the U.S. National Institute of Diabetes and Digestive and Kidney Diseases proposed that a genetic flaw accounted for at least some cases of hyperactivity. Their group located people with attention-deficit disorder who were unable to process thyroid hormone correctly, probably as a result of a defective allele of the thyroid-hormone receptor gene. This version of the gene might also cause alterations in the development of the brain. The population studied was identified by another development problem caused by defects in the thyroid-hormone receptor i.e., short stature. Of the group examined (22 children and 27 adults), 70 percent also were diagnosed with attention-deficit disorder. Note that this study began with people with the receptor disorder and found hyperactivity; a study going in the other direction, most experts think, would find that very few people with attention-deficit disorder also turn out to have defective thyroid-hormone receptors. If there were a one-to-one correspondence, physicians or school psychologists long ago would have learned to associate short stature with hyperactivity.

Depression

Loring J. Ingraham and Paul H. Wender, working at the NIMH, investigated depression (and the related problems of alcohol abuse and drug addiction) in data compiled concerning 67 people in Scandinavia who were both adoptive parents and hospitalized for severe depression (*see also* "Genes for Alcoholism?," p 61). Their report in January 1993 indicated that biological relatives of the 67 depressed *parents* were about twice as likely to be also depressed or to abuse drugs or alcohol. (Although it is not clear that depression causes addiction or even that addiction causes depression, there is a linkage in that a higher portion than normal of addicts are also depressed.) The adopted *children,* however, were no more likely to be depressed than the population at large. Thus, this small study indicates that heredity is more important than environment with regard to severe depression.

There are a number of reasons, however, to doubt the basis of the NIMH study. Not only were the number of parents involved in the study small, but also the actual number of depressed or addicted relatives of the parents was also very small. The risk of severe depression used in the study for the general population was one to two percent compared to a four-percent ratio found among relatives of the parents. It is not clear how drug or alcohol abuse was defined, since most studies report much higher incidence than four percent for those conditions alone. A more typical statistic finds a 15 percent chance of alcohol abuse in a given person's life.

Aggression and Violence

Just as scientists have long looked for a genetic basis for alcoholism or schizophrenia, they have also tried to understand aggressive behavior as a hereditary disease. One study, by workers at City of Hope Hospital in Duarte, California, for example, thought they could link the gene allele others have tried to connect to alcoholism (*see* "Genes for Alcoholism?," p 61) to aggression, although other researchers doubt there is such a connection.

In 1992 a report by the U.S. National Research Council of the National Academy of Sciences called *Understanding and Preventing Violence* recognized that although "evidence of a genetic influence specific to violent behavior is mixed," genetic and biological factors need to be considered along with environmental problems in understanding the causes of violence. On the other hand, a couple of months earlier a conference planned on "Genetic Factors in Crime," scheduled for October 9, 1992, had its funding removed by the U.S. National Institutes of Health because the sponsors were thought to accept too readily the idea that there is a genetic basis for aggression, violence, or crime. The prospectus for the conference had stated that eventually genetic markers might be found for such traits as impulsiveness, but that alone would not necessarily lead to criminal behavior.

In the 1960s inconclusive studies of prison populations tried to link the male-determining Y chromosome to aggression, since there is a history of anecdotal evidence back at least to Homer's time that ties fighting, rape, spouse-beating, and violent crime much more to men than to women. Most psychologists later rejected this work. In 1993 the first clear case of a genetic defect plausibly linked to violent behavior emerged—and it is linked to the "female" X chromosome, not the Y.

Although counterintuitive, this link should not have been surprising. Many genetic diseases are sex linked and most of them result from defects in the large X chromosomes and most of them primarily affect males. This happens as a result of two factors. First, the Y chromosome contains many fewer genes than does the X, so the opportunities for failure are much less. Second, a normal female human has two X chromosomes, while a normal male human has one X and one Y chromosome (different species use different mechanisms). Thus a "defective" gene on one copy of the X chromosome is usually covered in a female by a "good" gene on the other copy of the chromosome.

Note that no gene by itself deserves to be called "defective" or "good"; what is a defect in one situation may be an advantage in another. A gene for aggression, for example, might be advantageous for Viking raiders and a serious handicap to postal workers. Furthermore, no gene directly makes behavior: genes control the manufacture of proteins. What happens at the level of whole-body activity as a result of a particular protein is greatly influenced by the environment, by other proteins produced by other genes, and very likely by forces that are not well understood by scientists. Even drugs administered by doctors produce paradoxical results in some patients—as shown by the well known example of the drug Ritalin, which induces activity in most people but helps control it in hyperactive people. Active proteins produced in the cells can be even less predictable.

Thus the gene defect discovered by Hans G. Brunner of University Hospital in the Netherlands, Xandra O. Breakefield of Massachusetts General Hospital, and various coworkers in both the Netherlands and the U.S. cannot be accurately classified as a "gene for male violence." Instead it is a hereditary change in one base of thousands in a gene that controls the development of a protein called monamine oxidase A (MAOA). What MAOA does is consistent with the concept that a defective allele might lead to violent behavior, since its main function is to break down several neurotransmitters—dopamine, epinephrine, norepinephrine, and serotonin (see "The Ubiquity of NO in Life," p 305)—that are involved in the fight-or-flight reaction to stress. Thus, when possessors of this allele are stressed slightly, they might overreact, exhibiting actions that would be classed as violent or aggressive behavior.

MAOA also breaks down such "false neurotransmitters" as tyramine, which by fitting the same receptors alter the effect of true neurotransmitters. False neurotransmitters are found in such foods as chocolate, red wine, and some cheeses, and perhaps should be avoided by persons with defective MAOA. Similarly, the neurotransmitters that are degraded by MAOA are built in part from the amino acids phenylalanine and trytophan; foods rich in those might also be avoided to prevent neurotransmitter buildup. It should be emphasized, however, that it is unlikely that this genetic mechanism accounts for all, or even very many, instances of violent behavior. The allele involved is known so far from only one Dutch family.

An animal experiment has also shown that an allele of a gene for a particular cell chemical causes aggression in mice. René Hen and coworkers at the Institut de Chimie Biologique in Strasbourg, France, based their work on suggestions that levels of serotonin affect aggression—Prozac and similar drugs work by increasing availability of serotonin. Instead of attacking serotonin production, which could interfere with many biochemical functions, the French scientists worked with the gene for a chemical called the 5HT1b receptor, which is one of the means by which serotonin is brought into cells. Different receptors acquire serotonin for different purposes. The French researchers used genetic engineering to produce mice without the receptor. Such mice have as much serotonin in their brains as the wild type, but less of the chemical reaches the interior of cells.

The mice produced by eliminating the gene for 5HT1b are measurably more aggressive than those with the gene intact: they attacked other mice faster, more often, and more intensely. It is thought, however, that the particular serotonin receptor used is not at issue here. Instead, the research has been interpreted as confirming the role of serotonin itself in aggression.

TIMETABLE OF GENETICS AND THE MIND

1857	*Traité des Dégénérescences* contends that hereditary degeneration causes mental retardation, mental illness, alcoholism, and criminality.
1874	Richard L. Dugdale produces a study of an Irish family, given the name

"Jukes" for the study, showing that "hereditary crime" ran in the family; evidence for the 709 family members studied includes nearly 11 percent who had criminal convictions, about 30 percent who had been on relief at one time or another, 18 percent who were prostitutes, and almost three percent who were madams. Some of these groups overlap considerably.

1876   In *L'Uomo Delinquente,* Ceseare Lombroso [born Verona, Italy, November 6, 1835; died Turin, Italy, October 19, 1909] states that criminals are the products of heredity and can be recognized by physical features; thieves have small shifty eyes, he says, while sex criminals have bright eyes and voices that crack when they speak.

1883   Francis Galton's *Enquiries into Human Faculty* introduces the term *eugenics* and suggests that humans could be improved by selective breeding.

1901   The journal *Biometricka* is founded by psychologists to support the ideas of eugenics and hereditary influences on behavior.

1905   Alfred Binet [born Nice Alpes-Maritimes, France, July 8, 1857; died Paris, France, October 18, 1911], V. Henri, and T. Simon develop the first intelligence test.

1909   Cyril Burt [born Stratford-upon-Avon, England, March 3, 1883; died London, England, October 10, 1971] writes his first paper purporting to claim that intelligence is inherited; after his death in 1971 it was discovered that much of his data was made up or doctored to fit his thesis.

1921   Ernst Kretschmer's [born Wüstenrot, Germany, October 8, 1888; died Tübingen, Germany, February 8, 1964] *Physique and Character* suggests that mental state and personality are related to body build.

1926   *The Measurement of Intelligence* by Edward Lee Thorndike [born Williamsburg, Massachusetts, August 9, 1847; died Montrose, New York, August 9, 1949] describes how to use tests to develop numerical measures of intelligence.

1938   In September, the Nazi government of Germany institutes the Nuremburg Laws, forbidding Jews to become citizens or marry non-Jews, in the name of racial purity.

1968   Frank R. Ervin and coworkers at Massachusetts General Hospital in Boston determine that about 40 percent of the violence-prone people in a study of recurrently violent individuals have some form of brain damage, which Ervin thinks might be controlled by surgically removing the older parts of the brain.

In October, an Australian jury acquits a murderer on the grounds of insanity caused by an extra Y chromosome.

1969   Arthur R. Jensen writes in the *Harvard Educational Review* that genetic factors cause African-Americans to score poorly on standardized tests; this conclusion is widely disputed at the time.

1983   Sarnoff Mednick in an article in *Science* compares criminal records of 14,427 men adopted in Denmark with the records of their biological parents; he finds a hereditary pattern leading to property theft, but no evidence of hereditary violence.

Prime Minister Lee Kwan Yew of Singapore urges educated women to marry early and have more children to prevent the intelligence level of the population from decreasing.

(Periodical Sources and Additional Reading: *New York Times* 9-15-91, p I-1; *New York Times* 9-15-92, p C1; *New York Times* 11-13-92, p A12; *New York Times* 1-5-93, p C3; *New York Times* 4-13-93, p C3; *Scientific American* 6-93, p 122; *Science* 6-18-93, p 1722; *New York Times* 8-22-93, p I-27; *New York Times* 10-22-93, p A21; *Science News* 11-27-93, 366)

Depression UPDATE

Depression is the major mental illness in the U.S. and is rising throughout the world. Estimates vary widely, but about 2.5 million to five million Americans are thought to suffer from major or clinical depression, while another 8.5 million are depressed from time to time, although for most of those it is undiagnosed and untreated. A study of depression in the U.S. and Puerto Rico, Canada, Italy, Germany, France, Taiwan, Lebanon, and New Zealand as reported in *Journal of the American Medical Association* in December 1992, found that serious depression rates appeared to be rising in all the countries studied. In this study, several generations in each country were asked about bouts of depression. Although members of the youngest generation had lived many fewer years, they reported a higher incidence of depression. For example in Italy, people born before World War I had a lifetime incidence of depression of eight percent, but those born in the past 30 years had already experienced depression at a rate of 18 percent (and most would live for many years more, so the rate for this current generation would rise even higher in the future).

Not only is depression a major economic burden through lost work ($11.7 billion a year in the U.S.), impairment on the job (another $12.1 billion), and associated treatment costs (another $12.4 billion), but also depression is implicated in most suicides (15,000 men and 3400 women in 1990) and suspected in a large number of automobile accidents. The figures are from a study of costs of depression that used 1990 data and was reported in the December 1993 *Journal of Clinical Psychiatry.*

Considerable research suggests that women suffer from depression at a rate two to three times higher than men, with one study reporting as many as seven million depressed American woman. Women's depression has been attributed to environmental factors (poverty, abuse, and infertility) instead of physical factors (chemical imbalances or heredity).

Causes of Depression

As with all mental illnesses, the pendulum of informed opinion has recently swung toward physical, especially genetic, causes for depression. But a careful study by Kenneth S. Kendler of the Medical College of Virginia in Richmond, and coworkers, published in the August 1993 *American Journal of Psychiatry,* found that stressful events, including divorce, loss of a job, and serious illness, triggered most episodes of depression in their sample of 416 identical and 264 fraternal female twin pairs. All the pairs had lived together in the same Virginia households until at least the age of 16, and the participants averaged about 30 years in age. Nearly a third of the participants reported at least one episode of severe depression.

Background

Depression as a medical condition is more than simply being sad, but not all forms of depression are classed as the same.

Major (or clinical) depression (sometimes called "unipolar disorder"): Physical symptoms are often present, including insomnia and loss of appetite. Feelings of confusion, indecision, and lethargy can interfere with all aspects of life. Mental symptoms are often severe enough to interfere with work, sex, and other interpersonal relationships, and pleasure in general. Feelings of unworthiness, self-pity or self-blame, hopelessness, and agitation can lead to suicide. Between 2.5 and five million Americans are afflicted with major depression.

Mild depression As the name applies, this is sadness, but sadness that often lasts for months or years. Although any of the symptoms associated with major depression can be present, such as insomnia or loss of appetite, such effects are less severe. Sometimes mild depression can be associated with a specific cause, such as death of a loved one or loss of a job. About 4.1 million Americans are thought to suffer from mild depression during any one year.

Dysthymia This is a personality disorder that is essentially just personality. It includes a perpetual state of mild depression as well as generalized crabbiness along with such feelings as being insecure or being a malcontent. Usually there are no physical symptoms. Often dysthymia is not thought of as a disease, but it is sometimes successfully treated with antidepressants.

Bipolar disorder (sometimes still called "manic depression" or "manic-depressive disease") This condition is marked by periodic excursions between two poles of personality: a *manic phase* in which the person affected feels elated and superior, a phase marked also by grandiosity and bad judgment; and a *depressive phase* that is similar to a severe major depression, sometimes marked with psychosis. (In addition to the unipolar major depression, described above, clinicians recognize a unipolar manic state in some patients; in each case, the condition is simply half of the bipolar disorder.) About 1.8 million Americans suffer from bipolar disorder.

Seasonal affective disorder (SAD) Many physicians recognize a form of depression that occurs in winter outside the tropics. Similar in symptoms to mild depression, SAD is believed to result from insufficient production of hormones that need light for their manufacture, and thus the most common treatment has been to provide bright lights on a regular basis. More recently, some physicians have prescribed supplemental hormones.

Both major and mild depression tend to occur in episodes, but 80 to 90 percent of patients who have weathered one episode are likely at some time to have another.

The study was designed to examine the effects of heredity. While it demonstrated that genetic factors did contribute to susceptibility to depression, stressful events seemed to explain about half the depressive episodes even when considered with no relation to heredity. The study was unable to locate the cause of the other half of the depressive episodes, suggesting that further research is needed.

Depression is often associated with physical conditions, such as alcoholism or major illnesses, including heart attacks, cancer, and AIDS. The combination can be

TREATMENT FOR DEPRESSION

Most patients today begin with a drug that raises serotonin levels in the brain, of which the most common is fluoxetine (Prozac). These drugs work by inhibiting the re-uptake of serotonin by brain cells after the chemical has been released. Some 65 to 75 percent of patients respond to such drug treatments within two or three weeks. Although there are some side effects, most patients find the side-effects acceptable and often continue the drug for many years with no further depressive incidents. In many cases, some form of talk or self-help therapy is used in conjunction with the drugs.

Side effects for Prozac and related drugs include loss of sex drive, slow sexual response with delayed orgasm, impotence, inability to ejaculate, weight loss, and insomnia. Controlled studies have discounted early anecdotal reports of Prozac-induced suicides. Animal studies suggest the possibility that Prozac or similar drugs could cause cancer to progress more quickly.

Prozac and such related drugs as Zoloft and Paxil are also used to treat the eating disorder bulimia and obsessive-compulsive disorders.

Other antidepressant drugs are older than those that affect serotonin; these other drugs have more side effects because they produce a broad range of effects in the brain. These include the tricyclics and the monamine oxidase inhibitors, both of which were first introduced in the 1950s. While small doses of tricyclics are sometimes used along with Prozac or other serotonin re-uptake inhibitors to overcome sleep disorders, the combination of a monamine oxidase inhibitor and a serotonin re-uptake inhibitor is very dangerous and can even be fatal. All types of antidepressants are associated with increased miscarriages during the first trimester of pregnancy.

Major depression and bipolar disorder have long been treated with lithium salts, which were accidentally discovered by a physician trying to find a way to calm a unipolar manic state. Although side effects are a problem with lithium, it continues to be an effective treatment for conditions than are more severe that those usually treated with Prozac or similar antidepressants.

Patients who do not respond to drugs may be given electroconvulsive therapy (ECT), formerly known as shock treatment. One reason the name "shock treatment" is no longer used is that research has shown that it is the convulsions that actually remove depression, not *shock* in either the medical sense or in the electrical one. A combination of anesthesia and muscle relaxers are used to prevent any pain or damage from muscle spasms.

Estimates vary, in part because some patients do not want their ECT experience known, but the lowest estimate for use in the U.S. is that 30,000 persons a year undergo the treatment, while high estimates reach as many as 110,000. It is known that Medicare pays for over a hundred thousand treatment sessions a year, but each patient normally has from eight to 12 sessions.

No observable brain damage results from ECT, but there is generally some memory loss for events both before and after the treatment. Normally only memories of a few days are affected, but some patients claim to have lost years that have never come back. Slight memory loss is considered acceptable because ECT relieves depression for from 75 to 85 percent of the patients, most of whom were not previously helped by drugs.

---

lethal. Depressed alcoholics are frequent suicide victims, while depressed heart-attack survivors have three or four times the death rates of those without depression as reported in the October 1993 *Journal of the American Medical Association*. There is some evidence that depression's physical affects include promotion of blood clots and interference with heart action.

It is thought that *if* there is a genetic basis for depression or for alcoholism, *there may* also be some connection between the two conditions at a genetic level. Not everyone who is alcoholic is also depressed and certainly depression does not cause alcoholism, but it appears that more alcoholics suffer from depression than chance could explain.

A number of studies have connected depression to HIV, the virus that causes AIDS, but the exact interaction in that case is also elusive. In 1992 one team reported that depression in HIV-infected persons hastens the onset of AIDS and death, but a year later the same group said that further study showed that this is not the case after all, although they still found that depression affects the immune system adversely. Research by a different group failed to confirm any progression of disease or lowered numbers of immune cells in depressed HIV-infected persons.

Mysteriously, study after study has connected depression to cigarette smoking. Even people who once smoked, but since have stopped, are more likely to develop serious depression according to research reported in the January 1993 *Archives of General Psychiatry*. There seems to be a reciprocal relationship: people who had previously been depressed are also more likely to become addicted to nicotine upon first exposure. One thought by the scientists involved in conducting the studies was that a gene predisposing a person to nicotine addiction might be connected in some way to a gene for depression. This would tend to agree with the loose connection between depression and alcoholism, provided that there is, as many physicians claim, a generalized addictive personality.

(Periodical References and Additional Reading: *New York Times* 12-9-90, p I-31; *New York Times* 12-8-92, p C1; *Science News* 1-30-93, p 71; *New York Times* 7-19-93, p A1; *Science News* 7-31-93, p 79; *Science News* 8-14-93, p 102; *Science News* 10-23-93, p 263; *New York Times* 12-3-93, p A25; *Science News* 12-4-93, p 374; *New York Times* 12-13-93, pp A1, B8)

THE MYSTERY OF SCHIZOPHRENIA

Until recently, opinion had been sharply divided between those who thought schizophrenia was caused by events or environment and those who thought that it was an inborn error of metabolism. The latter theory got a big boost and schizophrenics benefitted greatly when an effective drug treatment for many patients was approved for use in the U.S. in February 1990.

Clozapine and the D4 Receptors

The new approved drug is clozapine, which binds to the D4 receptor for dopamine in the brain. Previously, few treatments had been very effective, although some of the major tranquilizers were commonly used and electroconvulsive therapy ("shock treatment") was sometimes tried. Clozapine does not cure schizophrenia, but it improves mental health well enough so that schizophrenics can function in the community. The D4 receptors are only one class of a group of molecules that take dopamine into cells. Other neuroleptic drugs — also known as antipsychotic drugs — affect the D2 receptors or have broad affects on dopamine or other neurotransmitters. Later studies have revealed that the effectiveness of clozapine varies with a person's allele of gene for his or her D4 receptor; clozapine is most effective when there are several repeats of a small section of the gene.

The dopamine connection to schizophrenia had been suspected since the 1960s, but it was difficult to prove. In September 1993, however, Canadian scientists were able to demonstrate conclusively that the brains of schizophrenics have about six times as many D4 receptors as people with no brain disease, people with Alzheimer's disease (which involves a different neurotransmitter from dopamine), and people with Parkinson's disease (known to be caused by dopamine insufficiency in particular regions of the brain).

Although clozapine has been a breakthrough drug for many, it has also had a side-effect with its own side-effect. The side-effect is a severe blood disorder called agranulocytosis, which results in a reduction of white blood cells with an AIDS-like loss of immune function. Although agranulocytosis stops shortly after clozapine is discontinued, the side-effect of the side-effect is the cost of continually monitoring the patient's blood to prevent death from agranulocytosis. This cost has made the drug among the most expensive treatment therapies. Protests eventually forced the manufacturer to permit varied monitoring arrangements for the blood disorder, which in the first ten months of use in the U.S. affected over two percent of the patients taking the drug. Prices for use of the drug dropped considerably with monitoring by hospitals or clinics chosen by doctors who prescribe the drug; earlier only one supplier, chosen by the drug manufacturer, did all the monitoring at a cost of $8944 per year for the drug and monitoring in 1990. Monitoring by clinics at that time ran about $800 annually, but Sandoz, the manufacturer, still planned to charge nearly $5000 annually in the U.S. for the drug (excluding monitoring costs), twice the cost in Germany and more than quadruple the British cost to patients.

Before the advent of clozapine, and even afterward, a common treatment for schizophrenia was the use of various neuroleptic drugs that affect dopamine receptors other than the D4. These drugs were not nearly so effective, and they produce in one out of five patients the side-effect *tardive dyskinesia,* characterized by rapid and involuntary twitching of the mouth, lips, tongue, limbs, or trunk, which becomes worse when treatment stops.

Schizophrenia and Life

Despite the evidence that changing dopamine uptake in the brain removes symptoms of schizophrenia in many patients, a Swedish study in 1992, published in the *Lancet,*

Background

It has been estimated that one person out of every hundred throughout the world develops schizophrenia. Another estimate is two to three persons per thousand. Before the advent of drug treatments, one out of every four or five admissions to a mental hospital was diagnosed as schizophrenia and, because it was not very treatable, more than half the residual population of mental hospitals were thought to be schizophrenics. The picture is confused in part because some researchers believe that there are several different diseases that are diagnosed as schizophrenia. This hypothesis would help explain the variable response to treatment.

Schizophrenia is often confused in the popular mind with multiple-personality disorder because a vernacular term for the latter is "split personality" and the root *schizo-* means "split." But the split in schizophrenia is not between parts of the personality, but between the personality and reality. Schizophrenics often hear voices that no one else hears and they sometimes see things that no one else sees. Around the beginning of the twentieth century, the German psychiatrist Emil Kraepelin (1856–1926) identified the syndrome, which he called dementia praecox to indicate that most people develop this "dementia" when they are otherwise healthy young adults.

Hearing voices is the hallmark trait of schizophrenia. Several studies in the early 1990s used brain scans to establish that auditory hallucinations originate in regions of the brain connected to speech, notably Broca's area. It is thought that the brain activity mimics actual speech as far as a schizophrenic's perception of it. There is also some indication that hearing is shut down when the voices are operating. The left temporal lobe of the brain, where meanings of sounds are located, may be physically altered in schizophrenics. Electrical stimulation of this lobe by physicians or by epilepsy also produces auditory hallucinations.

Other symptoms commonly associated with the disease, which may occur in varying combinations, include what psychiatrists call "low affect" (a lack of emotion); delusions (paranoia, the delusion of persecution, is especially common, as is a belief in great personal importance; schizophrenics are notorious for believing themselves to be Napoleon or God); and catatonia (striking motor behavior including both rigidity and limpness under the same heading).

The cause of schizophrenia has been identified many times in various contradictory or complementary ways. Some of the suggested causes include:

- genetic defects
- viral infections of schizophrenics or of their mothers while pregnant
- structural problems with the brain caused in fetal development or during changes caused by puberty
- improper receptors or numbers of receptors for various neurotransmitters, especially dopamine
- head trauma
- psychological stress

Some of these may work together. For example, an inherited immune disorder may make the fetal brain more susceptible to damage by the influenza virus during the second trimester of pregnancy (May 1993 *Schizophrenia Bulletin*).

found a strong environmental link to the disease. Men raised in cities in Sweden have a 38 percent higher rate of schizophrenia than men who grew up in the country, even after all other suggested factors are taken into consideration. Because of the unusually high quality of Swedish medical records, the researchers were able to follow nearly 50,000 young men who were in their 20s or early 30s throughout the period 1970-83 to establish which ones became schizophrenic and also to determine such background factors as parental divorce, drug use, family history of psychiatric disease, as well as the schizophrenic's early environment. Follow-up was planned to see if a specific facet of city life could be found that predisposed young men to schizophrenia.

Other studies have suggested that more schizophrenics are born during the winter. City life and winter might mean exposure to more viral diseases.

(Periodical References and Additional Reading: *New York Times* 12-6-90, p D3; *Science News* 5-11-91, p 293; *Science News* 7-18-92, p 44; *Science News* 5-29-93, p 346; *New York Times* 7-21-93, p C3; *New York Times* 9-22-93, p C12; *Nature* 9-30-93, pp 393, 441)

THE UBIQUITY OF NO IN LIFE

Recognition that nerves communicate messages from one part of the body to another was slow in coming; nerves were confused with tendons, for example. It took even longer to begin to understand the means of communication, which is complex in the typical way of living organisms. Ancient Greeks, impressed by their own aqueducts and canals, thought that the parts of the body communicated with hydraulics. For a time after the discovery of electric currents, it was believed that electricity provided all the answers. Although some chemicals used in nerve transmission were known in the 1920s and 1930s, word of these discoveries did not spread far for many years. It was still possible in the 1950s to write in a reputable publication that normal nerve messages were electric pulses "and nothing else."

Excitement over the role of the chemical messengers, called neurotransmitters, did not begin until the early 1980s, after some neurotransmitters were found to act like psychoactive drugs and some were implicated in chronic diseases of the brain and nervous system. The electrical currents in the nervous system were recognized as secondary. The currents were flows of electrically charged atoms induced by the neurotransmitters.

In the 1990s, it was appreciated that the simple inorganic chemical nitric oxide, known to chemists as NO, also forms another means of communication, although this was first discovered a few years earlier. Unlike the neurotransmitters that cause ion flow by binding to receptors in nerve cell membranes, however, NO crosses the membranes and interacts directly with proteins in the cell's interior. Nitric oxide mediates relaxation in blood vessels and in peristalsis (the muscular motions of digestion) and controls another important neurotransmitter, glutamate, in some of its operations.

Nitric Oxide's Many Roles

For some time scientists have recognized that an unknown chemical released in the lining of blood vessels causes the vessels to dilate. In 1987 scientists were surprised to

RADICALS AND FREEDOM

NO, although about as simple as a chemical can be—one atom of nitrogen joined to one atom of oxygen—actually occurs in three different forms in the body, with three different actions.

The basic molecule, NO, could also be called nitrogen monoxide. Nitric oxide when given a chance grabs another oxygen atom to become NO_2, or nitrogen dioxide. All medium-sized molecules "want" an outer shell with exactly eight electrons, which is why one atom combines with another in the first place. Nitrogen has five outer electrons and oxygen has six, so NO has one eight-electron shell with three electrons left over. NO_2 has a second eight-electron shell with only one electron left over, which is "preferred." A third combination of nitrogen and oxygen, nitrous oxide or N_2O, is the famous "laughing gas" used as an anesthetic. Since it has two fives from the two N's and a six from the one O, N_2O can arrange the 16 electrons to form two shells of eight each, which makes the molecule "content." N_2O is quite stable, but NO changes into or is incorporated into other chemicals within five seconds of its production in the body.

Chemical reactions of molecules depend on the number of electrons in the molecule's outer shell, which can vary from the number in the basic molecule. After NO is formed, the molecule often picks up an additional electron (in other words "is reduced"). The reduced form, symbolized as $NO^•$, has a different chemistry from NO. $NO^•$ is dangerous because it enters into chemical reactions readily. Research by Stuart A. Lipton of Harvard Medical School in Boston, Massachusetts, and coworkers, published in the August 12, 1994 *Nature*, indicates that $NO^•$ is toxic to nerve cells. Depending on other chemicals in the vicinity, however, NO can also lose one of those three outer electrons, becoming NO^+. While $NO^•$ participates in reactions that lead to toxic compounds, NO^+ is involved in reactions that protect nerve cells from damage.

Any group of atoms joined together that has a charge is called a *radical*. An extra electron produces a negative charge, while the lack of one results in a positive charge. Radicals are most "comfortable" in conjunction with each other, so that negative and positive charges balance, producing a neutral molecule. Left to their own devices (that is, not matched with a radical of the opposite charge) charged combinations of atoms are *free* radicals. Thus, both $NO^•$ and NO^+ are free radicals. But, as noted in the previous paragraph, not all free radicals are bad. Even though $NO^•$ is harmful, NO^+ is helpful. NO by itself acts as a weak free radical (*see* Background on p 307).

The reason for the generally bad reputation of free radicals is that they can combine with all sorts of other molecules, often producing substances in the body known to cause cancer.

discover that the mystery chemical was the same as the very simple compound nitric oxide, NO. This discovery was the beginning of the recognition that lack of NO might be the mysterious cause of several physical disorders. High blood pressure is an obvious suspect. Investigation into this possibility has been carried out by, among others, Julio A. Panza of the Cardiology Branch of the U.S. National Heart, Lung, and Blood Institute, but he has been unable to pin down the exact mechanisms involved.

Possibilities include impaired production of NO and too rapid a breakdown of NO produced in normal amounts. The importance of this work is underscored by the fact that 90 percent of all cases of high blood pressure have an unknown cause.

Less clearly, some researchers think that lack of NO in the blood vessels promotes atherosclerosis (blockage of arteries) and its complications by increasing cholesterol deposits or by allowing bloc clots to form more easily. The mechanisms for such a role are not nearly so clear as the possibility that lack of NO causes hypertension.

The only proven condition caused by too little NO production is impotence. Relaxation of arteries is necessary to permit the blood to fill spongy tissue in the penis, the cause of an erection. Iñigo Saenz de Tejada of Boston University School of Medicine and coworkers discovered that NO is needed for an erection and that oxygen is necessary to produce NO. Their work suggests that insufficiency of oxygen causes about 80 percent of biological impotence. It is thought that erections are needed to increase the oxygen supply, so in the total absence of erections, temporary impotence becomes persistent.

Although NO has essential purposes in the body, some forms of it—the free radicals—are among a class of chemicals that have had very poor reputations in the 1990s. Furthermore NO even acts like a free radical itself. As with other free radicals, when too much NO is produced, it damages cells. This can occur during septic shock, when macrophages use NO as a weapon against foreign invaders; during strokes, when NO caused by oxygen deprivation is one of the damaging chemicals produced; and as a part of progressive brain disorders, when NO destroys DNA in brain cells that have lost their essential protection against the compound.

The damage to neurons in a stroke is thought to be caused by a massive release of glutamate. Since NO controls glutamate, chemicals that inhibit formation of NO also

Background

Nitric oxide (sometimes called nitrogen oxide or nitrogen monoxide) consists of one atom of nitrogen combined with one atom of oxygen. NO is not found much outside the body, even though air is almost all nitrogen and oxygen. It takes a very high temperature (3000° C), such as that produced by lightning or an electric arc, to get nitrogen and oxygen molecules excited enough for nitric oxide to form. Then as soon as things cool down, the nitric oxide molecule, NO, quickly grabs another oxygen molecule to form the more stable nitrogen dioxide, NO_2.

Nitrogen and oxygen are elements 7 and 8 on the periodic table, which means that nitric oxide has 15 electrons, an odd number. Electrons pair up in molecules with even numbers of electrons. Some evidence suggests that in NO the unpaired electron, is bounced back and forth between the two atoms in the molecule. As a result NO acts as a part-time free radical, a type of chemical particle that has a very bad reputation for damaging cells, especially for altering DNA. Nitric oxide, however, is much less reactive than true free radicals. But it can still produce serious damage when too much of it is available in one region of the body. After all the ordinary free oxygen is grabbed, NO begins to combine with oxygen that has already lost an electron, resulting in two powerful free radicals that quickly damage nearby tissue.

prevent the deluge of glutamate and reduce damage from stroke. This effect has been shown to occur in clinical tests as well as in the test tube.

Recognition of Neurotransmitters

Because neurons use so many different pathways to communicate, listing all of the approximately 50 chemicals identified as neurotransmitters is neither easy nor straightforward. Early biologists entangled the concepts of hormone and neurotransmitter; and confusion between the two became complicated further because some substances that definitely act as hormones under some circumstances are neurotransmitters at other times in other places.

Not all neurotransmitters act as hormones, however. Other neurotransmitters were difficult to recognize because they are simple substances, such as amino acids and their derivatives. The single-amine derivatives of amino acids form an important group of neurotransmitters collectively called the monoamines. Combinations of amino acids, called peptides, form another class.

While the amino-acid-derived neurotransmitters form the bulk of the neurotransmitters, a few are simple chemicals, of which the simplest is nitric oxide. Two derivatives of adenosine, one of the four bases in DNA, also sometimes act as neurotransmitters.

Further complicating the understanding of neurotransmitters is that each one of them usually affects several different types of receptors. Receptors are protein complexes embedded in cell membranes that selectively snag chemicals and bring them into cells. The response of receptors expressed on one cell may be quite different from those on a different cell. For example, GABA receptors in one part of the brain respond to such tranquilizers as Valium, but the receptors in another part of the brain do not.

Finding the receptors is as important and potentially useful as knowing the neurotransmitters, and finding the receptor may come first or second. For example, the receptors for natural opium-analogues (endorphins and enkephalins) were not discovered until December 1992, nearly two decades after the discovery of the neurotransmitters. But the receptor for anandamine was mapped in the brain as early as 1988, several years before the discovery of the neurotransmitter.

Date	Neurotransmitters described or neuron function recognized	Notes on function
1921	acetylcholine (a simple amine)	Found at nerve-muscle connections for all voluntary muscles and some involuntary ones; slows down muscle contractions; also used as a neurotransmitter by the brain in conjunction with memory; lack of acetylcholine may be a factor in Alzheimer's disease; produces orgasm when directly administered to appropriate section of the brain.
1920s	epinephrine (a monoamine— also known by earlier name as adrenaline)	Recognized as a hormone early in the century, it became viewed as a messenger to other parts of the body in 1923.

Date	Neurotransmitters described or neuron function recognized	Notes on function
1930s	norepinephrine (a monoamine)	Used by sympathetic nerves of the autonomic nervous system to accelerate heart action and produce other "flight-or-fight" responses; also involved in memory.
1950s	various amino acids (GABA, glutamate, aspartic acid, glycine)	GABA seems to operate only as a major neurotransmitter in higher centers of the brain; glutamate (also known as glutamic acid) is the principal excitatory neurotransmitter in the brain and perhaps in the visual pathway, and seems to be involved in information storage and retrieval; glycine is an inhibitor of impulses in the spinal cord and brain stem. These transmitters work mainly by transmitting chloride ions.
1958	dopamine (a monoamine)	A major transmitter in the part of the brain involved in movement; lack of it is thought to be the primary cause of symptoms of Parkinson's disease, while an excess seems to be a factor in some mental illnesses.
1960s	substance P	Transmits pain from the skin to the spinal cord, but also occurs in the brain, gut, and sexual organs; the P stands for "powder," not "pain."
1970	serotonin (a monoamine)	Used by a discrete group of neurons in the brain; involved in regulating temperature, sleep, and some aspects of perception and memory.
1974	"hypothalamic-releasing hormones"—thyrotropin-releasing hormone (TRH), luteinizing hormone-releasing hormone (LHRH), and somatostatin (SRIF)	Somatostatin metabolism is involved in various brain disorders.
1975	enkephalins and endorphins (peptides)	A group of related chemicals that act on the same receptors as opiates do and are involved in pleasure.
1976	vasoactive intestinal polypeptide (VIP) and cholecystokinin (CCK—also a peptide)	CCK influences feelings of satiety.
1977	adrenocoorticotropic hormone (ACTH)	Known earlier as a hormone, it also is produced and used by neurons; different fractions of it involve memory and social interactions.
1978	other pituitary hormones, insulin, vasopressin, oxytocin, gastrin, and angiotensin	These proteins and peptides also were recognized as hormones first; vasopressin is involved in memory.
1979	glucagon (a protein)	Originally found mixed in with insulin, increasing the amount of sugar in the blood; also produced by islets of Langerhans in pancreas.
1981	corticotropin-releasing factor (CRF—a peptide)	Originally considered a hormone.
1982	growth-hormone releasing hormone	Originally considered a hormone.

Date	Neurotransmitters described or neuron function recognized	Notes on function
1987	nitric oxide (a very simple chemical)	Plays a central role in interactions of nerves and smooth muscles, in smell, and many other processes; found active in the brain as early as 1988; definitely labeled a neurotransmitter in 1992.
1992	anandamide (derived from arachidonic acid)	Resembles THC, the active agent in marijuana, in its effects; perhaps involved in appetite stimulation as well as in soothing feelings; discovered by William Devane, Raphael Mechoulam, and coworkers at Hebrew University in Jerusalem; *ananda* means "eternal bliss" in Sanskrit.
1993	carbon monoxide (a very simple chemical)	Involved in long-term memory and also protects against excess activity by neurons, possibly by countering effects of nitric oxide; also stimulates production of cyclic GMP, an intracellular messenger; suggested as a possible neurotransmitter in 1992.

In addition to those listed above, various other chemicals have at one time or another been identified as neurotransmitters: these include histamine (a simple chemical); adenoside and adenosine triphosphate (derived from adenine); galinin (causes fat cravings); lipotropin (acts in brain, spinal cord, guts, adrenals, and sexual organs); neuromedin (like substance P, transmits pain); neuropeptide Y (causes carbohydrate cravings); substance K (chemically similar to substance P); and substance S (sleep inducing).

(Periodical References and Additional Reading; *Science* 7-24-92, p 494; *Nature* 11-12-92, pp 106, 163; *New York Times* 1-26-93, p C3; *Science News* 2-6-93, p 88; *Nature* 8-12-93, pp 577, 626; *Sciences* 9/10-93, p 27; *Harvard Health Letter* 10-93, p 6; *Scientific American* 11-93, p 58)

BODY AND MIND

YOUR EMOTIONS CAN MAKE YOU ILL

There is considerable evidence that mental states affect illness. Women who suppress anger, for example, die three times as often during a given period as those who do not. One study of people followed from the age of 25 to the age of 50 found that the people ranking high in hostility died at five times the rate of those who ranked in the lowest hostility quartile. The exact mechanisms connecting emotions to disease and death are not always known, although stress has long been known to raise hormone levels.

Other mechanisms and recent results are described below.

Stress and the Immune System

Wife and husband Janice Klecott-Glaser and Ronald Glaser, a psychologist and an immunologist respectively, studied how arguing in 90 couples affected the immune system. Couples who showed the most hostility or negative feelings also showed a drop during the next 24 hours in immune-system responses. The couples in the study were not genuinely battling, either. They were just asked to resolve in a laboratory setting some issue on which they disagreed.

A study published in the August 29, 1991 *New England Journal of Medicine* confirms that the effect of stress on the immune system can actually increase risk of disease. Sheldon Cohen of Carnegie-Mellon University in Pittsburgh, Pennsylvania, David A. J. Tyrrell of the United Kingdoms's Medical Research Council, and Andrew P. Smith of the University of Wales studied 400 volunteers who were given either a sterile saline solution or a cold-virus cocktail of five different viruses in a nose swab. Although 74 percent of the exposed volunteers rated as in a low-stress group became infected, 90 percent of the exposed high-stress group showed signs of infection. More dramatically, when overt cold symptoms were counted, not just signs of infection, only 27 percent of the low-stress group showed them, but 47 percent of the high-stress group succumbed to cold symptoms.

Stress does not have to be unpleasant to have effects. David E. Phillips of the University of California in San Diego has conducted a number of studies of how regular important events such as birthdays and major holidays affect death rates. Men (but not women) tend to die more often just before birthdays. Women more often die just after birthdays and both sexes tend to die just after major holidays.

Stress and Cancer

In addition to suppression of the immune system, which may affect the course of cancer, stress has been shown to have other specific effects that can increase risk of cancer. And studies of stress in human beings have shown an actual risc in some types of cancer among the chronically stressed.

A Japanese study of stressed rats reported in the September 15, 1993 *Cancer*

Research has shown that such rats produce chemicals that can damage DNA, and the chemicals actually do damage DNA, in the livers of the rats. Although such damage is generally repaired by cell mechanisms, earlier work has shown that over a lifetime some of the damage fails to be corrected, and that damage can lead to cancer.

In 1991 Australian researchers reported that stressed people develop higher rates of colorectal cancer. A U.S. follow-up study reported in the September 1993 *Epidemiology* confirmed that even when other factors that cause cancer are taken into effect, people who report being particularly stressed at work for a period of ten years have 5.5 times the risk of developing colorectal cancer as the ones reporting low job stress over the same period.

Depression and Disease

Depression can itself be a disease with a physical cause and physical effects (*see* "Depression UPDATE," p 299), but it also can result from major traumas, including disease. As such, depression exacerbates other diseases, including diabetes and kidney failure. Nevertheless, a striking study by Jeffrey Burack of the University of California at San Francisco, reported in July 1992 at the Eighth International Conference on AIDS in Amsterdam, The Netherlands, that found that depressed men infected with HIV died sooner than those without depression was retracted by the same team after another year of study.

Even broken bones seem to heal faster when there is no depression over the break—at least the non-depressed patients were discharged earlier than the depressed ones by 8 days, according to a study by James Strain of Mount Sinai Medical Center in New York, New York, and coworkers, published in the August 1991 *American Journal of Psychiatry*. Furthermore, the elderly women in the study needed less physical therapy and were less likely to be readmitted to the hospital for further treatment.

Heart disease, often found to be affected by mental health (see below), is also made worse by depression. During the six months following a heart attack, depressed patients were three to four times as likely to die according to a study reported in the October 10, 1993 *Journal of the American Medical Association*.

Heart Disease, Personality, and Problems

Folk wisdom has for a long time suggested that anger could provoke a heart attack. In the early 1990s researchers demonstrated various physical mechanisms that could cause such a thing to happen. In the August 1992 *American Journal of Cardiology* Gail Ironson of the University of Miami in Coral Gables, Florida, and coworkers reported on what happened when people with coronary heart disease described incidents that had made them especially angry. Merely reliving the experience reduced the ability of their hearts to pump blood by five percent. It is thought that the effect on their hearts was probably much greater during the anger-provoking event itself. Specialists said that the reduction was enough to provoke heart attacks although none of the 18 patients in the study had such an attack while describing the anger-provoking experience. This research tends to confirm earlier studies that show that hostile people are more likely to have heart attacks.

Folk and comic-book wisdom also attributes a positive correlation between anger and high blood pressure. This too has been born out in scientific studies. Men seem to be more affected than women: at least in arguments where husbands tried to change their wives' minds on an issue, it was the husband's blood pressure that increased. One 1992 study showed that just listening to a speaker with whom one disagrees causes the listener's blood pressure to rise. A year later a study published in the November 24, 1993 *Journal of the American Medical Association* also showed that for middle-aged men (but not women) anxiety over a period of many years produces high blood pressure. High blood pressure is a well-known contributor to heart disease.

Another contribution to heart disease may come from a different mechanism. Stephen Manuck of the University of Pittsburgh observed that monkeys hostile to their cage-mates develop blocked arteries at a rate double those who get along. All the monkeys were followed over a two-year period in which they consumed a high-cholesterol diet. A study of teenagers showed that those with high hostility have higher blood cholesterol levels later in life according to Redford Williams and Ilene C. Siegle as reported at a 1990 meeting of the American Heart Association. Furthermore, the ratio of bad cholesterol to good (LDL to HDL) was also unusually high in the hostile people.

Stephen Manuck, graduate student Susan B. Malkoff, and coworkers also report that humans exposed to a stressful laboratory test almost immediately start to secrete adenosine triphosphate (ATP) in high amounts from their blood platelets. This could help trigger heart attacks, The men taking the test also had jumps in heart rate and blood pressure often associated with stressful situations.

Many of the studies just cited used only male subjects and those that involved both sexes often had different results for each. All in all, a number of studies have shown that the best personality indicators for heart disease in men are hostility, suspiciousness, aggressiveness, and a volatile temper. The relation between heart disease and emotions seems to be different for women. One long-term study of a small number of women, for example, showed that women who suffer patiently are more likely to die of heart disease than hostile women.

Beliefs and Death

Perhaps the most surprising recent result in the connection between mental and physical health has been the discovery that a strongly held belief that a particular condition will eventually cause death seems to affect the ultimate cause of death. For example, people who have a life long belief that they are more prone to heart disease die faster from acute heart disease than those who believe that they are likely to be susceptible to cancer, and vice versa. This conclusion is the result of a study of Chinese-Americans who traditionally associate certain birth years with specific bodily disorders. It is not just the birth year that creates the effect, since non Chinese who do not hold these beliefs are not affected. But the study in the November 6, 1993 *Lancet* by David E. Phillips (of the major events research results cited above) and coworkers found that Chinese believers die from 1.3 to 4.9 years earlier than Caucasian non-believers who are otherwise matched in birth year and disease.

(Periodical References and Additional Reading: *New York Times* 12-13-90, p B23; *New York Times* 8-29-91; *New York Times* 8-5-92, p C12; *New York Times* 9-2-92, p C12; *New York Times* 12-9-92 p C1; *Science News* 10-10-92, p 237; *Science News* 9-25-93, p 196; *Science News* 10-16-93, p 244; *Science News* 11-6-93, p 293; *New York Times* 11-7-93, p 27; *Science* 11-19-93, p 1211; *New York Times* 11-24-93 p C8; *Science News* 12-4-93, p 380; *Science News* 12-18/25-93, p 404)

CAN THE MIND HEAL?

Since bad thinking can aggravate disease (*see* "Your Emotions Can Make You Ill," p 311), it seems reasonable to believe that mental techniques can improve health. Rationalists suspect that mental healing is involved in all sorts of faith cures, religious and otherwise. It is also the rationale for using humor or meditation to promote healing.

Biofeedback is a special technique used to harness the mental powers in dealing with specific symptoms, especially those concerned with circulation such as high blood pressure or Raynaud's disease (a cause of impaired circulation in extremities). Sufferers with Raynaud's disease can train themselves to warm their hands by practicing thinking warm thoughts as a quick-response thermometer measures hand warmth. Biofeedback has also been used to improve symptoms of irritable bowel syndrome.

At least one recent theory, however, says that mental techniques cannot work for the same reason that it is difficult not to think of the left eye of a camel (or any other very specific concept). According to Daniel M. Wegner of the University of Virginia in Charlottesville, any thought that is consciously suppressed will eventually break through and then become impossible to eradicate, rather like a jingle that unbidden occupies a person's thoughts. Wegner's theory predicts that thinking away pain, such as painful work on teeth or gums by a dentist, is the worst way to avoid the pain. Tests of the theory with volunteers who try to think pain is gone by concentrating on pleasant scenes show that their pain becomes worse. But the pain is more easily tolerated by those who concentrate on facing it directly.

(Periodical References and Additional Reading: *Harvard Health Letter* 2-91, p 5; *Harvard Health Letter* 1-92, p 1; *Science News* 3-6-93, p 156)

IMAGE DISORDERS

A number of recognized disorders that affect women rather more than men can be classed as "image disorders." Some of these are body weight problems (*see* "Weight and Health," p 144), but others can be classed as neuroses that affect health, notably anorexia (full name—anorexia nervosa, meaning deliberate starvation in the search for a better body image) and bulimia (vomiting or purging after bouts of overeating).

Background

As early as the 1600s anorexia was described but not recognized. The first clinical description dates from 1873. At that time it was thought to be rare. Reported incidence began to rise about a hundred years later and was recognized as a serious problem in affluent nations in the 1980s. Estimates vary, but some sources claim there are about 300,000 Americans with the disorder, mostly teenage girls. Bulimia was noted in the 1980s. About one in 20 bulimics is a young man.

The health effects of eating disorders can be severe. Some teenage girls and even older women have effectively starved themselves to death. Bulimia may affect the throat or the digestive system, as well as the electrolyte balance of the blood. Even tooth enamel may be eroded by exposure to digestive fluid.

Similar disorders for men are less severe and less common, although in the early 1990s the emphasis on male muscular development through weight lifting or other body building exercise could sometimes lead to physical complications, especially when hormones were used to speed up the process.

Physical problems that arise from eating patterns, exercise patterns, or certain kinds of drug abuse—including the use of amphetamines to lose weight as well as steroid hormones to gain muscle—can be classed as image disorders. Ultimately the root of the problem is a poor self-image. Often a teenage girl with anorexia appears thin to all but her mirror.

One study published in May 1991 in the *Journal of Abnormal Psychology* demonstrated that teenage girls with eating disorders were the daughters of mothers who had a history of image disorders themselves. Other studies in 1993 found more sinister patterns. David B. Herzog of Massachusetts General Hospital in Boston and coworkers found that of 20 bulimic women studied, 13 had been sexually abused as children according to lengthy interviews with the women. But a more extensive study directed by Joel Yager of the University of California-Los Angeles, found that of 80 bulimic women compared to 40 non-bulimic controls, there was much more self-reporting of patterns of pervasive physical or psychological abuse in the women with current or past bulimia than in the controls. Sexual abuse did not emerge as a factor in Yager's research. Both Herzog's and Yager's reports were made at the 1993 annual meeting of the American Psychiatric Association.

(Periodical References and Additional Reading: *New York Times* 5-5-91, p I-37; *Science News* 6-5-93, p 366)

Infectious Disease

THE STATE OF THE FIGHT AGAINST INFECTIOUS DISEASE

An infectious disease is one caused by one or more kinds of parasite invading a susceptible human. The general name used in medicine for such parasites is *pathogen,* meaning "generator of suffering." Pathogens include viruses, bacteria, fungi, protozoans, worms, and sometimes the larvae of insects. A pathogen carries out part of its life in or on a human and in the process damages the human in some way. The pathogen only wants to eat and reproduce. As a by-product of eating and reproducing, however, the pathogen may release toxic chemicals or damage essential parts of cells or organs. The damage may also result from the human immune system trying to remove the pathogen.

A study by Will Kastens, a student at the Harvard School of Public Health, identified 412 different diseases caused by pathogens. While 180 of these diseases appear to be exclusive to humans, about the same number are also diseases of animals—118 human diseases that animals can catch and 62 animal diseases that sometimes affect humans. The remaining 35 diseases are uncommon results of encounters between a human and a pathogen from which a human disease can sometimes spring—not really an infectious disease at all in the normal sense of "infectious." Thus there are not quite 400 diseases currently considered infectious.

Diseases Rise and Fall

The number of diseases generally rises over time. New diseases are found or appear; notably in recent years scientists have discovered Lyme disease, Legionnaire's disease, and toxic-shock syndrome in the 1970s; AIDS and possibly chronic fatigue syndrome in the 1980s; and Four Corners disease in the 1990s. Stephen Morse of Rockefeller University has suggested that most of these new diseases began as animal diseases, including yellow fever, Marburg fever, Ebola fever, and AIDS viruses from monkeys; Rift Valley fever from livestock, which is transmitted to humans by mosquitoes; and various hantaviruses, including Four Corners disease, from rodents. In the 1990s new prospective studies of ecological changes, such as roads into rain forests and clearing of islands, are expected to yield new insights into how diseases transfer from animals to humans.

Other diseases rise and fall in incidence with time, as has occurred recently with measles, cholera, and tuberculosis. A highly dangerous strain of the streptococcus bacterium called M-type-1, which causes streptococcal toxic shock when it invades the bloodstream, was first recognized in 1987, rose to a peak in the U.S. in 1989 (it followed somewhat different curves in European counties and in New Zealand), and fell to fairly low levels by 1991.

Only one disease—smallpox—is known to have been completely eradicated, but several have been beaten back considerably, especially in industrialized countries. For example, polio is virtually gone from the New World—the first completely polio-free year in the Western Hemisphere was between August 23, 1991 and August 23, 1992. The World Health Organization hopes that polio will go the way of smallpox by the end of the 1990s.

Sometimes scientists know or think they know the reason for a major change in incidence of a disease. Changes in measles and the eradication of smallpox are almost entirely the result of patterns of vaccination; people caused the change directly. The rise of Lyme disease is thought to be a result of new practices in forest management and suburbanization. In other instances, the disease may have origins that are suspected but not proven, such as the effect of weather on the Four Corners disease.

The Asian tiger mosquito carries a number of viral diseases not previously common in the U.S. This "vector" (carrier of pathogens) entered the U.S. in 1985 as larvae in water in recapped tires shipped from Japan. Since then the mosquito has spread throughout warmer regions and even into the upper Midwest.

As for AIDS, there are many conflicting theories on its origin. Although the hypothesis that it was originally a disease of monkeys is considered strongest, it is also not clear whether or not it was introduced to humans by some form of social contact (e.g., keeping monkeys as pets), by predation (e.g., killing monkeys to eat), or by some rare mishap (e.g., infection of cultures used in a vaccine trial is one suggestion).

Diseases Become Harder to Treat

It is thought that sometimes a disease mutates in a way that makes it more virulent or less virulent. Smallpox was known throughout human history, but it suddenly began to kill people much more frequently in the eighteenth and nineteenth centuries. More recently, toxic shock syndrome appeared as a result of a toxin produced by an otherwise less troublesome staph bacterium. And the variety of *E. coli* that caused a widespread epidemic of food poisoning in 1993 was unknown before 1955.

Work by John J. Mekalanos and coworkers at Harvard University promises a better way of understanding how such change in virulence can arise. They reported in the January 29, 1993 *Science* that they had located the "virulence genes" from typhoid and salmonella organisms. The genes are those that are only activated when the bacteria invade their hosts (mice, in this study). It is thought that knowledge of such genes will aid in developing vaccines or antibiotics as well in helping to understand the differences between human reactions to the same bacteria. Some people fight off the disease, others become ill, and some die, but the difference is in the people and not in the bacteria causing the disease.

Forms of the bacteria that cause gonorrhea, tuberculosis, or other diseases have evolved so that they now resist the medicines previously effective against those diseases. Some estimate that for the cost of such antibiotic resistance in the U.S. alone is $100 million annually—and some people die as a result of bacterial resistance.

New approaches are helping to solve this problem. For example, the drug of choice for bacteria that are not susceptible to penicillin and related drugs—and also the drug used with persons allergic to penicillin—is vancomycin. In the 1980s it was observed that bacteria were becoming resistant to vancomycin in Europe, and the resistance quickly spread to become worldwide by 1990. The gene that causes this resistance in bacteria was located and cloned by 1993. From the gene it was possible to determine how the bacteria actually resist the disease, leading to a way around the resistance.

NEW OR NEWLY NOTICED DISEASES

Year	Place	Type of agent	Name of disease or agent	Remarks
1961	Brazil	Virus	Oropouche	First found in a dead sloth in 1960 when a new road was opened in the rain forest; caused human epidemic in Bélem in 1961; transmitted by midges.
1975	Old Lyme, Connecticut	Spirochete bacterium	*Borrelia burgdorferi*	Disease identified in the U.S. in 1975, but perhaps known earlier in Europe; found to be borne by tick *Ixodes dammini* in 1978; spirochete identified in 1983.
1977	Japan	Retrovirus	HLTV-1 (or adult T-cell Leukemia)	Virus found first in the U.S., but Japanese researchers were first to connect it to a disease; 15 percent of population of southwestern Japan infected, but only two to four percent of population develops disease symptoms.
1983	Uganda	Retrovirus	AIDS (HIV-1)	Acquired immunodeficiency syndrome.
1986	—	Rickettsia	*Ehrilchia chaffeenis*	Systemic infection with fever, headache, low white-blood-cell count.
1987	—	Bacterium	*Streptococcus* M-type-1	Deadly and quick form of Group A strep; caused sudden death of puppeteer Jim Henson in 1990.
1989	—	Virus	Hepatitis C	Previously part of non-A, non-B hepatitis; transfusion related and sporadic.
1990	—	Virus	Hepatitis E	Acute hepatitis, water-borne epidemics and sporadic.
1991	Venezuela	Virus	Hemorrhagic fever	Severe internal bleeding.
1992	India	Bacterium	*Vibrio cholerae* 0139	New variant of cholera.
1992	Kenya	Virus	Yellow fever	New location; severe hepatitis and internal bleeding.
1993	New Mexico	Virus	Hantavirus	New syndrome in which lungs suddenly fill with fluid; sometimes called Four Corners disease.

(Periodical References and Additional Reading: *New York Times* 7-24-92, p A10; *New York Times* 9-11-92, p A24; *New York Times* 10-21-92, p C12; *Nature* 3-95-93, p 340; *Science* 7-16-93, p 308; *Science* 8-6-93, p 680; *Natural History* 12-93, p 6; *American Scientist* 1/2-94, p 52; *Harvard Health Letter* 3-94, p 3; *New York Times* 5-10-94, p C3)

TIMETABLE OF FIGHT AGAINST INFECTION TO 1990

1345   Plague spread by fleas on rats, endemic in parts of central Asia, breaks out as trade between Asia and Europe increases, and spreads to Astrakhan (in Russia) on the Volga and Caffa (Feodosiya, Ukraine) in the Crimea; it is the beginning of the epidemic known as the Black Death.

1347   Plague spreads to Mediterranean ports and begins to terrorize people all over Europe as they hear of its terrible symptoms and many deaths.

1348   Black Death is imported to England from France by ships carrying claret wine and flea-infested rats.

1352   The Black Death reaches northern Europe, including Scandinavia and northern Russia.

1701   Giacomo Pylarini, considered by some the first immunologist, inoculates three children with smallpox in Constantinople in the hope of preventing them from developing more serious cases of smallpox when they grow older.

1713   Emanuel Timoni describes to the British Royal Society the Turkish practice of inoculating young children with smallpox to prevent more serious cases of the disease when they get older.

1717   Lady Mary Wortley Montagu [born London, 1689; died London, August 21, 1762] brings back to England the Turkish practice of inoculation and has her own two children vaccinated against smallpox.

1721   Zabdiel Boylston [born Brookline, Massachusetts, March 9, 1679; died Brookline, March 1, 1766] introduces inoculation against smallpox into America during the Boston epidemic.

1796   Physician Edward Jenner [born Berkeley, England, May 17, 1749; died Berkeley, January 26, 1823] performs the first inoculation against smallpox by infecting a boy with cowpox (vaccinia virus).

1797   The Royal Society rejects Jenner's inoculation technique for smallpox.

1800   Chlorine is used to purify water by William Cruikshank [born Edinburgh, 1745; died June 27, 1800] in England.

        Benjamin Waterhouse [born Newport, Rhode Island, March 4, 1754; died Cambridge, Massachusetts, October 2, 1846] is the first American physician to use smallpox vaccine (on his son).

1840   *Pathologischen untersuchungen* (Pathological Investigations) by German pathologist and anatomist Friedrich Gustav Jakob Henle [born Fürth, July 19, 1809; died Göttingen, May 13, 1885] expresses his conviction that diseases are transmitted by living organisms, although he offers no hard evidence.

1843   Oliver Wendell Holmes [born Cambridge, Massachusetts, August 29, 1809; died Boston, Massachusetts, October 7, 1894] advises doctors to prevent spreading puerperal fever (a common disease of mothers after childbirth at the time) by washing their hands and wearing clean clothes.

1844   The Commission for Enquiring into the State of Large Towns establishes a connection between dirt and epidemic disease in England.

1847   Hungarian physician Ignaz Philipp Semmelweiss [born Budapest, July 1, 1818; died Vienna, August 13, 1865] discovers that puerperal fever (childbed fever) is contagious; he has doctors working for him wash their hands in the hopes of reducing the number of cases of the disease in his hospital.

1854   John Snow [born York, England, March 15, 1813; died London, June 16, 1858] shows that removing the pump handle of a well contaminated by sewage reduces the incidence of cholera in the vicinity of the well.

1865   Joseph Baron Lister [born Upton, England, April 5, 1827; died Walmer, Kent, February 10, 1912] introduces phenol as a disinfectant in surgery, thus reducing the surgical death rate from 45 percent to 15 percent.

1866   William Budd [born North Tawton, England, September 14, 1811; died Clevedon, Somerset, England, January, 1880] demonstrates in Bristol, England, that limiting the contamination of a town's water supply can stop a cholera epidemic.

1876   Robert Koch [born Klausthal-Zellerfeld, Hanover, Germany, December 11, 1843; died Baden-Baden, May 27, 1910] discovers that the microorganism responsible for cattle anthrax can be grown in culture.

1877   Louis Pasteur [born Dole, France, December 27, 1822; died Saint-Cloud, September 28, 1895] notes that some bacteria die when cultured with certain other bacteria, indicating that one bacterium gives off substances that kill the other; 60 years passed before this observation is put to use, when René Jules Dubos discovers the first antibiotics produced by a bacterium.

1879   Louis Pasteur discovers by accident that weakened cholera bacteria fail to cause disease in chickens and that chickens previously infected with the weakened virus are immune to the normal form of the virus, thus paving the way for the development of vaccines against many diseases, not just smallpox.

1880   Louis Pasteur's "On the Extension of the Germ Theory to the Etiology of Certain Common Diseases" develops the germ theory of disease; he also demonstrates his findings on vaccination to the Academy of Medicine.

1881   Louis Pasteur develops the first artificially produced vaccine; the vaccine is for anthrax, a deadly disease that affects both animals and humans. On May 5 he successfully demonstrates that vaccination of sheep and cattle against anthrax prevents their falling ill with the disease after injection with live bacteria; unvaccinated animals die when given the same amount of live bacteria.

1882   Paul Ehrlich [born Strehlen, Silesia, March 14, 1854; died Bad Homburg, Rhenish Prussia, August 20, 1915] introduces his diazo reaction for diagnosing typhoid fever.

    Robert Koch discovers the bacterium that causes tuberculosis, the first definite association of a germ with a specific human disease.

1885   Louis Pasteur develops a vaccine against hydrophobia (rabies) and uses it to save the life of a young boy, Joseph Meister, bitten by a rabid dog.

1886   Ernst von Bergmann [born Riga, Latvia, December 16, 1836; died Wiesbaden, Germany, March 25, 1907] introduces steam sterilization of surgical instruments in his Berlin clinic.

1890   Emil von Behring [born Deutsch-Eylau, Germany, March 3, 1854; died
             Marburg, Rhenish Prussia, March 31, 1917] develops a vaccine against tetanus
             and diphtheria and introduces the concepts of passive immunization and
             antitoxins.

             Paul Ehrlich standardizes the diphtheria antitoxin, establishing the field of
             immunology.

             Surgeon William Halsted [born New York, September 23, 1852; died Baltimore
             Maryland, September 7, 1922] introduces the practice of wearing sterilized
             rubber gloves during surgery at Johns Hopkins Hospital in Baltimore.

             Robert Koch announces the discovery of tuberculin as a cure for tuberculosis.

1891   Paul Ehrlich uses methylene blue for treating malaria.

1892   Russian biologist Dmitri Ivanovsky [born Gdov, November 9, 1864; died
             U.S.S.R., June 20, 1920] shows that viruses exist.

             Robert Koch introduces filtration of water for controlling a cholera epidemic
             in Hamburg, Germany.

1893   Physician Niels Finsen [born Faeroe Islands, Denmark, December 15, 1860;
             died Copenhagen, September 24, 1904] claims that red light reduces the
             symptoms of smallpox; although this idea was later abandoned, Finsen goes on
             to establish that ultraviolet light kills bacteria and to cure the skin disease
             lupus vulgaris with ultraviolet light.

1897   The English bacteriologist Almroth Wright [born Middleton Tyas, Yorkshire,
             England, August 10, 1861; died Farnham Common, Buckinghamshire, April 30,
             1947] introduces a vaccine against typhoid.

1905   Robert Koch of Germany wins the Nobel Prize for Physiology or Medicine for
             his tuberculosis research.

1906   German bacteriologist August von Wasserman [born Bamberg, February 21,
             1866; died Berlin, March 16, 1925] begins to develop his famous test for
             syphilis when unexpected destruction of red blood cells appears in his work.
             Although it is initially very sensitive to the skills of the bacteriologist
             performing the test, the test is gradually refined into a reliable test after several
             international "Wassermann conferences" arranged by the League of Nations as
             well as various improvements by workers in the field.

1910   Paul Ehrlich and Sahachiro Hata introduce "salvarsan" (arsphenamine), also
             known as 606, as a "magic bullet," or cure, for syphilis, the beginning of
             modern chemotherapy.

             Major Frank Woodbury of the U.S. Army Medical Corps introduces the use of
             tincture of iodine as a disinfectant for wounds.

1917   Alice Evans discovers the organism causing brucellosis, a microbe that
             develops in the udders of infected cows.

             Ralph Parker [born Malden, Massachusetts, February 23, 1888; died September
             4, 1949] develops a vaccine against Rocky Mountain spotted fever.

1919   Louise Pearce [born Winchester, Massachusetts, March 5, 1885; died August
             10, 1959] discovers a compound, which becomes known as tryparsamide, that
             cures sleeping sickness.

1921   Alexander Fleming [born Lochfield, Scotland, August 6, 1881; died London,
             March 11, 1955] discovers the antibacterial substance lysozyme in saliva,

mucus, and tears. As with his later discovery of penicillin, a fortuitous accident was involved; he had a cold and some of his mucus dripped onto a culture plate, where it dissolved the bacteria present.

1923   Albert Calmette [born Nice, France, July 12, 1863; died Paris, October 29, 1933] and Camille Guérin [born Poitiers, France, December 22, 1872; died Paris, June 9, 1961] develop the tuberculosis vaccine BCG (Bacillus Calmette-Guérin).

1928   Alexander Fleming discovers penicillin in molds; its clinical use in therapy starts only in the 1940s, when Howard Florey and Ernst Chain further develop it, and it is learned how to manufacture it in quantity.

1930   Infants in Lübeck, Germany, develop tuberculosis when disease-producing tuberculosis bacteria are given to them as a vaccine instead of attenuated bacteria of the BCG type.

        Hans Zinsser [born New York, New York, November, 1878; died September 4, 1940] develops an immunization against typhus.

1931   Ernest Goodpasture [born Montgomery County, Tennessee, October 17, 1886; died Nashville, Tennessee, September 20, 1960] grows viruses in eggs, making the production of such vaccines as polio vaccine possible for viral diseases.

1935   Elizabeth Hattie Alexander develops an antiserum that cures some cases of meningitis, previously 100 percent fatal in children.

1937   South African-American microbiologist Max Theiler [born Pretoria, South Africa, January 30, 1899; died New Haven, Connecticut, August 11, 1972] introduces a vaccine against yellow fever.

1939   René Jules Dubos [born Saint-Brice, France, February 2, 1901; died February 20, 1982] searches for and finds two compounds produced by a soil bacterium that kill other bacteria—i.e. antibiotics. These are the first antibiotics to have been deliberately sought for this property.

1940   Howard Florey [born Adelaide, Australia, September 24, 1898; died Oxford, England, February 21, 1968] and Ernst Chain [born Berlin, June 19, 1906; died Ireland, August 11, 1979] at Oxford University obtain penicillin in a purified form and show that it can be used as an antibiotic.

1941   Scientists create sulfadiazine, the fourth sulfa drug.

        Russian-American microbiologist Selman Abraham Waksman [born Priluki, Russia, July 22, 1888; died Hyannis, Massachusetts, August 16, 1973] coins the term *antibiotic* to describe substances that kill bacteria without injuring other forms of life.

1942   After the yellow fever vaccine used to inoculate thousands of U.S. Army personnel is shown to have caused hepatitis B in many of them, a new vaccine is developed that does not require the use of human blood serum.

        Dorothy I. Fennel discovers a powerful new penicillin species, *Penicillium fennelliae.*

1943   Selman A. Waksman discovers the antibiotic streptomycin, produced by a mold that grows in soil; previous antibiotics worked only against Gram-positive bacteria, but streptomycin is effective against Gram-negative bacteria.

1944   Benjamin Minge Duggar [born Gallion, Alabama, September 1, 1872; died New Haven, Connecticut, September 10, 1956] and coworkers discover the antibiotic Aureomycin, the first of the tetracycline family of antibiotics, as a result of checking many soil samples for antibacterial action.

1945   Sir Alexander Fleming, Sir Howard W. Florey, and Ernst Boris Chain [born Berlin, June 19, 1906; died Ireland, August 12, 1979] of England win the Nobel Prize for Physiology or Medicine for the discovery of penicillin and research into its value as a weapon against infectious disease.

1947   Chloramphenicol, a powerful antibiotic, is discovered; its use is now restricted because of dangerous side effects.

1948   John Franklin Enders [born West Hartford, Connecticut, February 10, 1897; died 1985], Thomas Huckle Weller [born Ann Arbor, Michigan, June 15, 1915], and Frederick C. Robbins [born Auburn, Alabama, August 25, 1916] learn how to grow mumps viruses in chick tissue using penicillin to prevent bacterial contamination; the same technique works for the polio virus.

Elizabeth Hazen and Rachel Brown discover the antibiotic Nystatin, which is the first safe fungicide; it has a wide field of applications, including treatment of athlete's foot and the restoration of books or paintings attacked by fungus.

1952   A polio epidemic strikes in the U.S., affecting 47,665 persons.

Jonas Edward Salk [born New York, October 28, 1914] develops a killed-virus vaccine against polio; it is used for mass inoculations starting in 1954 and successfully prevents the disease, although it is later superseded by a live-virus vaccine developed by Albert Sabin.

1955   Some lots of "killed-virus" Salk vaccine intended to prevent cases of polio are produced with the virus incompletely deactivated, resulting in 100 cases of paralysis in children who have received the vaccine; the flawed vaccine was produced by Cutter Laboratories and no other bad batches are known to have been produced.

On January 11, Lloyd H. Conover [U.S., born 1923] patents tetracycline, the first antibiotic made by chemically modifying a naturally produced drug; it soon becomes one of the most useful antibiotics for treatment of a number of infectious diseases.

Niels K. Jerne [born London, December 23, 1911] suggests that antibodies against all sorts of foreign proteins are regularly made, but that the immune system selects those stimulated by an antigen and produces more of them. This theory is later shown to be correct and accounts for the success of vaccination in preventing disease.

1957   Polish-American microbiologist Albert Bruce Sabin [born Bialystok, Poland, August 26, 1906; died Washington, D.C., March 3, 1993] develops a polio vaccine based upon live, weakened viruses.

Frank Macfarlane Burnet [born Traralgon, Australia, September 3, 1899; died Melbourne, August 31, 1985] and, independently, David W. Talmage hypothesize that individual lymphocytes (white blood cells) carry just one type of antibody, which they display on their surfaces.

Alick Isaacs [born July 17, 1921] and Jean Lindenmann discover interferons, natural substances produced by the body that fight viruses.

1963   The first vaccine against measles is introduced; it uses a killed virus and is not reliably effective.

1964	Baruch S. Blumberg [born New York, July 28, 1925] discover the Australian antigen, which is the key to the development of a vaccine for hepatitis B.
1965	On July 13, Benjamin A. Rubin [born New York, September 27, 1917] patents the bifurcated vaccination needle, useful mainly for delivering smallpox vaccine in small doses with little difficulty; it becomes one of the main tools used in the worldwide eradication of the disease.
1971	In the United Kingdom, the first completely sterile hospital units are introduced to protect patients at special risk from infection.
1977	The last recorded case of smallpox found in the wild is in Somalia; after this the smallpox virus is believed to be extinct in the wild, although the virus is retained for research purposes in several laboratories.
1980	Scientists at the New York Blood Center develop a successful experimental vaccine against hepatitis B.
1981	Ruth and Victor Nussenzweig [born Sao Paulo, Brazil, November 2, 1928] of New York University applies for a patent on a malaria vaccine; subsequent trials show that the vaccine is ineffective.
1983	Luc Montaigner at the Pasteur Institute isolates the AIDS virus; a sample of it, supplied to Robert Gallo and his team at the National Institutes of Health, leads to the infection of cultures and the unjustified claim by Gallo in 1984 of being the first to isolate and grow the virus. Gallo later withdraws his claim for priority of the discovery.
1986	Six persons in the U.S. and Jamaica are diagnosed with a new disease of the lymph system, which is later found to be caused by a previously unknown herpesvirus (known as HHV-6) that primarily infects children under the age of four.
1987	Michael Zasloff announces in August that he has discovered potent new forms of antibiotics, which he termed magainins, in the skin of the African clawed frog.
1988	The U.S. Food and Drug Administration approves alpha interferon as a treatment for genital warts.

Vaccine UPDATE

The U.S. Centers for Disease Control and Prevention (CDC) in Atlanta, Georgia, declared on October 28, 1993 that vaccination had, for the *second* time in 40 years, virtually eliminated measles, mumps, and rubella ("German measles"). Despite this declaration, in 1992—the previous year—there were about 2000 cases of measles and about the same number of cases of mumps in the United States.

On the other hand, pertussis (whooping cough) made a comeback in the U.S. in the 1990s as a result of falling vaccination levels. In 1993 the number reached about 5500, the highest number of cases since 1967. One factor in a lack of vaccination for pertussis was a persistent series of reports that the vaccine could cause nerve damage of various kinds. After several studies found no permanent effects except immunity, a panel of the Institute of Medicine of the U.S. National Academy of Sciences ruled in 1991 that there was no evidence to support nerve damage from pertussis vaccine. The panel also gave a clean bill of health to rubella vaccine, which to a lesser degree had been suspected of nerve damage. Some allergic reactions do occur with both vaccines.

Polio has largely been eliminated in the U.S., but the live vaccine that has been generally so successful has produced about 260 cases of paralysis in people who either received the vaccine or were in close contact with people who had been vaccinated.

The general success of vaccination in eliminating childhood diseases in the U.S., with exceptions noted above, has come even though only 56 percent of U.S. children had the required vaccinations, according to the American Academy of Pediatrics. The U.S. is the 70th nation from the top in rankings of preschool immunization rates.

Smallpox, completely eliminated in the wild as early as 1977, has caused infection since then only from a laboratory escape. At the end of 1993 there were still some smallpox viruses in the U.S. and in Russia, although the World Health Organization recommended in 1990 that all stocks be eliminated. A last-minute hold was put on destruction of smallpox reserves at the end of 1993 so that scientists could reconsider the possible beneficial uses of the dangerous virus one more time.

New vaccines continue to emerge. In the August 13, 1991 *New England Journal of Medicine* there was a report of a successful vaccine for hepatitis A, a communicable liver disease that causes serious illness and occasional death. Further testing will be needed before the new vaccine is authorized for general use in the U.S.

Measles

Measles is the most serious of the three viral diseases inoculated against in the combined measles-mumps-rubella vaccine. The 1993 announcement of virtual elimination concluded an outbreak in the late 1980s and early 1990s in the U.S. that had involved more than 50,000 cases of measles, resulting in 132 deaths. In the first three years of the 1990s, however, the rate of measles infections reported had fallen to 1.25 percent of its peak, dropping from 14,000 cases in the first six months of 1990 to 175 reports in the same period of 1993. By the end of 1993 the CDC was able to announce a three-week stretch of no new measles cases in the U.S. CDC spokesperson William L. Atkinson declared that a major concerted effort by state, local, and federal health agencies had reduced the incidence of measles in the U.S. in 1993 to the lowest level in history.

Although after this most recent outbreak medical personnel no longer contemplated the complete eradication of measles in the near future, the drop by 1993 was interpreted as demonstrating that an aggressive vaccination program could reduce levels of a disease to barely noticeable levels.

Because of its frequent complications, doctors have long recognized measles as more serious than other common childhood diseases. But before a measles vaccine was developed in 1963, nothing could be done to prevent measles and there was little to treat the disease. With four to five million U.S. cases per year, most of them in children, measles was considered a normal risk of living, like crossing a street. After an effective vaccine was introduced, an aggressive vaccination program cut the number of measles cases down to a previous low of 1500 a year in 1983.

Vaccination Programs in U.S.

But by 1983 a combination of social factors—ranging from poverty, rising health care costs, and immigration—resulted in a deterioration in the vaccine rate. For the measles-mumps-rubella combination, coverage had fallen to 65%. The number of instances of all infectious diseases previously prevented by vaccination was on the rise. The CDC estimates that current (1993) preschool vaccination coverage for once-common childhood diseases in the U.S. is as follows:

PERCENTAGE OF CHILDREN VACCINATED

Disease	Percent of children covered by vaccination
Chicken pox	0%
Diphtheria	45%
Tetanus	45%
Pertussis (whooping cough)	45%
Polio (three doses of oral vaccine)	55%
Mumps	80%
Rubella	80%
Measles	80%

Vaccination has had singular successes with most of these diseases, though smallpox is omitted from the list because its complete elimination is the biggest success of all. Polio, which struck 33,000 in 1950, reached the zero-reported-case level by 1990 and medical workers believe that complete elimination worldwide is attainable. Pertussis, with over 120,000 cases in 1950, infected only a couple of thousand a year in the early 1990s. Rubella reached only about a thousand reports annually in the early 1990s after being over 50,000 a year as recently as 1970.

In a time when individuals and governments are struggling to meet rising medical expense, vaccines are cost effective. The measles-mumps-rubella (MMR) series of shots provides $3 worth of medical protection for every $1 spent on the vaccine—that is, the cost of treating the diseases if they had not been prevented would be three times the cost of the vaccine and its administration. When indirect costs are included, such as days lost from work by parents or by adults with the disease, the amount of expense covered by each $1 spent on MMR vaccine rises to $14.40, according to a study commissioned for the CDC and released in June 1993. Even the more specific (one disease only) *Hemophilus influenzae* Type B vaccine provides $2.40 in direct benefits ($2.80 with indirect benefits added) for every $1 spent on the vaccination program.

On August 10, 1993, the U.S. government established a new program to provide free vaccines to poor or uninsured children in the hopes of raising the vaccination rate in the U.S. Drug companies that manufacture the vaccines opposed the program, primarily because they saw it as a government attempt to control fast-rising prices they charge for the vaccines. Although industry opposition continued into 1994, the government also proceeded with plans to implement the new policy.

Collapse of Communism and Rise of Infectious Disease

The collapse of communism in Eastern Europe has been seen as involving political, economic, and environmental causes and consequences. In addition to harmful environmental effects on health, communist policies on provision of medical care have had large effects in the past, and the abrupt end of those policies has also produced unpredicted problems. Diseases usually thought of in conjunction with undeveloped countries have been on the rise there. Cholera, for example, went from two cases in Russia in 1991, to five in 1992, to 22 in the first six months of 1993. Tuberculosis was up 26 percent (*see also* "The Return of Tuberculosis," p 363), while there were also outbreaks of typhoid fever and anthrax in Russia in 1993.

Diphtheria epidemic   In the early 1990s an epidemic of the deadly disease diphtheria struck both Russia and Ukraine, and cases were also reported in other parts of the former Soviet Union. Although the total number of cases at the end of 1992 was probably only about 6000, (about 4000 in Russia and about 1300 in Ukraine), this was more than ten times previous levels. The case load stayed about the same in 1993, killing more than 100 Russians. Furthermore, because of the vast region of the former Soviet Union, epidemiologists were not hopeful about quickly reducing the number of infected persons to previous levels.

The epidemic developed because of policies in the immunization program. Too many children were allowed to escape initial vaccination, so only 47 percent had been immunized in 1991 at the start of the epidemic, down from 80 percent in earlier years. Adults were not given follow-up shots, and the unvaccinated population of all ages was as high as 32 percent. The social unrest in the former Soviet Union has also caused more people to move from one place to another, spreading the disease. As a result of these policies and social changes, most of the victims in the current epidemic have been adults, although diphtheria is usually thought of as a childhood disease. Fatalities have included both adults and children, although 70 percent of the fatalities were adults. Because of continuing governmental problems, steps to correct the situation have been slow.

Diphtheria immunization in the Soviet Union was late in coming. Although the first vaccines for diphtheria date from 1890, the practice did not start in the Soviet Union until the 1960s. At that time there were over 50,000 cases a year, by the 1970s there were fewer than 200 cases a year.

Outside of the former Soviet Union, diphtheria has been largely eliminated by vaccination. There were four cases in 1992 in the U.S. In 1991 there was one report of diphtheria in France, one in Italy, two in Germany, and none in Spain.

Chicken Pox Progress and Dilemmas

In the early 1980s the Japanese began trials of an experimental live-virus vaccine for chicken pox. Chicken pox is mainly a mild viral disease of children. The virus that causes it is known to lurk in the body for years, only to re-emerge as the painful and

Background

Causes and symptoms of some of the diseases prevented by vaccines are listed below.

Chicken pox Contagious disease caused by virus of the herpes family. Usually the main symptoms in children are a rash and a fever, with few complications in otherwise healthy children. Virus often hides in the nerve cells for many years after the first attack, however, and can emerge when the immune system is compromised by age or other factors to cause a second set of extremely painful symptoms known as shingles. About 90 to 95 percent of Americans develop chicken pox as children or as adolescents, while another 2.5 percent develop a more severe form of the fever and rash as adults.

Diphtheria Disease caused by airborne bacteria that produce a toxin that causes inflammation of the nervous system and heart, which can cause it to be fatal in a short period of time. Antitoxin can be used to treat a disease once it has taken hold, but vaccination against the bacterium is preferred. Sometimes misdiagnosed as a sore throat or as angina.

***Hemophilus influenzae* type B** A bacterial complication of influenza, colds, or other respiratory diseases. Illness persists for a long period of time unless treated, making it seem as if the "flu" just won't go away. More seriously, this bacterium is one of the most common causes of meningitis, a potentially deadly inflammation of the lining of the brain.

Hepatitis A and B *See* "Through the Alphabet with Hepatitis," p 345.

Influenza A viral disease characterized by fevers, aches and pains, and lethargy (not to be confused with various other diseases nicknamed "flu," such as "stomach flu," which may involve diarrhea or vomiting). Influenza has a high mutation rate, so different vaccines must be prepared for the strains expected to infect the population each year. There are two main types, however, known as A and B, of which type A is the most dangerous. Influenza occurs almost entirely in the winter (although sometimes there is a secondary peak in the spring). Influenza can lead to serious complications, often involving a secondary infection by bacteria, and causes about 20,000 deaths in the U.S. each year, mostly among the young, elderly, infirm, or immune system-compromised.

Measles Highly contagious disease caused by virus, characterized by high fever, followed after a couple of days by white spots on the lining of the mouth, and followed by a characteristic rash. There is a high rate of respiratory complications.

Mumps Viral disease that infects the salivary glands and often the testes or ovaries, causing sterility in rare cases. Not as contagious as most other childhood diseases.

Pertussis Disease caused by bacteria. Commonly known as whooping cough or sometimes as the 100-day cough for its primary symptom, an uncontrollable cough that last for several weeks, comes in uncontrollable bursts, and ends with a deep, wheezing sound (the "whoop"). Infants are most severely affected, and about 0.5 percent of infant infections result in death from pneumonia, seizures, or inflammation of the brain. Whooping cough, like many infectious diseases, runs in cycles that peak every three or four years.

Polio (poliomyelitis, or infantile paralysis) Viral disease that in a small number of cases causes permanent paralysis. Although the disease has largely been eliminated by vaccination, a few persons who developed the disease in the time before the vaccine was developed (in 1952 and 1955) have had a mysterious recurrence of symptoms in the 1990s.

Rubella (German measles)   Mild disease caused by a virus; the main concern is that it can cause damage to an unborn child if the mother becomes infected.

Tetanus (lockjaw)   Serious disease caused by bacteria that normally live in soil but that can grow if they reach a human bloodstream by way of a wound. Because the bacteria are killed by oxygen, a deep wound or a puncture is more dangerous than a shallow wound that is exposed to air. Muscles become rigid and go into painful spasms, which can lead to death.

sometimes devastating disease called shingles. Thus there was a great deal of concern about the possibility for harm to some persons who might receive the vaccine or who might be exposed to others who had been vaccinated. A live-virus vaccine is a strain of the disease that confers immunity but still invades the cells, mingles with DNA, and spreads to other people. The live polio virus, which has almost eradicated polio, has also caused a few people to become paralyzed, including some who did not themselves receive the vaccine. (The live virus more often confers immunity on people in contact with the person vaccinated, increasing the effectiveness of the vaccine in preventing the spread of the disease.)

Of course the difference between polio and chicken pox lies in the severity of the symptoms. A risk taken with a live virus for polio can easily be deemed worth it—although some doctors would like to see a turn to a recently available and more-effective killed-virus polio vaccine—but the dangers of a live-virus vaccine for the much milder chicken pox scared off most U.S. doctors. The Japanese persevered, however. Their tests showed that the vaccine is safe and 97 percent effective. The fear that it might result in shingles years later also abated with experience. Today all children in Japan receive the vaccine, as do those in South Korea.

In the U.S., the CDC is expected to decide whether or not to approve the vaccine sometime in 1994.

U.S. VACCINE RECOMMENDATIONS

Vaccine	Diseases covered	Vaccination schedule
DPT	Diphtheria Pertussis Tetanus	at 2 months; at 4 months; at 6 months; between 15 months and 18 months; school booster; separate tetanus booster (often including diphtheria) at 14 to 16 years; tetanus when possible exposure if not in past 10 years.
Tetramune	Diphtheria Pertussis Tetanus *Hemophilus influenzae* type B	at 2 months; at 4 months; at 6 months; at 15 months; school booster.
Hib CV	*Hemophilus influenzae* type B	at 2 months; at 4 months; at either 6 months or 12 months; at 15 months.

Vaccine	Diseases covered	Vaccination schedule
Hepatitis B	Hepatitis B	Birth, between 1 month and 2 months; between 6 months and 18 months.
MMR	Measles Mumps Rubella	at 15 months; school booster or at entry to middle or junior high school.
OPV (oral)	Polio	at 2 months; at 4 months; between 12 months and 16 months; school entry booster.
Polio (injected)	Polio	at 2 months; at 4 months; followed by OPV at 12 months.

(Periodical References and Additional Reading: *Harvard Health Letter* 9-90, p 5; *New York Times* 7-5-91; *New York Times* 11-1-91, p A16; *New York Times* 1-29-93, p A8; *Harvard Health Letter* 3-93, p 1; *New York Times* 5-29-93, p 5; *New York Times* 7-7-93, p A1; *New York Times* 8-11-93, p C11; *New York Times* 8-16-93, p A1; *New York Times* 8-22-93, p I-8; *Harvard Health Letter* 9-93, p 8; *New York Times* 10-29-93, p A14; *New York Times* 12-3-93, p A30; *New York Times* 12-7-93, p A34; *New York Times* 12-10-93, p A25; *New York Times* 12-25-93, p A1; *Science News* 5-26-94, p 344)

VIRAL DISEASE

THE YUPPIE FLU BECOMES RESPECTABLE

In the 1950s doctors and patients began to describe a condition that seemed something like depression, something like flu, something like mononucleosis or polio, and something like overwork—but the problem did not seem to be exactly any of those previously well-characterized conditions. By the 1980s, localized outbreaks of a condition that matched this melange had become more common and had started to make newspaper pages in addition to medical journals. The breakthrough breakout was in the Lake Tahoe area of California. Uncertain as to the cause of the condition, doctors who believed in the reality of the problem assigned the noncommittal name "chronic fatigue syndrome." Doubters, claiming that most of the "victims" were young, urban professional women and men ("yuppies"), dubbed it the "yuppie flu."

By either name, the condition persisted into the 1990s, becoming a background diagnosis across the U.S. while dropping from the newspaper pages for the most part.

News stories on the subject were revived in 1991 and 1993 when the U.S. Centers for Disease Control and Prevention (CDC) announced revisions of previously issued standards for identifying the syndrome, by then known as CFS, an abbreviation of "chronic fatigue syndrome." In England the disease is called myalgic encephalomyelitis. In Japan, it is the low natural killer cell syndrome. CFS is also more neutral as to cause or symptoms than either of these.

The newer standards, replacing those first set in 1987, were the major factor in demonstrating that CFS is a real condition with an unidentified cause instead of a catch-all for any vague problems troubling middle-class and upper-class patients. A survey of "fatigue" cases in four urban areas established that more than a quarter of them, amounting to two to seven percent of the total population, met the new CDC

Background

CFS is defined as debilitating fatigue that does not go away with bed rest and that reduces or impairs daily activities by half for at least six months. Other known causes of similar fatigue must be ruled out. Physically, the observable signs are low-grade fever, inflamed throat without discharge, and tender lymph nodes. The patient must report, in addition to the observable signs, muscle weakness and pain, generalized headaches, joint pain, and such psychological problems as forgetfulness, irritability, confusion, lack of concentration, and sleep disturbances. CFS is not reported as ever having progressed to the point of causing death.

There is no specific treatment for such a poorly understood syndrome, although mild exercise, such as walking, seems to help. Symptoms, such as pain, depression, or sleep disorders, can be attacked by conventional medicines, although these do not get at the largely unknown cause. As with other chronic diseases, a number of unproven, unlikely treatments are offered outside of conventional medicine.

standards, a much higher number than expected. The average patient was a white female whose illness started at age 30. At the time of the survey, the average patient had been ill for 7.5 years.

CFS Causation Theories

Although a number of viral agents have been proposed as causing CFS, notably the Epstein-Barr virus identified with mononucleosis, none have proven to be the culprit after rigorous testing. Furthermore, although CFS often occurs in clusters, the syndrome does not seem to be contagious in the way that mononucleosis or AIDS is. Finally, CFS does not seem to be removed by the immune system in the way that influenza is. CFS is possibly caused by a virus that hides in the brain the way that chicken pox and herpes hide for years in the nerves.

Recently a number of chronic diseases, including forms of arthritis and diabetes, have been thought to be the result of an immune system activated by a viral infection. Although the infection is suppressed, the immune system fails to calm down and itself causes the chronic condition. Immune system chemicals such as interleukin and tumor necrosis factor are known to produce as side effects fatigue, muscle aches, and bouts of fever. Anthony L. Komaroff, director of general medicine and primary care at Brigham and Women's Hospital in Boston, Massachusetts, suggests this viral/immune etiology for CFS, although the identity of the original virus is not clear.

More conventionally, but without a complete rationale, two small British studies in 1991 showed that a magnesium deficiency might also be involved in CFS in some way.

Some doctors are still holdouts for the theory that there is no CFS. Most patients who claim CFS, they think, actually have chronic depression (*see* "Depression UPDATE," p 299).

(Periodical References and Additional Reading: *New York Times* 12-4-90, C1; *New York Times* 4-20-91; *Harvard Health Letter* 9-93, p 1)

A NEW DISEASE AT THE FOUR CORNERS

In the spring of 1993, several suspicious deaths occurred around the Four Corners region of the U.S., the place where Colorado, Utah, Arizona, and New Mexico borders meet at right angles. Although quite mysterious at first, the infection was soon found to be a previously unknown virus from a viral family known as hantaviruses.

The hantaviruses had been discovered in Asia, where they infect rodents and also cause illness or death in humans. Like its Asian relatives, the American hantavirus has an alternate rodent host, the deer mouse, *Peromyscus maniculatus*. Since deer mice are found throughout the U.S., it was no surprise when hantavirus infection in humans was soon found in parts of the country away from the Four Corners, including Louisiana, California, Idaho, and Montana. More than 60 cases had been reported by the end of 1993 with more than 25 deaths.

The first known death preceded the spring 1993 outbreak by several months; it was in Arizona in November 1992. The second known death and first of the spring series occurred at a medical center in Gallup, New Mexico, in May 1993. At that point the

Background

Hantaviruses are named for the Hantaan River in South Korea. In 1976, scientists found near this river a virus that caused deadly Korean hemorrhagic fever. The symptoms of that disease are different from those of the Four Corners hantavirus. In Korean hemorrhagic fever, blood leaks from the blood vessels while a high fever rages; death is caused by kidney failure. Other hemorrhagic fevers, also deadly, are found in Africa. None, however, are nearly so deadly as the Four Corners disease, which killed more than half the persons known to have been infected.

The Four Corners disease kills when blood plasma, not whole blood, leaks into the lungs. After death, the plasma-filled lungs can weigh twice as much as normal. Other symptoms include high white blood cell counts, low platelet counts, fever, and a cough, so that the early symptoms resemble the viral diseases people usually group as "the flu." Perhaps as many as 50,000 cases of unexplained "adult respiratory distress syndrome" occur in the U.S. each year, and an unknown number of these cases are probably caused by hantaviruses.

Scientists have known since 1982 that rodents in the U.S. also harbor hantaviruses, but no instances of infection in humans had been found in the U.S. before 1992. Hantaviruses are members of the largest family of animal viruses, called the Bunyaviridae, which has more than 200 species. These species are capable of rearranging their DNA easily to cross from one species to another.

illness was still being given the descriptive term "adult respiratory distress syndrome," a catch-all designation used when no causative agent is known. On May 14, 1993 at the same medical center in Gallup, another deadly case of the unknown syndrome alerted officials that they might have something more than just an isolated puzzle. Furthermore the latest victim's fiancée had also died with the same symptoms just five days earlier, although not at the Gallup center. Both had been healthy young adults, and the man was locally well-known as a track star. In each case the disease began as a flu-like fever and cough but was followed after a couple of days with a sudden collapse of breathing and then death.

By May 24, 1993, doctors determined that the cause of the mysterious respiratory collapse was no known infection and thus alerted all physicians in New Mexico to the unusual symptoms. By then six persons were known to have died and one other had experienced the symptoms but recovered. A newspaper broke the story three days after the physicians' alert. The U.S. Centers for Disease Control and Preventions (CDC) in Atlanta, Georgia, then became involved. By June 9, 1993, CDC scientists had used antibodies and DNA analysis to recognize the cause of the outbreak as the previously unknown form of hantavirus. U.S. varieties of hantavirus had been known to virologists for over a decade but were considered harmless to humans before the development of Four Corners disease. By November 1993, two groups of scientists were able to isolate the specific disease virus. This feat is expected to lead to better diagnosis in the future.

Meanwhile the hantavirus disease appeared in a number of Western states after the spring outbreak of 1993. During 1993, the disease struck 45 people in California, Oregon, Nevada, Idaho, Arizona, Montana, Colorado, New Mexico, both Dakotas,

Texas, and Louisiana. Of these, 27 died. Over 70 percent of all the cases, however, were in the Four Corners region, although none were reported in the Four-Corner state of Utah.

Like many phenomena around the world, the hantavirus outbreak has been blamed on the weather, and specifically the weather phenomenon named El Niño. Although the El Niño weather pattern was first noticed off the coast of Peru, it directly involves the whole Pacific Ocean and indirectly weather around the world. In the U.S. Southwest, El Niño brings rain to a usually arid region. One result in 1993 was a large increase in the number of deer mice, which some ecologists have claimed to be the origin of the hantavirus outbreak at the Four Corners.

(Periodical References and Additional Reading: *New York Times* 5-31-93, p 8; *New York Times* 6-3-93, p D3; *New York Times* 6-5-93, p 1; *New York Times* 6-6-93, pp I-23, IV-2; *New York Times* 8-13-93, p A12; *Science* 11-5-93, p 850; *New York Times* 11-21-93, p I-24; *Discover* 12-93, p 82; *Discover* 1-94, p 86; *Science* 12-24-93, p 1961)

THE CALAMITY OF A VIRAL MEDICINE

In 1993, reports were released that an experiment medical treatment had misfired and taken the lives of five patients, a third of those in the test. The patients were using comparatively high levels of a drug intended to cure the viral disease hepatitis B. Later examination of deaths in earlier trials using lower levels of the drug or a related drug suggested that the experiments might have caused an additional five deaths. Although critics of the trials attacked the researchers because of the fatal results of the medication and their failure to recognize the first symptoms, some medical researchers stated that the small number of deaths, all among persons already suffering a serious disease, demonstrated that procedures to protect the general public from dangerous drugs are effective. Other fatal experimental drugs in modern times have killed hundreds to thousands of people before doctors recognized what was going on. Nevertheless, the U.S. Food and Drug Administration (FDA) announced that it would improve procedures to prevent further calamities in drug testing.

A Side Effect Worse than the Disease

The deaths came to light as Jay H. Hoofnagle, director of the Division of Digestive Diseases and Nutrition of the National Institute of Diabetes and Digestive and Kidney Diseases, one of the U.S. National Institutes of Health (NIH), and coworkers were conducting their second trial of an experimental drug called fialuridine or FIAU. The drug had originally been developed by Oclassen Pharmaceuticals of San Rafael, California, which had sold its rights to Eli Lilly & Company, who partly funded the NIH trials. Tests of the drug on dogs and mice had shown good tolerance and indications of benefits against virus diseases. An earlier trial of four weeks on 24 human patients at a low dose had also shown some effectiveness for FIAU and seemed to reveal only easily tolerable side effects of the types commonly experienced with antiviral medicines. Therefore a second test was begun at a higher dosage, an experiment planned for 24

ANTI-VIRUS MEDICINES

Until recently no drug was available to cure or even treat any disease caused by a virus. Modern medicine began with drugs for bacterial diseases, potent dyes, and even more effective antibiotics. None of these had any effect on viruses.

Bacteria are living organisms, creatures that feed, move, grow (somewhat), and reproduce. Given some food and any reasonable environment bacteria perform these functions on their own. Although their mode of reproduction by division makes bacteria theoretically immortal, in practice bacteria, like other living organisms, can be killed and, in fact, die regularly. Bacteria can be deprived of food or water, poisoned, or killed with heat or radiation. All of these methods are used to rid parts of our environment or our bodies of harmful bacteria.

According to the criteria most scientists use, viruses are not living organisms. They do not feed. A virus has no way to move through the environment on its own. Instead of growing, a virus is assembled. Instead of reproducing in almost any environment, a virus is reproduced by the genetic material of another living being. Technically, a virus cannot be killed, only inactivated; inactivating a virus is like decaffeinating coffee, only simpler. But once a virus has reached a place within a cell where it can use the cell's DNA to assemble more copies of itself, it is almost impossible to devise a way to remove the virus without damaging the cell's DNA.

Despite this formidable barrier, scientists have found a limited number of ways to treat a few diseases caused by viruses. In the 1960s the related compounds amantadine and rimantadine were found to be helpful in treating influenza A, a viral disease, in clinical trials. Another drug, ribavirin, also was tested, although with mixed results. The 1970s saw the development of chemicals that interfered with the development of the herpes viruses. FIAU was among the drugs synthesized at this time, but was not very effective against herpes. The drug vidarabine was the first drug licensed for treatment of a herpes disease, and was also shown in clinical trials to reduce mortality from encephalitis. Later the drug acyclovir was shown to be safer and more effective. Acyclovir works by inhibiting viral replication. Because it does nothing to cells unless they are infected with herpes, acyclovir has few side effects and is the first ever antiviral drug to become widely used.

The basic idea of FIAU and several of the related anti-virus drugs, including AZT, ddI, and ddC (all used to combat AIDS symptoms), is to trick DNA into poisoning itself by incorporating the drug into its spiral molecule instead of a natural compound that belongs there. The drugs resemble DNA building blocks (FIAU is similar to thymidine, the T of the familiar CTGA code) but are not functional. Some of the chemicals, once incorporated into a DNA molecule, cause the replication process to halt when the building-block mimic is reached. (DNA replication involves making copies of the molecule by starting at one end and proceeding along like a monkey climbing a rope.) Others, including FIAU, allow the first replication to complete itself, but then will not link up with the appropriate complementary base, needed for the helix to become double.

A virus is nearly all DNA (or in some cases RNA) and preventing DNA duplication effectively kills the virus. The trick, of course, is to stop viral DNA duplication while allowing normal DNA processes to proceed. One way to do this is to take advantage of any differences that exist between viral DNA's method of replication and that of human DNA. FIAU is incorporated into DNA by an enzyme that is not the same as either of the enzymes that are used in normal cell division. Thus FIAU attacks the virus but not the DNA already in the cell's nucleus.

Since 1989, however, it has been known that some drugs that work by poisoning DNA not only prevent viral reproduction but also prevent reproduction of a type of DNA that is used in the production of cellular energy. The small bodies that normally produce energy in cells, which are called mitochondria, have their own DNA that is separate from the DNA in the nucleus. The enzyme that incorporates a base into mitochondrial DNA is essentially the same as the one that incorporates a base into viral DNA. (A highly plausible theory is that mitochondria were once free-living creatures that became symbiotes with all higher life forms early in evolution, perhaps accounting for their different type of DNA.) There are between 300 and 1000 mitochondria in a cell, so the slow poisoning of each would account for the weeks it takes for FIAU to become lethal.

Furthermore, if the mitochondria are poisoned, one of the chief symptoms would be the build-up of lactic acid in the body. Lactic acid results from using the cellular energy pathway that does not rely on mitochondria, a pathway normally used only in rapid exercise that requires energy beyond that provided by mitochondrial oxidation. This symptom was observed in all the patients who died and in survivors as well.

Finally, the poisoned mitochondria could not recover because FIAU lodges itself in the heart of DNA where repair mechanisms, especially weak mitochondrial mechanisms, cannot reach.

A number of medicines have been developed in hopes of combating the HIV virus that causes AIDS. These are discussed further in the article "AIDS Prevention and Treatment" on p 353.

---

weeks, starting March 24, 1993 with ten patients and adding another five at the beginning of June.

On June 26, 1993, when one of the 15 experimental participants in the new test developed severe liver failure, the test was abruptly terminated and the other patients taken off the drug. This was not soon enough, however. By July 9, 1993 two more patients were dead. Other subjects who had been in the experimental group developed severe and unrelenting liver failure weeks after they stopped using FIAU. Although liver transplants saved the lives of two of the seven whose livers failed as a result of FIAU, five of the original ten in the experimental group died. Among the other eight patients, some developed severe nerve pain (neuropathy) in their feet and legs as much as four months after the trials were ended.

There were other symptoms as well, including tingling and pain in the extremities from irritated nerves and nausea. A serious cause of general illness and debilitation was a build-up of lactic acid in all the tissues of the body.

The participants in the study all began the trial with damaged livers from their hepatitis B, a viral disease of the liver that is often transmitted by the same pathways as is AIDS and is therefore most common among male homosexuals and intravenous drug users, though it is certainly not limited to those groups. Furthermore, all the patients had been previously using alpha interferon as an antiviral drug but had found it ineffective or intolerable.

FIAU, though too deadly to ever be used again, was extremely effective against the virus. At some point an analog may be developed that will work against the virus and not against the patient.

Unsuspected Deadly Effects

One result of the deaths in the high-dosage trial was a re-examination of the results of the earlier low-dosage experiments and of even earlier experiments with a related anti-viral medicine fialcytosine (FIAC). Three different trials on humans were involved before the March 1993 high-dosage experiment, involving a total of 79 patients. The review showed that 23 of the 79 had developed unreported symptoms of liver toxicity during the trials. The symptoms were not described in original reports of the experiment in part because there were alternative reasons why the patients in the tests might have high levels of liver enzymes.

Five of the 79 persons in the earlier trials died under circumstances that in retrospect suggest that the drug may have been a factor. Another five persons were hospitalized. In only one instance was the possibility even raised that the drug test might have accounted for a death, and that one possibility was finally attributed to side effects of surgery instead.

Nearly six months after the trial was terminated it was revealed that one subject, after taking only a few doses of the same drug in a different trial by Eli Lilly & Company, had also displayed the sudden rise in liver enzymes that often indicates damaged liver cells. The patient was an alcoholic, among whom high liver enzymes are common, and he was hospitalized voluntarily for 13 days to keep him from drinking during the test, which his doctors thought would complicate any liver problems aroused by the drug. Soon another patient in the Lilly test, which was primarily designed to determine if the FIAU would be more effective as a pill or in liquid form, developed severe liver poisoning and was hospitalized for four weeks, beginning March 17, 1993.

Some critics of the way this problem was handled consider the dates of the two tests crucial. In the Lilly test, the patient with liver poisoning was hospitalized a week before the NIH experiment began, the experiment that led to the five deaths. Since Lilly was also involved financially in the NIH trial, critics argue that the company should have alerted the NIH and stopped further testing.

The author of the retrospective study of the various tests, Roger L. Williams, noted that deaths were overlooked because there was no reason to expect them, because they occurred weeks or months after the experimental drug had been administered, and because the symptoms caused by the drug were similar to those of the disease being treated.

As a result of the review, David A. Kessler, Commissioner of Food and Drugs, proposed policy changes on experimental drug use. All deaths, serious side effects, and reasons why patients stop taking an experimental drug must be reported to the FDA along with an analysis of the possible involvement of the drug in the death or other changes. Furthermore, autopsy reports would be passed along to the FDA.

Different Deadly Drugs

This is not the first time that an effort to handle a viral illness has resulted in deaths. In the 1960s, for example, a trial vaccine intended to protect babies against the virus called respiratory syncytial virus, which for most infants produces symptoms similar to a cold but which is deadly for a few, turned disastrous. Instead of protecting babies, the vaccine made the disease worse and resulted in several deaths.

The antibiotic Omniflox, manufactured by Abbott Laboratories, reached the market in January 1992, but was withdrawn on June 8, 1992 after the FDA received reports of more than 50 adverse reactions. There were also reports of three deaths associated with Omniflox.

On November 2, 1993, Merck & Company terminated its U.S. trials of a Swedish drug intended to treat schizophrenia when it learned that eight patients in European tests of the drug had developed aplastic anemia, a severe blood disorder, and that one of those eight had died. About a hundred patients in the U.S. had been taking the drug, which Merck planned to market under the trade name Roxiam. Merck had applied to the U.S. Food and Drug Administration in January 1993 for approval to market Roxiam in the U.S.

(Periodical References and Additional Reading: *New York Times* 6-9-92, p D4; *New York Times* 7-9-93, p A10; *New York Times* 9-1-93, p A11; *New York Times* 10-23-93, p 9; *New York Times* 11-3-93, p D5; *New York Times* 11-16-93, p A1; *Discover* 3-94, p 56)

PRIONS REVISITED

A number of mysterious diseases of animals and humans around the world have been connected to an agent sometimes identified as a "slow virus" because of a long period spanning several years between infection and symptoms, a phenomenon better known in AIDS which is not, however, caused by a slow virus. This agent is sometimes identified as a prion (PREE-on), a quasivirus that is actually a protein. If prions exist—which has been hotly debated for the better part of a decade—they are the only infectious agents that contain neither RNA nor DNA.

One of the diseases known to be caused by slow viruses is Creutzfeldt-Jakob disease (CJD), which can take 35 years to develop after exposure to the infectious agent. CJD in recent years has been transmitted by tiny amounts of a virus that contaminated some batches of human growth hormone which had been collected from the pituitary glands of cadavers. In the U.S. and Britain such contamination became apparent in 1985, although all the exposures were plausibly from before 1977. When the fatal cases appeared in 1985, however, human growth hormone was available in a genetically engineered form. Both the U.S. and Britain immediately stopped using the hormone collected from cadavers and switched to the safe version.

In France, for reasons that are not clear, however, the authorities decided to continue to use human sources of growth hormone, but to treat the pituitary extracts with urea, which had previously been shown to eliminate 99 percent of the agent that causes scrapie in sheep, another disease caused by a slow virus. By 1993, however, one new CJD case a month was emerging in France and there was talk of indicting with murder the scientists who decided not to use the gene-engineered hormone. CJD is incurable, brain destroying, and fatal.

The Prion Hypothesis

The idea that prions can transmit disease without nucleic acids was first proposed for scrapie in the 1960s by J. Griffith of Bedford College in London, but did not become popular until rediscovered by Stanley Prusiner of the University of California at San Francisco in the early 1980s. There has been a lot of resistance to prions because: (1) if there is no nucleic acid (RNA or DNA) in prions then it is difficult to see how the number of prions can increase after transmission; (2) recognized prions appear to be normal proteins that are present in all brains; and (3) some suspected prion-induced diseases, including some instances of CJD and a dementia called Gerstmann-Sträussler-Scheinken syndrome (GSS), are inherited. Also, prions clearly come in different varieties, called strains, that have somewhat different symptoms; this variation seems unusual for anything other than a living creature or virus that contains a nucleic acid with which to transmit the variation.

Although scoffed at, prions were shown to exist in animal models through genetic engineering in an experiment by Prusiner and coworkers in 1990.

The prion concept received a rehearing in London on September 22-23, 1993, in

---

Background

Diseases known to be associated with slow viruses or prions include scrapie (a neurological disease of sheep that was the first clearly identified disease of this type), kuru (a rare brain disease of humans found in an isolated part of New Guinea), Creutzfeldt-Jakob disease (known as CJD; another rare human brain disease that, like kuru, can be transmitted by contact with infected brain tissue), and mad cow disease (officially bovine spongiform encephalopathy or BSE, a form of scrapie that began to infect cattle in Britain starting in 1986). Known slow-virus diseases are quite rare in humans. During the past decade, however, there has also been evidence that something like prions are a part of or perhaps the cause of the common human brain disease known as Alzheimer's disease, but this is far from certain. For one thing, a different protein from PrP is involved in Alzheimer's.

The protein PrP is produced by the gene *PRNP* which is located on the short arm of chromosome 20. Different alleles of the PrP, known generically as PrP^c, cause such hereditary diseases as Gerstmann-Sträussler-Sheinker syndrome (GSS), CJD, or the very recently discovered (in 1992) fatal familial insomnia. The latter two diseases were traced in 1992 by a large team of researchers to specific point mutations of the PrP gene.

part as a result of new research that followed the outbreak of mad cow disease (BSE). Although some scientists continued to argue that only nucleic acids could produce the observed results of experiments with mad cow disease and other animals, even the people arguing for this point of view were unable to find any nucleic acids in their own preparations. Belief that there are nucleic acids in slow viruses was more a matter of faith, which was too much for Prusiner, who stuck by his previous views at the London conference.

Prusiner also has shown that prions are recognizably different from the normal protein present in all brains, which is known as PrP. In 1991 he had been able to demonstrate that the disease causing version of PrP, known as PrP^c, is resistant to chemicals that break down ordinary PrP.

Charles Weissmann of the University of Zurich, who has long been investigating slow viruses, and coworkers reported to the London conference that they had produced mice in which the protein PrP was "knocked out." Mice that lack PrP are unable to be infected by slow viruses, which suggests that the prion version of PrP, or PrP^c, somehow transforms the normal protein over a long period of time. While this explanation would account for all the data, it still lacks a convincing mechanism by which the transformation could take place. The one favored by Prusiner is that PrP^c is just a different conformation of the protein. Somehow the PrP^c causes PrP to change to the other conformation, which many think requires proteins to behave in an unexpected way for a chemical, even a protein.

In another transgenic mouse experiment, Prusiner's group showed that mice given the gene for the form of the PrP^c protein that leads to GSS dementia develop the disease. More telling, when the brain tissue from the GSS mice is transplanted into wild-type mice, the recipients soon develop GSS dementia.

The London locale for the conference where the re-evaluation of the prion concept took place is no surprise. People in beef-loving Britain are afraid that mad cow disease, or BSE, could spread to humans who consume meat and, especially, brains from contaminated calves or steers. BSE has been traced in its initial outbreak to cattle feed contaminated with sheep meat (presumably infected with scrapie) and a change in the way the feed was processed. After new policies started in 1988 to insure that no sheep meat could be mixed into cattle feed, BSE began to abate somewhat. But then there was a second wave, ultimately traced to meat from cattle that had been used in place of sheep meat. In the meantime, the disease has spread via beef products in pet or animal food to cats and zoo animals. While there is no evidence that any humans have contracted BSE, the possibility seems too serious not to investigate. Although there is no question of experimenting on actual humans, tests with mice that have human genes will be completed soon and should reveal to what extent humans might be susceptible to mad cow disease.

A reassuring fact is that humans have been eating scrapie-infected sheep and even sheep's brains for hundreds of years, but apparently have not been infected.

(Periodical References and Additional Reading. *Harvard Health Letter* 11-90, p 1; *Science* 10-30-92, p 806; *Science* 12-4-92, p 1571; *Science* 7-30-93, p 543; *Nature* 9-30-93, p 386; *Science* 10-8-93, p 180)

Virus UPDATE

You haven't felt well for several days, so you visit the company nurse or some other medical advisor. The report: "It's just that virus that's going around. Get some rest and you'll be better in a day or two." No drugs prescribed. No blood tests. No cultures taken. What's going on?

No drugs are prescribed because almost no drugs are effective against viral agents. A blood test could reveal only that your immune system had been activated, since a virus is too small to see except in special preparations in an electron microscope. No cultures are taken in part because of the impossibility of growing a virus except in living cells.

Although scientists have known that viruses exist and cause disease almost as long as they have known the same information about bacteria, viruses are ultimately much more of a puzzle. Although a vaccine for a viral disease—rabies—was among the first developed, it has been only in the past 50 years that any understanding of how a virus infects or causes disease has been reached. But progress is being made rapidly on all fronts today (*see also* "The Calamity of a Viral Medicine," p 335). A few medicines have become available to treat viral diseases, and more are likely on the way.

Infection

Although the main purpose of a virus is to produce more copies of itself, it has to get into the interior of a cell and often into the nucleus of the cell to achieve that goal. As scientists began to understand viruses better in the early 1990s, some of the surprising ways that viruses have developed in order to infect became known.

First the virus must attach itself to a suitable cell, which it does by being grabbed by a cell receptor. The receptor molecules have evolved to bring specific proteins or other chemicals through the cell membrane and into the cell for the cell's own uses. Some varieties of virus have evolved to have a part of their outer envelope resemble molecules that the receptors are intended to grab. As a result, a receptor takes hold of a virus as the germ passes the cell, wraps the virus in a nice bit of cell membrane, and pulls the package into the interior of the cell as sort of a gift-wrapped letter bomb. Other viruses have their own mechanism for attaching to a cell's outer membrane.

Another problem solved by viral evolution is getting the virus out of the membrane wrapping or through the outer membrane and into the part of the cell where it can take over. In the May 21, 1993 issue of *Cell*, researchers reported on how the influenza virus manages the first part of this task. Certain peptides (short chains of amino acids) in the viral envelope act as springs. After the virus is carried into the cell by a receptor, conditions within the membrane wrapping become more acidic. The acidity loosens the hold on the peptide springs, and part of the coat springs into a new configuration, pushing it against the membrane and allowing the part of the virus adapted for getting through the membrane to do its work. The AIDS virus, which also is taken into cells by a receptor, is thought to use a similar mechanism.

Viruses and Sex

Until recently, when one thought of sexually transmitted diseases (STDs to health workers), one thought of bacteria. The best known STDs were syphilis and gonorrhea,

Background

A virus is a far cry from the obvious complexity of the organism that causes malaria or from the less-obvious complexity of the bacterium that causes cholera. A virus is so simple that it would not be classified as alive by most criteria, being only an order of magnitude or two more complex than a protein such as insulin. Some viruses are known almost atom for atom and artificial viruses have been constructed.

It helps to begin to understand viruses by thinking about crystals. Crystals are formed by most simple chemicals, including elements and simple compounds such as sodium chloride (table salt). A given crystal has a definite structure that develops from interactions among atoms or molecules of the same material, usually even when the arrangement was previously unstructured. In some cases, however, a "seed" crystal needs to be present to provide the initial structure.

Some compounds arrange themselves into a different crystal form to match a given seed crystal. Thus crystals grow and reproduce a particular form, although crystals are not alive.

Although a virus is more alive than an inorganic crystal, a virus is such a simple organic chemical that it too can be crystallized, with all the ordinary properties of a crystal. The differences between a virus and an inorganic crystal grade into each other and do not have a sharp division. For example, certain kinds of inorganic crystals in clay have been shown to evolve following rules of natural selection. Proteins, somewhat higher on the chain of being, not only evolve, but as prions (*see* "Prions Revisited," p 339) appear to replicate their structure and cause disease in animals. Both crystals and proteins, however, need to have very specific components available for replication. Viruses have evolved to become expert in using available mechanisms to assemble more of their own kind from varied precursors.

Most viruses consist of a strand or two of genetic material (the genome, which is a nucleic acid polymer) along with a protein *envelope* (sometimes called a *coat*) to enclose the genetic material. There is a basic division between viruses based on RNA and those based on DNA, the two different types of nucleic acid that are used as genetic material. All viruses use their genetic material to take over part of a living cell, which they then direct to produce more copies. A typical virus has just enough instructions on its genome to produce copies of the genome and the envelope and to provide for a mechanism for bringing them together. No further instructions are needed.

The taxonomy of viruses is not as well developed as that of plants and animals, but viruses can be classified into eight groups that have related structures within a group. Here is a brief description of these classes with examples of human diseases that viruses in each class (except the last two) cause:

- Unenveloped plus-strand RNA (many colds, poliomyelitis)
- Enveloped plus-strand RNA (some cancers, AIDS, yellow fever)
- Minus-strand RNA (flu, mumps, rabies)
- Double-stranded RNA (Colorado tick fever)
- Small-genome DNA (viral hepatitis, warts)
- Medium- and large-genome DNA (herpes, chicken pox (shingles), some cancers, smallpox)
- Bacteriophages (infect bacteria only)
- Viroids—single-stranded unenveloped RNA (infect plants only)

both caused by bacteria. But antibiotics greatly reduced the risk of each, although gonorrhea is still widespread and has developed antibiotic-resistant forms. The most common STD in the U.S. is still a bacterial disease: the disease is chlamydia, which although it can also be cured with antibiotics, has run rampant through the sexually active population largely because it is often symptomless (especially in women) and because until the past few years it was unrecognized by many physicians.

For the past quarter of a century, however, much of the concern about STDs has focused on the one in five infections caused by one or another of four different sexually transmitted viruses. Now that syphilis can be controlled by antibiotics in most cases, some viral STDs are the most deadly sexually transmitted diseases, with the most famous, AIDS, still invariably (or nearly invariably) fatal (*see* "The State of the AIDS Epidemic," p 349, and "AIDS Prevention and Treatment," p 353). AIDS aside, the most common viral STD, known as human papilloma virus, or HPV, is thought to cause cancer. The next most common, genital herpes, can kill or blind newborn babies. The third most common viral STD, hepatitis B, can cause chronic liver disease and is thought to lead to liver cancer in some instances.

Treatment options for all viral diseases are limited.

For HPV it is possible to remove the warts by chemicals, freezing, or laser or conventional surgery. Often, however, the most damaging warts for women are located where they can go unnoticed until they produce cancer.

The epidemic of genital herpes that preceded AIDS in quelling sexual activity also led to the first successful medicine against a viral disease. Medical treatment does not cure herpes, which can retire to a hiding place in nerve cells for long periods of time, but it does alleviate symptoms.

Hepatitis B is usually "self-limiting," which means that, like such viral diseases as the common cold, it eventually succumbs to the immune system. However, until that happens—it can take weeks or months—the disease is acute and only symptoms can be treated, not the disease itself. In some cases, the immune system cannot rid the body of the virus and the infection becomes chronic.

STD INCIDENCE IN U.S.

Disease	Cause	Annual incidence
Chlamydia	Bacterium	4 million cases
Trichomoniasas	Parasite	3 million cases
Gonorrhea	Bacterium	1.1 million cases
AIDS and HIV	Virus	1,000,000 infected with virus (HIV) of which about 80,000 have AIDS symptoms
HPV	Virus	50,000 to 1 million cases
Genital herpes	Virus	200,000 to 500,000 active cases (chronic infection in 31 million)
Hepatitis B	Virus	100,000 to 200,000 active cases (chronic infection in 1.5 million)
Syphilis	Bacterium	120,000 cases

(Periodical References and Additional Reading: *New York Times* 4-1-93, p A1; *Science* 5-29-93, p 340)

THROUGH THE ALPHABET WITH HEPATITIS

There is a disease that was unknown until a few years ago; examination of stored blood samples suggests that the disease did not even exist to any observable extent 50 years ago. The disease is caused by a virus that was not identified until the 1980s. No one who contracts this disease ever recovers from it, although it may take many years for the symptoms to appear. When the symptoms do appear, the disease can be fatal. Among the common ways the disease can be contracted are by shared needles for intravenous drug use and contaminated blood transfusions, but it is a disease of poverty in any case. There is not a very good treatment available and little hope of developing a vaccine.

This disease is *not* AIDS. Indeed, the disease in question, now known as hepatitis C, is three times as prevalent as AIDS, according to one survey of patients admitted to hospital emergency wards.

Liver Disease Through the Ages

The ancients could not help but be aware of the liver, since it is the largest internal organ in humans. Livers of nonhumans were important as food items and for use in foretelling the future. Ancient writers such as Galen recognized three principal organs—the heart, the brain, and the liver—and often the liver seemed to be the most important. Indeed, a well-functioning liver is essential to health.

Like other organs, the liver can become infected. For unknown reasons the infections that are specific to the liver are all viral. The Latin term for "inflammation of the liver" is *hepatitis,* so that is the general name for such diseases, although more careful physicians speak of "acute viral hepatitis."

The history of modern medicine is marked with a persistent feeling that previously identified causes must account for current diseases. The germ theory of disease recognized that disease could be spread by infected substances, as polluted water may carry cholera; or through the air for diseases such as measles; or by direct physical contact with ill people, as smallpox was often spread. Thus there was a natural predisposition to assume that hepatitis was similarly transmitted, especially since there were sometimes outbreaks that could be linked to such a transmission route.

During World War II, however, a major outbreak of serious hepatitis quickly led to discovery of another mode for transmission of the disease. A newly developed vaccine intended to protect U.S. troops against yellow fever had to be withdrawn quickly when the vaccine was found to be the cause of the hepatitis outbreak. The vaccine had been made from human blood products. Research into this kind of hepatitis after the war—as well as deliberate exposures to radioactive substances, experimental nontreatment of syphilis, and administration of psychedelic drugs to unsuspecting personnel—can be counted as one of the serious abuses of research in the name of science. Children with Down's syndrome and prisoners were deliberately injected with infected blood to determine the cause and progress of the newly discovered form of hepatitis.

As a result of these experiments, however, physicians realized that there were two different viruses that infected the liver by different routes, so they designated them as

Background

The earliest symptom of hepatitis for many infected persons is jaundice, a yellowish cast to the skin or whites of the eyes caused by poor liver function. Other symptoms include those similar to various "flus," such as nausea, loss of appetite, vomiting or diarrhea, and fatigue. As with most viral illnesses, after a time (often about six weeks for hepatitis) the immune system wins and all the symptoms go away.

But sometimes the disease takes a sharp turn for the worse. Acute hepatitis (from any cause) is known as fulminant hepatitis and may affect the brain, resulting in coma or even death. (*Fulminant* means that it occurs suddenly and intensely.)

In other instances, the disease symptoms go away, but the virus continues to infect liver cells, a condition called "chronic." In some cases, the chronic hepatitis has no further effect on the human host, but it is able to spread to other humans by its particular transmission route. In other instances, chronic hepatitis can lead to the scarring of the liver called cirrhosis. Severe cirrhosis interferes with liver function, which causes death.

Hepatitis A   This virus is transmitted enterically to people who have previously developed no immunity against the disease, so there are frequent outbreaks caused by a single source of contamination. ("Enterically" means that an infected person sheds the virus in fecal matter, which contaminates water supplies or food, directly or indirectly via the water; drinking the water or eating the food passes the virus on to a new host.) In 1991 about 29,000 cases of hepatitis A were reported in the U.S., but it is thought that many cases go unrecognized. The main therapy is bed rest, although sometimes a mixture of antibodies taken from donated blood and known as gamma globulin may be injected in the hopes of mitigating symptoms or preventing transmission. Hepatitis A can be identified with a commercial blood test.

In 1992, tests indicated that a new vaccine was effective against hepatitis A.

Hepatitis B   This virus is usually transmitted by blood or blood products or by sexual contact, although mothers sometimes transmit it to newborns shortly after birth. Infection with hepatitis B can be mild and fairly short-lived, as it is in many cases. Half of all infections cause no symptoms at all. Some estimates are that one out of 20 Americans will have hepatitis B at some time in their lives, but more than half of these will not notice it. But the B virus can lead to various serious symptoms or complications. Hepatitis B can become fulminant, or occur as an acute attack. When hepatitis B fails to go away, it becomes chronic (five to ten percent of all patients). Finally, hepatitis B is thought to cause liver cancer in a fairly high percentage of cases. It can be identified by a commercial blood test.

Vaccines have been developed for this disease; the one currently used is manufactured by genetic engineering, so it cannot infect the person vaccinated. Once suggested for high-risk individuals only, the vaccine is now part of the standard series of vaccinations for infants.

Hepatitis C   Primarily spread by blood products, it is also thought that there is a slight chance of transmission of hepatitis C by sexual contact, though it is not proven. About 70 percent of those who test positive for the virus have no symptoms at all. Nearly everyone becomes chronically infected. About 60 percent of those chronically infected have enough inflammation that the disease can be detected by a commercial blood test. Tests for carriers who do not have an inflamed liver are used only by specialists. Although very high among poverty-stricken people tested, the virus shows up only about one in 200 times among healthy blood donors. Nevertheless, it is estimated that about 150,000 new cases of hepatitis C occur each year in the U.S., leading to 8000 to 10,000 deaths.

Hepatitis D, or the delta factor   In this case, the infectious agent is more like a viroid (a plant pathogen that consists almost entirely of nucleic acid) than like a virus. The hepatitis D virus needs to use the envelope from hepatitis B to infect cells, so it is a "co-factor" of that disease. For a person with both the B virus and the delta factor, the probability that fulmination or cirrhosis will occur is enhanced, as compared to a person with B only. A person without a hepatitis B infection cannot contract hepatitis D, however. A commercial blood test is available for hepatitis D as well.

Hepatitis E   A viral disease transmitted by the same paths as hepatitis A, largely through what physicians have called "enteric means." In addition to being caused by a different virus than hepatitis A, which can be determined only with advanced blood tests, hepatitis E is known primarily from outbreaks in developing nations of Africa and Asia. Although there were two outbreaks in Mexico in 1986, it has not been detected in the U.S. except sporadically in travelers.

infectious hepatitis and serum hepatitis. More experience with the diseases demonstrated that "serum" hepatitis was spread in other ways as well, and it was also "infectious." The names of the two liver diseases were changed to the noncommittal hepatitis A (formerly "infectious") and hepatitis B (formerly "serum").

Hepatitis B is not only transmitted by blood products, but it is also a sexually transmitted disease (STD). It was found to be rampant in the male homosexual community during a period when there was a great deal of promiscuity in that community.

Then in 1975 some patients who got blood transfusions in hospitals developed yet another form of hepatitis, which came to be called nonA, nonB. This virus appeared to be transmitted only in blood. The virus became known as hepatitis C after it was isolated in 1987. Since 1990, when a blood test for hepatitis C became available, physicians have learned that C is by far the most common hepatitis, infecting about 20 to 40 percent of people coming for treatment to inner city hospitals and about 80 percent of intravenous drug users. For a virus whose only definitely known method of transmission is via blood, these figures are amazingly high.

Recognition that there were more than two viruses soon led to the identification of hepatitis D, also known as delta, and hepatitis E. At this point, the possibility of a "Hepatitis F" cannot be ruled out. The old "nonA, nonB" hepatitis was recognized in three forms: long incubation, short incubation, and enterically transmitted. The first of these is now hepatitis C, while the last is hepatitis E. Thus short-incubation, nonA, nonB hepatitis may someday become F.

Hepatitis C, New Kid on the Block

Although the existence of hepatitis C has been officially recognized since 1975, and the infection is now very common, there is evidence that hepatitis C did not exist or was at least rare only 50 years ago. Stored blood samples from World War II fail to test positive for the disease. Work with hepatitis B in the 1960s found many puzzling cases of liver disease that seemed to be something different from B, and these are now largely assumed to be hepatitis C. Thus the disease became widespread in the 1950s. This period coincides with the first wave of intravenous drug use in the U.S., and that may not be a coincidence.

Although hepatitis C is known to be transmitted by blood only, about 30 percent of those with the disease have no record of transfusions or recollection of intravenous drug use. It is believed that subtler forms of blood transfer may have taken place, such as use of the same toothbrush. There is no evidence that sexual contact is a factor. For example, only a few homosexual men have hepatitis C (about twice the rate of healthy blood donors), while hepatitis B is endemic to homosexual men, reaching perhaps as much as 80 percent of the population, suggesting that hepatitis B may be sexually transmitted.

Since February 26, 1992, treatment of hepatitis C with genetically engineered alpha interferon has been approved by the U.S. Food and Drug Administration. It is a long-term treatment, not a cure. The drug must be given three times a week for six months, providing symptomatic improvement without a relapse in about 25 percent of the patients. Alpha interferon is also helpful in restoring liver function in patients with hepatitis B.

The good news concerning hepatitis C is that in one study of those permanently infected with the virus, the death rate over 20 years was no higher than the background rate of the population who were not infected.

(Periodical References and Additional Reading: *Harvard Health Letter* 10-90, p 3; *New York Times* 2-26-91, p D1; *New York Times* 8-13-92, p D19; *New York Times* 12-31-92, p A20; *New York Times* 1-19-93, p C1)

THE STATE OF
THE AIDS EPIDEMIC

AIDS is the Acquired Immune Deficiency Syndrome that has taken almost 300,000 lives in the U.S. and probably about 2 million worldwide. Unknown to medicine before 1980, the existence of AIDS is one of the central facts of medicine and life in the early 1990s. In 1985 it was possible to summarize the state of the AIDS epidemic for people who were not homosexual nor intravenous drug users as follows (from the 1986 *Facts on File Scientific Yearbook):*

> Soon, many Americans feared AIDS more than they had feared any recent deadly disease. It was not clear at all, however, that these fears made sense for most of the population. . . . There were some indications that the rate had been slowing down since the first recognition of the disease . . . there were many signs that the average American did not need to fear the disease. Most of the people with the disease were homosexual, and some authorities pointed to evidence that the disease was unlikely to spread by typical heterosexual contacts. . . . [F]or people not in one of the high-risk groups, the chance of contracting AIDS is calculated as less than one in 1,000,000. . . . So far, no one has recovered from AIDS. . . .

The situation was not well understood then and is quite different today.

In 1985, the U.S. government could virtually ignore heterosexually transmitted AIDS. The raging epidemic among heterosexuals in sub-Saharan Africa had been barely recognized even there. The similar occurrence of heterosexual transmission in Haiti was noticed, but American medical authorities downplayed news of AIDS in general among Haitians in the U.S. and in Haiti, thereby trying to counteract claims that the authorities were discriminating against Haitians.

Careful statistics reveal that in the early 1990s the group most at risk for AIDS in technologically advanced nations consists precisely of young people practicing heterosexual sex. For example in England and Wales, though new AIDS cases among homosexuals rose to nearly 5000 at the peak of the homosexual epidemic in 1983, new AIDS cases among homosexuals fell to a tenth of that amount by the early 1990s. In the meantime, new heterosexual AIDS cases increased at a steady rate, and by the early 1990s the cases reached an incidence level three times that of the homosexual population.

The experience of the past ten years shows how difficult it is to say where all this is going. One thought has been to compare the incidence of AIDS to that of other sexually transmitted diseases. One somewhat comparable statistic comes from the records of London's maternity wards. Genital herpes, which has been recognized as epidemic for about twice as long as AIDS has and which spreads by similar mechanisms, appears to have reached about seven to ten percent of pregnant white women in their late 30s in London. If this is extrapolated to other populations in other developed countries, it suggests that the increase in the heterosexual population can still continue.

AIDS in the U.S.

Echoing the "reassuring" reports of 1985, however, on February 4, 1993, a panel of the National Research Council of the U.S. National Academy of Sciences reported that AIDS continues to have little impact on the daily life of most Americans. Instead, the disease has from the beginning injured primarily socially disadvantaged or poor people, including homosexuals and intravenous drug users, but also the very poor and the less educated heterosexuals who do not abuse drugs. Middle- and upper-class Americans in the "mainstream" continue to escape the epidemic. On the other hand, the panel recognized a major impact among what they termed "marginalized" Americans.

Despite the opinion of the National Research Council, the U.S. Centers for Disease Control and Prevention (CDC) reported on July 23, 1993, in their *Morbidity and Mortality Weekly Report* that "infection with HIV is spreading slowly, but relentlessly, into all sectors of our society."

By the end of the first quarter of 1993, for example, the CDC's new definition of AIDS was doubling the number of reported American cases. Even under the old definition, the increase in American cases was 21 percent. All told, the number of new cases reported to the CDC in 1992 was 47,095 with perhaps as many as 100,000 expected for 1993 using the new definition. Although more and more cases continued to be reported each year, the amount of growth was slowing down somewhat, at least under the older definition. It was thought that AIDS itself would reach about 600,000 Americans by the end of 1995, including about 350,000 who would die from the disease by that year and 250,000 with manifest symptoms. About the same number with AIDS (that is, an additional 600,000 people) will have HIV infection and no symptoms at that time.

But even when the illness does not directly infect self, family, or close friends, AIDS still affects everyone. For example, AIDS and even HIV infection without AIDS has produced financial strains on the U.S. health establishment. The official figures at the start of 1993 claimed that two cents out of every hospital dollar was spent on AIDS. One study released in the May 12, 1993 *Journal of the American Medical Association* found, however, that costs of AIDS treatment were underestimated because additional hospital costs associated with HIV positive individuals had been omitted.

AIDS—A Worldwide Epidemic

The World Health Organization's (WHO) international AIDS conference in Berlin in June 1993 included a WHO prediction of 40 million AIDS cases worldwide by the year 2000. This figure can be compared with the current figure that was commonly used in 1993, which estimated that 14 million around the world had the disease. AIDS infection is so heavy in sub-Saharan Africa (six million or so infected in the early 1990s) that the disease may completely halt the swift population growth of the region, population growth that has characterized Africa since the 1960s. It is now generally recognized that the AIDS epidemic got its start in Uganda and it is still most pervasive in that country and in its neighboring countries. At the end of 1993 almost 70 percent of all the people in the world infected with the HIV virus were in Africa.

Although Africa has long had more than its share of the disease, the early 1990s found AIDS becoming common in regions around the world where it was rare or unknown in the 1980s.

In the East, the governments of India, Japan, and Myanmar denied the possibility of AIDS right until they found that their own countries had become a big part of the epidemic. By the end of the 1990s it is expected that Asians will surpass Africans as the main population victimized by the AIDS epidemic, mainly because there are just more people in Asia than there are in Africa, or anywhere else for that matter. Three quarters of the spread of AIDS from person to person in Asia is thought to be from heterosexual relations.

Denial also has fueled a worsening situation in Latin America. From fewer than 10,000 cases in the mid-1980s, the number of people with AIDS in Latin America has soared to more than 60,000 cases in the early 1990s. The number infected with HIV who have not yet developed AIDS is startlingly high. Brazil, for example, is thought to have as many HIV-infected persons as the U.S., but the total population of Brazil is only two-thirds that of the U.S.

The collapse of communism and its organized health care has helped the rise of AIDS in Eastern and Central Europe, another region in which the official line had been that AIDS would not penetrate their nations very deeply because their citizens did not engage in promiscuous sex.

Around the world, half of the new infections in the early 1990s were occurring in people younger than the age of 25; in Africa, young people are about 60 percent of those infected. Furthermore, as the epidemic has progressed, AIDS has affected women more than it did previously, so that by 1992 the number of newly infected women worldwide was about the same as the number of new cases in men. In the U.S., the number of AIDS cases among women was increasing at a rate four times faster than the men's rate.

Efforts to Stop the Epidemic

While most of the reports concerning treatments or vaccines have been discouraging—even those scientific advances that at first appeared to be breakthroughs usually were found to be useless or at least not very useful—there have been a few signs of hope. One such beacon has been the discovery of people who are regularly exposed to the HIV virus and yet fail to become infected. Another has been a small group of people who are known to have been infected by HIV for eight or more years, but who show no signs of developing AIDS. While there is a small, but highly vocal, group of iconoclastic scientists who say that this latter result means that HIV does not cause AIDS at all or is only one of many causes, very few scientists think that these critics are correct. But if it is true that HIV causes AIDS, then it would appear that at least some human immune systems are capable of preventing the transition from quiet infection to active and deadly disease.

Health experts, however, do not think that for the near future any medical breakthroughs in developing new medicines, vaccines, or understandings will be as helpful as prevention through education. For example, it is thought that if a vaccine of ordinary effectiveness were available in 1995, it would be 15 years or more before it affected the rate of AIDS deaths. But if people do not themselves contract AIDS because they do not engage in behavior that causes AIDS—e.g.; unprotected sex, sharing needles—then they also cannot spread the disease. This is the multiplier effect of prevention. Prevention in women is particularly important, not only because women are the fastest-growing group in the epidemic, but also because they can pass the disease on to children. In developing countries, as many as 25 to 30 percent of women with AIDS pass the disease on to their children, while figures are only slightly less in the developed nations.

Education can make a difference. Haiti was one of the first nations to be hit hard by AIDS, but efforts in the 1980s to give away condoms for prevention were met with indifference by most Haitians. An educational campaign that uses Haitian culture as its basis, however, has made condoms a part of life in the nation in the early 1990s.

An Animal Model for AIDS

AIDS research has been hampered by lack of a good animal model. The only known animal that can be infected with HIV is our close cousin, the endangered chimpanzee, but so far chimpanzees infected with the virus do not become ill.

Mike McCune and Jerome Zack of Systemix Corporation in Palo Alto, California, have apparently filled the need for an animal model by using human tissue, but in another species. Mice without an immune system, or naked mice, were given cells from the human immune system, specifically liver cells (which are the stem cells of the fetus) and thymus cells. The naked mice, also known as SCID mice because they are born with what in humans is called Severe Combined Immunity Deficiency (SCID), then become the variant SCID-hu.

Early experiments with SCID-hu mice show that they can be infected with HIV and that the human immune system in the mice eventually begins to disappear, as happens in AIDS.

Among the advantages of the SCID-hu mice is that they are not endangered, expensive, and slow-breeding primates. Furthermore, they are now the only animals other than humans that can develop a form of AIDS.

The Non-HIV Scare

In 1985 the first general screening of the blood supply for the recently discovered virus now known as Human Immunodeficiency Virus 1 (HIV-1) was just getting under way. The "AIDS virus" had been identified by teams in France and the U.S. during the period 1983-84. Later a related virus, HIV-2, was found to cause AIDS in some parts of Africa. Although a few scientists have to this day claimed that HIV-1 and HIV-2 are not the cause of AIDS, nearly everyone thinks that the case against the two viruses is closed.

The issue revived, however, when headlines in 1992 proclaimed that instances of AIDS, the syndrome, were occurring around the world without accompanying infection by HIV-1 or HIV-2, the virus. The commotion began on July 21, 1992 at an international AIDS conference, when Jeffrey Laurence of Cornell University Medical School claimed five cases of AIDS-like illness had been caused by a different virus. Sudhir Gupta of the University of California at Irvine also claimed a different virus had caused two cases of AIDS. David Ho of the Aaron Diamond AIDS Research Center in New York City, New York, reported that he had identified 11 cases of AIDS without HIV infection. Other researchers reported up to a half-dozen such cases in their own clinical practice. By the end of the day the number mentioned at the conference was about 25 or 30, depending on how some reports were counted. A few of these non-HIV illnesses had also been reported earlier, but had received no public response.

The flurry of concern mounted for a few days. Eventually about a hundred cases of AIDS around the world with no noticeable HIV infection were identified. By the end of September 1992 it was generally agreed that something other than the HIV virus could cause immune deficiencies of unknown origin, but that this situation was not a major cause for public concern. On February 11, 1993, there were six reports in the *New England Journal of Medicine* that discussed the syndrome, which had been labeled "idiopathic CD4-positive T-lymphocytopenia," or ICL. Not only did scientists still not know what caused ICL, but they could not predict the clinical course of the disease. Some with ICL, unlike anyone known with AIDS, simply recover—but others die. ICL does not appear to be contagious by any known route.

(Periodical References and Additional Reading: *New York Times* 6-22-92, p A8; *New York Times* 7-21-92, p C3; *New York Times* 7-22-92, p A1; *New York Times* 7-23-92, p B8; *New York Times* 7-28-92, p C3; *New York Times* 11-8-92, p I-13; *New York Times* 1-15-93, p A12; *New York Times* 1-25-93, p A1; *New York Times* 2-5-93, p A15; *New York Times* 2-7-93, p I-30; *Science News* 2-20-93, p 119; *New York Times* 4-8-93, p A2; *New York Times* 4-30-93, p A18; *New York Times* 5-13-93, p A18; *Nature* 6-3-93, pp 393, 466; *New York Times* 7-6-93, p 10; *New York Times* 6-15-93, p C1; *New York Times* 7-15-93, p A4; *Science News* 7-31-93, p 68; *New York Times* 12-13-93, p B8; *Discover* 1-94, pp 46, 48)

AIDS PREVENTION AND TREATMENT

At the end of 1993, U.S. Secretary of Health and Human Services Donna E. Shalala announced at a news conference that "the sad fact remains that not a single new drug application for an anti-retroviral drug" was pending at that time. Almost six months earlier, the chairperson of the experts at a U.S. National Institutes of Health AIDS symposium made comments such as "we are in the infancy, I hope, of being able to treat this disease effectively" (Merle A. Sande of the University of California at San Francisco). He said that AIDS was a long way even from being controlled, much less cured.

Viral diseases are difficult to treat. Until recently, there were no drugs that attacked the virus itself, in the way antibiotics attack bacteria. Earlier drugs for viral diseases relieved a few symptoms only. Even today, the number of effective viral drugs can be numbered on one hand without using all the fingers (*see* "The Calamity of a Viral Medicine," p 335). Nothing like an antibiotic has surfaced, which suggests that bacteria, molds and other fungi, and other living creatures have failed as much as humans have in creating simple chemical antidotes to viral diseases. (Antibiotics, of course, were first found among chemicals produced by molds and so forth to protect themselves against bacteria.)

AIDS Vaccines

Fortunately for humans, most viral diseases can be fought and eventually conquered by the body's system of defenses that collectively form the immune system. One of the main problems with AIDS is that its point of attack—i.e., certain leukocytes—are key elements in this line of defense. Thus AIDS, unlike a cold, does not simply "go away" after a week or so.

Vaccines are often able to improve the odds against viral diseases. The purpose of any vaccine is to shore up the immune system for facing a particular challenge, so it is far from impossible for an AIDS vaccine to accomplish such a goal.

The first really positive results of AIDS-vaccine trials in humans that were reported and generally accepted came in the summer of 1993, but at that time the results only involved 28 people unlikely to be exposed to AIDS for one reason or another. Although nine of the ten humans who received a higher dose of the vaccine developed changes in their blood that suggested immunity to AIDS, no one was willing to take the dangerous step of challenging those humans deliberately by infecting them with the HIV virus. Instead, a new trial was planned that administered the AIDS-vaccine to persons whose lifestyles might cause them to encounter the HIV virus in a natural setting. Few would be willing to believe that the vaccine really was effective until either direct challenges were made or massive field trials showed general protection. This experimental vaccine was genetically engineered to resemble the outer coating of the HIV virus.

Later in the year, however, there had been no other glimmer of hope for any of the experimental vaccines (see below), all of which failed laboratory tests, which were not human trials. Defenders claimed the tests were at fault.

The Unending Saga of gp160

Any legislation affecting AIDS is controversial. One of the more striking examples recently has been the flap about testing the experimental vaccine against HIV known as gp160, a name derived from the weight of the glycoprotein fragment on the HIV envelope that the vaccine uses as an antigen. When the U.S. National Institutes of Health refused to give a developer of a gp160 vaccine special considerations, the developer, MicroGenSys of Meriden, Connecticut, took its problems to congresspersons Sam Nunn (Democrat-Georgia) and John Warner (Republican-Virginia). At that time both were prominent in supervision of the U.S. military. In 1992, the U.S. Congress appropriated $20 million for the military to conduct human trials of the MicroGenSys vaccine.

Some members of the House became suspicious of the test, however. The House Energy and Commerce subcommittee began to study whether or not there was a valid reason for the armed forces to be involved in the testing of a vaccine for a disease that has primarily affected civilians. All during 1993, the issue went back and forth in the U.S. National Institutes of Health, the House, and the Army. At the end of 1993, the House Energy and Commerce subcommittee arranged for an additional six-month extension for government scientists to study the circumstances of the gp160 trials. Presumably the fate of the vaccine trial will be settled sometime in 1994.

Background

The Smallpox Story   Long before the first vaccines, people noted that some diseases strike a person only once during a lifetime, although others recur. Among the more noticeable examples of a one-time-only disease was smallpox, a common childhood disease that became epidemic among adults in a deadly form in Eurasia during the sixteenth century. Like many childhood diseases of the past, smallpox had been considered a regular part of growing up, albeit more unpleasant in that smallpox left scars that tended to be permanent. Otherwise, a case of smallpox while a child was lifesaving, for although adults often died from the disease, those who had contracted smallpox as children could not be infected with the disease a second time.

Chinese doctors are credited with being the first to learn how to keep the relatively happy event of childhood smallpox from being left to chance. They collected the crusts from smallpox pustules and blew the powder into nostrils of healthy youngsters to provide protection against later bouts of the disease. The children then developed smallpox at a time in their life when it seldom caused complications, and thereafter were immune for life.

When the epidemic of a form of smallpox with a high mortality rate began in Asia and spread west, the concept of infecting children with mild cases of the disease spread along with the epidemic. Methods for infecting children with smallpox became common in Turkey and Africa.

The disease continued to move west, however. By the start of the eighteenth century, about one in ten deaths in London was due to smallpox. Boston also experienced the virulent epidemic at this time. In both cities courageous leaders pushed for adoption of the Turkish or African procedures for protection. Although these leaders were assailed and even bombed for such "barbaric proposals," it soon became clear that the practice, known as *inoculation*, was effective.

Inoculation slowly became recognized in England and the U.S. during the eighteenth century. By 1793 the country doctor Edward Jenner had found an even safer way to induce immunity based upon a disease called cowpox or *vaccinia* (possibly smallpox in a different form, and certainly a close relative of the smallpox virus). Although Jenner also had difficulty getting his method adopted, it soon prevailed in Western nations, who then spread it around the world. Jenner's basic method was so successful that it resulted in the complete elimination of smallpox as a disease in less than 200 years; the last case in the wild occurred in October 1977.

Other Viral Vaccines   Various strategies exist for development of vaccines. The first successful vaccine, the vaccinia virus (cowpox), is unique in being a virus that causes a mild illness that also provokes a strong reaction in the immune system, a reaction powerful enough to protect against a different virus. The next successful viral vaccine was for rabies, produced on the model of early bacterial vaccines; Louis Pasteur, the inventor, created this vaccine mostly through intuition, as Pasteur worked long before there was any clear concept of what a virus was. Working by what amounted to trial and error, Pasteur produced a form of the virus that provoked immunity but that did not cause disease. A hundred years later, these two approaches were melded when genetic techniques were used to attach part of a rabies virus to a vaccinia virus, resulting in a powerful oral vaccine for rabies that could be used in the wild.

In 1953 Jonas Salk attained lasting fame by developing a vaccine for polio based on viruses that had been "killed" by formaldehyde. "Altered" or "inactivated" is more accurate than "killed," since it is not clear that any virus is alive in the same sense as such organisms as bacteria, plants, or animals.

In 1961 and 1962 another approach was taken by Albert Sabin, whose polio vaccine used "live" viruses that had been "attenuated." Although both types of vaccine were successful, the explanation of their preparation in terms of living and dead and attenuated was hardly clear. It was still too early in medical understanding of viruses to know exactly what was producing the immune reaction or why some live viruses cause mild, self-limiting diseases along with immunity, but other live viruses of the same general type cause severe illness or death. Even with present-day knowledge of viruses, the "live" Sabin-type vaccine causes a serious disease about one time in each 4 million doses as a result of differences in the immune system of the persons receiving the vaccine.

Since 1962, both "killed" and "live" viruses have been developed, with the "live" form generally preferred as longer lasting and more effective generally. This was the case with the vaccines developed for measles, for example.

Recently some vaccines have been created from the chemistry set, or at least from the genetic engineering vat. These artificial vaccines, of which the most successful has been one for hepatitis B, do not contain either "live" or "killed" viruses. One of the main advantages of such a genetically engineered product is that it can never induce the illness it is intended to prevent—which has happened in a few cases with "killed" vaccines and often with "live" ones.

A virus consists of two parts: a complex outside known as the viral coat or envelope and an inner core that is a DNA or RNA molecule. (In HIV it is RNA.) Artificial vaccines consist of parts of the viral envelope, which are produced by genetic engineering. Most AIDS vaccines are based on using the envelope proteins of the HIV-1 virus, especially the ones known as glycoproteins (protein-sugar complexes) or parts of proteins, which are called peptides.

There are still a few holdouts who believe that AIDS is caused by something other than the direct action of the viruses named HIV-1 or, more rarely, HIV-2. The evidence, however, continues to mount that AIDS is a standard viral disease with a particularly deadly target. Just as the herpes virus preferentially attacks skin cells and lives safely and quietly in nerve cells, HIV resides mainly in certain cells of the types previously lumped together as "white blood cells," killing some of these leukocytes (Latin for white cells) while merely infecting others. Thus there is some hope for using parts of the HIV-1 virus (and perhaps of HIV-2 as well) to prevent infection with AIDS.

Vaccines on Trial

In mid-1993 at least 16 HIV vaccines were being tested on humans and others on animals, but no one expected any of them to be available before the twenty-first century. These vaccines require extensive tests to insure that there will be no harm from coming close to infection with so deadly a disease.

Candidate vaccine	Developer(s)	Description	Study history
"Killed" whole viruses	Jonas Salk	"Killed" whole viruses	Salk claimed positive immune response in 70 HIV-infected humans.
gp 160 (rpg160)	MicroGenSys ImmunoAG 160 Pasteur-Merieux, Connaught	Genetically engineered version of protein from viral coat	Administered to more than 200 HIV-negative humans before 1991 and some HIV-infected humans; no data released on effectiveness.
gp 120 (rpg120)	Genetech, Inc. Biocene	Different coat protein made by genetic engineering	Protected chimpanzees from HIV infection; a trial with 28 humans resulted in good antibody production in nine of ten who received high doses.
Vaccinia-gp160	Bristol-Myers, Squibb	Vaccinia virus genetically altered to display gp160	
Canarypox-gp160	Pasteur-Merieux, Connaught	Canarypox virus genetically altered to display gp160	
MAPS-V3-Octomers	United Biomedical	Multiple antigenic peptides	
V3 loop unconjugated	Pasteur-Merieux, Connaught		
HGP 30	Viral Technologies	A peptide sequence of an HIV protein named *gag*	
Ty, p24, VLP	British Biotech	A segment of the *gag* protein arranged in the shape of a virus	
V3 loop-purified protein derivative	Swiss Serum and Vaccine Institute		
Vaccinia-gp160 + five envelope products	Various companies	The vaccinia virus re-engineered and various chemicals made by the envelope	
Vaccinia-gp160 + gp160 + three envelope peptides	G. Beaud and coworkers	Re-engineered vaccinia and a glycoprotein and parts of other envelope proteins	

Medications for AIDS

In February 1993, there was a great media celebration of a new strategy for treating AIDS using a combination of three drugs, zidovudine (AZT, tradenamed Retrovir), dideoxyinosine or didanosine (ddI), and pyridinone. "Drug Mixture Halts H.I.V. in Lab, Doctors Say in a Cautious Report" was about the mildest front-page headline.

Part of the attraction to the story was that the person who found the approach,

Yung-Kang Chow, was a Harvard graduate student. Yung-Kang Chow, principal investigator Marvin S. Hirsch, and coworkers at Massachusetts General Hospital in Boston, Massachusetts, reported in the February 18, 1993 *Nature* that the drug combination prevented the HIV virus from infecting cells in the test tube (*in vitro*) because the virus needed too many mutations to adapt to all three of the medications. By end of the year, however, a number of other researchers had found that the HIV virus had additional mutational arrows in its quiver. As a result even *in vitro,* the virus could accommodate the combination of medications. Furthermore, it became apparent that the original research was hurried and sloppy. A trial with 400 human volunteers using the combination continued, however.

In April 1993, Merck Research Laboratory and 14 other pharmaceutical companies signed an agreement to cooperate in the development of drugs for AIDS, especially so that the newest drugs could be tested in various combinations. Among the reasons for using combinations of drugs is that early in 1993 the HIV virus was already showing the ability to evolve resistance to the drug AZT. AZT was first licensed in 1987 and still is the principal drug against the HIV virus. By the end of the year scientists observed that drug-resistant strains tripled the chance of a patient dying in any given time interval.

A European study of AZT, known as Concorde and summarized in *Lancet* on April 3, 1993, caused a considerable stir when it reported that AZT fails to delay the onset of AIDS when administered to HIV-positive individuals before AIDS itself develops. Later in the year, a study in Australia directly contradicted the Concorde results (July 29, 1993 *New England Journal of Medicine*).

Another drug for HIV treatment, zalcitabine (ddC), is already approved and originally was used only in combination with AZT. Tests early in 1993 indicated that it might also be used alone. The media also touted oral alpha interferon, which, under the name Kemron, was supposed to be having success in Africa. Although skeptical, the U.S. National Institutes of Health said on October 26, 1992 that it would sponsor a test of the approach. One of the reasons cited was underground use of the drug. Alpha interferon is legally used in high doses to treat several cancers, including Kaposi's sarcoma, which is a common complication of AIDS.

Even though no new HIV medicines reached application-for-approval stage at the end of 1993, a few new approaches were at earlier stages. Nearly all researchers hoped to emulate the action of penicillin, which works because: (1) it interferes with something needed for a bacterium to reproduce, and (2) that something is not needed by human cells for any function. For the HIV virus a typical promising target has been the gene known as *tat* or perhaps a protein made by *tat*. However, *tat* is probably too similar to human genes for this strategy to be effective without serious side effects.

Surprisingly, an actual antibiotic has been found to block HIV reproduction *in vitro*. Neomycin (and related antibiotics called aminoglycosides) kill bacteria by preventing them from making proteins, thereby interfering with the operation of RNA. Michael Green of the University of Massachusetts noted that the messenger RNA (*see* "The State of Genetic Medicine," p 19) used by HIV and other RNA-based viruses (*see* "Virus UPDATE," p 342) needs a protein called Rev to accomplish its tasks. Blocking the action of Rev with neomycin would be similar to the way antibiotics attack bacteria without killing humans, since humans do not use the Rev-RNA mechanism to make proteins. Green and coworkers reported in September 1993 in *Cell* that neomycin and other aminoglycosides were effective *in vitro,* but the possible side effects in humans were too serious for clinical testing. The scientists hope to produce a modification of the basic antibiotic type that would be safer and yet still do the job. If they succeed, this class of antibiotics might also be used against such viral disease as influenza and the common cold.

Another class of drugs being tried are called protease inhibitors because they block the enzyme protease, used by the HIV virus. Also potent *in vitro,* they tend to bind with blood proteins, which may make them unworkable in clinical practice.

Researchers are trying almost every possible approach. For example, finding that thalidomide affects the immune system, it has also been used in *in vitro* studies against HIV. (Thalidomide, you will recall, is the notorious drug that stops proper development of the limbs of the fetus.)

Treating Secondary Infections

Some of the most effective treatments for an AIDS patient do not attack HIV, but instead are aimed at the various infections or cancers that invade when the immune system is lost. Death is a result of one of these other infections in most cases, and a lot of the misery of terminal AIDS also comes from these infections. These infections may come from bacteria, viruses other than HIV, fungi, or protist parasites.

Bacteria   Among the new drugs used to treat infections in AIDS patients is the antibiotic clarithromycin (trade name, Biaxin), used to treat mycobacterium avian complex, known more often as MAC. MAC is a deadly respiratory infection that spreads rapidly in the body of a person with AIDS, though it is seldom harmful to other persons. MAC strikes about one in four AIDS patients.

Viruses   The cytomegalovirus infections in AIDS patients often attack the eyes, producing CMV retinitis. Ganciclovir, an early anti-virus medication, was used intravenously as a treatment, but study data released late in 1993 showed that an oral form was as effective (foscarnet is also used intravenously for treatment).

Fungi   The anti-fungal medicine fluconazole was shown in another study around the same time to delay *Candida albicans* infection and also the more dangerous and invasive fungal disease cryptococcal meningitis.

Other Treatment Concepts

One of the first unusual treatment concepts was the idea of Jonas Salk and coworkers in 1987 to use a vaccine to slow the progress of the disease rather than to prevent its development outright. Early in the nineteenth century, Almroth Wright experimented with using vaccines of a sort on people already infected with disease. Despite his limited success, he was knighted and has become known to historians of medicine as "Sir Almost Right," which reflects present thought on using a vaccine as a treatment. Results of the use of the Salk vaccine in this way, announced in June 1993, suggested that this approach had small benefits, but not enough for anyone to become very excited at the time. As few other treatments showed any benefit, however, AIDS researchers became more intrigued with the results: the virus, which increased 56 percent a year in HIV-infected controls, increased only 14 percent in patients receiving the vaccine. Another disease marker changed by five percent in a year in the controls, but hardly changed at all in treated patients. And AIDS researchers began to look toward larger and longer trials of the Salk vaccine approach that were scheduled to start near the end of 1994.

In March 1993, the well-known mathematician Leonard Adleman calculated that a new approach to forestalling AIDS might be to remove some of the T cells. This paradoxical idea is based on the observation that HIV only infects and destroys a population of T cells known as CD4s because they have a receptor called CD4 on their surface. The other population of T cells has a different receptor, known as CD8, which cannot be used by HIV to enter the cell. HIV infection turns to AIDS as the number of CD4 T cells becomes very low, but the total number of T cells does not change. It is easy to think that this happens because the body makes CD8 cells to replace the CD4s it is losing. Adleman calculated, however, that the body turns out T cells in the same CD4/CD8 ratio as before, but HIV kills the CD4s while the CD8s live on. The calculations suggest that removal of ten to 15 percent of the body's CD8 cells every six months would restore the CD4/CD8 ratio to normal. Since it is loss of the CD4 cells that ultimately causes AIDS, a person should be able to be maintained on such a regime indefinitely. For this method to succeed, however, researchers must first develop a method of selectively removing the CD8 cells and leaving the CD4s, a method which has not yet been found.

In the July 10, 1992 issue of *Science,* researchers from the Fred Hutchinson Cancer Center in Seattle, Washington, and coworkers reported that they could "train" leukocytes to attack a specific virus. The virus in question was not HIV (it was a virus known as cytomegalovirus), but it was thought that the same technique could be used against HIV and AIDS.

At the end of 1993 Gene M. Sherer of the U.S. National Cancer Institute and coworkers reported in the December 10, 1993 *Science* that interleukin-12 (IL-12), an immune-system chemical (or cytokine) discovered in 1991, could restore certain immune system functions to HIV-infected T-lymphocytes *in vitro.* Specifically, cells from HIV-infected people that previously did not mount a defense against influenza virus or synthetic HIV-envelope proteins did defend themselves after exposure to IL-12. Safety tests for IL-12 in humans were scheduled to begin in the summer of 1994. Effectivity tests would follow if humans are shown to tolerate IL-12.

(Periodical References and Additional Reading: *New York Times* 6-30-92, p C3; *New York Times* 7-10-92, p A15; *New York Times* 1-1-93, p A18; *New York Times* 1-24-93, p I-24; *New York Times* 2-28-93, p A1; *New York Times* 3-9-93, p C3; *New York Times* 4-2-93, p A1; *New York Times* 4-30-93, p C10; *New York Times* 6-6-93, p I-20; *New York Times* 6-10-93, p A16; *New York Times* 6-12-93, p 5; *New York Times* 6-29-93, p C3; *New York Times* 7-1-93, p A13; *New York Times* 7-22-93, p A1; *New York Times* 7-27-93, p C3; *New York Times* 7-29-93, p A20; *Nature* 8-5-93, p 489; *Science News* 10-2-93, p 214; *New York Times* 11-16-93, p C10; *New York Times* 12-1-93, p A21; *New York Times* 12-10-93, p A22; *Science* 12-10-93, p 1721; *New York Times* 12-12-93, p IV-3; *New York Times* 12-17-93, p A28; *New York Times* 12-21-93, p C7; *New York Times* 12-30-93, p A17; *Science* 6-3-94, p 1402)

DISEASE CAUSED BY BACTERIA

ANOTHER CHOLERA EPIDEMIC

Cholera is an ancient terror that is thought to have originated in India, where it is endemic to this day. Chinese records show that it reached China from India in 1669. Cholera epidemics were, to a lesser extent, the "Black Death" of the nineteenth century, with several waves of pandemics that covered much of the world. The first pandemic, from 1817 to 1825, spread from India throughout Asia and into Russia. The second wave started in India the next year (1826) and spread through Europe and into North America, halting around 1838. Two years later another pandemic began in India, and lasted in parts of the world until 1873. During the wave from 1879 through 1883, Robert Koch identified and studied the bacterium that causes the disease, *Vibrio cholerae*. His studies would eventually aid in halting the massive pandemics, although there were two more before World War II.

Although the great pandemics of the nineteenth century were not to be repeated in the twentieth, there was a serious scare near the end of the century. First, an epidemic began in Peru in January 1991 that swept through much of Latin America despite efforts to close borders to the disease. More than 600,000 Latin Americans were infected and more than 5000 of these people died in 1991 and 1992. In February 1992, the disease spread via a single air flight from Argentina to the U.S. A contaminated seafood salad aboard the Argentine plane caused 75 of the passengers to become ill. Another 20-some people, also mainly travelers, were treated for cholera in the U.S. in 1992, which gave 1992 the greatest number of reported cases in the U.S. of the disease since 1961—by far, since there were only ten American cases over the 30 years between 1961 and 1992.

The year 1992 also marked the discovery of a new cholera strain sweeping through India and into neighboring countries of Asia to the east. Known as O139, the new mutant attacked people who were immune to older versions of the disease.

And in July 1994, cholera swept through the Goma, Zaire, camp of refugees from the Rwandan civil war. As of this writing, more than 10,000 people died, most infected with cholera from contaminated water.

Modern medical treatment for cholera consists mainly of oral or intravenous rehydration—i.e., replacement of the fluids lost through diarrhea and vomiting. If promptly administered, it can keep the patient alive until the immune system fights off the disease. In the 1970s scientists discovered the toxin produced by the bacterium. This toxin is the root cause of the symptoms through its effect on the cells of lining of the human gastrointestinal tract. It was not until 1991, however, that enough of the toxin could be produced in a laboratory for detailed studies of the chemical. It is hoped that such studies will eventually result in an antitoxin, which could stop cholera symptoms more quickly than the human immune system.

(Periodical References and Additional Reading: *New York Times* 6-4-91; *New York Times* 4-19-91, p A3; *New York Times* 9-11-92, p A16; *New York Times* 8-13-93, p A2)

BACTERIA, ULCERS, AND CANCER

Chronic stress has been closely linked in the popular mind with stomach or duodenal ulcers (also called gastrointestinal ulcers or peptic ulcers). The duodenum is the part of the small intestine that is closest to the stomach. The "theory" behind the linkage of peptic ulcers to stress is that stress causes the stomach to release digestive juices, including hydrochloric acid; although the lining of the digestive tract is supposed to deal with such juices, the mucous barrier becomes overwhelmed and the juices penetrate in spots to the inner lining, where they begin to digest the walls of the stomach or duodenum, producing the raw spots known as ulcers; once such ulcers form, the same area continues to be susceptible to attack by the digestive juices.

Bacterial Infection Causes Ulcers

Given the popular link between stress and ulcer, it came as a surprise to everyone, even physicians and biomedical researchers, that ulcers often are symptoms of an infectious disease caused by a corkscrew-shaped bacterium *Helicobacter pylori* (formerly known as *Campylobacter pylori*). This astonishing discovery was made in Australia by Barry J. Marshall and J. Robin Warren in 1983, but it took more than a decade to be officially recognized. During that decade, study after study found the *H. pylori* bacteria living in the gastrointestinal tract of almost everyone with duodenal ulcers and in 80 percent of those with stomach ulcers.

Finally a research group in Texas reported in the May 1, 1992 *Annals of Internal Medicine* on their experimental treatment of stomach ulcers with antibiotics to kill the *H. pylori.* The complete treatment regime also included the standard acid-repressing ulcer medication (ranitidine, trade-named Zantac) and the familiar bismuth subsalicylate (trade-named Pepto-Bismol). The patients in the trials not only had stomach ulcers, but all were known to be infected with *H. pylori* before the treatment began. After two weeks of the combined medications, only the Zantac was continued until the ulcers healed.

Over the next two years, only 12 percent of patients who followed the antibiotic treatment regime suffered another ulcer attack. But 95 percent of the control group had another attack during this period. Repeat studies found approximately the same cure rate: 15 percent of the ulcers treated with antibiotics did not recur, but 85 percent or more of the ones treated with other medicines recurred.

Research in 1993 indicated how the bacterium affects the walls of the stomach or duodenum. After *H. pylori* bores through the mucous layer that protects the wall of the stomach or duodenum from gastric juices and stomach acid, the bacterium attaches itself to the inner wall. This calls the immune system to observe that an invader is present, so the immune system mounts an attack. However, the attack is more harmful on cells in the wall than it is to the bacterium.

By early 1994 the U.S. National Institutes of Health endorsed the use of antibiotics to aid in curing gastrointestinal ulcers. But, the panel emphasized that both ulcers and *H. pylori* must be established as present before administering the antibiotics.

HOW MANY ARE AT RISK?

Estimates of the number of people infected with *Helicobacter pylori* vary, and rates are thought to be quite different from country to country. Some estimates of *H. pylori* infection in the U.S. are 20 percent (Thomas Boren in 1993) and 30 percent (Julie Parsonnet in 1991). Worldwide, Boren thinks that some Third World nations may have infection rates of 80 percent.

A Cancer-Causing Bacterium?

Early in 1991 the first report linking *H. pylori* with stomach cancer surfaced in the *Journal of the National Cancer Institute*. Later in the year two other studies found from 23 to 37 percent more infections with the bacterium among those with stomach cancer than among the controls. Yet nearly 70 percent of the controls also had *H. pylori* inhabiting their stomachs, a high percentage that may result from the populations in the study being chosen from groups known to have high stomach cancer rates.

Since clearly not everyone with the bacteria gets stomach cancer, infection is not the sole cause as it is for, say, measles, which takes hold in almost anyone not previously infected. But *H. pylori* seems to be a contributor to stomach cancer. Infection with *H. pylori* acts more like tobacco smoke does in preparing a person for lung cancer; nonsmokers can develop lung cancer, but nearly all cases of lung cancer develop in smokers.

The process of binding to the stomach wall or duodenal explains a long-standing mystery of gastrointestinal science. People with blood type O are 150 per cent to 200 per cent as likely to develop peptic ulcers or stomach cancer as people with other blood types. At least one binding site for the bacterium to the cells of the wall is the same as the carbohydrate chains of the O blood type; there is no similar binding site for the A or B blood types. A second binding site, however, seems to have no connection with blood types, which is consistent with the observation that many people with A, B, or AB blood get peptic ulcers or stomach cancer. Knowing the binding sites suggests that a chemical blocker might be developed that would prevent the bacterium from attaching itself to the stomach wall, though the blocker would have to get through the mucous layer on its own.

(Periodical References and Additional Reading: *New York Times* 5-7-91, p C5; *New York Times* 10-17-91, p B10; *Harvard Health Letter* 3-93, p 2; *New York Times* 12-17-93, p A29; *Science* 12-17-93, pp 1817 & 1892; *Harvard Health Letter* 6-94, p 1)

THE RETURN OF TUBERCULOSIS

Tuberculosis was once called the "white plague" as well as "consumption." We still familiarly call it by the initials TB. It was the resident scourge of the nineteenth century, as opposed to cholera, which came and went. At the turn of the twentieth century, a third of all adult American deaths from infectious disease were caused by TB.

During the twentieth century, however, the epidemic slowly abated. With the invention of X-rays, it was possible to observe the hardened parts of lungs or other organs built by the body to wall off TB infections. Before fear of radiation and diminishing returns took over, mass X-ray screenings for TB were common. Sometimes a train with the equipment and medical personnel would pull into a town railroad station; the population would stream forth in long lines to get their TB X-rays. In conjunction with these screenings, schools and other institutions would also give skin tests (tuberculin tests). If the skin turned red, the person had been or was infected with TB; then it was off for X-rays and other tests to find out if the infection was active.

The public health measures made a difference. Newly discovered drugs helped even more. Early in the 1980s, public health officials announced that TB could be eliminated in the U.S. by the year 2010.

Resurgence in the U.S.

Until quite recently the landscape of the U.S. was dotted with large, forbidding buildings known as TB sanatoriums, or just sanatoriums—as if they were simply places to be healthy, which the word *sanatorium* suggests. In the decades after World War II, however, TB seemed to be under control and the sanatoriums were closed or turned to other purposes. The drug isoniazid controlled the disease and antibiotic courses were found that could cure it. Tuberculosis was simply not a big problem in the U.S. anymore. The low point of the disease was in the U.S. in 1985, following a steady decline for 30 years since 1955.

In 1981, however, there was the first recognition of AIDS. With the loss of immune function, people with AIDS became more vulnerable to TB, which had never completely vanished. During the 1980s, as AIDS spread through the population, so did tuberculosis. Other changes in U.S. life, such as homelessness and immigration, also encouraged the spread. Gradually the isolated reservoirs of the disease merged, and a new infestation—although not an actual epidemic—began. The number of cases began rising, and the annual number of new cases was 20 percent higher by the 1990s than in 1985 (about 27,000 in 1992 as opposed to about 22,000 in 1985). Since many more harbor the germ than show the symptoms, a total of about 15 million people in the U.S. were thought to be infected at any one time during the early 1990s.

When widespread tuberculosis reentered the medical scene in the early 1990s, the giant institutions that had been developed to deal with the disease were gone. Urban areas were hard hit by the renewed disease. In New York state the number of cases doubled in the years between 1985 and the early 1990s, with nearly all of the increase in the large cities. The highest rate in the country in the early 1990s was in Atlanta, Georgia, however.

In New York City in the early 1990s, the City Health Department began to consider reopening the now closed sanatoriums. Tuberculosis wards had to be reopened in city hospitals, rooms with a separate air-conditioning system to keep the air from spreading the disease.

Background

Despite *Camille* or its opera version, *La Traviata,* or John Keats or any of the other men and women who died young from tuberculosis, there was never anything romantic about TB. It was and is an infectious disease caused by a bacterium. The human body can, when well nourished and with a strong immune system, keep TB at bay for long periods of time. An undernourished or otherwise unhealthy person, a person under stress, or a person with a compromised immune system cannot, and the disease destroys the organs it infects—most often the lungs, but also the brain, bones, or kidneys. The most likely victims are the poor, prisoners and people in institutional settings of all kinds, and those already suffering from another disease.

Robert Koch discovered the cause of the disease and announced it to a stunned audience of physicians on March 24, 1882. Tuberculosis is caused by an airborne bacterium that can be passed through the air by sneezing or coughing, which helps explain its prevalence in crowded institutions. Most people when they first contract the disease develop a dormant and noninfectious version; the bacterium moves into the large white blood cells called macrophages, and just stays there. Later—often years later—the bacterium may emerge, having multiplied enough for the person to become a carrier, spreading the germ easily. (One shipyard worker in Maine over a period of eight months in 1989 and 1990 spread the disease to 417 coworkers and three patrons of his favorite tavern.) Ninety percent of the people infected, however, never reach the contagious stage. But when a person is contagious, he or she also will become ill from the disease.

For most patients, the illness begins as a nagging cough: because the bacterium likes oxygen and is airborne, it tends to settle in the lungs. Other early symptoms often include fatigue, weight loss, low-grade fever, night sweats, and blood in the sputum.

In 1873 the U.S. physician Edward Livingstone Trudeau discovered that his own TB symptoms abated during a vacation to Saranac Lake, New York, in the Adirondack Mountains, an observation that led to the first sanatoria, places where it was believed that the sunlight, clean air, and mild exercise might cure the disease.

Over 40 years ago, streptomycin (discovered in 1943 by Selman Waksman), was found effective in killing the bacterium. In the 1950s the drug isoniazid (isonicotinic acid hydrazide), synthesized as early as 1912, was found to be a successful treatment for TB, and has been used since. The drug rifampin also proved useful. Other antibiotics combined with isoniazid or rifampin therapy can rid the body of the bacterium, but six to nine months of steady treatment is needed for effectiveness. After a few weeks of treatment, the patient is no longer contagious, but still carries the bacterium. The poor or homeless often fail to complete the treatment, which helps account for the rise of resistant strains of the bacterium.

An Epidemic Worldwide

Tuberculosis continues to be a deadly disease in undeveloped countries. The World Health Organization (WHO) declared tuberculosis a global emergency in April 1993, noting that it killed more *adults* than all other infectious diseases combined, almost three million a year. About eight million new cases occur annually around the world, so that one person in every three on the earth is infected with the bacterium.

WHO was campaigning, unsuccessfully in the U.S., for more funds with which to fight TB. One telling argument from WHO is that nations have contributed nearly five times as much money to fight leprosy, which kills about 2000 persons a year, as they do to fight tuberculosis in developing countries, which kills a thousand times as many people annually as leprosy.

It is not just developing countries that have a TB problem. Among those with worse increases in incidence than the U.S. are Switzerland (a third more cases in the 1990s than at its low point), Denmark, and Italy (each up about 30 percent).

TB and Drug Resistance

Ever since the introduction of effective antibiotics, it has been apparent that after a time the organisms that are supposed to be killed by the antibiotics can develop resistance. Furthermore, for bacteria, resistance can be spread from bacterium to bacterium by exchange of DNA rings called plasmids. But tuberculosis was thought to be different in that resistant strains developed in some patients, but did not spread from those patients to others. Thus although TB drug resistance was a problem for individuals, it was not a problem for society.

Infectious cases of TB drug resistance continued to be rare throughout the 1980s, but in the early 1990s there appeared more than a dozen locations in the U.S. where resistant strains of tuberculosis were found to pass from person to person. As early as 1991, about 14 percent of all new cases of TB in the U.S. were resistant to at least one drug; nearly a quarter of those were also resistant to at least one other drug as well. In New York City, the center of drug resistance for TB in the U.S., more than a third of all cases were resistant. Even with treatment about half of those people would die from the resistant strain of the disease.

The main cause of drug resistance, experts say, is that poor or homeless patients begin to feel better after a few weeks of medication, so they stop treatment. At that point, the population of bacteria is low, but those that remain are the ones resistant to treatment. When the disease breaks out again in the patient, the bacteria are all descendants of the remaining resistant group. Thus the second course of treatment must be longer, stronger, and use different drugs.

When *Mycobacterium tuberculosis,* the cause of TB, began to develop resistance to drugs in the early 1990s, the newly resistant bacteria presented several challenges to the system and to the patient:

- Infections could not be easily cured.
- The risk of dying became 50 percent greater when the drug-resistant bacteria were involved.
- Successful treatment replaced the two drugs normally used with four or even seven, and doubled the length of time needed for effective treatment.
- Costs of control skyrocketed.
- More people stopped treatment before a cure was reached.
- Half-treated people increased the rate at which the disease spread to new patients.
- The version of the bacterium being spread was drug resistant.

FIGHTING TUBERCULOSIS

The following quotations are all taken from published contemporary accounts for the years indicated.

1937   As a first step in the detection of tuberculosis, the tuberculin test has been applied to more than a million persons throughout the United States in 1937. . . . Whole cities inaugurated tuberculosis control programs through publicity in newspapers and over the radio. . . . Hospital beds for the isolation and treatment of the tuberculous have been increased by the construction of new sanatoriums in such States as Florida and North Carolina. The total capacity of such institutions in 1937 was approximately 80,000. General hospitals are admitting about 35,000 tuberculous patients annually. . . .

1946   During the past few years slipshod and short-cut methods of diagnosis resulted in a large number of diagnostic errors. As many as 15%-25% of the patients admitted to sanatoriums were found to have some other disease, or if tuberculosis was present it had already been controlled by nature. . . . About 2% of the six-year-old white children reacted to tuberculin . . . slightly more than 10% by the age of 18 years. Among Negro children the incidence of tuberculin reaction was three times as high. . . . The division of tuberculosis of the United States public health service estimated a sanatorium bed deficiency of 44,388. . . .

1956   Despite progress, tuberculosis remained in 1956 the most destructive infectious disease. . . . As of 1956, this survey program was averaging about 1,000,000 routine chest X-ray film inspections annually, and approximately 2,000 active cases were being found each year. . . . Because of the decrease in the number of new cases of tuberculosis . . . the demand for sanatorium beds had decreased. Three public and two private tuberculosis hospitals were closed in upstate New York. Sanatoria were also closed in other states, although many physicians regarded their closing as premature. . . . As the number of persons with contagious tuberculosis decreased, certain groups, such as recalcitrants and alcoholics became more conspicuous. . . . The only generally accepted method of preventing tuberculosis consisted of protecting against tubercule bacilli so as to avoid their initial invasion.

1962   Those who had set extermination of tuberculosis as a goal were encouraged in 1962 because the word "eradication" appeared in medical writings much more frequently than at any previous time. . . . The goal was set to eradicate tuberculosis so that by 1973 no child entering school would react to tuberculin. Some health authorities felt that eradication is possible not only in the United States but all over the world. . . .

1966   Although tuberculosis no longer ranked among the leading causes of death, it still constituted a serious health problem. . . . Mortality from the disease was increasingly concentrated at the older ages, particularly among men. The current level of mortality from tuberculosis among nonwhites was at about the level of that of the white population a decade earlier.

1967   Long-continued dosage with isoniazid was recommended for prevention of relapses in tuberculosis and for the protection of personnel in TB sanatoriums. . . .Tuberculosis remains a scourge in poor countries. . . .

The preceding quotations were from various issues of *The Brittanica Book of the Year*. In the early years, separate articles each year were devoted to tuberculosis. Later, TB was mentioned in reviews of medicine. By the 1970s, there are no mentions of the disease at all.

A team comprised of Stewart Cole from the Pasteur Institute in Paris, Ying Zhang, Bryan Allen, and Douglas Young from Hammersmith Hospital in London and Beate Heym in France discovered (and reported in the August 13, 1993 *Nature*) at least one way in which *M. tuberculosis* becomes resistant to isoniazid: it deletes one of its normal genes so that the drug no longer has a point of attack. This resistance by an unexpected mechanism can be transferred to other bacteria. Knowing how the trick is done may help devise new drugs that attack at a different vulnerable point. More immediately, it enables physicians to identify a drug-resistant case earlier, changing the way that the disease will be treated. Another method for spotting a resistant germ was developed in 1993 by a team from the Albert Einstein College of Medicine in the Bronx, New York. They found a way to make resistant bacteria glow in the dark.

(Periodical References and Additional Reading: *New York Times* 7-10-91, p B1; *New York Times* 8-1-92, p 1; *Science News* 2-6-93, p 90; *Science* 5-7-93, pp 750 & 819; *New York Times* 8-13-92, p A1; *Nature* 8-13-92, pp 538 & 591; *Sciences* 9-10-93, p 14; *Science* 9-10-93, pp 1390 & 1454; *New York Times* 10-8-93, p A23; *New York Times* 10-11-93, p I-1; *New York Times* 10-12-93, p A1; *New York Times* 10-13-93, p A1; *New York Times* 11-16-93, p C8; *New York Times* 12-26-93, p A13)

Lyme Disease UPDATE

Lyme disease has been recognized as problem for about 20 years. It is a bacterial disease spread by the bite of a tick associated with the white-tailed deer.

Although Lyme disease is seldom if ever fatal, it remains a great cause of concern to citizens in regions where the disease is endemic. It is not clear whether or not this concern is excessive, perhaps a result of the relative novelty of the illness, or perfectly reasonable. In any case, anxiety has produced considerable alteration in behavior brought on by fear of the deer tick that carries the disease. Suburbs in the U.S. northeast and midwest are rife with residents who refuse to go into the woods, who douse their children with the insect repellent DEET, and who dress in long-sleeved shirts and long pants to go into their own backyards on a hot summer day.

Some Reasons for Reduced Concern

The number of persons known to be infected with Lyme disease in the U.S. is small, only 9667 in 1992 (up from about 500 when the media first noticed the disease in the early 1980s). Because of the small numbers involved, some have suggested that the economics of fighting the disease show an overreaction. In 1989, medical laboratories in Wisconsin tested about 94,000 suspected cases of Lyme disease at a cost per test of about $100. They found only 545 cases that year, so the cost of testing per established instance of disease was nearly $18,000.

It is also frequently unclear whether or not the disease has been contracted. Lyme disease has always been difficult to diagnose, and there is considerable evidence that it has been misdiagnosed in some situations—one study reported that 77 percent of purported cases were "over-diagnosed" at some medical centers. That is, mild and self-limiting viral diseases, arthritis with other causes, or even spider bites were mistaken for Lyme disease.

There are good reasons why Lyme disease is often misdiagnosed. It is difficult to persuade the Lyme bacterium to grow in a culture. Present tests identify antibodies to the bacterium and are prone to false positive results. The symptom considered the best indicator of the disease is a bull's-eye rash, red with clearing at the center (where the tick bit), after exposure in a suitable environment, but the characteristic rash fails to appear or to be noticed in many cases. New tests for Lyme disease, based on using monoclonal antibodies to find proteins on the surface of the bacterium or on looking for strands of bacterial DNA, are under development. If these succeed, diagnosis will be both more accurate and quicker.

It also may be more difficult to contract the disease than people think. Some research suggests that as few as 1.2 percent of the persons bitten by deer ticks, even ticks known to carry the Lyme disease bacterium, become infected with the bacterium. The tick may have to remain attached to the host for over a day to transmit the bacterium. If so, failure to contract the disease could be either because of an ineffective mode of transmission from tick to human or it could be because most people have encountered the disease earlier and developed an immunity or partial immunity to it. In any case, it is not as easy to contract Lyme disease as many suppose.

Chronic Problems

Furthermore, although everyone agrees that most cases of Lyme disease promptly caught are easily cured with antibiotics, there is considerable controversy over whether or not long-term consequences occur in some patients whose disease is not cured. Patients who still have symptoms attributable to Lyme disease—chronic arthritis, the facial spasm known as Bell's palsy, chronic fatigue, and mental disorientation—often yield no detectable bacteria. Many other symptoms of purported chronic Lyme-disease victims are subjective or vague, such as loss of libido, personality changes, intolerance to noise, or depression.

Scientists who believe that these patients have Lyme disease have suggested that the reported symptoms are caused by a very few Lyme bacteria dwelling in the joints, central nervous system, or even inside cells. The small number of bacteria are enough

Background

In the early 1970s, parents and pediatricians in a suburban region of Connecticut along Long Island Sound began to notice a characteristic group of symptoms in children from the region. The illness began with a localized rash and continued with fever, chills, and muscle aches. Some of the children also developed a form of juvenile arthritis.

One of the parents pursued the problem and in 1975 Allen C. Steere described the new disease, which he named Lyme disease after the community of Old Lyme, which was a focus of the disease. Proximity to Yale University in nearby New Haven, Connecticut, aided in research on the disease. The disease was found in 1978 to be borne by tick *Ixodes dammini*; in 1982 the bacterium that was the cause was tentatively identified. The next year the bacterium was identified and eventually it was named *Borrelia burgdorferi*. Eventually it was recognized that Lyme disease was the same disease as one that had previously puzzled authorities in Scandinavia.

The tick in question is called a deer tick because it usually mates on deer, so it is not present unless deer are also present. The main hosts for the ticks, however, are field mice. Furthermore, other *Ixodes* ticks with different hosts, including birds, have been shown in some instances to carry the disease.

For the most part, the disease is concentrated in suburban regions in the U.S. northeast (e.g. Connecticut, southeastern New York state, Long Island, Massachusetts, and northern New Jersey), the upper midwest (e.g. Wisconsin and Minnesota), and on the west coast (e.g. parts of California). Large regions, such as the Wyoming, seem to be free of the disease.

Borrelia burgdorferi is a spirochete, the corkscrew type of bacterium whose cousins are the cause of syphilis and yaws. The Lyme bacterium is very difficult to isolate from patients and to culture, which has led to problems in diagnosis. There is some concern that such a disease could damage the unborn child of a pregnant woman who became infected. Scientists who claim long-term chronic Lyme disease point out the similarity of *B. burgdorferi* to *Treponema pallidum*, the cause of syphilis. Syphilis is known to survive for many years in untreated victims, damaging various organs and eventually causing death.

to provoke an attack by the immune system, and the attack itself causes the other symptoms.

Scientists who disagree with this theory think that the purported Lyme patients have some different disease or, in some instances, no disease at all. One study by the New England Medical Center concluded that of patients who had been identified with intractable Lyme disease, fewer than a quarter of them really suffered from Lyme disease.

There are consequences of the chronic Lyme-disease dilemma. Long-term treatment of the disease is not just an economic burden, although treatment costs can run as high as $17,000 per month. Intravenous antibiotics, often used for cases thought to be chronic Lyme disease, are dangerous. Children under such treatment have sometimes had to have their gall bladders removed because of antibiotic-induced gallstones (14 instances in the U.S. according to a report by the Centers for Disease Control and

Prevention at the end of 1993). More often, the young patients have had bloodstream infections. These side effects might be more acceptable if it were clear that the patients actually had Lyme disease, but that as always is difficult to prove.

Vaccine Hopes

Whatever concern individuals have about Lyme disease may soon be relieved by a vaccine. Tests of promising vaccines were conducted on Block Island, Rhode Island (off Long Island and Connecticut), in Westchester County, New York, on Nantucket Island, Massachusetts, and in similar high-incidence areas in Europe. Both vaccines being tested target the same protein on the cell wall of the spirochete, a protein known as O.S.P. -A, which is the most common protein on the outer surface of the germ. The gene for O.S.P. -A is known, so genetic engineers were able to insert the gene into the bacterium *Escherichia coli,* the workhorse of genetic engineering, which then churns it out.

There is good reason to hope for success with the vaccines. Clinical observations suggest that people who have once had Lyme disease develop at least a partial immunity to the bacterium, though the difficulty of diagnosis makes it impossible to be certain. Furthermore, animal tests of the vaccines have shown the shots to be remarkably successful. Not only did the vaccines prevent infection in mice, but the mouse blood ingested by ticks contained enough antibodies to kill the bacteria living in the tick.

If the vaccines have continued success in the human trials, a course of three shots over three months will become recommended for people in heavily infected areas or for people planning to camp or hike in infected woods.

The main concern about possible dangers from the vaccine stems from the theory that an immune reaction to Lyme disease is the cause of the symptoms attributed to the chronic version. For this reason, researchers concentrated on using a protein rather than a whole killed bacterium for the vaccine. The protein O.S.T. -A has not produced arthritis or other side effects in mice and so far has not shown such effects in humans.

(Periodical References and Additional Reading: *New York Times* 12-17-92, p B18; *Nature* 3-25-93, p 340; *New York Times* 6-15-93, p A1; *New York Times* 8-24-93, p C1; *New York Times* 8-25-93, p C10; *New York Times* 9-21-93, p C1; *New York Times* 1-4-94, p A1)

BACTERIAL SURPRISES

Bacteria are the most common form of life on the planet Earth and, as far as we now know, in the universe. Although humans have found ways to tame bacteria (e.g., to make vinegar and human growth protein) and to subdue or render ineffective many of the bacteria that produce human disease, the little creatures did not obtain ubiquity without having a great many tricks tucked into their cell walls.

Staph and Strep

Two of the most common causes of death from bacterial disease today are unique because the bacteria involved are not exactly the cause of any specific disease—the way that, say, *Mycobacterium tuberculosis* causes tuberculosis. At the same time, they produce suites of symptoms that are identified as some of the most destructive infections people face in this almost antiseptic age. Between them, the two somewhat similar bacteria cause a wide range of diseases: toxic shock syndrome, abscesses, blood poisoning, a form of pneumonia, the heart inflammation endocarditis, and some food poisoning (*Staphylococcus*); as well as scarlet and rheumatic fever, blood poisoning, a different form of heart disease, some cases of kidney inflammation or tonsillitis, and possibly some cases of toxic shock syndrome (*Streptococcus*). The two types of bacteria are so familiar that nearly everyone calls them by their nicknames, staph and strep.

Not all newly discovered diseases have been connected to a specific cause (*see* "The State of the Fight Against Infectious Disease," p 317). One of the most mysterious has been Kawasaki disease, so named because it was first identified in 1967 by Tokyo pediatrician Tomisaku Kawasaki. It has been attributed to a retrovirus (like the HIV virus), allergies to dust mites, and various bacteria. In the December 4, 1993 *Lancet* the disease was tied to toxins produced by a newly discovered strain of staphylococcus and by a streptococcus and was thought to be caused by the immune-system response to the bacteria or the toxins.

Kawasaki syndrome is similar to scarlet fever in that it has a high fever followed by a characteristic rash (including a rash on the tongue, known as strawberry tongue). Like scarlet fever, it tends to attack children, although children who are the main victims of Kawasaki are most often younger than two. Like scarlet fever, it can produce heart disease as a complication, although the form of the heart disease—aneurysms of the coronary arteries—is different. There are about 5000 cases annually in the U.S. and it occurs around the world.

Strep has been in the news recently for other diseases as well. Researchers have found that antibodies to the strep toxin may be a cause of movement disorders in susceptible children. It has long been known that strep-induced rheumatic fever can cause a movement disorder that results in legs and arms flailing about uncontrollably.

Group A *Streptococcus* became famous early in 1994 as the cause of a moderately rare group of blood and skin diseases in which the toxins kill cells at such an accelerated rate that surgery to remove the infected part of the body is the only effective treatment. Although the syndrome was not new, tabloid journalists focused on the gruesome symptoms and managed to cause considerable public concern over "deadly, flesh-eating bacteria." The strep A bacteria might better be described as "carrion-eating," since they live on dead flesh that has been killed by the bacterial toxins. Physicians call the strain "necrotizing," meaning that it kills cells.

When the necrotizing process has advanced, the living bacteria are safe from treatment because they are in the killed flesh, which has been abandoned by the bloodstream that might carry antibiotics. Meanwhile, the bacteria continue to produce the toxin, which seeps from the dead flesh into the living, where it kills adjacent cells. Physicians have no recourse except surgery to remove all the dead flesh and with it the infection. Failure to take this drastic measure can lead to death. The

Background

The coccus family of bacteria is characterized by the spherical shape of individual bacteria. *Staphylococcus* describes those in which the spheres form clusters; *Streptococcus* describes those in which the spheres connect in lines, like a string of beads. Because bacteria are so small and featureless, scientists have had a difficult time determining evolutionary relationships, but DNA studies are expected to cast light on these diseases.

Infection by either staph or strep causes damage by two main mechanisms—toxins produced by the bacteria destroy flesh, and immune reactions to either of the bacteria or the toxins can also attack parts of the body.

Glomerulonephritis A particular kidney infection that is most often a consequence of an untreated strep throat. The actual damage is thought to be caused by antibodies directed against the bacteria, not by the bacteria themselves. With proper treatment most victims (usually children) recover completely, although permanent kidney damage can occur.

Rheumatic fever A strep infection, such as strep throat, that invades the joints and heart is called rheumatic fever. Although the disease has been reduced in incidence recently, probably because of antibiotics, children and young adults are still susceptible. The name stems from the pain and swelling in the joints, but the permanent damage comes from an infection of the valves of the heart, which occurs in about three infections out of five. Sometimes the bacterium also affects the brain, but the damage there is not permanent.

Scarlet fever A now rare strep-induced childhood disease characterized by a high fever and a distinctive rash. Although most children recover, it can lead to either glomerulonephritis or rheumatic fever, which are more serious than the original disease.

Septicemia, septic shock, or blood poisoning These very general terms apply not only to staph or strep infections that multiply rapidly in the blood, but are also used for any bacterial infestation of the bloodstream that produces a harmful toxin (the "poison" of the common name). Septic shock caused by gram-negative bacteria, such as *E. coli*, are more difficult to treat than shock caused by staph or strep, which can be more easily eliminated by antibiotics.

Staph also causes many less serious conditions, including boils, sties on the eye, impetigo, and bloody diarrhea. Similarly, strep causes the skin disease known as cellulitis or erysipelas.

infection proceeds very fast, so it is important that any hint of a rampant infection, especially combined with high fever, be treated with powerful antibiotics while the bacteria are still in the living part of the flesh.

Because the necrotizing strep bacterium thrives in dead flesh, it usually attacks damaged areas, such as wounds or sores. But it is seldom capable of infecting another healthy person, unlike a different strep strain, which causes strep throat and which can move from person to person in confined settings.

Both staph and strep seem to run in cycles. Staph seems to have a ten-year-cycle for each particular strain of the bacterium. The destructive strains of strep A were at a high level in the 1940s, but incidence fell until about 1980. Since then the numbers of cases of necrotizing strep have been rising. The U.S. Federal Centers for Disease and

Prevention analyzed incidence of this nonreportable infection (when a disease is "reportable," doctors treating it must prepare a written report, ensuring that exact statistics are available) for the years 1989 and 1990, concluding that there were about 10,000 to 15,000 incidences in the U.S. each year, a higher level than past experience would suggest.

New Outbreaks of Bacterial Diseases

Despite antibiotics, other bacterial diseases continue to pose serious risks.

Plague   Although we tend to think of plague as a former disease, the cause of the Black Death that terrorized Europe from the fourteenth through the seventeenth centuries, it is actually endemic in several parts of the world, including the western U.S. Plague is a disease with several alternate hosts, including rodents, fleas, and humans. The most common form is the one that spreads from a reservoir of infected, but usually not very ill, rodents via flea bites to humans, but plague has always been able to be transmitted from person to person through the air, the same route as many respiratory diseases. Plague spread by a flea bite is generally *bubonic,* attacking the lymph nodes; plague spread through the air is usually *pneumonic*, attacking the lungs. When plague moves into the bloodstream, it can be *septicemic,* the general name for a bacterial infection of the blood.

There are a dozen or so cases of plague in the American West most years, but 1992 brought the first reported death in five years. A man in Tucson, Arizona, developed pneumonic plague, probably caught from breathing air previously breathed by a cat, who also died from the disease. The cat is thought to have caught it from a rodent, most likely a chipmunk.

Syphilis   Like many diseases, syphilis can pass from an infected pregnant woman to a fetus she is carrying. A child born with syphilis, which is then termed *congenital syphilis,* can often be spotted by an enlarged spleen and liver and peeling skin on the palms and on the soles of the feet. Blindness and deafness are common, and the fetus often dies before or at birth. But symptoms of congenital syphilis vary greatly and sometimes cannot be observed until years later. Although it is thought that brain damage in congenital syphilis can be prevented by early treatment, there has been not enough experience so far to be certain. The more common sexually transmitted syphilis goes through three stages, including a second stage in which the disease works quietly in the body and a third in which organs are destroyed by action of the germs. Congenital syphilis, however, always skips the first stage, and proceeds directly to the second or third.

Congenital syphilis was almost forgotten in the U.S. after the introduction of penicillin. Expectant mothers could be tested for syphilis and, if the disease was found, treated with antibiotics. Treating the mother also cured the fetus. By the early 1980s, the rate of congenital syphilis as based on reports of children born with disease symptoms fell to about 200 annually by the early 1980s. Then the numbers began to increase.

As the incidence of recognizable disease in newborns tripled in 1989, the U.S. Centers for Disease Control changed its reporting requirements. Instead of reporting only symptomatic newborns, doctors were required to report all births to mothers who were found to have untreated syphilis. With the new requirements, cases rose even faster, reaching 4322 in 1991.

The swift rise was apparently a consequence of drug addiction. Addicted women do not always seek out doctors when they become pregnant. Trades of sex for drugs have contributed to the spread of all sexually transmitted diseases.

Anthrax   The bacillus that causes anthrax has been studied longer than any other disease causing bacterium. It has proven capable of relatively easy modification, as Pasteur demonstrated in the nineteenth century. The bacterium can survive under all sorts of conditions in an inactive form, so it can be stored in a warehouse for years with no special attention. Among the modes of infection for anthrax is airborne distribution; for example, in dust or another light powder. When contracted by an unvaccinated person via inhalation, death follows quickly and surely. If exposure is expected, humans can be protected by vaccination.

Thus anthrax has been viewed by the military of many countries as a perfect agent for biological warfare.

It is known that the U.S. has experimented with the disease. For most countries, including the former Soviet Union and Iraq, strong suspicions of anthrax biological weapons have to suffice because of secrecy.

So when 68 to 300 persons contracted the now rare disease of anthrax in what was then Sverdlovsk (now Yetkaterinburg) in Siberia, many observers concluded that the Soviet Union had been experimenting with biological warfare and that the agent had escaped—as in Michael Crichton's *Andromeda Strain*. The Soviets denied it: they said that the anthrax came from a batch of contaminated meat.

In the March 14, 1993 *Proceedings of the National Academy of Sciences,* however, a team of six American and Russian doctors concluded that the deaths of 42 of the

---

Background

Anthrax was the first disease for which a bacterial origin was definitely established (by C. J. Davaine in 1863) and the first bacterial disease for which a vaccine was developed (by Louis Pasteur in 1881). It is a deadly disease that attacks humans, their domestic animals, and also wild animals. Anthrax can be transmitted in a variety of ways in part because it can exist for years in a dormant state. Dormant bacteria are called *spores,* although they are quite different from the reproductive spores formed by fungi, mosses, and ferns. Dormant *Bacillus anthracis* spores can last for years in soil. They can enter the body through the skin, in breathed air, or in food. Contaminated wool or fur or even animal hair used in shaving brushes (which caused a widespread epidemic among soldiers in World War I) also can spread the spores.

When spores enter the body, they reactivate and give off toxins that can result in sores (if localized) or death (if the infection is general). Epidemics sometimes sweep through animal populations, but infection of humans tends to be sporadic. In former times, anthrax sores were common among butchers, who became infected from handling infected meat. Pulmonary anthrax, almost invariably fatal, struck people who sheared sheep or processed wool. Widespread vaccination of domestic animals has reduced the incidence of this once widespread disease.

victims, whose records they were able to obtain (including tissue samples and preserved organs), had come as a result of airborne spores. The symptoms of the victims, most of whom died within four days and who were most often diagnosed initially as having pneumonia, strongly suggest that an accidental release of an airborne biological weapon was the cause of the epidemic.

Mycoplasma

Pneumonia is not a disease, but a symptom. Various bacteria are associated with the symptom, which is an acute or chronic inflammation of the lungs, but it can also be caused by a virus or even by inhaled chemicals. Bacterial pneumonia is often connected to "Pneumococcus" or "Pneumonobacillis," although the actual germs involved are classed more specifically by bacteriologists—Pneumococcus might be *Diplococcus pneumoniae* or Pneumobacillis might be *Klebsiella pneumoniae*.

In the early 1990s, however, there was an outbreak of pneumonia in the U.S. that was caused by an entirely different bacterium. Mycoplasma form a separate phylum among bacteria from the ones associated with familiar diseases. They are not well understood. At one time, the mycoplasma were said to be "in between" true bacteria and viruses.

Well understood or not, the bacterium *Mycoplasma pneumoniae* emerged as a part of a cycle similar to the one for influenza and began infecting people around the U.S. and causing pneumonia in the winter of 1993-94 with outbreaks reported in Texas, Ohio, and New York. Although the disease is seldom fatal and can be treated with antibiotics, the similarity of its symptoms to those of influenza (which cannot be treated) often cause the pneumonia to be overlooked.

Mycoplasmas cause other diseases that resemble those caused by more ordinary bacteria as well. Inflammations of the genito-urinary system are commonly caused by the two most widespread sexually transmitted bacteria, *Chlamydia trachomatis* and *Neisseria gonorrhoeae,* whose infections are known as chlamydia and gonorrhea. But the urethra can develop an inflammation that culturing shows is not caused by either bacterium. Mycoplasmas are difficult to culture, but it now appears that many instances of urethritis of previously unknown cause are actually the result of infection by *Mycoplasma genitalium.* Although the bacterium was discovered as long ago as 1981, it was not until a report in the September 4, 1993 *Lancet* that it was definitely linked to the disease. (Often a bacterium is present in a diseased organ for reasons unconnected with the disease symptoms.) However, the methods used in the 1993 research only provided a statistical linkage—rather like the relationship between lung cancer and tobacco smoking. Further study is needed to establish a mechanism by which the mycoplasma causes the symptoms.

Learning from Your Teeth

Dental amalgam, using commonly for fillings, has long been suspected as a possible source of mercury poisoning (*see* "Danger from Mercury," p 250). Bacterial resistance to antibiotics has long been known to be caused in part by inadequate dosages of the medicines. A bacterial surprise in 1993 was the possibility that at least some bacterial resistance comes not from direct exposure to antibiotics, but from the influence of the mercury in fillings.

Anne O. Summers of the University of Georgia and her coworkers wrote in *Antimicrobial Agents and Chemotherapy* that the genes for antibiotic resistance, although different from those for resistance to mercury poisoning, are next to each other in many types of bacteria. The researchers gave a half dozen monkeys mouths full of mercury amalgam-filled molars. Within five weeks bacteria harbored in the guts of the monkeys became resistant to mercury, penicillin, streptomycin, kanamycin, chloramphenicol, and tetracycline, which had not previously been the case. Indeed, for some forms of bacteria that had a nine percent resistance rate before the fillings, the number rose to 70 percent after the fillings. When the amalgam fillings were subsequently removed, the resistance rate for these bacteria fell to 12 percent.

Bacteria multiply and are shed so rapidly that populations of resistance evolve or are lost within a few days or weeks. Suspicion of dental fillings came in part because about 60 percent of humans harbor resistant intestinal bacteria even when many have not recently taken antibiotics. Resistance to either mercury or antibiotics is eliminated from most of a bacterial population by natural selection unless there is continuing presence of the chemical that is being resisted.

(Periodical References and Additional Reading: *New York Times* 2-14-91, p A1; *New York Times* 8-28-91; *New York Times* 10-9-92, p A19; *New York Times* 11-21-92, p A13; *New York Times* 3-15-93, p A6; *New York Times* 4-27-93, p C1; *Science News* 7-17-93, p 39; *Science News* 9-11-93, p 166; *New York Times* 12-3-93, p A28; *New York Times* 12-10-93, p A23; *New York Times* 6-14-94, p C3)

THE STATE OF THE WAR
AGAINST PARASITES

Long ago it was noted that "great fleas have little fleas/ upon their backs to bite'em; little fleas have lesser fleas/ and so on, *ad infinitum.*" Technically, all the little and lesser "fleas" are parasites, so our littlest—the viruses—and not quite so little—the bacteria—are examples of human parasites. But long tradition restricts the use of the word *parasite* in medical usage to more complex creatures than bacteria—the protists, fungi, and animals. (Plants do not seem to become parasites of animals, only of other plants.)

Some authorities have found it convenient to separate human parasites into the *microparasites,* which include all the creatures so small that they reproduce within the human body, including viruses, bacteria, protists, and fungi, and the *macroparasites,* which reproduce outside the human body. Of the macroparasites, the ones that produce conditions we recognize as "diseases" are often worms of one kind or another, such as the agents of schistosomiasis (sometimes called bilharzia), trichinosis, and filariasis. Other worm infestations are known primarily by the name of the worm: pinworms, roundworms, whipworms, hookworms, and flukes. Larger worms also produce disease conditions, although they are often thought of as infestations instead of infections: tapeworms of various types and the agent of river blindness.

Perhaps because of their complexity, disease-causing parasites are often more difficult to handle than bacteria. (Viral diseases are difficult to treat because of the simplicity of viruses.) Some parasites can be poisoned without severely infecting the host.

Anti-fungal compounds have improved greatly in recent years, especially. Topical (meaning applied directly to the fungus infection) creams and ointments have been successful in handling most fungal infections on the skin. New systemic (meaning throughout the whole body) anti-fungal agents not only can be used to treat surface infections (which include, but are not limited to, ringworm, athletes foot and jock itch, and *Candida* yeast infections), but may be helpful in the more serious internal infections. The rise of AIDS, which leaves its victims susceptible to all manner of fungal infections, has spurred research in this area.

Attempts to devise a vaccine to protect against microscopic parasites have produced some positive results, but no actual successes. Often the best way known to control the incidence of a parasitical disease is through elimination or reduction in numbers of alternate hosts, such as mosquitoes, flies, or snails. Such diseases are limited by the range of the alternate host, which is often tropical. A frequent question U.S. physicians ask during routine examinations or when confronted with unusual symptoms is: "Have you been out of the country recently?" They are especially looking for a "tropical disease," which most likely would be caused by a parasite. Thousands of Americans and Europeans were exposed to leishmaniasis (sand-fly fever) for the first time during the Persian Gulf War of 1991.

Protists

Leishmaniasis is one of several diseases caused by a protist that has a fly as an alternate host. African sleeping sickness, caused by the organism known as a trypanosome

(*Trypanosoma brucei*) and hosted by the famous tse-tse fly, is another. So is malaria, since to a biologist a mosquito is a species of fly. All are major scourges of humankind.

Progress Against the Trypanosome The early 1990s saw the first progress in 40 years in treatment for and understanding of African sleeping sickness. Near the end of 1990 the U.S. Food and Drug Administration gave its important, although largely symbolic, approval to Ornidyl, a new drug that often results in full recovery from the disease. The previous treatment was so toxic that it killed one out of 20 who used it. Because Ornidyl is used intravenously for two weeks, however, it is far too expensive for routine use in the parts of Africa where it is most needed.

Understanding the trypanosome that causes sleeping sickness may eventually provide better answers. The reason that the body cannot rid itself of the trypanosome is that the protist is able to change the proteins on its outer coat into thousands of different shapes. Even its DNA has evolved an unusual structure to produce this ability to escape detection by the immune system. Early in 1991, however, scientists reported that they had demonstrated a method to modify the parasite with genetic engineering. It was hoped that further work with the genetics of the trypanosome would lead to a cheaper medicine and perhaps someday even a vaccine.

Another experimental approach has been aimed at finding a bacterium that might kill trypanosomes in the tse-tse fly itself.

Malaria Vaccine Problems and Progress Malaria is one of the main diseases around the world. It is estimated that one person out of every 20 on the Earth, or about 300 million people, are infected with malaria. Perhaps as many as two million of them die each year, while most of the remainder are debilitated by the disease. Resistance to the older drugs used to treat the disease has been rising at an increasing rate for the past quarter century. Although new drugs, notably mefloquine, have been introduced in the 1990s, the parasite already has shown resistance to them as well. Thus much of the hope in the early 1990s for improvement in the malaria situation rested on a variety of vaccines that were under development.

The possibility of a vaccine might seem remote, since humans do not naturally develop immunity to new attacks of malaria. People who are cured of the disease by drugs often leave the hospital and are infected all over again. But for three of the four types of malaria (each caused by a different species of *Plasmodium*), many people survive for years with the disease, suffering recurrent attacks of fever and illness. Over a period of years, such attacks become less frequent, which suggests that there is some form of mild immunity to the disease.

In an early research effort, volunteers exposed themselves to the bites of hundreds of mosquitoes that had been irradiated to kill any *Plasmodium* in the bites. After hundreds of mosquito bites, the subjects became fully immune to all forms of malaria. Unfortunately, it was not clear how to achieve this effect without the hundreds of mosquito bites.

In the late 1980s, scientists discovered that one protein on the coat of one stage of the parasite did lead to antibodies against it. Although they were able to produce a vaccine based on that protein, it did not work very well. Eventually nearly 20 different vaccines were under development at one time or another in the early 1990s. Only one has gone to large-scale field trials, however. In Colombia, Manuel Elkin Patarroyo's entirely synthetic vaccine known as SPf66 has been from 40 to 60 percent effective in preventing the deadliest form of malaria, caused by *Plasmodium falciparum* (re-

Background

Protists can be defined as one-celled or colonial (many identical cells in clumps or strings) organisms other than plants or fungi that have a membrane around their genetic material. Other one-celled and colonial organisms, without the enclosed DNA to form a cell nucleus, are generally classed as monerans (bacteria, archaebacteria, and blue-green algae). Different taxonomists have used different schemes, so sometimes most protists are grouped with animals and a few are called plants. Sometimes protists are also called by an older name, *protozoa*. There are about 35,000 different species of protists, including *Paramecium,* dinoflagellates, amoebas (some of which produce dysentery), euglenas, and slime molds, as well as the disease-causing protists discussed in this article. Sometimes algae are classed as protists, but often they are classed as plants.

African sleeping sickness   Caused by a trypanosome; the modifier "African" is needed to separate the disease from various forms of encephalitis that are also known as "sleeping sickness." Carried only by the tse-tse fly, this trypanosome attacks cattle as well as humans and has restricted the range of cattle in Africa, eliminating for grazing purposes a region larger than the continental U.S. In addition to fever and general malaise, the human host is sleepy during the day and an insomniac at night, a stage of the disease always followed by seizures and death. The trypanosome multiplies until it consumes all the glucose in the body, so there is none left as an energy supply for cells. It infects about 10,000 persons in central Africa annually.

Cryprosporidiosis   Caused by *Cryptosporidium* (*see* "Don't Drink the Water," p 383).

Giardia   Both the organism and the disease have the same name. Unlike most of the protists listed here, *Giardia* lives freely in water until ingested by a mammal. It is common in mountain streams and has been reported among beavers, sheep, and mountain goats. It has been recognized as a public health problem only since the early 1980s, but since then outbreaks have occurred in Washington state and upstate New York.

Leishmaniasis   Caused by *Leishmania;* there are various forms of the disease or disease group, including kala-azar (common in India, where it is often fatal) and sand-fly fever, which results in skin sores.

Malaria   Caused by several species of *Plasmodium,* which have as an alternate host mosquitoes of the genus *Anopheles;* most common in the tropics and subtropics. Initial symptoms may include headache, bone and muscle pain, and delirium; anemia is also common. Comas, liver damage, brain hemorrhage, and mental disturbance are more serious symptoms that often affect younger victims. Symptoms vary with the life cycle of the parasite, which reproduces in waves in the liver and blood. One species, *Plasmodium falciparum,* bursts forth from an infected liver all at once; it is the deadliest form of malaria, causing 95 percent of all malaria deaths.

Trichomonas   Caused by *Trichomonas,* this is a common sexually transmitted disease that is irritating and painful, but not thought to be dangerous.

ported in the March 20, 1993 *Lancet*). It is not effective on the other species of malaria, however. Further trials are underway.

Although some researchers continued to look for a better vaccine, others looked for different approaches. One concept is to "vaccinate" the mosquitoes. Genes were located that could cause mosquitoes to resist the parasite. The problem with this approach is that no one has shown a way to introduce these genes into the mosquito population. The discovery of the early 1990s that for fruit flies at least there are transposable genes that can spread through the species suggests that perhaps a transposable element can be found for mosquitoes that would carry the gene for parasite resistance into the population.

Worms

Much of the misery for impoverished people in about 70 percent of the world comes from various parasitical worms. In developing countries, about a third of the population is infested to one degree or another with helminths (another name for the smaller parasitical worms, especially the nematodes and flukes). Entire communities have been blinded by *Onchocerca volvulus*. Long-term infection in children can lead to lowered mental abilities. For adults, parasitic worms typically induce morbidity instead of mortality, with individuals gradually growing weaker as the parasite population harbored increases and becomes a drain on the economy. Lack of industry in other populations is associated with the physiological burden of harboring a large population of parasites.

Parasitic worms are difficult for the body to handle, producing only slight immune responses even after long periods of infestation. Thus although most viral or bacterial diseases that are not fatal are self-limiting—symptoms and infectious agents are eliminated after a few days or weeks—infestation of parasitical worms can last for years or for life. Despite this apparent lack of immune response, in most communities a minority of individuals harbor a majority of the parasites, suggesting some ability in the others to repel or expel the invaders.

Gradually researchers are learning how the worms evade the human immune system. In 1992, for example, James H. McKerrow of the University of California in San Francisco and coworkers found that *Schistosoma mansoni,* one of the worms that causes schistosomiasis, uses a part of the immune system to locate its favorite place in the body to live and that the human immune system provokes the worm to lay eggs. The part of the human immune system involved is a chemical called tumor necrosis factor, which normally is present in the veins that carry blood from the small intestine to the liver. The reason that tumor necrosis factor is present is that it is produced by white blood cells called macrophages, which recognize toxins from bacteria in the venous blood (many of the bacteria die in the small intestine and release the toxins) and flock to that part of the body on a regular basis. Tumor necrosis factor is "the sex chemical of the schistosome," causing mating couples to lay eggs. In its absence, they still mate, but with no issue. Some of the eggs penetrate (and damage) the walls of the intestine or bladder and are then excreted, but others are carried to the liver where they lodge. The immune system then turns on them and causes permanent walls to be built around them. Eventually the liver is impaired by the buildup of the encased eggs.

(Periodical References and Additional Reading: *New York Times* 11-30-90, p D19; *New York Times* 2-12-91, p C1; *New York Times* 3-19-91; *New York Times* 8-4-92, p C3; *New York Times* 9-22-92; *New York Times* 3-23-93, p C1; *Science News* 4-3-93, p 220; *Science* 7-30-93, p 546; *Nature* 10-28-93, p 797)

Background

To most people, the word *worm* conjures up, first, an earthworm and then, perhaps, nondescript, small white or red wiggly things. Biologists use the word *worm* as a very general term covering what in some classification schemes amount to about 15 different phyla. Among the many different creatures are worms that cause trichinosis, the whipworms, hookworms, pinworms, roundworms, and the worms that cause filariasis.

Often the parasitic worms are called *helminths,* from a Greek term that means "parasitic worm," though this is not a biological classification. To confuse matters, medical writers sometimes speak of "parasitic helminths."

The parasitic worms cause nearly as much misery as malaria. Schistosomaisis leads the list with 200 million cases annually worldwide; a pork tapeworm is also a major problem, with 50 million cases annually. The International Task Force for Disease Eradication declared in March 1992 that the pork tapeworm, which produces the disease taeniasis-cysticercosis, could potentially be eliminated in humans. Other serious diseases include hookworm, which causes about 60,000 deaths each year, and roundworms (ascariasis), which cause about 20,000 deaths annually.

PARASITIC WORMS

Disease or name of worm	Parasite	Size (in.)	Location in infected person	Mode of transmission
Bladder fluke	*Schistosoma haematobium*	1.2	Blood vessels of bladder	Water inhabited by snails contains larvae that enter through skin
Filariasis	*Wuchereria bancrofti*	3.6	Lymph system	Mosquito bites
Hookworm	*Ancylostoma duodenale* *Necator americanus*	0.5 0.4	Small intestine	Larvae in soil penetrate skin
Pinworm	*Enterobius vermicularis*	0.4	Colon	Eggs in fecal matter are transmitted to food or objects that are put in mouth
River blindness	*Onchocerca volvulus*	16	Beneath skin	Bite of blackfly
Roundworms (ascariasis)	*Ascaris lumbricoides*	8	Small intestine	Eggs in fecal matter are transmitted to food or objects that are put in mouth
Schistosomiasis	*Schistosoma mansoni* *Schistosoma japonica*	0.8	Veins, especially of abdomen	Water inhabited by snails contains larvae that enter through skin
Trichinosis	*Trichinella spiralis*	0.04	Adults in small instestine; larvae form cysts in muscles	Eating infected pork
Whipworms	*Trichuris trichiura*	1.2	Cecum in large intestine	Eggs in fecal matter are transmitted to food or objects that are put in mouth

DON'T DRINK THE WATER

In September 1993, the U.S. Natural Resources Defense Council announced at the end of a two-year investigation that as many as 900,000 Americans become ill from drinking water contaminated with microbes each year. Of those becoming ill, about 900 die, mostly people already weakened by age or other diseases. The report was published during a year that dramatically illustrated the problem described. A major outbreak of water-borne disease in Milwaukee, Wisconsin, was followed by scares in New York City and Washington, D.C.

There are 59,000 community water systems in the U.S. serving about 92 percent of the population. In April 1993, a report by the U.S. General Accounting Office, the investigative arm of Congress, suggested that state inspection programs for such supply systems were far behind schedule and often used untrained or inadequately trained inspectors in any case.

Milwaukee

In the spring of 1993 people in Milwaukee, Wisconsin, began to develop abdominal cramps and diarrhea. About one out of ten cases required medical treatment and one in 100 was severe enough to lead to hospitalization. Eventually nearly 400,000 persons developed the problem. Milwaukee's Health Department determined that of nine deaths of persons known to be infected with the mysterious disease, one death of a 71-year-old woman probably occurred as a direct result of the disease. Most of the other victims were already so ill from other diseases that determining the influence of the water-borne disease would be impossible.

On April 7, 1993, the cause of the disease was identified—a parasite called

Background

The protist genus *Cryptosporidium* was discovered in 1907 in a mouse at Harvard. The intestinal parasite is about two ten-thousandths of an inch (five microns) in diameter, about half the size of an amoeba. Since then, it has been found in the intestines of cattle and other animals; however, it was not recognized as a cause of human disease until 1976. Unlike most bacteria, *Cryptosporidium* is not killed by the chlorine amounts added to water supplies. Although invisible to the naked eye, the parasite is large enough to be removed from water by filtration.

The disease caused by *Cryptosporidium,* called cryprosporidiosis, commonly consists of pains and cramps in the abdomen, nausea and vomiting, and flu-like symptoms, such as fever and fatigue. It is rarely fatal except when the immune system is compromised by AIDS, other illnesses, or old age. Treatment is largely to prevent loss of fluids, using anti-diarrhea drugs. After a time the normal immune system succeeds in ridding the body of the parasite and symptoms vanish. Symptoms disappear before the parasite is completely ousted, however, so care needs to be taken for several more weeks to avoid spreading the disease to others.

Cryptosporidium. A 1991 study of water around the U.S. found that 87 percent of untreated water sources and 27 percent of treated water contains some *Cryptosporidium* parasites, although apparently not enough individual organisms to cause healthy people to become ill. *Cryptosporidium* is evidently in most surface water. Although it is resistant to chlorination, enough parasites are removed by normal water treatment to prevent many people developing symptoms caused by the parasite; however, the last U.S. outbreak before Milwaukee occurred in Jackson County, Oregon, and sickened as many as 15,000 people.

There is some evidence that there was *Cryptosporidium* in Milwaukee's water in November 1992. As part of another study, cryprosporidiosis (infection with *Cryptosporidium*) was sampled in AIDS patients in several large cities. Milwaukee had double the number of cases found in Los Angeles, the largest city in the sample; indeed, Milwaukee had 26 cases, while cities such as Boston, San Francisco, and Philadelphia had fewer than half as many. The most likely source of the contamination in Milwaukee was cattle feces that had been washed into the Milwaukee River, which empties into Lake Michigan near a water-treatment plant.

New York and Washington

The Milwaukee experience was still on official minds when problems developed in Washington, D.C. and northern Virginia. Heavy rains had caused contamination from sewer and farmland runoff at a treatment plant run by the U.S. Army Corps of Engineers. For the first time in its history, the plant was producing water that failed to meet turbidity standards. The Corps told the U.S. Environmental Protection Agency (EPA), which on December 8, 1993 advised two hundred thousand people who normally use the water not to drink it unless they boiled it first. The main concern cited by the EPA was that the dirty-looking water might also be contaminated with *Cryptosporidium,* the villain in Milwaukee.

Testing and analysis of the water took four days, but on December 11, 1993 the water was found to be free of parasites and drinkable. The Corps of Engineers advised users to run their water taps for at least three minutes to clear any water that had been left standing during the alert.

The Corps decided that the problem would never have occurred if workers had increased the amount of aluminum sulfate when turbidity started to rise. Aluminum sulfate causes particles in water to fall to the bottom of tanks (precipitate), leaving clearer water. Although it does not directly kill parasites, it removes food sources and often the parasite along with the mud. In Milwaukee, there was some reason to suspect that a switch to a different chemical intended to precipitate smaller particles may have contributed to the outbreak of cryprosporidiosis.

Earlier in 1993, some New York neighborhoods had a similar alert and were told to boil their water for a few days. In that case, the problem was not *Cryptosporidium,* but the common intestinal bacterium *Escherichia coli.* About 35,000 New Yorkers were affected by the call for home water treatment, but no one was identified as ill from the bacteria.

In 1993 Adrian Parton suggested to his employer, Scientific Generics, a new approach to testing water for *Cryptosporidium* and *Giardia,* another common and troublesome water-borne parasite. The approach, which is being tested by the Severn Trent water utility in the United Kingdom, captures the microbes by first using a monoclonal antibody to attach a microscopic bead to the parasite found floating in water. A rotating electric field then spins the bead-microbe combination, which produces a signal that is also detected electrically. Even a few parasites can be detected and identified by this method, which is far more sensitive than any previous way of recognizing microbes in water.

(Periodical References and Additional Reading: *New York Times* 4-9-93, pp A1, A15; *New York Times* 4-10-93, p 6; *New York Times* 4-20-93, p C3; *New York Times* 4-25-93, p I-40; *Scientific American* 7-93, p 103; *New York Times* 12-8-93, p B17; *New York Times* 12-12-93, p 30; *Discover* 1-94, p 86)

Chronic Diseases

THE STATE OF THE FIGHT AGAINST CHRONIC DISEASE

The dictionary definition of *chronic* is not very helpful in categorizing "chronic" diseases as opposed to other kinds. Dictionaries define it as "of long duration, prolonged, frequently recurring, lingering, ..." and so forth.

Some infectious diseases, such as hepatitis, can be either acute or chronic, in which case the dictionary definition works. Even diseases caused by parasites, such as malaria and schistosomiasis, once contracted often linger for life, perhaps flaring up in recurring episodes. But infectious diseases are usually not intended when diseases are grouped as "chronic."

Hereditary diseases are also not usually labeled "chronic," provided that they are known to be purely genetic in origin. Sickle-cell anemia would fit easily into a class of disease that includes asthma, diabetes, and multiple-sclerosis—except that it has long been known that sickle-cell anemia is caused entirely by one recessive gene that obeys Mendelian laws. There may or may not be a genetic component to asthma, diabetes, and multiple sclerosis, but if there is some hereditary factor it is not the whole story. Some diseases have been moving gradually from classification as "chronic" to "genetic": Alzheimer's is one. Many forms of cancer are also becoming known to be at least partly hereditary.

The tradition of linking such diseases as cancer, heart disease, and Parkinson's disease in a single group labeled "chronic" dates from when very little was known about the causes of the disease. We now know for sure that all cancers are diseases of DNA, although the exact instigator of the disease and even the exact changes in DNA are not often known. The most common forms of heart disease result from cholesterol deposits that are affected by genetics, diet, exercise, and probably other factors. Although it is far from clear what starts Parkinson's disease, it is now certain which neurotransmitter, brain regions, and so forth have changes that cause the symptoms.

The diseases here labeled "chronic" are more like Parkinson's in that the ultimate cause is not well understood. A classic example would be "essential" hypertension, for which the word *essential* means—to physicians at least—that the cause is completely unknown. The same is true for much hearing or eyesight loss.

Here is a list of diseases not mentioned above that to one degree or another have poorly understood causes and last for a substantial period of time or recur: acne (skin), Addison's disease (adrenal glands), allergies, amyotrophic lateral sclerosis (ALS, or "Lou Gehrig's disease"), aneurysm (blood vessels), angina (heart), ankylosing spondylitis (joints), arteriosclerosis, atherosclerosis, atrial fibrillation (heart), Bell's palsy (tic), benign prostatic hyperplasia (*see* "Prostate Problems," p 230), Buerger's disease, bursitis, carpal tunnel syndrome (wrist and hand), cataracts (eyes), Crohn's disease (intestines), Cushing's disease (adrenal glands), diabetes insipidus (pituitary), diverticulitis (intestines), eczema (skin), emphysema (lungs), endometriosis (uterus), epilepsy (brain), farsightedness (eyes), fibroids (tumors), gallstones (gall bladder), glaucoma (eyes), gout (joints), hemorrhoids (intestines), hyperthyroidism (high hormone levels), hypoglycemia (metabolic), hypothyroidism (low hormone levels), irritable bowel syndrome, kidney stones, macular degeneration (eyes), Meniere's disease (ears), migraine (headaches), Myasthenia gravis (muscles), myopia (eyes), osteoarthritis (joints), osteoporosis (bones), polymytosis (muscles), polyps, pre-eclampsia (see "New Uses for Aspirin," p 527), psoriasis (skin and joints), purpura (blood vessels), pylelonephritis (kidneys), Raynaud's disease (circulation), retinal detachment (eyes), rheumatoid arthritis, sarcoidosis (lungs and other organs), sciatica (a nerve inflammation caused most often by ruptured disk in spinal column), scleroderma (skin), stroke (blood vessels in brain), systemic lupus erythematosus (SLE, an autoimmune disease), temporal arteritis (arteries in cranium), tendonitis (tendons), and ulcerative colitis (intestines).

As you can see, "chronic" diseases range widely. They include some such as ALS that cause death invariably, usually within four years of onset, to others such as myopia that are easily treatable and more of an annoyance than an actual disease. Most on this list are in between these extremes—diseases that persist as a major disability throughout life or diseases that in some forms are mildly debilitating and in other forms are deadly. The reason for this great spread is that the category is a "catch-all" formed mostly by lack of knowledge. As the causes of these disease become more clear, they move into different categories.

The two main causes of death in the U.S. are included in the "chronic" category, although all too often they are fatal rather than chronic in the dictionary sense. Heart disease can strike without warning and kill in a matter of minutes. Often someone with this "chronic" disease dies without ever feeling a symptom until the acute attack. Nevertheless, conditions for the heart attack have been building for years, and the deceased had heart or circulatory disease all during that time. Cancer can seem very swift, usually a matter of months, but it too has existed in the body for a long period before the symptoms have become evident, perhaps as a slow-growing cancer or as a pre-cancerous lesion of some kind.

A third large group of diseases in the "chronic" category are moving toward a major category of their own. Autoimmune diseases are similar to cancers in that they are linked by one ultimate cause but have many occasions and attack many different parts of the body in different ways. The immune system was barely known 50 years ago and only recognized as a complex body system in the more recent past. As its parts and methods of operation have become known, many diseases that once appeared mysterious and disparate are recognized as being the effects of an attack by a person's immune system on the person's organs.

Diabetes mellitus illustrates better than most conditions the complexity. As long ago as the ancient Greeks, this disease could be recognized by sweet urine (the other diabetes, by coincidence also involving the pancreas, has as a symptom excessive urine also, but the urine is not sweet). Gradually, physicians recognized that there were two types of diabetes mellitus as well, and that different mechanisms of sugar metabolism were at work. In type I diabetes (formerly called juvenile), possible factors of initiation were genes and infections, but the ultimate cause was an attack by the immune system on certain cells in the pancreas. In type II diabetes (formerly called adult), possible factors of initiation were genes, lifestyle (diet and exercise), and something unknown. Type II diabetes may or may not be an autoimmune disease. Furthermore, there is a third category of diabetes for which the ultimate cause is one of several other chronic diseases that have diabetes mellitus as one of their occasional symptoms.

The more physicians learn about chronic diseases, the more they turn out to be like diabetes. Arthritis, for example, was once thought to be simply wear and tear on the joints as an inevitable result of old age. Then rheumatoid arthritis was recognized as sharply different from osteoarthritis, and later the rheumatoid form was found to be an autoimmune disease. Osteoarthritis was still considered mostly mechanical, but more recently genetic factors have become suspect.

Advances in Treatment

Because of the complex nature of the causes of the "chronic" diseases, advances are most always restricted to specific conditions. Among the newer therapies that are being attempted for several of these diseases is fetal cell transplantation (*see* "Cell Transplantation: Fetal Tissue and More," p 511). There have also been some general approaches to autoimmune disease through the use of monoclonal antibodies that attack the unfriendly antibodies attracting the organs; through a new technique called oral tolerization; and through the reduction of antibody-producing cells (white blood cells). Reduction of white blood cells has the side effect of lowering overall immunity to disease, making this a treatment reserved for people with serious illness. (*See also* "Autoimmune UPDATE," p 447.) Listed below are some new treatments or experimental treatments of the 1990s:

Gallstones   In the late 1980s a new drug and a new treatment seemed to bring an end to gall bladder removal as a treatment for gallstones. Nevertheless, the stones kept coming back after the new treatment, lithotripsy (the use of sound waves to break up the stones), and after ursodial (the main new drug). In 1990, however, laproscopic removal of the gall bladder was developed as a truly effective treatment.

Migraines   These headaches are periodic and often accompanied by disturbed vision or nausea. No one knows exactly what causes them. A disturbance to blood flow in the brain is the immediate cause of the headache pain, however; thus they are sometimes alleviated if high blood pressure is brought under control. In March 1993, an injectable drug called sumatriptan (tradenamed Imitrex) that is said to stop a migraine in progress began to be marketed in the U.S. One study found that 70 percent of those who tried the drug got relief and that nearly half the patients felt no symptoms after the injection. Sumatriptan works by acting on serotonin receptors in the brain. It is expensive and not recommended for patients with atherosclerosis. An oral form may be coming.

Polyps   Benign growths in the lining of the large intestine are a major form of polyp for which surgery is usually recommended. Such polyps are likely to change over into colon cancers. In April 1993 the National Polyp Study reported that after intestinal-polyp surgery, follow-up examinations by colonoscope (an uncomfortable, costly, and slightly dangerous procedure) are needed at three-year intervals instead of the one-year intervals previously thought necessary.

Osteoporosis   This condition is a general weakening and thinning of bone that is usually associated with aging. While nearly all news about osteoporosis has focused on diet, exercise, and estrogen, two studies in 1990 demonstrated that it can also be caused by even a slight excess of thyroid hormone.

Psoriasis   This disease is most often confined to the skin, where it can pose a lifelong problem, although it is even more serious when it moves into the joints and causes arthritis. It may have both genetic and autoimmune causes, perhaps in tandem. Treatment with cortisone compounds sometimes helps but fails to cure. Ultraviolet light, by itself or combined with the photosensitive drug psoralen, has also been used.

An accidental observation in Japan, where a compound was being tested for its effect on osteoporosis, has led to a new and remarkably successful psoriasis drug. The drug is the familiar vitamin D, but as an ointment whose major ingredient is an active form of the vitamin called calcitriol (or 1,25-dyhydroxyvitamin). First tested in the U.S. in 1988, the ointment moved slowly into clinical practice because of fears that calcitriol would increase the amount of calcium circulating in the blood, causing stones in the urinary tracts or other kidney complications to develop. After several years of testing, however, calcitriol became available for regular use in the U.S., where it quickly found fans among long-term psoriatics.

Scleroderma   In this disease, the skin thickens and hardens; similar changes inside the body can also disrupt organs, which can be life-threatening. Scleroderma is thought to be an autoimmune disease in which the protein collagen, an important structural protein in skin and elsewhere, is attacked. The disease became better known to the general public when scleroderma was among the diseases thought to be induced by silicone breast implants, though there never was conclusive evidence of this connection (*see* "Implants and the Immune System," p 223).

Tests were ongoing at the end of 1993 on the use of the drug penicillamine as a possible control for scleroderma; if the drug is found to be effective, it will be the first treatment that works. Other new therapies are also being tested in about 30 different centers around the U.S. and in other trials in other countries.

(Periodical References and Additional Reading: *Harvard Health Letter* 2-91, p 7; *Harvard Health Letter* 3-91, p 7; *Harvard Health Letter* 4-92, p 1; *Harvard Health Letter* 7-93, p 8; *Harvard Health Letter* 11-93, p 8; *New York Times* 3-19-93, p D3; *Harvard Health Letter* 5-94, p 6)

TIMETABLE OF PROGRESS AGAINST CHRONIC DISEASE TO 1990

1670	Thomas Willis [born Great Bedwyn, England, January 27, 1621; died London, November 11, 1675] rediscovers that the urine of people with diabetes tastes sweet, which had also been known to ancient Greeks.
1683	Thomas Sydenham [born Wynford Eagle, England, September 10, 1624; died London, December 29, 1689] produces a careful description of the symptoms of gout.

1726   Stephen Hale [born Bekesbourne, England, September 17, 1677; died
        Teddington, England, January 4, 1761] makes the first measurement of blood
        pressure of a horse.

1733   *Haemostaticks* by Stephen Hale relates his experiments on blood pressure
        with notes on the mechanical relations of the pressure to conditions, the
        velocity of blood flow, and the capacity of the different blood vessels.

1801   Thomas Young [born Milverton, England, June 13, 1773; died London, May 10,
        1829] discovers the cause of astigmatism.

1864   Franciscus Cornelius Donders [born Tilburg, North Brabant, Netherlands, May
        27, 1818; died Utrecht, Netherlands, March 24, 1889] rediscovers that
        astigmatism is caused by an uneven curvature of the lens or cornea of the eye.

1889   Oskar Minkowski [born Kaunas, Lithuania, January 13, 1858; died Fürstenberg
        an der Havel, Germany, July 18, 1931] discovers that urine from dogs whose
        pancreas has been removed contains excess sugar, suggesting that absence of
        pancreatic function causes diabetes mellitus, recognized since ancient times by
        the presence of sugar in urine; according to some, the dogs' urine attracted
        flies and Minkowski was impelled to taste the urine to find out why.

1903   Surgeon Georg Perthes [born Germany, September 17, 1869; died 1927]
        discovers that X rays inhibit the growth of tumors and proposes X-ray
        treatment for cancer.

1910   Francis Peyton Rous [born Baltimore, Maryland, October 5, 1879; died New
        York, February 16, 1970] discovers that sarcomas in chickens are caused by a
        virus.

1912   In Chicago, James Bryan Herrick [born Oak Park, Illinois, August 11, 1861;
        died Chicago, Illinois, March 7, 1954] for the first time teaches other
        physicians how to recognize heart attacks in the living; previously, heart
        attacks had only been diagnosed after death.

1936   George Richards Minot [born Boston, Massachusetts, December 2, 1885; died
        Brookline, Massachusetts, February 25, 1950] and William B. Castle publish
        Pathological Physiology and Clinical Description of the Anemias.

1948   Philip Showalter Hench [born Pittsburgh, Pennsylvania, February 28, 1896;
        died Ocho Rios, Jamaica, March 30, 1965] discovers that cortisone can be used
        to treat rheumatoid arthritis.

        Paul Dudley White and other heart specialists start the Framingham Heart
        Study, which provides the first solid evidence of the relationship between
        lifestyle and heart disease; data from the study—which began with 5200 men
        and women, added another 5000 sons and daughters starting in the 1970s, and
        was still ongoing 50 years later—have also been used in many studies of
        illness other than just heart disease.

1960   Surgeon William Chardack and electrical engineer Wilson Greatbatch develop
        the "permanent" implantable pacemaker, which operates on long-life,
        replaceable batteries.

1968   French-American physiologist Roger Guillemin [born Dijon, France, January 11,
        1924] and Polish-American biochemist Andrew Victor Schally [born Vilnius,
        Lithuania, November 30, 1926] discover a simple substance produced by the
        brain that affects the hormones produced by the pituitary gland.

1971   Chemists at the Research Triangle Institute in North Carolina isolate the active ingredient of a powerful anti-cancer drug made from the bark of Pacific yew trees; they name this ingredient taxol. The anticancer activity of extracts from the bark had been known since the 1960s.

U.S. President Richard M. Nixon on December 23 signs the National Cancer Act, popularly known as the "war on cancer."

1976   John Michael Bishop [born York, Pennsylvania, February 22, 1936] and Harold Elliott Varmus [born Oceanside, New York, December, 1939] recognize that a viral gene that causes cancer in chickens is essentially the same as a normal gene in most animal cells; this is the first recognition of a specific proto-oncogene, a normal gene that with a slight mutation could become an "oncogene," or a gene that causes cancer by promoting excessive growth.

1982   Swedish physicians attempt to cure Parkinson's disease with dopamine generated by the patients' own adrenal glands; however, implanting tissues from the gland in the brain produces either temporary or no improvement.

1985   The U.S. Food and Drug Administration approves the implantable cardiac defibrillator, a mechanical device used to prevent the heart from beating too rapidly or from fibrillating (quivering instead of beating); it is implanted in the patient's chest where it is powered for five years by a lithium battery.

Bert L. Vallee [born Hemer, Germany, June 1, 1919] and coworkers find the tumor angiogenesis factor first predicted by Judah Folkman in 1961; it stimulates the growth of new blood vessels. They rename the factor angiogenin.

1987   Murray B. Bornstein reports on a two-year study of the drug Cop 1, which he finds is successful in slowing the early stages of multiple sclerosis.

Ignacio Navarro Madrazo announces that surgery implanting a cell from a person's adrenal gland in the brain can cure or alleviate Parkinson's disease; earlier experiments along the same general lines had been unsuccessful, but Madrazo changes the location of the implant.

DISEASES OF THE CIRCULATORY SYSTEM

CHEMISTRY AND HEART ATTACKS

The most common cause of death in the U.S. is heart disease. Although deaths from almost all diseases of the circulatory system have fallen dramatically ever since the 1950s, when it was popularly recognized that cholesterol and fat contribute to heart disease, the death rate from heart disease is still about 40 percent higher than the next group of causes, cancers. About one death in three is attributed to heart disease.

There are, no doubt, many causes for the continuing drop in heart-disease deaths. Increased exercise and healthier diets are certainly important. So is the reduction in smoking in the U.S.

But physicians know that lifestyle changes are not the whole story. A very important part of the decline in heart disease results from the use of new drugs to prevent or treat heart disease. (And there are other factors, too. *See* "Heart Disease and Strokes UPDATE," p 400.) Of these chemicals, the best established and perhaps the most beneficial so far are compounds that reduce high blood pressure (*see* "High Blood Pressure UPDATE," p 407). Other drugs are newer, less widespread in use, and in some cases controversial. But these chemicals are also having an impact on heart disease now, and some look as if they will become even greater factors against heart disease in the future.

Cholesterol and Drugs

Cholesterol is implicated in the build-up of plaque inside arteries, a condition known as atherosclerosis which is the basic cause of most heart disease. Although many people succeed in lowering cholesterol levels in their blood somewhat by diet (often combined with exercise), it is extremely difficult to make a major impact on cholesterol levels that way. Diets must be extremely restrictive, not just "replace butter with margarine and stop at only one egg a week and cut down on red meat." For many individuals, not even a low-fat vegetarian diet makes enough difference. But drugs have been shown to be successful in reducing cholesterol, especially in conjunction with diet improvement. The combination has reduced serum cholesterol levels in Americans from an average of 220 mg/dl in the early 1960s to an average of 205 mg/dl at the start of the 1990s.

In 1992, more than 26 million prescriptions were filled for cholesterol-lowering drugs, mostly lovastatin (tradenamed Mevacor—also available as Zocor or Pravachol) at 47 percent of all prescriptions and gemfibrozil (Lopid) at 29 percent. Lovastatin works by causing the liver to make less cholesterol. Gemfibrozil speeds up removal of lipoproteins from the blood. Another pair of medicines cause more cholesterol to be used up in the manufacture of bile acids, so the cholesterol does not get released into the blood. For those who find such drugs too "chemical," there is the well-known B vitamin niacin, which has been shown to be moderately effective in reducing cholesterol.

Background

The problem chemicals in the blood for heart disease occur when levels of substances variously labeled as cholesterol, fatty acids, triglycerides, trans fats, lipids, and low-density lipoproteins (LDLs) are too high. There is also frequent mention of high-density lipoproteins (HDLs), which are thought to be beneficial. Anyone without a background in organic chemistry is bound to be confused by it all.

Lipids are fats; the three main nutrients are carbohydrates, proteins, and lipids, all necessary for life. When fats are consumed, the body uses enzymes to break some of the complex fats into free fatty acids and glycerol, known to many as an ingredient in antifreeze.

Fatty acids are sometimes classed as lipids, and sometimes considered to be sister chemicals. They are best known from the omega-3 fatty acids found mainly in fish and thought to be a protective factor for the circulatory system.

Fatty acids aside, there are two kinds of simple lipids: triglycerides and sterols.

As the name suggests, a *triglyceride* is a chemical derived from the familiar sweetish solvent glycerol by binding it to a fatty acid. Triglycerides are what we normally think of as fats, including the saturated, monounsaturated, and polyunsaturated kinds, although it is actually the fatty acids in triglycerides that are or are not saturated. By themselves, triglycerides are probably not harmful to the circulatory system, even in large amounts. High blood levels of triglycerides can inflame the pancreas, or the triglycerides can be deposited as fat on the back or buttocks.

A *sterol* is classed as an alcohol, with *cholesterol* being the principal sterol in vertebrate physiology, being one of the main ingredients in the membrane that surrounds each cell.

A *lipoprotein* is a simple protein that has been combined with a fat or a fatlike substance. Lipoproteins are used to transfer lipids through the blood. Dietary fat from the intestine is packed into one kind of lipoprotein, while fat manufactured from leftover carbohydrates and proteins in the liver is packaged into another kind of lipoprotein along with cholesterol that is also made in the liver. The packages made in the liver are called very-low-density lipoproteins.

As the very-low-density lipoproteins travel through the body, they gradually give up their triglycerides to various fat cells, but the cholesterol remains. When the triglycerides are gone, the package becomes what is called *low-density lipoprotein* or LDL. Each LDL aggregation contains about 1500 molecules of cholesterol loosely packed in a bag that is similar in composition to a cell membrane. Cholesterol by itself is insoluble in blood and needs such packages to get around. The LDL bag has a handle. The handle is a protein projecting through the bag. This protein is the target for a receptor that is in all cells. If all goes well, the LDL receptor snares an LDL package as it floats through the blood and brings it into a cell for disassembly so that the cholesterol molecules can be used. People who do not have enough of the receptor molecule as a result of their particular alleles of the gene for that receptor develop very high levels of LDL in their bloodstreams, because not enough LDL is being picked up by the cells.

Tighter packaging of cholesterol results in *high-density cholesterol*, which contains approximately equal parts of lipid and protein. HDL is thought not to cause the build-up of plaque in arteries, or to clog them the way that LDL does, but no one is certain why. Prominent theories are that HDL removes excess cholcstcrol from blood-vcssel walls and transports it back to the liver for reprocessing; and that high HDL levels are simply a marker for good metabolism of fats, and not themselves active in protection against heart disease. Experiments in 1993 suggest, however, that HDL is most likely active in protecting against atherosclerosis by some means or another.

Trans fats are unsaturated fats that have been straightened by the addition of hydrogen. This stiffens the fats and keeps them from melting at room temperature. "Solid" vegetable oil margarines all maintain their partial solidity with trans fats. The closer to solidity the margarine is, the more trans fats it contains. Recent research has suggested that trans fats also raise the amount of cholesterol circulating in the blood.

CHOLESTEROL-LOWERING DRUGS

Drug	Tradenames	Number of prescriptions	Comments
Nicotinic acid	Niacin	Over the counter	Inexpensive but effective at doses of at least 1.5 g per day, which can produce abnormal liver function in one out of 20 patients.
Lovastatin	Mevacor, Zocor, Pravachol	15,000	Inhibits liver enzyme that initiates cholesterol production; used mainly for people with hypercholesterolemia; lowers LDL as well as total blood cholesterol.
Gemfibrozil	Lopid	8000	Reduces triglycerides and elevates HDL; may cause gallstones with long-term use.
Cholestyramine	Questran, Questran Light, Cholybar	3000	Reduces total and LDL cholesterol, but may elevate triglycerides; often constipating, as it works by combining with bile in intestines, promoting excretion of the combination.
Probucol	Lorelco	500	Reduces total and LDL cholesterol, but may elevate HDL; not for use in patients with abnormal heart rhythms; mode of action unknown.
Colestipol	Colestid	250	Similar in action to cholestyramine.

Some studies also showed that oat bran and later rice bran oil lower cholesterol. For women, an unexpected side effect found in a large-scale test of the drug tamoxifen on breast cancer was a reduction in LDL cholesterol (*see also* "Breast Cancer," p 216). For men, Per Bjorntorp of the University of Gothenburg in Sweden found that smearing a testosterone gel on the arms and shoulders not only reduced serum cholesterol levels but also promoted weight loss, muscle strength, resistance to diabetes and perhaps prostate cancer (*see also* "Prostate Problems," p 230).

Monkeying with mice   Keith R. Marotti and a team from Upjohn reported in the July 1, 1993 *Nature* that a protein changes the way cholesterol affects heart disease.

In their study, mice bred to be susceptible to heart disease developed much larger and more serious atherosclerotic plaques in the aorta when the mice also had high levels of a protein known to reduce the ratio of HDL cholesterol to LDL cholesterol.

All the mice in the study had been confronted with what the researchers termed a "high-fat, high cholesterol semi-synthetic diet." The diet was actually comprised of ingredients of which a half were sugar, a fifth protein from cheese, a seventh butter, and somewhat more than a tenth vitamin-and-mineral-enriched cellulose, with only one percent cholesterol—a diet apparently modeled on one of the special meals at a fast-food restaurant.

The specific protein involved is known as simian cholesterol ester transfer protein (CETP)—simian because it is a monkey protein genetically inserted into the strain of mice. Its normal task is to turn triglycerides in the blood into LDL cholesterol. Mice with a lot of CETP also develop large amounts of LDL cholesterol. The total amount of cholesterol in the blood is not affected, but more of the cholesterol is LDL and less therefore is HDL. True to expectations, the mice with the high LDL levels also get heart disease.

Nature suggests that Upjohn's research might eventually be directed toward development of a way to reduce CETP levels in humans as a way of reducing heart disease. It would appear that this might work for humans exposed to a diet similar to that of the experimental mice.

TIMETABLE OF LIPIDS AND THE HEART

1939	Carl Müller of the Oslo Community Hospital in Norway identifies familial hypercholesterolemia, a hereditary disorder of metabolism in which high cholesterol levels lead to an early death from heart disease.
1951	Robert Burns Woodward synthesizes cholesterol.
1973	Michael S. Brown and Joseph L. Goldstein of the University of Texas Health Center at Dallas discover how cholesterol gets from the liver, where it is manufactured, to the cells. They recognize low-density lipoprotein and find the receptor for it.
1978	Yoshio Watanabe of Kobe University in Japan finds a strain of rabbits that have very high-cholesterol levels and develop human-like coronary heart disease as a result.
1983	A panel of the U.S. National Institutes of Health (NIH) finds that triglycerides are markers for lipid conditions that could lead to coronary heart disease. They recommend diet or drug intervention to lower triglycerides below 250 mg/dl.
1984	A ten-year study using drugs demonstrates that reducing cholesterol levels in blood protects against heart attacks. An NIH panel recommends that aggressive diets be used to lower both total cholesterol and LDLs.
1985	The National Heart, Lung and Blood Institute of the NIH sets up the National Cholesterol Education Program (NCEP).
1987	The Adult Treatment Panel of NCEP suggests to physicians and the general public that a serum (blood) cholesterol level less than 200 mg/dl is a desirable goal for everyone. Also, LDL levels below 130 mg/dl and HDL levels above 35 mg/dl are desirable.

1990   Dutch researchers find that trans fats in hydrogenated vegetable oils, even when the oils are polyunsaturated, raise serum cholesterol levels.

1993   Various animal researchers demonstrate that different forms of HDL vary greatly in their effects on heart disease, with Type A-I HDL cholesterol being the "good" lipoprotein. Aldons J. Lusis, Craig H. Warden, and coworkers of the University of California-Los Angeles, for example, find that Type A-I HDL cholesterol stops plaque but type A-II fails to protect against heart disease (in mice). Meanwhile, laboratory studies show that a different low-density lipoprotein, known as lipoprotein(a) and not counted as LDL, also may be a cause of heart disease.

Other Heart Failure

Heart attacks are sudden emergencies, but many people live for years with "bad tickers." Multiple heart attacks, chronic valve disease, or viral illnesses such as pericarditis and rheumatic fever can interfere with heart action in various ways. Although sometimes open-heart surgery can repair valves or solve other problems, often the heart is beyond repair and needs to be replaced (*see* "Organ Transplant Proliferation and Problems," p 505). But sometimes the waiting list for a suitable new heart is too long or the patient is too weak for a transplant, and death eventually comes from another heart attack or complications of heart failure.

Drugs have now been successfully used to treat these kinds of coronary problems by lowering the blood pressure within the heart itself first and later lowering pressure and body fluids in a more conventional way. For the most part the drugs are the same as those used to control blood pressure and angina, but the drugs are administered through a catheter that has been threaded through a neck artery and into the heart. Such procedures are only appropriate on those whose hearts are failing, and even then they are successful in only two out of three patients in improving the quality of life. For those for whom this procedure does work, however, relief is apparent within 24 hours. Breathing improves and they feel stronger. Soon patients are walking one or two miles a day, which, along with oral or transdermal administration of the same drugs, often keeps the patient relatively healthy until a transplant heart is available. Then as another benefit, the patient is stronger and better able to survive the rigors of the transplant operation and a new heart.

Other Chemical Causes of Heart Attacks

Cholesterol and other lipids are not the only contributors to heart attacks, though they may be the main villains in the atherosclerosis that is the primary cause of nearly all heart disease. The kidney hormone renin when present in high levels in the blood is associated with a heart attack rate that is five times that of people with low renin according to a paper in the April 18, 1991 *New England Journal of Medicine.* Both beta blockers and ACE inhibitors (*see* "High Blood Pressure UPDATE," p 407) used to treat hypertension also lower renin levels. Indeed, high renin levels are one of the main immediate causes of high blood pressure. This is because renin calls up another hormone, angiotensin, from the body; it is the angiotensin that closes up blood vessels and raises blood pressure. The ACE that is inhibited is a chemical called angiotensin converting enzyme. Animals that have been injected with angiotensin develop heart attacks or strokes.

Similarly, a 1992 study found that men who had two particular alleles for the gene that manufactures natural ACE have a 34 percent higher risk of developing heart disease. These alleles, known as deletion polymorphisms (which does NOT mean that the gene is deleted, as some popular accounts of this research suggest), cause the level of angiotensin II in the blood to be twice what it is in individuals with the more common alleles of this gene. Another gene, this one for the precursor of angiotensin, has also been shown to possess alleles that contribute to high blood pressure, a known risk factor for heart disease.

Levels of blood chemicals in the renin-angiotensin system vary rapidly and it is difficult to be certain how changes in the various chemicals in this system might cause heart disease or heart attacks. A number of individuals experience heart attacks without high cholesterol or other known risk factors, but this array of evidence implicates the renin-angiotensin system in at least some of those cases.

In 1981 Jerome L. Sullivan of the Veterans Affairs Medical Center in Charleston South Carolina proposed that high levels of iron in the body could cause heart disease. Although Sullivan's theory was rejected by the *New England Journal of Medicine* and

---

THE RENIN-ANGIOTENSIN SYSTEM

Renin (pronounced REE-nin) and several forms of angiotensin work together with ACE in a typical biological fashion. The apparent role of a protein called angiotensinogen is to wait around in the blood for something to happen. The kidneys make the hormone called renin in response to such factors as blood pressure. Kidneys clean the wastes from blood and they need a constant and plentiful of blood supply to do their work. If the kidneys require higher-pressure blood, they call it up with a messenger, which is the hormone renin. Renin interacts with the waiting angiotensinogen to change it into a peptide (small amino-acid chain) called angiotensin I. Angiotensin I also does not do anything but sit around and wait, although not for long. Also circulating in the blood is another chemical, angiotensin-converting-enzyme or ACE, which interacts with angiotensin I and produces angiotensin II.

Angiotensin II is the real worker in this story. Its primary purpose, from the kidneys' point of view at least, is to constrict blood vessels, raising the blood pressure. As with other active biochemicals, angiotensin II may also have other physiological effects, which at present are not well understood.

ACE has other known actions in addition to conversion of angiotensin. Among these is the degradation of certain chemicals called vasodilator kinins. In laboratory studies, ACE is produced in larger amounts by tissue involved in heart attacks. There is a suggestion that ACE could be involved in the overall stiffness of blood vessels.

ACE inhibitors are several chemicals that interfere with the action of ACE. Some of these have been shown to reduce the risk of both heart failure and heart attack. Although ACE inhibitors lower high blood pressure, studies with humans have shown that ACE by itself does not cause high blood pressure.

by the *Journal of the American Medical Association,* it was published in *Lancet.* Even with Sullivan's warning, physicians were taken by surprise when a Finnish study in 1992 by Jukka T. Salonen of the University of Kuopio showed that high levels of ferritin, the protein most often measured to determine iron levels in the body, correlate positively with heart attacks in at least in Finland. Epidemiological studies also correlate high iron levels with heart disease. One possible way that iron could cause heart disease is by combining with LDL cholesterol to form plaque.

Stopping Heart Attacks

The American Heart Association estimates that 2.3 to three million persons in the U.S. each year experience what are commonly called heart attacks or heart failure. Not all heart failure is an "attack," but about 1.5 million heart failures are "attacks," mostly as a result of sudden blockage of an artery in the heart by a blood clot. Only about 340,000 of the heart attack victims die, so there are somewhat more than three nonfatal heart attacks for every fatal one.

One reason that many survive heart attacks has been the ability of various drugs to bolster patients chances. Standard treatment now is a three-pronged attack: aspirin to reduce blood clotting (*see* "New Uses for Aspirin," p 527), an injected clot-dissolving drug such as streptokinase, and a beta-blocker, which both lowers blood pressure and steadies heart beat. Some new drugs are being tested or used as a part of the highly successful regimen.

A large-scale study of the new drug vesnarinone was described in the July 15, 1993 *New England Journal of Medicine.* The drug was used with 477 men and women undergoing heart attacks who were failing to respond to standard therapy. The death rate from all causes in these patients was reduced to 62 percent of what happened in a matched group who received a placebo. Vesnarinone is controversial, however, for two reasons: (1) no one knows how it works and (2) the safety window for dosage is unusually narrow. Heart attack victims who receive slightly too much of the drug die as a result of the overdose. Further studies will be needed, both to try to discover the cause of its effectiveness and to become more familiar with the safe level for administering the drug. But its success rate in the first round of tests was two to four times greater than that of other drugs for preventing death during heart attacks.

Although several new drugs have been helpful in improving the survival rate for heart attacks, doctors have continued to look for additional drugs that could boost that rate even further. Three promising ideas were to use nitric oxide to relax blood vessels (*see* "The Ubiquity of NO in Life," p 305), to use a second blood-pressure drug (in addition to the beta blocker) that has a different mechanism (*see* "High Blood Pressure UPDATE," p 407), and to use injectable magnesium. All have been tried sporadically for several years, but only in 1993 have there been large-scale trials to determine effectiveness.

Nitrogen and heart attacks   In the 1990s it has become clear that nitroglycerine helps overcome angina and heart-attack pain by increasing the supply of nitric oxide, which in turn relaxes blood vessels. Various nitrates have also been used for the same purpose. Two double-blind studies tested whether or not the same concept would also reduce death rates. In both studies the death rate with the nitrogen was statistically the same as with the placebo. Nitrogen compounds are safe and still have an important place in reduction of pain, but are not useful in improving survival.

Magnesium Physicians often inject magnesium after a heart attack to stimulate the heart's pumping ability and to reduce arrhythmia. Low magnesium in the diet is suspected of causing heart disease. A 1993 study of 27,413 patients conducted by researcher from Oxford University in England, however, shows that intravenous magnesium does not help when compared to a placebo. On the other hand, an earlier report by researchers from the U.S. National Heart, Lung and Blood Institute and also the Oxford University study found that magnesium improved chances of survival by 55 percent.

ACE inhibitors Angiotensin-converting-enzyme (ACE) inhibitors are successfully used to lower blood pressure, although their mechanism is poorly understood. One of these, captopril, has been aggressively tested for other possible uses in the U.S. Another drug of the same class is lisinopril. The two drugs were tested as an add-on to standard heart-attack treatment by the Oxford group and in China (captopril) and in Italy (lisinopril). Although the ACE inhibitors reduced death rates slightly (about seven percent), captopril at least also produced more instances of kidney failure than the placebo did. An earlier study using a different ACE inhibitor, enalapril (trade-named Vasotec), with heart attacks was halted when it showed no benefit and possibly some harm.

On the other hand, a different earlier study of enalapril found that hospitalizations and death from heart failure were both reduced with older patients who had been diagnosed with chronic heart failure.

(Periodical References and Additional Reading: *Harvard Health Letter* 5-90, p 2; *New York Times* 1-15-91; *New York Times* 4-18-91; *New York Times* 8-1-91; *Harvard Health Letter* 6-92, p 6; *Harvard Health Letter* 8-92, p 8; *New York Times* 9-8-92. p A1; *Nature* 9-10-92, p 107; *Nature* 10-15-92, pp 588 & 641; *New York Times* 10-15-92. p B14; *New York Times* 10-20-92. p C3; *Science News* 1-30-93, p 77; *Harvard Health Letter* 3-93, p 1; *Science News* 3-6-93, p 150; *Science News* 6-12-93, p 375; *New York Times* 7-16-93, p D21; *Science* 7-23-93, p 469; *Science News* 7-24-93, p 55; *New York Times* 9-1-93, p C10; *Statistical Bulletin,* 10/12-93, p 10; *New York Times* 11-8-93, p B10)

Heart Disease and Strokes UPDATE

At the beginning of the 1990s an estimated 70,020,000 Americans had some form of a circulatory disease, which includes high blood pressure as well as heart failure and strokes. Not all of these Americans were elderly: one out of every six men and one of every nine women in the 45–64 age bracket suffered from these heart diseases. The circulatory diseases resulted in death for 930,477 persons in the U.S. in 1990, with about one victim in six under the age of 65.

From one point of view, however, this is good news. That is because the 1990 death rate from heart diseases in the U.S., which was 152 deaths per hundred thousand in population, marked another reduction in a sequence of annual death-rate declines that began in 1968, when the American rate was 270 deaths per hundred thousand. Even before 1968 the rate had an overall tendency to decrease—it had been over 300 per hundred thousand in 1950. From the 1920s to the 1950s, however, death rates from heart disease had been on the rise in the U.S.

The cause for the reduction in deaths is not entirely known, but such risk factors as high serum cholesterol and tobacco smoking also declined during this period, while exercise, which offers protective benefits, increased. Treatment for heart disease and heart attacks has also improved, with new drugs, better uses for old drugs, new surgical procedures—including heart transplants—and better emergency transportation.

More and more people try to prevent that first heart attack with surgery—e.g. heart bypass operations or some form of angioplasty. More than 550,000 Americans opted for one or the other annually in the early 1990s. The older procedure is bypass surgery in which blood is routed around blocked coronary artery, using an artery taken from elsewhere in the patient's body. Angioplasty is the mechanical opening of the arteries. By far the most common form of angioplasty uses a long narrow balloon that is inflated inside the artery, pushing plaque against the vessel walls. Lasers are sometimes used to clear plaque from arteries and other mechanical means have also been tried. Research conducted in 1993 demonstrated that the less physically demanding angioplasty is just as effective as bypass surgery for blockage in a single artery, although deposits in more than one artery are better treated by a double, triple, or even quadruple bypass operation.

Improved treatment has had a high price—hospitals, nursing homes, doctors, and nurses cost $93.1 billion in 1990. Initial costs for bypass surgery average about $24,000 and $18,000 for balloon angioplasty, but both procedures often must be repeated, especially the angioplasty. Even when a heart-attack victim apparently has been lost after emergency treatment seems to have failed, additional efforts are often made in a hospital setting to resuscitate the victim. The added cost of the hospital effort is from $2000 to $3000 per patient, but few of such victims are successfully revived. Reviving patients already in hospitals after their hearts have stopped results in hospital expenses of about $150,000 per survivor, but even then only one in 20 becomes well enough to be discharged from the hospital. Thus, most recent efforts have focused on getting doctors, nurses, or more often paramedics to where a heart attack has occurred as quickly as possible and administering standard cardiopulmonary resuscitation (CPR) on the spot.

Heart Disease in the Industrialized World

Heart disease is not confined to industrialized nations, but in the developing world so many die from infectious disease at younger ages that fewer are left for the chronic diseases of middle and old age. In the most advanced nations, however, heart disease mortality ranges from a low of 104 (women) or 206 (men) per hundred thousand in Japan to a high of 569 per thousand for men in Finland and Scotland. (All figures in this section are age adjusted to match the distribution of the U.S. population in 1940 and cover only the ages from 35 through 74.)

In this group of nations the U.S. falls above the middle for both women's and men's deaths.

The high men's death rates in Finland and Scotland are 41 percent higher than those in the U.S., and rates for men are also higher in Northern Ireland (37 percent),

England and Wales (13 percent), Norway (five percent) and Denmark (one percent higher than the men's rate in the U.S.). In Japan the men's death rate is 51 percent of what it is in the U.S. Other nations with lower men's rates than the U.S. include Germany (98 percent of the U.S. rate), Sweden (89 percent), the Netherlands (86 percent), Iceland and Canada (tied at 75 percent), Switzerland (71 percent), and France (53 percent, although France traditionally classes more heart-attack deaths as "other" than most countries do).

U.S. women's rates look slightly worse internationally, but only because both Denmark and Norway have lower women's rates than American women's rates. Otherwise the distribution by nation is about the same as for the men, although both French and Swiss women beat out Japanese women for the lowest rates.

The low French rates for both men and women led to suggestions that red wine and foie gras, both popular in France, might protect against heart disease. Further study suggests that the red wine may contain chemicals in the grape skins that offer some protection, but that the same chemicals are in the grape skins when eaten fresh. No chemical connection for foie gras that might lower heart disease has been located so far.

What Prompts a Heart Attack?

Many remember the dramatic beginning of the movie *Private Benjamin* in which a new groom dies immediately after the wedding reception as he begins to have sex with the bride. High emotions, over-indulgence in food and drink, physical activity, and sex are commonly thought of as instigators of heart attacks for those so predisposed. But recent research has suggested some additional occasions for heart attacks—that is dreams, birthdays, and waking up in the morning.

The common view that heightened physical activity often leads to heart attacks among those with heart disease is indeed correct. Studies in 1993 showed that the risk during exertion can be two to six times as great as it is when a person is sedentary. In fact, it is the sedentary person who is at highest risk while engaging in activities to which he is unaccustomed, such as pushing a car, shoveling snow, or taking up jogging in an effort to get back in shape all at once. Physically fit people who regularly exercise or work at active jobs are less likely to have heart attacks from bursts of effort, even if they have heart disease. (One German study showed that people with known heart disease were not at greater risk because so many in the control group had undiagnosed heart disease.)

Although a disproportionate number of heart attacks occur during heightened activity, the amount of time spent in such activity is a lot less than the amount spent sleeping, eating, resting, watching television, or engaging in low-level physical activity, such as washing dishes or carpentry. Thus when all heart attacks are considered, only about one in 20 occur during strong exertion. The other 19 occur while sunbathing, doing desk work, driving, walking slowly to work, cleaning windows, or fishing—that is, during periods of low physical activity.

Actually, several studies since 1985 have shown that three times as many heart attacks and strokes occur during the first two or three hours after waking up in the morning than during the rest of the day. Here are some other "hazardous times":

For men:
- Heart attacks are 21 percent higher on birthdays than on other days in the year.

For women:
- Birthday heart-attack risk is only nine percent higher.

Both men and women:
- During sex (according to a 1993 study by James E. Muller of New England Deaconess Hospital in Boston, Massachusetts, and coworkers, sex doubles heart attack risk).
- During emotional dreams or REM sleep. A 1993 study found that sympathetic nervous system activity doubled during REM sleep, when dreaming takes place.
- On the day after a holiday (Easter Monday leads with 28 percent excess over other days of the year).
- Upon wakening during the night.
- On getting out of bed.
- During cold weather.
- Mondays.

Despite the above list, it is probably not a good idea to stay awake and avoid sleep, especially on Mondays after a holiday in the winter. Sleep deprivation may also lead to heart attacks.

In the May 21, 1992 *New England Journal of Medicine*, JoAnn E. Manson of Harvard University and coworkers listed some of the ways that people can prevent heart attacks from occurring, ways which range from lifestyle changes to medical intervention. They also give their estimate of the average reduction in risk. Although the percentages add to more than 100 percent (and not because of rounding), combinations of factors do provide somewhat greater risk reduction than any one of these taken separately.

Quit smoking: Reduces risk by 50 to 70 percent. Maximum risk reduction takes about five years for the body to become readjusted.

Exercise: Brings a 45 percent risk reduction to the previously sedentary.

(For women) Use estrogen replacement after menopause: Reduces risk by 44 percent.

Maintain an ideal weight: Compared with people who are 20 percent or more overweight, risk of a heart attack can be lowered by 35 to 55 percent.

Take low-dose aspirin: 33 percent lower risk.

Drink one or at most two alcoholic drinks each day: This can bring a 25 to 45 percent risk reduction compared to nondrinkers. The researchers did not report the risk of alcoholism, but excessive drinking can lead to a condition called nutritional cardiomyopathy, which may result in heart failure or stroke.

Treat high blood pressure: Can reduce risk on the average from 10 to 20 percent, but individual cases vary a great deal. Figure two to three percent reduction for each whole number less in the bottom number of the reported blood pressure (*see also* "High Blood Pressure UPDATE," p 407.)

Reduce blood cholesterol: Reduces risk about ten percent with the best improved diet and 20 percent with drug therapy combined with diet. There is a two to three percent decline in risk for each one percent reduction in total cholesterol up to these limits (the report did not estimate risks on the basis of HDL/LDL ratios).

There has also been a suggestion in the early 1990s that viral infections by herpes simplex I or cytomegalovirus might cause clots and plaque to form more easily in arteries. Since these infections are hard to avoid and so far virtually impossible to get rid of, this concept is more interesting than useful.

Fighting Heart Attacks

A heart attack occurs when the blood supply to the cardiac muscles are blocked, most often by a clot. Normally this occurs only after arteries in the heart (*coronary arteries*) have been narrowed by fatty deposits as in atherosclerosis, a condition known as coronary artery disease. Quick action and drastic steps are needed to prevent death of the muscle cells. If patients do not respond in short order to emergency paramedics' treatment however, the chances are good that they will not respond at all.

Among the treatments administered for heart-attack victims are clot-busting drugs and balloon angioplasty to clear up blocked arteries. Two studies late in 1992 looked at combining these treatments. Both found that it was unwise. In one instance, the clot-busting drug was given shortly before angioplasty for some patients and not for others. The ones receiving the drug had more complications and longer hospital stays than the ones who got the angioplasty alone. In the other study, some patients who had clot-buster therapy as a first line of defense got angioplasty several days later,

---

SYMPTOMS OF AN ATTACK

Both heart attacks and strokes can often be mitigated considerably if they are treated early. If treated later, muscle cells or brain cells have died, and dead cells can't be revived. If you think you are having a heart attack or have had a stroke, you should seek medical attention as soon as possible, but do not try to travel to a physician. Let the emergency workers or ambulance come to you.

Common symptoms of a heart blockage
- Uncomfortable pressure, pain, or squeezing sensation in the center of the chest, especially if it lasts more than two minutes (pain may also be in neck, jaw, or stomach)
- Sweating or chills
- Vertigo (dizziness or fainting)
- Nausea
- Shortness of breath

Common symptoms of a cerebrovascular accident (stroke)
- Sudden weakness or numbness on one side of the body
- Sudden loss of vision; or blurred or double vision
- Loss of speech
- Unexplained severe headache
- Confusion or dizziness

---

while the controls did not. After one year, five times as many in the angioplasty group had second heart attacks. In both studies, very small numbers of patients and even smaller numbers of second heart attacks were involved. Large-scale research sometimes shows that effects in such small studies were caused by chance.

The clot-busting drugs were in the news during the early 1990s. First of all, one of them gained initial fame during the late 1980s by being among the first drugs to be produced by genetic engineering. This drug is tissue plasminogen activator, known as TPA (tradenamed Activase). Two years before TPA came to the market in 1987, a small trial showed that it worked twice as fast as streptokinase, the clot-buster then in use, which had been around for decades. Three years after its introduction, two-thirds of the heart attacks in the U.S. were being treated with TPA, despite the fact that TPA at that time cost $2200 per dose and streptokinase could be had for as little as $70 a dose in some instances (at $240 a dose in most situations). Most other countries in 1990, however, continued to rely on streptokinase.

Studies were launched comparing the expensive drug with the relatively cheap one. After two studies showing no significant difference in effectiveness and better safety for streptokinase, a combination of TPA, aspirin, and the blood thinner heparin was found in 1993 to be about 14 percent more effective in saving lives than several combinations, including one that had TPA, aspirin, heparin, *and* streptokinase. The study was financed by five pharmaceutical companies with various stakes in the outcome, including Genentech, the U.S. manufacturer of TPA.

A third clot-buster, known as Eminase, became available in 1990. Like streptokinase, it is manufactured from bacteria. TPA, on the other hand, is manufactured by genetically engineered animal cells. Many other genetically engineered drugs are produced by bacteria.

Strokes

One of the mysteries of strokes in the U.S. is that they strike disproportionately in the Southeast. For men and women, above average rates are found in the contiguous and largely southeastern states of Virginia, North and South Carolina, Georgia, Alabama, Tennessee, Kentucky, Indiana, Mississippi, Louisiana, Arkansas, and Oklahoma. Lower than average stroke rates for both men and women are also found in a contiguous region that is largely in the Great Plains: Minnesota, Iowa, Kansas, Nebraska, North and South Dakota, Montana, Colorado, New Mexico, Arizona, and Nevada (lower rates are also found in the outlying states of Alaska and Hawaii). Although national stroke rates are declining as a part of the overall U.S. reduction in heart disease, the Southeast is maintaining its position above below the falling national average.

Explanations of this distribution based on diet, race, or poverty do not hold up to close examination. In 1992, however a rural Georgia physician proposed a theory that many find makes sense. The states with more cerebrovascular accidents are the same ones with less selenium in the soil. Around the world, selenium is absent or nearly so in northern China, southern Finland, New Zealand, and the southeastern United States. These regions in China and Finland are well known for high levels of heart disease. Selenium is thought to help prevent damage to blood vessels by aiding anti-

Background

When a blood vessel in the brain is blocked by a clot formed there as a result of atherosclerosis (cerebral thrombosis) or by a clot from elsewhere in the circulatory system (cerebral embolism), or when a blood vessel in the brain leaks or bursts (cerebral hemorrhage), the illness is called *stroke.* About 70 to 80 percent of strokes are caused by thrombosis or embolism, while the remainder is caused by hemorrhage. The death rate is much higher for strokes caused by hemorrhage, with more than half of the people who experience such a cerebral accident dying as a result.

Stroke can be a terrifying disorder because, in most cases, it comes silently and without warning, causing sudden effects such as paralysis, loss of one or more senses, or unconsciousness, frightening observers in some cases even more than the victims. (For example, a person whose speech has been distorted by a stroke may not recognize the defect, though it is clear to the listener.)

oxidants. If this theory proves to be true when studies in Georgia, Mississippi, and South Carolina are completed, adding selenium to people's diets in that region may become a major lifesaver.

Stroke of the cerebral-embolism variety can be caused by a common heart condition called *atrial fibrillation,* which in turn is most often yet another bad result of atherosclerosis. The fibrillation, which is an abnormality in heart rhythm, can cause clots that then head directly for the brain. People with this heart-rhythm abnormality are five or six times as likely to experience stroke as people with regular heart beats. In some instances the irregularity is a result of an overactive thyroid, which can be treated. Aspirin can help prevent the clot formation that causes stroke (*see also* "New Uses for Aspirin," p 527) when the fibrillation has some other cause.

Many physicians in the early 1990s have prescribed a low dose of the anticoagulant warfarin to patients with atrial fibrillation. Studies completed in October 1993 suggest that warfarin therapy can prevent two-thirds of the strokes in people with atrial fibrillation, a result so dramatic that the trials were stopped and all the controls taking placebos or patients using aspirin (also tested in the same trial) were given warfarin instead. Andreas Laupacis, a Canadian researcher who worked on the study (which also involved physicians from Denmark and the U.S.), noted that "for every 33 atrial fibrillation patients who are treated with warfarin for one year, one stroke will be prevented."

(Periodical References and Additional Reading: *Harvard Health Letter,* 5-90, p 1; *New York Times* 6-30-91, p I-1 *Harvard Health Letter,* 3-92, p 1; *New York Times* 7-22-92, p C12; *New York Times* 8-5-92, p C12; *Harvard Health Letter,* 9-92, p 1; *New York Times* 10-27-93, p C3; *New York Times* 1-19-93, p C6; *New York Times* 2-4-93, p B8; *Science News* 2-6-93, p 95; *Harvard Health Letter,* 3-93, p 5; *New York Times* 3-19-93, p A12; *New York Times* 3-21-93, pp I-27 & IV-7; *Science News* 4-3-93, p 216; *Harvard Health Letter,* 5-93, p 8; *New York Times* 5-1-93, pp 1 & 7; *New York Times* 9-22-93, p A23; *Statistical Bulletin* 10/12-93, p 19; *New York Times* 11-11-93, p A19; *Science News* 11-20-93, p 332; *New York Times* 12-2-93, p A18)

High Blood Pressure UPDATE

High blood pressure, or *hypertension* as it is more formally known, is a common condition that is frequently treated with diet control; exercise; other lifestyle changes, such as quitting smoking and stopping alcohol use; and drugs. About one American in ten is hypertensive according to some surveys. Unlike most conditions that are considered diseases, most high blood pressure has no symptoms that the person with the condition can detect, although it is easily measured with special equipment. Only extremely high pressure is associated with such noticeable signs as headaches or a general feeling of ill health. But high blood pressure wreaks damage on the heart, blood vessels, and kidneys, leading to increased incidence of heart attacks, stroke, and serious kidney failure. If pressure is so high that the kidneys fail, that failure induces even higher pressure that can affect the brain or other organs, such as the eyes.

For the most part, physicians do not know what causes some people to have high blood pressure and what allows others to escape. In less than ten percent of individuals can a cause (such as kidney disease) be located; for the rest, the label is *essential hypertension*. But a French research team reported in the October 2, 1992 *Cell* that two specific alleles of the gene for angiotensinogen (*see* "Chemistry and Heart Attacks," p 393) are associated with high blood pressure. Most likely the cause of essential hypertension is a combination of heredity; lifestyle choices such as diet, exercise, smoking, or drinking; and stress.

In 1973 the U.S. government launched a major attack on high blood pressure. As part of the attack the National High Blood Pressure Education program was instituted, which among other activities provides reports from time to time advising physicians on how to test for or treat high blood pressure. The 1992 report, for example, suggested for the first time testing all children over the age of three every year, although that may have been in error; the recommendation for adults, who are far more likely to have high blood pressure since risk increases with age, was a test every two years. Treatment recommendations at that time were also on the conservative side, suggesting that only diuretics and beta blockers be used to treat high blood pressure resistant to lifestyle changes and that only a single drug be tried on the patient at the beginning of treatment. Newer drugs, though already popular with physicians and patients (in part because of fewer side effects), were thought to be unproven in terms of reduction of heart disease or strokes or in terms of increase of lifespan.

The report also instituted a new way of classifying blood-pressure readings. Although blood pressure today is often measured with electronic devices that produce digital read-outs, the units used for measuring are based on the older device, which measures the height of a column of mercury. Pressure in the blood, transmitted by air through a tube, keeps the mercury from falling. The idea is an adaptation of the mercury barometer, which also uses a column of mercury to measure air pressure.

A cuff is placed around a person's arm and air is pumped into the cuff. When the air in the cuff has raised the mercury above what the blood pressure is expected to be, air is allowed to escape and the physician or nurse listens to a vein below the cuff to see if the contraction of the heart is enough to stop the mercury which provides a number known as the *systolic*, presenting pressure during a heart contraction. When the pressure sinks enough for the blood to flow during relaxation of the heart, the physician or nurse is given the other number, the *diastolic*. Since the height of the mercury column is measured in millimeters, both the high systolic and the lower diastolic are actually lengths—but they represent pressures. Often the pressure is written as something like 120/80, read as "120 over 80," which means a systolic pressure of 120 mm of mercury and a diastolic pressure of 80 mm of mercury.

Here is the system of classifying blood pressure instituted in 1992. The possibility of low blood pressure is not considered, though in some physical crises, the body will have blood pressure low enough that steps must be taken to raise it.

BLOOD PRESSURE CLASSIFICATIONS

Range of blood pressure	Classification
Less than 120/80	Optimal; very low readings may have clinical significance depending on other factors
Less than 120 over 80-84 120-29 over less than 80 120/80 to 129/84	Normal
Less than 120 over 85-89 130-39 over less than 80 120/85 to 139/89	High normal
140/90 to 159/99	Stage 1 hypertension
160/100 to 179/109	Stage 2 hypertension
180/110 to 209/119	Stage 3 hypertension
210/120 or over	Stage 4 hypertension

In the August 11, 1993 *Journal of the American Medical Association* the results of the Treatment of Mild Hypertension Study revealed that medication (any medication, it seems) for high blood pressure reduces the risk of heart attacks or other cardiovascular troubles by 31 percent in people with moderately high pressure (diastolic pressures between 90 and 99 millimeters of mercury). A total of 902 persons in this category were tracked for five years. Among the drugs that some of the 902 took were a diuretic, a beta blocker, a calcium-channel blocker, an alpha blocker, and an angiotensin-converting-enzyme (ACE) inhibitor. It did not matter which drug was taken, so long as it was successful in lowering the blood pressure into the normal range (considered to be below 130/80 millimeters of mercury in this study). All the participants in the study watched their weight, eliminated excessive fat and salt from the diet, and exercised—but the ones who took no drugs still had a higher rate of heart problems than those who were medicated.

In the December 23, 1993 *New England Journal of Medicine* members of the long-term Framingham Heart Study announced that they had determined people with a systolic blood pressure between 140 and 159 are almost twice as likely to develop full-fledged high blood pressure at some later time than those with systolic pressures in the normal range. The Framingham researchers did not advise treatment of such

PROLIFERATION OF PILLS

In the early 1950s the first truly effective drugs for the treatment of high blood pressure was introduced, based on the ancient use of a herbal drug in India, which the Indians called "snake root" and biologists call *Rauwolfia*. (This was not the same plant as the snake root that came to be associated with bogus herbal medicines—as in "snake oil"—in the U.S. during the nineteenth century). While *Rauwolfia* successfully reduces blood pressure, its side effects have limited its use. But since that introduction, a number of different drugs that act by essentially different mechanisms have come into being. With the present array of drugs, most patients can control their blood pressure with few side effects, though it may be necessary for an individual to try several different remedies before finding the right one.

Here is a list of some of the drugs available recently. Many are also marketed in combinations with a different tradename from any of those given here.

DRUGS TO CONTROL BLOOD PRESSURE

Class	Year introduced	Generic names	Trade names
ACE inhibitors	1979	captopril	Capoten
	1981	enalapril	Vasotec
	1988	lisinopril	Prinivil
			Zestril
alpha adrenoceptor agonists	1969	clonidine	Catapres
		guanabenz	Wytensin
	1980	guanfacine	Tenex
alpha-1 receptor blockers	1987	terazosin	Hytrin
	1970	prazosin	Minipress
beta blockers	1973	acebutolol	Sectral
	1973	atenolol	Tenormin
	1983	carteolol	Cartol
	1978	labetalol	Normodyne
			Trandate
	1974	metoprolol	Lopressor
	1976	nadolol	Corgard
	1976	penbutolol	Levatol
	1972	pindolol	Visken
	1966	propranolol	Inderal
			Inderide
			Ipran
	1972	timolol	Biocadren
			Timoptic
calcium channel blockers	1977	diltiazem	Cardizem
	1984	nicardipine	Cardene
	1972	nifedipine	Adalat
			Procardia
	1967	verapamil	Calan
			Isoptin
diuretics	1967	amiloride	Midamor
	1983	bumetanide	Bumex

Class	Year introduced	Generic names	Trade names
diuretics (continued)	1960	chlorthalidone	Hygroton Hylidone Thalitone
	1964	furosemide	Lasix
	1974	indapamide	Lozol
	1974	metolazone	Diulo Microx Zaroxolyn
	1959	spironolactone	Aldactone Alatone
	1964	triamterene	Dyrenium
guanethidine		guanethidine	Ismelin
hydralazine	1950	hydralazine	Alazine Alpresoline
methyldopa	1963	methyldopa	Aldomet
minoxidil	1972	minoxidil	Loniten Minodyl
reserpine	1953	deserpidine rauwolfia reserpine	Serpasil
thiazide diuretics	1957	cholothiazide	Diachlor Diurigen Diuril
	1959	hydrochlorothiazide	Esidrix HydroDIURIL Oretic Thiuretic Zide
	1960	methyclothiazide	Aqutensen Enduron

It is not known exactly how most of these drugs work. ACE inhibitors reduce the action of angiotensin converting enzyme, which is one of the steps in the sequence of hormones and enzymes used by the kidneys to regulate blood pressure. Alpha andrenoceptor agonists stimulate the part of the brain stem that controls blood pressure and reduce control of the nerves on blood pressure. Alpha-1 receptor blockers similarly block a type of receptor that is at the junction of the nerve cells and blood vessels. Beta blockers are more formally known as "beta adrenergic blockers"; they clog up certain receptors in the sympathetic nervous system, slowing down the transmission of nerve impulses, which in turn slows down the heart and reduces contraction of blood vessels that is stimulated by nerve signals. Calcium-channel blockers (or calcium antagonists) interfere with transmission of signals between cells by blocking passage of calcium ions through cell membranes in nerve and muscle cells. Since movement of calcium ions is a major mode of electrical transmission in the body, this also slows down the electrical conduction in heart muscle and reduces the stress-related contraction of blood vessels. Methyldopa decreases the activity of the part of the brain that controls blood pressure. Diuretics and thiazide diuretics increase elimination of salt and water through the kidneys, which also reduces the total blood volume and sodium in the blood. Hydralazine acts directly on artery walls to relax them by an unknown mechanism. Minoxidil also relaxes artery walls, especially those of the smaller arteries—and it grows hair as a side effect. As Rogaine, minoxidil It Is used directly to grow hair. Reserpine depletes the neurotransmitter norepinephrine, reducing the ability of nerves to signal blood vessels to constrict. Terazosin also blocks the ability of nerves to cause the blood vessels to contract.

In the October 21, 1993 *Nature* a team of researchers from Hoffmann-La Roche in Switzerland announced a new potential drug, an endothelin-receptor-antagonist. Clinical trials have not taken place, as the effect has only been noted *in vitro*.

---

borderline or Stage 1 hypertension, but suggested frequent follow-up testing for increases in high blood pressure. Physicians have long considered the other number, the lower or diastolic reading, the best measure of danger from borderline hypertension. The Framingham report reinforces the results of a 1991 study demonstrating that treatment lowering a high systolic reading in elderly people also results in fewer instances of stroke or heart disease. The Systolic Hypertension in the Elderly Program was able to cut the incidence of stroke by 36 percent and of heart attacks by 27 percent using the drug chlorthalidone to lower systolic pressure.

Another discovery in 1991 was more surprising in that it found that the amount of increase in the mass of the heart muscle was a better measure of damage from high blood pressure than the pressure itself. Higher death rates are better correlated to an enlarged left ventricle in the heart than to blood pressure. The meaning of this finding is problematical; while blood pressure can be lowered safely with life style changes and with drugs, it is not certain what can be done after a heart has already developed excess muscle.

A study in the November 14, 1993 *Journal of the American Medical Association* revealed what many have suspected all along: anxious middle-aged men are more likely to develop high blood pressure than those who are serene. The surprise was that anxious women or anxious elderly men did not show any increased risk.

(Periodical References and Additional Reading: *New York Times* 6-26-91; *Harvard Health Letter* 8-91, p 7; *Harvard Health Letter* 3-92, p 2; *Science News* 10-10-92, p 230; *Harvard Health Letter* 3-93, p 4; *Science News* 8-14-93, p 100; *Nature* 10-21-93, p 759; *New York Times* 10-31-93, p 5; *New York Times* 11-3-92, p C3; *Science News* 12-4-93, p 380; *New York Times* 12-23-93, p A15; *Harvard Health Letter* 3-94, p 3)

CANCER

REPORT FROM THE WAR ON CANCER

On December 23, 1971, the United States declared war on cancer—then, as it is now, the second leading cause of death in the U.S. By 1973 the statistical measures that tell as much as anything how that continuing war was progressing had been put in place. Consequently, progress in fighting cancer is most often reported using 1973 as a base year. By 1993, 20 years of statistics had accumulated, but the situation was still murky. Some could argue that cancer was simply winning the war and that doctors who have been fighting against it have been beaten at every turn. Optimists, however, could claim that a flood of new knowledge and new treatments promise that, just around the corner, most cancer will be classified as a preventable and treatable disease, with death rates from this cause dropping dramatically.

Some of the following data are extrapolated from statistics that are only available through 1990 or another recent year, but changes historically occur so slowly that broad statements made on the basis of 1990 data almost certainly apply to 1993 as well. Much of the data comes from the U.S. President's Cancer Panel, which issued the report *Evaluating the National Cancer Program: An Ongoing Process* on September 22, 1993. Another useful source is *Cancer Facts and Figures—1993* from the American Cancer Society.

First, the Bad News

When all the data are known, they are expected to show that about 526,000 deaths in the U.S. in 1993 had cancer as the primary cause. While this is still only somewhat more than two-thirds of those who died from heart disease, the trends are that heart disease deaths are declining steadily and cancer deaths continue a slight rise, an increase totaling somewhat more than seven percent since 1973 if changes in population size and age composition are taken into account. If only deaths per 100,000 population are considered, cancer deaths rose almost 25 percent during that 20 years, but nearly all of this is accounted for by the increased age of the population. Age adjusted figures show no rise. Nearly all of the unadjusted rise in number of cancer deaths is caused by lung cancer, while the death rate from other cancers has remained remarkably steady over the 20-year period. Lung cancer in 1993 accounted for more than 25 percent of cancer deaths in the U.S.

Lung cancer is not, however, the only form of cancer for which death rates are rising. Rises in death rates since 1973 have occurred in melanomas, liver cancer, multiple myeloma, prostate cancer, non-Hodgkin's lymphoma, and cancers of the esophagus, kidney, breast, and brain.

Looking even earlier than 1973, the climb in the death rate seems worse, since there was a somewhat steeper rise in the 20 years before 1973 than in the 20 since. The following U.S. death rates are age adjusted to reflect the age-distribution in the population in 1940. Thus, none of the rise in death rate comes from our aging population.

DEATH RATES FROM CANCER

Year	Cancer death rate per 100,000 population (age adjusted)
1950	124.4
1955	125.8
1960	125.8
1965	127.9
1970	129.9
1975	130.9
1980	132.8
1985	133.6
1990	135.0
1991	134.5
1992 (est.)	133.2

Death rates are the bottom line of disease treatment, but by themselves death rates could mean all sorts of failures. For example, if incidence of a disease is rising rapidly and death rates only rise a little bit, then treatment is probably improving; but if death rates and incidence are rising at about the same rate, there are other possibilities. It is not necessary at this time to consider the case that incidence is falling, and death rates are rising, for that is not happening for cancer. Indeed, the true situation is that incidence is rising somewhat faster than deaths are rising. Taking population size and age composition into account, cancer incidence has risen about 18 percent since 1973, a higher rate than the similarly adjusted figure of 7 percent for death rates.

As with death rates, incidence varies by type of cancer. The greatest concern is lung cancer in women, which has doubled since 1973, almost certainly because many more women than previously began to use cigarettes in the period between 1920 and 1950. Another significant increase in incidence is the skin cancer melanoma, which has gone up over 80 percent since 1973. Since the 1930s the increase has been from one in 1500 persons to one in 1200 persons, which seems to be too high for sunbathing alone to account for, especially since fewer people now work outdoors. This increase is thought to be connected to exposure to sunlight, although that is difficult to prove for a large population—the relationship seems clearer in individual cases (see also "Ultraviolet Rays from the Sun," p 189). A third cancer that has risen greatly in incidence affects only men; prostate cancer has risen at about the same rate as has melanoma. The reason for such a rise is not completely clear.

Cancer in children is also rising in incidence, especially acute lymphocytic leukemia and brain or nervous-system cancers.

Despite these statistics, the state of the war against cancer remains unclear, in part because changes in diagnosis or even in autopsy practice can strongly affect both incidence and death rate numbers. Figures that are not adjusted for age (most of the data given above were adjusted for age) cannot be used for long-term trends because of the great increase in collective lifespan since the beginning of the twentieth century, an increase that continues at a slower rate today. In 1900 fewer than one death out of 25 was attributed to cancer and today the number is almost one death in four, but in 1900 the leading causes of reported death were pneumonia, influenza, and tuberculosis. Childhood infectious diseases were also rampant in 1900, accounting for a large part of the lower mean lifespan.

And Now the Good News

Not only has the age-adjusted death rate remained nearly unchanged for 20 years and has even declined thus far through the 1990s, also both the death rate and incidence of some specific cancers have declined since 1973. These specific cancers include cancers of the cervix, uterus, and stomach. Death rates, but not incidence, have declined for colorectal cancers, bladder cancer, some bone cancers, gall bladder cancer, and cancer of the testis. Incidence alone fell for cancers of the pancreas and mouth, Hodgkin's disease, and some leukemias.

Although statistically swamped by the much larger number of deaths of adults from cancer, better treatment had reduced the death rate for children with cancer to nearly half of what it was in 1973. In fact, the death rates since 1973 have declined for people under the age of 50, although they are rising for older people.

Death rates are far from the whole story. People are living significantly longer after cancer is diagnosed. The following data comes from the U.S. National Cancer Institute. It was developed by combining data from five different studies of Americans.

SURVIVAL RATES OF CANCER PATIENTS

Period of diagnosis	Survival rate
1960 to 1963	38.0 percent alive 5 years after diagnosis
1970 to 1973	42.0 percent alive 5 years after diagnosis
1974 to 1976	49.0 percent alive 5 years after diagnosis
1977 to 1980	49.4 percent alive 5 years after diagnosis
1981 to 1986	50.7 percent alive 5 years after diagnosis

While only 51 percent of the people diagnosed with cancer in 1981 were alive five years later, the fall-off after the first five years was slight. In 1991, 44 percent of the persons diagnosed with cancer in 1981 were still alive.

Of course, cancer is really a collection of different diseases of unrestricted growth of cells, and survival rates differ widely by the type of cancer. In the 1981-86 period, survival after five years was only 3.1 percent for pancreatic cancer 4.5 percent for liver cancer, and 8.0 percent for stomach cancer. But survival rates for some other cancers were high: cancer of the thyroid, 94.2 percent; of the testis, 92.1 percent; of the uterus, 82.6 percent. Skin melanoma also had a high rate of survival, 81.1 percent.

Another difference in survival rate is race. During the 1981 to 1986 period, U.S. whites survived five years or more at a rate of 52 percent, while U.S. blacks only survived that long 36.2 percent of the time.

Other articles in *Handbook of Current Health and Medicine* deal with the specific good news of better treatment (*see* "Genes Against Cancer," p 73, "Molecular Biology Against Cancer," p 419, and "Chemicals Against Cancer," p 425). The discussion below includes general information about changes in cancer diagnosis, treatment, and prevention. Improvements in prevention, diagnosis, or treatment depend largely on better understanding of the disease, which is coming largely from genetics, discussed in "Genes for Cancer," p 54.

Diagnosis

There is a considerable question as to whether or not the increase in cancer incidence comes from improvements in diagnosis. One expert, John C. Bailar III of McGill University, has stated that many tumors are now diagnosed as non-life-threatening cancer, but these tumors also would be largely unnoticeable if it were not for modern diagnoses. In particular, Bailar thinks that the increase in the incidence of both lung and prostate cancer is an artifact of diagnosis.

There is evidence from a clinical study by Marie Desmeules of Health and Welfare Canada to support the concept that modern methods of diagnosis make a difference. She removed all evidence obtained by CT imaging or MRI from patients' charts, thereby prompting doctors to reclassify brain cancer as other diseases.

Prostate cancer is now commonly diagnosed in several stages, usually beginning with a blood test that shows an elevated hormone that often signals prostate cancer, followed by a sonogram. If the patient still appears to have cancer, a biopsy (or sometimes surgery, followed by a biopsy) is in order. Before the blood test and sonograms were available, the first indication of prostate problems was either physical symptoms or observation of prostate enlargement during a rectal examination. It is not totally surprising that the new tests are finding more cancers.

But the death rate from prostate cancer as well as its incidence is rising. One possibility is that coroners in the past were less likely to observe prostate cancer as a cause of death, often noting cancer deaths as "site unknown." The main cause of death from prostate cancer occurs when the cancer migrates to the skeleton. Although the cancer is now in the bones, the cells that are cancerous are still prostate-cancer cells, which might not have been easily recognized in the past.

Treatment

Since it seems that every week a new or improved treatment for cancer is announced in the media, it seems surprising to many observers that death rates are not decreasing at a greater rate when measured against cancer incidence. Often what is not noticed is that the new and improved treatment often works for a form of cancer that strikes relatively few persons. In the United States, the major problems are lung, colorectal, breast, and prostate cancer, only one of which has seen a significant improvement in cure rate. Early diagnosis and better surgery have led to higher survival rates for colorectal cancers; the discovery of a genetic basis for many colorectal cancers (*see* "Genes for Cancer," p 54) may very soon result in tests that will lead to earlier diagnosis. But the high and still increasing death rates for lung, breast, and prostate cancer skew statistics against success in treatment.

But there has been success for many of the less common cancers. Hodgkin's disease is very often curable, as are the similar leukemias. Almost 90 percent of people with Hodgkin's disease experience remission after radiation or combined radiation/chemotherapy; two-thirds of those are completely cured. Thyroid and testicular cancer are also frequently cured. Non-Hodgkin's lymphoma survival rates have greatly increased, and treatment with bone-marrow transplants has resulted in what appear to be cures in several dozen cases. Early diagnosis seems to be aiding the fight against cancers of the uterus and bladder. Many of the cancers for which the cure rate has improved affect children.

Treatment itself can be a major problem. Chemotherapy has been notorious for its adverse effects, ranging from nausea to baldness. Radiation may cause one cancer while being used to diagnose or treat another cancer. Chemotherapy can also cause development of a different cancer from the one being treated. Surgery in the past often involved removal of large parts of the patient, often parts that are needed for normal life.

Today as a whole, fewer breasts, legs, or bowels are being removed; doctors try to remove the minimum necessary to get rid of the disease. For example, breast cancer is not the only cancer for which lumpectomy is replacing a radical operation. In the early 1980s, bladder cancer was treated by removal of the bladder, with a consequent need for an external bag to collect urine—although nowadays even those whose bladders must still be removed can get artificial ones installed in their abdominal cavity. A study based on ten years of research and published in the November 4, 1993 *New England Journal of Medicine* showed that bladder lumpectomy combined with chemotherapy and radiation was as effective as removal of the bladder.

During and after treatment, research has shown that support groups, modeled somewhat on Alcoholics Anonymous and similar self-help organizations, have been shown to increase survival rates. One study of breast cancer showed that people who took part in the support sessions lived twice as long as matched members of a control group—three years after diagnosis as opposed to a year and a half for the control group.

Prevention

Cancer is caused by genes, but it is not usually a purely hereditary disease. Even when genetic heritage predisposes a person for a particular kind of cancer, some other event is usually required to produce the tumor. Often that other event is something in the environment—a chemical, radiation, a virus. In other cases it may simply be aging, which causes humans to lose some ability to repair damaged DNA. When the damage is repaired, no cancer results, but older people have less of the enzyme that is needed for such repairs.

A lot of effort and publicity have gone into identifying and promoting information that some behaviors or situations are to be avoided in order to prevent cancer. Smoking or chewing tobacco is behavior that causes several types of cancer, possibly even including leukemia (a 1993 study suggested a 30 percent increase in leukemia among smokers). Stopping smoking is the main decision to be made in cancer prevention. Heavy drinking of alcoholic beverages is also known to cause cancer of the mouth or esophagus, pancreas, and liver. The following table shows one rough estimate of the relative roles of causative factors:

Chemicals that naturally occur in foods	35 percent
Tobacco	30 percent
Sex and reproductive history	7 percent
Occupational hazards, mainly chemical	4 percent
Alcoholic beverages	3 percent
Food additives	1 percent

The percentages for these possible causes do not add up to 100 percent because no one knows what causes most instances of cancer.

A couple of items from the list above need explaining, although it is clear what is meant by tobacco, alcoholic beverages, and food additives.

Chemicals that naturally occur in foods   One of the chief cancer villains recently has been fat (*see* "Fat UPDATE," p 171), but hundreds of other substances or chemicals in food have been named as cancer promoters. Only a few are proven to cause cancer, such as chemicals from the aflatoxin molds that infect grains and peanuts. The National Cancer Institute, however, estimates that more than a third of cancers may be caused in part by diet.

While most dietary cancer concerns revolve around eating too much of a dangerous chemical, people also have come to believe that eating more of certain chemicals can prevent cancer. These include vitamins such as C, A, or E, along with beta carotene, a precursor of vitamin A (*see* "Vitamin UPDATE," p 160). The mineral selenium is also thought to help ward off cancer (*see* "Mineral UPDATE," p 168).

Sex and reproductive history   In this case, "sex" is not so much the act of sex than it is the differences in sex between a male and female. Statistically, however, some cancers are associated with the act of sex in one way or another; for example, genital warts spread sexually can become malignant. The increases in cancer associated with reproductive history are also largely statistical, with actual causes unexplained.

Occupational hazards, mainly chemical   Dioxins have long been known to cause cancer in animals, but only recently has there been any good evidence that these chemicals, which contaminate pesticides and are produced by burning, cause cancer in humans (*see* "Dioxin UPDATE," p 260). On the other hand, the evidence for cancer caused by asbestos is strong. Other chemicals, such as benzene, are under suspicion as well. Farmers have higher cancer rates than the rest of the population, and pesticides may be the reason (*see* "Pesticides: Insecticide and Herbicide UPDATE," p 265).

The list of potential causes of cancer is so long that people say that "even drinking water causes cancer" to ridicule fears. But drinking water does cause cancer! Chlorinated water raises the risk for rectal and bladder cancers slightly (about 21 to 38 percent higher), although the risks of infection from untreated water are far greater than the added cancer burden.

Farmers are among the persons with high rates of melanoma. This deadly cancer seems to occur more often in people who are exposed to ultraviolet radiation from the sun. Good sunscreens are thought to help protect against melanoma. (*See also* "Ultraviolet Rays from the Sun," p 189.) One theory suggests that newborns exposed to bright fluorescent lights in hospital wards have a higher incidence of leukemia later in their lives.

Some causes that did not make the list   Radiation from X rays or radioactive elements is so powerful a cause of cancer that most of the early workers with radiation developed the disease. Although today steps are taken to reduce exposure to X rays, and despite the fact that people have learned how to avoid the most obvious sources of radioactive elements, there is little one can do to escape radon, a colorless, odorless radioactive gas that escapes from granite or other rocks and enters people's homes through the basement. It can contribute to lung cancer unless air in basements is exchanged with outside air on a regular basis (*see* "Radon and Other Danger from Radioactivity," p 269). Some also think that another form of radiation, electromagnetic fields, causes cancer, especially fields from high-voltage, long-distance transmission lines. This contention has been tested in court (in May 1993) and rejected by a jury, but it still has many advocates (*see* "Is EMF a Cause of Disease?," p 280).

In some cases infections are known to be a causative agent of cancer, and thus these forms of cancer can be prevented by vaccination or by effective treatment. Liver cancer, for example, can be induced by hepatitis B, but there is a vaccine available that prevents the original disease from developing. The bacterium *Helicobacter pylori,* now known to be the chief cause of stomach and duodenal ulcers, is also implicated in stomach cancer. Known cases of infection with this bacteria can be cured with antibiotics. Since both liver and stomach cancer have exceptionally low survival rates, preventing their occurrence is the best defense.

Even stress has been linked to cancer. In 1991 Australian researchers found that stress increases risk of colorectal cancers. This finding was confirmed in the U.S. according to a report in the September 1993 *Epidemiology.*

International Comparisons

Mortality figures from various nations have especially suggested that dietary differences affect cancer incidence. The wide range in cancer incidence and mortality from nation to nation not only suggests specific causes of cancer but also suggests that changes in lifestyle can improve mortality rates. It is clear that heredity does not completely account for these differences because immigrants from one country to another soon achieve cancer rates similar to those of their new country.

Here is some of the basic information, using a standardized age distribution for persons between the ages of 35 and 74 (that is, rates for each decade are weighted so that every country acts as if it had the same age distribution the U.S. did in 1940, preventing skewing in data from different distributions). All figures are numbers of deaths from cancer per 100,000 members of the population as adjusted for age distribution. The figures for Finland are for 1989 instead of 1990.

NUMBERS OF DEATHS FROM CANCER

Country	WOMEN			MEN		
	1990	1980	Change	1990	1980	Change
Japan	143.4	165.9	−22.5	278.5	283.4	−4.9
Sweden	189.1	208.4	−19.3	221.6	243.2	−21.6
France	169.6	177.3	−7.7	390.1	389.5	+0.6
Finland	170.5	182.6	−12.1	280.6	323.3	−42.7
Switzerland	185.3	199.7	−14.4	294.6	317.4	−22.8
West Germany	207.9	217.4	−9.5	323.2	329.2	−6.0
England/Wales	251.7	253.2	−1.5	322.6	348.2	−25.6
Scotland	279.9	276.0	+3.9	367.6	383.2	−15.6
U.S.	228.0	223.1	+4.9	315.3	319.1	−3.8
Norway	200.5	195.5	+5.0	258.1	246.1	+12.0
Netherlands	209.0	203.1	+5.9	328.9	361.6	−32.7
Canada	222.7	215.0	+7.7	311.3	307.4	+3.9
Denmark	287.9	279.0	+8.9	343.2	338.8	+4.4
Northern Ireland	249.7	239.1	+10.6	324.4	313.2	+11.2
Iceland	256.3	197.1	+59.2	265.2	205.6	+59.6

(*See also* "Breast Cancer," p 216; and "Prostate Problems," p 230.)

(Periodical Reference and Additional Reading: *Harvard Health Letter* 6-90, p 1; *New York Times* 2-4-91, p A1; *Science News* 2-27-94, p 135; *Harvard Health Letter* 7-92, p 5; *New York Times* 7-1-92, p A18; *New York Times* 7-29-92, p C12; *New York Times* 2-23-93, p C3; *New York Times* 5-2-93, p I-42; *New York Times* 6-2-93, p C12; *New York Times* 9-15-93, p C13; *Science News* 9-25-93, p 196; *New York Times* 11-4-93, p A14; *Science News* 11-6-93, p 294; *Scientific American* 1-94, p 130; *Statistical Bulletin,* 1/3-94, p 2)

MOLECULAR BIOLOGY AGAINST CANCER

Cancer is a disease primarily of DNA, which not only controls heredity but also directs the manufacture of all the proteins produced by the varied cells in the body. Specific proteins then instigate the rest of the body's chemistry, such as lipid metabolism or utilization of such inorganic chemicals as nitric oxide. The damaged or aberrant DNA that causes cancer, therefore, acts via various proteins or the other chemicals they produce.

Cancer treatment today often includes in addition to surgery other interventions based on proteins and their products. More traditional radiation and much chemotherapy is simply directed at killing cancer cells (*see* "Chemicals Against Cancer," p 425). But as the 1990s have brought increased understanding how the body works at the level of individual molecules there has been a development of more subtle ways of diagnosing, treating, and even preventing cancer.

Diagnosis, Molecule by Molecule

Cancer would be a much less deadly disease if tumor cells stayed near their place of origin. Recognition of cancer cells that have moved from the original site to another site (a process called *metastasis*) is an increasingly important part of diagnosis. For example, after prostate cancer has been treated by removal of the gland, there is still the possibility that cells have metastasized to the bones or other organs. These cells, wherever they are in the body, are still prostate-cancer cells. Thus the chemical test for prostate-specific antigen (PSA) that may have detected the cancer originally can also detect the metastasized cells. (*See also* "Prostate Problems," p 230.)

Cancer cells produce molecules in profusion, molecules that are normally in short supply in the body. Some of these react with the immune system, which views these chemicals as foreign molecules. Antibodies are produced just as they are with prostate-specific antigen, and tests can detect these antibodies by their reaction to the original antigen, supplied from a standard source. One cancer test, for example, recognizes the tumor-associated antigen produced by melanoma. It can tell whether or not treatment for melanoma has been successful, since the test is capable of detecting both the antibody and also the antigen itself. Although such a chemical test cannot indicate the location of missed cells, a negative test means that no cells were missed and the cure is complete. Not only is this reassuring to the person who is now cured of melanoma, but it has a practical effect as well. Insurance companies, reluctant to insure persons who have been treated for melanoma (for which the treatment is successful nearly 90 percent of the time), will issue insurance to people who pass the tumor-associated antigen test.

Better tests to predict risk of cancer are also being developed by molecular biology. The early 1990s saw the identification of genes that are known to be involved in several cancers, including different forms of colorectal cancer. In all cases, when the gene is known, it is theoretically possible to test any individual for an allele of the gene with cancer-causing potential. At this time, however, for nearly all cancer-promoting genes such tests are not practical. It is unusual for a gene to have a 100-percent probability of causing cancer, as environmental or other factors will influence whether or not the potential turns into reality. Furthermore, many of the "cancer genes" have hundreds of alleles, some of which predispose for cancer and some of which do not. It is generally necessary to test for each allele separately.

Biologists at the end of 1993 found a way to get around these problems for an uncommon form of colon cancer called familial adenomatous polyposis (*see also* "Genes for Cancer," p 54). This disease produces intestinal polyps that almost invariably turn into cancer, often when the individual is in his or her 20s or even younger. The alleles that cause the polyps all affect the protein produced by the gene in ways that have a recognizable similarity. The protein is shorter than normal. Protein size is easily evaluated by standard biochemical methods. Therefore, the blood test for this form of potential colon cancer starts by cloning the gene for the protein, which is always the same gene whatever the allele. The gene is then produced in many copies using the polymerase chain reaction or a similar method. The resulting supply of the gene can then be encouraged to manufacture reasonably large amounts of protein, which can be examined for length. If the protein is too short, the person being tested is almost certain to have the characteristic intestinal polyps.

Tests like the one for familial adenomatous polyposis are helpful in alerting physicians and patients to watch for cancer. But they become vastly more useful if they can lead to prevention of cancer in the first place. One idea being tested is to use anti-inflammatory drugs to treat a person with the gene for this form of colon cancer even before the polyps develop. Although not yet established, such a treatment might prevent such polyps, which would also keep the patient from developing cancer later.

Treatment: Co-opting the Immune System

Since cancer cells produce tumor-associated antigens, why doesn't the immune system destroy cancers before they grow beyond single cells? It is believed that most potential cancer cells are in fact destroyed by the immune system. But the problem is that *most* is not *all*. When for some reason the cancer escapes the immune system, the single cell can produce daughters, and a tumor begins to develop. In some cases, the immune system then fights the cancer to no avail (as in melanoma), while in others it seems to give up the fight (some cancers found typically in the neck).

A report in the December 11, 1992 *Science* casts light on how some tumors escape the immune system attacks. Augusto C. Ochoa and coworkers at the U.S. National Cancer Institute found that colon cancer in mice does something mysterious that causes the immune system white blood cells known as T cells to malfunction. Affected T cells have a biochemical defect in the T-cell receptor molecule, the protein that is supposed to recognize foreign invaders and call out the immune calvary for a full-scale attack. The researchers also found preliminary evidence of the same unknown mechanism in human colon cancer.

The most plausible explanation is that the tumor releases some chemical that degrades parts of a protein connected with the T-cell receptor, since T cells that are not in direct contact with the cancer also lose parts of this protein. Either the chemical is not produced until late in the cancer's growth or else the degradation of T cells proceeds very slowly, since the effect is not noticed when cancer is just starting. If a chemical does cause the immune-system defect, there is hope that some way could be found to turn it off (*see, for example,* "Symmetry and Drugs," p 534).

A team from the United Kingdom Medical Research Center's National Institute in London has found an ingenious way to immunize against a specific tumor. Working with mice, they removed tumor cells, inserted genes that manufacture heat-shock proteins into the cells, and returned the altered cells to the mice. The heat-shock proteins made the tumor cells unable to reproduce, so no new cancers arose from them. But the cells alerted the mouse immune system to attack the other cancer cells in the body. Eighty percent of the treated mice survived for a year. The same technique should, in theory, work in humans and be safe. The British experiments were reported in June 1993 in the *Journal of Experimental Medicine*.

About the same time, several teams reported *in vitro* successes with novel molecular approaches for stopping uncontrolled multiplication of cancer cells based on stopping the action of the gene *ras*, perhaps the most famous of the "oncogenes" involved in most cancers. The oncogene *ras* in about a fifth of all human cancers is turned on and promotes cell division. Other cancers also have as one of the defining characteristics of the disease rapid cell division, but 80 percent of the time the cause of the unrestricted cell division is some gene other than *ras.*

These new molecular approaches all focused on preventing the protein produced by *ras,* known as Ras, from attaching to the cell membrane, which it needs to do in order to be a receptor for growth-stimulating hormones. The specific part of the protein molecule that makes this attachment is one of those biochemical parts that all organisms use over and over, just as humans tend to use paper clips for a variety of attachments. Within this attachment group, there is a small part called the CAAX box, consisting of four amino acids, which is the part of the molecule that is the attachment point. Without the CAAX box, Ras cannot be attached to the place where it can do its work. By introducing a fake CAAX box, which *ras* mistakes for a real one and inserts the appropriate part of Ras, the whole growth and division process can be sabotaged.

At least three different fake CAAX boxes were shown to work when introduced into the cytoplasm, so that *ras* uses the fakes instead of a real one. The problem is that the fakes are hard to get into the inside of the cells, where *ras* lurks. Not only do the fakes find it difficult to penetrate the cell membrane, but once inside, mechanisms within the cell break them apart, since the fakes are made from amino acids, just like the real CAAX box. (The initials "C A A X" stand for a cysteine amino acid, two aliphatic amino acids, and one other amino acid, represented by the variable X.) Finally in the June 25, 1993 *Science* two groups announced ways to modify their fake CAAXs with inorganics to permit passage through the membrane and protection once inside; a third group was reported to have found yet another solution to the same problem. So far, however, the products were still being tested only in cell cultures — where they worked, by stopping *ras*-induced cancer from growing. Nevertheless, the same fake-CAAX chemicals failed to stop normal growth of noncancerous cells in cultures, suggesting few undesirable side effects. Tests in animals will be next.

Some of the receptors produced by cancer cells in great profusion to enable the cancer to take in added nutrients for its fast growth are not common to other cells in the body. Monoclonal antibodies can be created that attach to these particular receptors. The antibodies block the receptors from recepting. Without the extra nutrients it needs, the cancer shrinks and dies. This approach was somewhat success-ful with animals in the late 1980s and was applied to humans starting in the early 1990s. So far this has not led to dramatic breakthroughs, but all of the approaches to cancer therapy work together to some degree. In the case of monoclonal antibodies, the success may have come when the technique was combined with chemotherapy.

The aim of most chemotherapy (*see* "Chemicals Against Cancer," p 425) is to find a way to target cancer cells and deliver a poison to them. Since 1975, when César Milstein announced the discovery of monoclonal antibodies, molecular biologists have been trying to hitch these antibodies to poisons that would be transported to where cancers are in the body. Monoclonal antibodies are uniquely suited to the delivery task since they can be selected to latch onto any specific antigen. The use of antibodies to a tumor-associated antigen causes delivery of the drug. Unfortunately, most early attempts failed to work.

In 1993, however, there was a promising new combination. A monoclonal antibody named BR96 homes in on an antigen on the surface of carcinomas (cancers derived from epithelial tissue, such as most lung and colon cancers) as well as on some noncancerous epithelial cells of the esophagus, stomach, intestine, and pancreas. When BR96 binds to this antigen, the combination is wrapped in a bit of cell membrane and transported into the interior of the cell.

A group led by P. A. Trail at the Bristol-Myers Squibb Pharmaceutical Research Institute has created a compound molecule that consists of the powerful chemotherapeutic agent doxorubicin (DOX) linked to BR96 by a bond that remains stable in the blood. After the combination, known as an immunoconjugate, is inducted through the cell membrane into the cell, the region inside the small envelope of cell membrane quickly becomes more acidic. This always happens within such bubbles in the cytoplasm and is an effect used by various natural processes to initiate chemical changes. For the immunoconjugate of DOX and BR96, the acidity breaks the chains that keep DOX from activity. Freed in the cytoplasm, the DOX proceeds to kill the cell. Use of the immunoconjugate can cause complete tumor regression in rats and mice at one-twentieth of the high dose that is often needed to achieve similar effects. Thus the immunoconjugate makes the chemotherapy much more effective and causes fewer side effects. So far this particular combination has not been tried in humans. Earlier attempts to use monoclonal antibodies, however, have been attempted in humans with results that are not nearly as good as one might expect from prior work with animals.

One similar approach that was tried in humans was described in the August 12, 1993 *New England Journal of Medicine*. The physicians were performing safety trials of a radioactive monoclonal antibody. The subjects were nine lymphoma victims who had failed to respond to chemotherapy. The physicians were surprised when the lymphoma disappeared in four of the patients during the safety trials, and when the lymphoma diminished in two of the others. After more than a year, the lymphoma reappeared in two of the four that lost all signs of the disease during the safety trials. Three out of the nine patients were not helped or harmed by the treatment. Further studies are being conducted to determine optimal dose sizes. The normal pattern for medical tests would be then to conduct a double-blind Phase 3 trial with a substantial number of patients and controls.

Vaccines Against Cancer

Vaccines can sometimes prevent cancer in what might be termed the ordinary way: by preventing a viral disease that can lead to cancer. But the cancer vaccines that have been in the news in the 1990s are not for prevention at all; instead, they are aimed at existing tumors. The reason they are called *vaccines* is that they are intended to do the same job that traditional vaccines do—mobilize the immune system. Some of the vaccines even use the old familiar cowpox (*vaccinia*) virus that was the basis of the original vaccine, the one that beat smallpox. But in one of these cases, the vaccinia has been genetically altered to express a tumor-related antigen known as the carcinoembryonic antigen (CEA). In another, the vaccinia virus is used to break apart melanoma cells into pieces. The virus then incorporates the pieces onto its surface. The virus expressing the pieces of cells can then be used as a vaccine against melanoma in the person who contributed the original cells.

Although some vaccines use viruses, many of the most modern cancer vaccines are more like the modern genetically engineered vaccines against infectious organisms: the vaccines are pure chemicals that carry the particular antigen but that are not now and never have been alive.

Some of the cancer vaccines are intended to stimulate the antibody system to attack the cancer, primarily to block growth and metastasis. Others try to induce the white blood cells known as T lymphocytes to attack and kill tumor cells. One new approach tries to do both at once.

One of the earliest attempts at producing a cancer vaccine was based on melanoma cells that had been screened to find cells that expressed antigens thought especially to provoke the immune system. These were killed with radiation and then injected into the patient, with the response enhanced by using the tuberculosis vaccine BCG to further stimulate the immune system. Very early reports suggested that the vaccine makes a difference, but further study found benefits in only 25 percent of the patients. Another study that made the news in 1992 used cancerous B cells from a person with lymphoma. The outer coats of these B cells were removed; the detached coats were injected back into the same person from whom the cells were removed along with a chemical to stimulate the immune system. Small trials showed some success with this method as well.

Results from this and other early trials of cancer vaccines were difficult to evaluate because generally there were only a few patients involved and often no controls. But gradually a baker's dozen or more of cancer vaccines have begun or are moving through the phases now expected of newly developed medical treatments: Phase 1 for safety; Phase 2 for dosage and response; and Phase 3 to determine whether or not it really works, usually with a double-blind trial in which neither the patients nor the doctors know who is getting the new treatment and who is not until after the trial is completed. (However, there are always watchers who know the truth so that they can stop the trial if something is going wrong or if the results are spectacularly good; in that latter case, everyone—even the controls—is put on the new treatment.)

Here is a brief summary of the studies ongoing at the end of 1993. The numbers add to more than the 13 vaccines being tested because three of the vaccines are being tried against more than one cancer.

SUMMARY OF CANCER STUDIES

Cancer	Number of vaccines	Remarks
Melanoma	8	One of the vaccines uses genetically engineered antigens; one uses a synthetic antibody; six of the vaccines use all or parts of melanoma cells that have been killed.
Colorectal	4	Three of these are genetically engineered or use purified antigens; the other uses cells from the patient's own colon tumor with BCG added to stimulate the immune system.
Breast	2	Both are based on ways of presenting specific antigens to stimulate antibody or T cell production.
Pancreatic	2	These are the same as the two breast cancer vaccines.

Cancer	Number of vaccines	Remarks
Clinical lymphotic leukemia	1	Uses synthetically assembled short chains of amino acids based on leukemic white blood cells.
Gastric	1	Uses a specific antigen presented on vaccinia virus (also used for colorectal, pancreatic, and breast cancers).
Lung	1	Uses a cloned antigen; same vaccine as one of the above colorectal vaccines.
Ovarian	1	Uses a specific antigen; also among the colorectal vaccines.

In addition to these trials on humans, other research is being conducted with animals. One leukemia vaccine that combines a product of B cells with a growth factor (technically, granulocyte-macrophage colony-stimulating factor) worked exceptionally well on mice at the start of 1993. Like some of the other vaccines being tested, it needs to be custom made to match each (mouse) patient's tumor.

(Periodical References and Additional Reading: *New York Times* 5-7-91, p C1; *New York Times* 7-31-92, p A10; *New York Times* 9-20-92, p III-6; *New York Times* 10-22-92, p A18; *New York Times* 12-11-92, p A30; *Science* 12-11-92, pp 1732 & 1795; *New York Times* 4-27-93, p C9; *New York Times* 6-22-93, p C3; *Science* 6-25-93, pp 1877, 1934, & 1937; *New York Times* 7-9-93, p A10; *New York Times* 8-12-93, p A17; *Science* 11-5-93, pp 841 & 844; *New York Times* 12-30-93, p A12)

CHEMICALS AGAINST CANCER

Chemotherapy and the Environment

Among the chemicals used against cancer, Taxol gained considerable fame in part because it was an issue connected to attempts to preserve old-growth forest in the Pacific Northwest. About the time that the northern spotted owl was becoming the main symbol of this conservation effort, results showed that Taxol, a chemical then derived entirely from the bark of the Pacific yew tree, is a potent anticancer drug. But loggers were destroying the Pacific yews with clear-cutting, even though the yew was not valued for its lumber. In the meantime, six separate studies during 1992 demonstrated that Taxol caused remission of both breast and ovarian cancers; a comparison with the standard chemical treatment (chemotherapy, often called simply "chemo") showed that Taxol was more effective in the treatment of ovarian cancer.

Eventually other sources were found for Taxol, thereby blunting its environmental message but improving in some cases the cancer-fighting potential of the chemical. A drug similar to Taxol, called taxotere, was found in the European yew tree and shown in 1992 to be effective against cancer, although with many of the typical side effects of chemotherapy. Taxotere could also be harvested from needles of yew trees, so the yew tree does not have to be killed, which is required for obtaining Taxol from yew bark.

Background

Chemotherapy, or "chemo," is simply the use of chemicals, typically administered intravenously, to fight cancers. The first chemotherapy was used in 1941 on prostate cancer. Many years passed before chemotherapy became an accepted cancer treatment along with surgery and radiation. After World War II, chemicals that had been developed as poison gases for war purposes were found to destroy white blood cells, so they were tried out on cancers of such cells, such as Hodgkin's disease and leukemias. Success, however, was quite limited. Ten years later, as scientists searched for new antibiotics, they discovered that while one known familiarly as DON was not much good against bacteria and worthless against viruses, it caused remission of several forms of cancers in rats and mice. A decade later, in the late 1960s, scientists realized the chemotherapy was going to be as important as radiation in cancer treatment, although they still knew how to treat only a few rare cancers with the method. At that time the chemical 5-fluorouracil, or 5-FU, was an experimental drug being tested on the less dangerous skin cancers.

By the early 1990s, chemotherapy was almost routine for all sorts of cancers, often combined with radiation and surgery. Advanced rectal cancer, for example, kills more than half of the people who have it, despite surgery followed by radiation. About 36 percent of those can be saved by using the old chemotherapeutic drug 5-FU, which long ago moved from the "experimental" to the "traditional" treatment category. As with most chemotherapy, the patients also suffered nausea, vomiting, diarrhea, and abnormally low numbers of white blood cells, but over a period of seven years 36 percent fewer of them died.

Cancer cells are notable and destructive largely because they reproduce themselves much more quickly than other cells in the body. Most chemotherapy is directed at this rapid-division aspect of cancer cells, using chemicals that interfere with cell division throughout the body. The idea of such conventional chemotherapy is that since the cancer cells divide more rapidly and often than any others, the chemicals will stop that process. Many adult cells, such as nerve cells, have long ago stopped reproducing themselves. But many normal body cells divide and grow with some rapidity, such as bone-marrow stem cells (which produce red and white blood cells) and hair cells. The result is that typical side effects of such chemotherapy include anemia, depressed immune function, and hair loss, as well as other effects caused by generalized interference with cell division.

In 1993 chemists from The Scripps Research Institute in La Jolla, California improved Taxol by creating chemicals they called protaxols. Unlike Taxol itself, some of the protaxols were easily soluble in blood. The protaxols turned to Taxol at rates that could be specified by the chemist, making it easier to use protaxols to reach the site of the cancer. Other scientists found that adding a phosphate group to chemo agents also improved their ability to dissolve in blood; the phosphate groups essentially act as a detergent.

Taxol was approved for general use by the U.S. Food and Drug Administration on December 29, 1992. A year later, many physicians and patients were not so excited about it as they had been. While Taxol caused remission of ovarian cancers, they soon began growing again. Studies did not find gains in life expectancy. And Taxol treatment (usually in combination with another chemotherapeutic drug) was expensive. Still, many physicians and researchers hoped that with more experience, the right techniques would be found to make Taxol or one of its close relatives a significant advance in cancer treatment.

Preventing Chemo's Side Effects

In 1991 physicians learned that granulyte colony-stimulating factor could help suppress some of the unpleasant side effects of chemotherapy. This led to testing a number of similar growth factors as a way of reducing loss of bone-marrow function, digestive problems, and hair loss—all associated with chemo because the cells involved are actively dividing. Sometimes this strategy seemed to work and sometimes not. When growth factors were used to reduce bone-marrow problems in people being treated for lung cancer, the cost of treatment was increased by a factor of six but the survival rate for the patients was unchanged. When human stem-cell factor was given to breast cancer patients, it aided the cells in bone marrow that produce blood cells, but it also produced allergic reactions.

Somewhat better results were obtained by combining granulocyte-macrophage colony stimulating factor with the cytokine interleukin 3. Like the other treatments cited, the aim of the combination was to stimulate cell growth in bone marrow, which it did much better than the growth factor did by itself.

The Breast Cancer Prevention Program

In 1992 the U.S. National Cancer Institute started a trial of the chemotherapy agent tamoxifen in 8000 healthy women who for one reason or another were thought to be at high risk of developing breast cancer. The Breast Cancer Prevention Program (BCPP) was intended to show that this powerful drug would also prevent the disease in the first place, presumably by killing the first few cancerous cells and thereby keeping them from proliferating.

The tamoxifen used in the BCPP is the first instance of a powerful chemotherapeutic agent used to prevent, rather than to treat, cancer. Tamoxifen is thought to occupy the sites on cancer cells that would otherwise be taken up by estrogen. The estrogen seems to spur breast cancers to grow, but tamoxifen does not.

From the beginning the trials were controversial because tamoxifen, like estrogen, increases risks of cancer of the uterine lining (endometrium) and may encourage formation of blood clots in some women. In September 1993 several studies emerged that showed that the endometrial cancers induced by tamoxifen were more potent than previously thought.

Tamoxifen has many effects on the body. Among these is a decrease in the cholesterol levels in the blood, presumably helping to prevent heart disease as well as cancer. Thus the BCPP was expected to prevent 62 cancers and 50 heart attacks among the 8000 women during the course of the trial. But an outside analysis published in *Epidemiologic Reviews* in September 1993 claimed that only 52 cancers and 13 heart attacks would be prevented, while producing perhaps 39 to 57 endometrial cancers. According to this review, the BCPP might, by causing more blood clots, inadvertently cause 17 more strokes than lowering cholesterol prevented. Furthermore, it might also cause ophthalmic complications. All in all this review, by Trudy L. Bush and Kathy J. Helzsouer of Johns Hopkins University in Baltimore, Maryland concluded that BCPP would cause as many as 31 to 57 more adverse situations than the number of benefits.

Bad news continued to roll in about tamoxifen. In the September 1, 1993 *Cancer Research* a long-standing rumor was confirmed; tamoxifen increases the amount of liver cancer in rats to rates that are 25 to 30 times that of normal rates, even at low doses. But only two human cases of liver cancer have occurred among humans using tamoxifen, despite 24 years of experience with the compound.

Further studies in 1994 continued to reveal similar cancer-causing potential in tamoxifen.

Chemo Activated by Light

In April 1993 Canada approved the first cancer chemotherapy that combines a chemical attack on recurrent bladder cancer with activation by laser light. The chemical is Photofrin II, which is a modification of a porphyrin used in handling oxygen in blood. Unlike earlier photochemicals, Photofrin II is activated by fairly long waves of light that can penetrate body tissues. Also unlike the other photochemicals, Photofrin does not affect DNA; instead it breaks oxygen molecules apart, producing the very active single atoms. These loose oxygen atoms combine with whatever is around, destroying most chemicals with which they come into contact and resulting in quick cell death. But this happens only when Photofrin II is activated by light. In the dark, Photofrin II is thought to be relatively harmless. The photochemical is now being evaluated for use in other cancers, including cancers of the lung, stomach, cervix, and esophagus.

However, Photofrin II takes a long time to accumulate in tissues and even longer to dissipate. As a result a person undergoing treatment must stay out of direct sunlight for about two months, or the destructive oxygen reactions will be initiated. Newer porphyrin-based compounds are being developed that will both accumulate and clear quicker, removing this block to wider use of the technique.

Japanese scientists have combined the light-activation of porphyrins with light-emitting properties. Used against lung cancer after conventional treatment, the Japanese chemical concentrates in any remaining cancer cells. These can be identified by the light the cells emit. Then the porphyrin can be activated by beaming light of the proper frequency at it, killing the left-over cancer cells.

More and More Chemicals Found

The continued search for new chemicals that are active against cancer provides additional choices for physicians. Some of these are used before cancer starts, mainly in situations for which the likelihood of cancer is great.

Bowman-Birk inhibitor A mouthwash based on soybeans used to prevent precancerous lesions in the mouth from turning into cancer. This mouthwash is now

Background

Since the time of the ancient Egyptians, physicians have known that some chemicals are only effective as a treatment when activated by light—the Egyptians doctors used a herb growing along the Nile to treat skin disorders. The active ingredients in the herb, chemicals called psoralens, were modified by chemists in the 1970s to form the basis for a common treatment for psoriasis that uses a psoralen called PUVA and ultraviolet (UV) light to treat psoriasis. The advantage of photochemotherapy is that once a chemical has accumulated in tissues, only those tissues that require treatment are illuminated with a laser. Thus, side effects are reduced.

Psoriasis, like cancer, is a disease in which some cells multiply rapidly; chemicals that work on one disease can also be effective on the other. PUVA could not be used for most cancers, however, because the ultraviolet light needed to activate it does not penetrate very far through body tissues. One experimental treatment for leukemias got around the low penetration of UV light by channeling blood outside the body, exposing it to light, and then putting the blood back into the circulatory system (somewhat as blood is handled in dialysis).

Psoralens act directly on DNA, which can be inactivated by the psoralen-light combination, stopping unrestricted growth in either psoriasis or cancer. This can be a disadvantage, however; since it modifies DNA, psoralen can be activated by components of sunlight in parts of the skin not being treated. Partial activation can damage DNA rather than stop it from working, leading in some cases to skin cancer.

The chemicals known as porphyrins have also been known to medical science for a long time. A hereditary disease known as porphyria (sometimes thought to have affected George III and George IV of England and some of their descendants) is a defect that causes accumulation of porphyrins. Hemoglobin is also a porphyrin, but not one of the ones that cause porphyria. The chemicals that accumulate in porphyria are activated by various environmental factors, including light. There are a number of different types of the disease, depending on the specific porphyrins and the particular alleles of the genes involved.

being tested in humans, although many years may be needed to determine effectiveness.

Byrostatin 1 Obtained by grinding and purifying the bryozoan (moss animal) *Bugula neritina*, a tiny colonial marine animal. Previously shown to be effective *in vitro* and in mice, safety trials were started in humans with various cancers late in 1993. Although only safety trials, several of the tumors shrank. The main side effect was muscle pain, somewhat different from the difficulties causes by most chemotherapeutic agents. The success of this drug tends to confirm what many environmental scientists have said about the importance of preserving obscure species because no one knows which ones will harbor a "cure for cancer."

Caffeic esters Honey-derived compounds that inhibit precancerous conditions in rat colons.

Limolene A chemical found in orange peels shown to be effective against breast cancer in mice. Six humans have also tried limolene, but results are not in.

Perillyl alcohol A chemical from the fragrant herb lavender is even more successful than limolene on breast cancer in mice. The actual chemical is not the effective agent. Instead, perillyl alcohol is broken down by the body into chemicals that actively attack the cancer cells.

RU-486   Because the famous "abortion pill" (*see* "Terminating Pregnancy," p 102) RU-486 blocks the action of the hormones progesterone and cortisol, it could be used in the treatment of breast cancer as well as of endometriosis (caused when tissue from the uterine lining grows in the wrong place) or Cushing's syndrome (an excess of cortisol).

Shark cartilage   In 1993, *60 Minutes* reported that sharks do not get cancer and that shark cartilage prevents blood vessels from forming and bringing blood to tumors. Without the extra blood supply the tumor is starved to death. None of this is true. Sharks have not only been found with cancers of the kidney, liver, and blood cells, but even with cancers of the cartilage. Scientists who study how blood vessels form to supply cancers with blood say that there is nothing special about shark cartilage and that whatever inhibitors of blood vessels in cartilage that are present are in such short supply that one would have to consume hundreds of pounds of cartilage to get any effect whatsoever. This time *60 Minutes* apparently got it wrong.

Tretinoin   This strange story begins when scientists found that 13-cis retinoic acid, also known as isotretinoin and tradenamed Accutane when used as an acne medicine, kills cancer cells *in vitro*. This was not a total surprise since retinoic acid, a close relative of vitamin A, has powerful effects on cells. Word of this discovery spread to China in 1986, but the Chinese researchers could not obtain Accutane. So they used the related compound all-*trans*-retinoic acid, known as tretinoin, on 24 humans who had acute promyelocytic leukemia, a fatal cancer of the white blood cells. All 24 patients went into remission; their cells, which had been unable to mature because of a chromosome defect, matured. Meanwhile back in the U.S., researchers found that although Accutane works *in vitro* it does not cure cancer in humans. (Later, however, a combination of Accutane and alpha interferon was successful on 16 of 26 patients with squamous cell carcinoma, a common skin cancer, of the head and neck.) After learning of the Chinese success, Raymond P. Warrell, Jr. of Memorial Sloan Kettering Cancer Center in New York City tried tretinoin on 11 patients with leukemia. Nine went into remission, about the same percentage as could be obtained with conventional intravenous chemotherapy. But not only is tretinoin an oral drug, it also does not have the side effects of conventional chemotherapy.

(Periodical References and Additional Reading: *New York Times* 5-21-91, p C3; *Science News* 6-1-91, p 341; *Harvard Health Letter* 3-92, p 1; *Discover* 1-93, p 52; *Science News* 1-9-93, p 28; *Science News* 5-29-93, pp 341 & 344; *Nature* 7-29-93, p 464; *Science News* 9-18-93, p 181; *Science News* 9-25-93, p 207; *Scientific American* 10-93, p 24; *Science* 10-1-93, p 32; *New York Times* 11-7-93, p I-1; *Science News* 11-27-93, p 358)

AUTOIMMUNE DISEASES

ALLERGIES AND ASTHMA

An estimated one out of five Americans is allergic to something. The most serious common allergic response is asthma, a chronic condition in which the bronchial tubes and other airways become narrowed as a result of allergic reactions. About five to ten percent of children in the U.S. have asthma, which may disappear during adolescence; but about the same number of adults develop asthma later in life (sometimes in their 80s) or have childhood asthma resurface, keeping the total asthma population fairly stable. Another major group of allergies is less serious, but more common. Allergic rhinitis, more commonly known as hay fever, affects about 15 percent of all Americans with sneezing, wheezing, and irritated airways. Food allergies, although self-diagnosed by one out of four Americans, probably actually are present in only one or two percent of the population. Like asthma and some food allergies, reactions to a few other ingested or injected substances, including penicillin and insect venom, can produce death as a result of an overwhelming allergic reaction known as anaphylactic shock. Contact allergies, such as skin inflammation in response to certain detergents or perfumes, are probably common, but are less serious and usually treated by avoidance.

The allergic responses are all part of the immune system, the main protection humans have against invading viruses, bacteria, other parasites, and some toxic chemicals. There are good reasons to think that the particular parts of the immune system involved in allergic reactions are those evolved originally to protect humans from such parasites as protists and worms (*see* "The State of the War Against Parasites," p 378). People who live in regions where those parasites are common have fewer allergies, perhaps because their immune reactions are fully occupied in dealing with the parasites. Biochemical studies have shown that the same cells and immune-system chemicals that are involved in allergic reactions are also used in defense against invading protists and worms. Different parts of the immune system commonly are employed against bacteria or viruses.

Asthma

Asthma is defined as a chronic inflammatory disease characterized by periodic attacks. These may consist of shortness of breath or more serious wheezing and panic from reduced air intake. Air passages may become completely blocked, which can result in death. Although asthma is generally thought to be caused by allergic reactions, there may be another cause in some instances. Persons prone to asthma may have attacks brought on by viral infections, such as the common cold, for example, or by medications prescribed for other ailments.

Asthma attacks begin when the B cells are stimulated to release immunoglobulin E (IgE) antibodies, stimulating the mast cells and basophils to release such chemicals as histamines and leukotrienes. Later the tissues of the air passages are invaded by

Background

Although immunologists often date the discovery of the immune system to the discovery of antibodies by Emil von Behring and Shibasaburo Kitasato (independently) in 1890 and the discovery of blood types by Karl Landsteiner in 1900 (and a case could be made for earlier work by Ilya Mechinkov, Louis Pasteur, or even Edward Jenner), the system did not get respect until 1983. That was the year that AIDS, the syndrome featuring loss of the immune system that was first recognized in 1981, became widely feared after the first well-known people died from the disease. It was also the year that physicians learned how to turn off parts of the immune system deliberately, using the drug cyclosporine to stop immune-system rejection of transplanted organs.

The immune system is a complex and effective defense against all manner of ills, with important roles played by skin, thymus, spleen, lymph system, and bone marrow. But the main soldiers in the war against foreign invaders of the body are the individual cells often lumped together as "white blood cells" and the chemicals that they produce or respond to.

White Blood Cells

B cells Lymphocytes that produce antibodies.

basophils White blood cells involved in allergic reactions that invade tissues after a lesion and orchestrate with chemicals the late response in allergic reactions.

eosinophils White blood cells involved in allergic reactions that invade tissues after a lesion.

granulocytes Granular leukocytes, including basophils, eosinophils, and neutrophils.

leukocytes The more formal name for "white blood cells."

lymphocytes About a quarter of the leukocytes—the B cells, including natural killer cells, and T cells—are known as lymphocytes.

macrophages Large cells that engulf foreign bodies and signal T cells to make lymphokines by presenting antigens to them in combination with MHC molecules.

mast cells Large cells that gather near source of infection and produce histamine and other chemicals important in allergic reactions.

memory cells B or T cells that wait for an antigen to come again.

monocytes Relatively large leukocytes with one nucleus; large monocytes are called macrophages, especially if they resemble amoebas.

natural killer cells Lymphocytes that release gamma interferon and are more like B cells than T cells.

neutrophils White blood cells that invade lesions to combat invasion by bacteria.

phagocytes A general term for any white blood cells that engulf and destroy foreign cells or particles.

T cells There are several kinds: helper T cells (CD 4 cells) coordinate various disease-fighting functions; cytotoxic (killer or CD8) T cells cause cells they attack to die; suppressor cells inhibit antibody production by B cells when stimulated by gamma interferon.

Immune-System Chemicals

antibodies Proteins that attach to foreign chemicals or cells, interfering with their operation and signaling phagocytes to ingest the foreigners; antibodies are actually soluble parts of B cell receptors for antigens.

antigens Not part of the immune system, but any chemical that sets it into action.

complement Proteins that bind to other proteins and then signal phagocytes to engulf the bodies on which the combination resides; they also kill cells by punching holes in cell membranes.

cytokines Any small proteins used as cell messengers, including interferons.

granulocytic macrophage colony stimulating factor (GM-CSF) A cytokine made by macrophages and other cell types that facilitates migration of eosinophils and basophils into damaged tissues and helps prolong the cells' lives.

histamine A chemical that is released in allergic reactions; it stimulates mucus production, causes smooth muscles to constrict in the lungs and intestines, and dilates and increases the permeability of small blood vessels.

immunoglobulin E (IgE) antibodies A class of antibodies secreted by B cells that have been matured by interleukin 4; IgE antibodies that are involved in protection against parasites and in allergic reactions.

interferons Three main types are known as alpha (20 members), beta (one kind), and gamma (one kind); there are also omega and tau interferons, which are much like alpha interferons, but somewhat larger; alpha interferons are primarily antiviral, but also arouse the immune system to attack tumors; gamma is involved in orchestrating the immune-system attack in part by activating macrophages; beta inhibits gamma and generally turns down the immune system.

interleukins Lymphokines that stimulate B cells to make antibodies or that the macrophages make to stimulate the liver to produce chemicals used in identifying bacteria.

leukotrienes Cytokines released by mast cells and basophils; constrict airways and increase permeability of small blood vessels.

lymphokines Cytokines that stimulate B cells to make antibodies and cytotoxic T cells to attack; produced by helper T cells.

MHC molecules Proteins produced by the Major Histocompatibility Complex of genes that cause various self-peptides and foreign peptides (when a cell has been invaded) to be displayed on the cell surface for inspection by helper T cells.

platelet-activating factor A cytokine released by mast cells and basophils; constricts airways and dilates blood vessels.

prostaglandin D A hormone-like chemical released by mast cells and basophils; constricts bronchial airways.

RANTES A cytokine made by T cells that regulates migration of eosinophils from the blood into injured tissues.

tumor necrosis factor The cytokine produced by cytotoxic T cells that is used to kill cells of various kinds, not just tumor cells.

eosinophils that produce, in addition to leukotrienes, prostaglandins and various proteins that are used in fighting foreign substances by promoting inflammation.

Asthma is diagnosed with increasing frequency in the U.S. The number of asthmatics was estimated at about 12.4 million Americans in the early 1990s as opposed to only 6.8 million in 1980. The number of deaths has doubled, reaching 4650 in 1992, nearly twice the 2598 deaths in 1979, the low point. Much of this increase has been among Americans of African descent, who are three times as likely to die from asthma as American whites. Prior to 1979, the asthma death rate had been much higher, ranging from more than four per 100,000 in the early 1950s down to less than one per 100,000 in the late 1970s. Around the world, death rates from asthma were even higher than those in the U.S.

Late in the 1980s and in 1990 studies implicated leukotrienes as the main culprits in asthma and drugs were developed to block them, just as antihistamines block the allergic chemical histamine. Among the drugs that are still experimental were zileuton, which interferes with an enzyme needed in leukotriene production, and venzair. The anticancer drug methotrexate was tried during 1990 and 1991 in hopes of preventing inflammatory cells from proliferating. Asthma treatment in Europe, South America, and Canada in the early 1990s began to develop the theory that inflammation of air passageways was a major problem and that anti-inflammatory medicines, such as steroids like cortisone, could be inhaled and applied directly to the inflammation in the lungs.

In the 1991 the U.S. National Heart, Lung and Blood Institute (NHLBI) recommended that asthma be treated with inhaled steroids daily to prevent inflammation, which was just being recognized as the root of many asthma problems, rather than just simple contraction of air passages. Bronchodialators, intended to open those air passages, should be used only during actual asthma attacks. Despite these guidelines, the chief of the allergy section of the U.S. National Institute of Allergy and Infectious Diseases in April 1993 announced that most primary-care doctors failed to treat asthmatics properly, providing only prescriptions for symptomatic relief through bronchodialators.

In 1994 a major NHLBI study, the Childhood Asthma Management Program, was started to compare treatment with the steroid budesonide, with a nonsteriodal anti-inflammatory agent called nedocromil, and with a placebo. All participants in the study, however, could use the inhalant albuterol to relax airways when needed.

There are two other diseases that are, in their symptoms, like a perpetual asthma attack: emphysema and chronic bronchitis, sometimes grouped together as chronic obstructive pulmonary disease. The same treatments that help deal with asthma are also useful in the chronic obstruction pulmonary diseases.

Allergy to Shrimp

Oddly, although thousands of substances are known to cause allergies, the exact chemical in the food, on the airborne particle, or even in the sting is rarely known. This situation changed for one of the common food allergies in 1993 when two teams of researchers discovered that the protein tropomyosin is the causative factor in shrimp. Like most proteins, tropomyosin is found in slightly different forms in a variety of animals. The version in shrimp was shown to bind to immunoglobulin E (IgE) antibodies, setting off itching in the mild cases and attacks similar to asthma in more serious instances. Shrimp can also set off anaphylatic shock, which can lead to death.

Proteins change shape somewhat during cooking. In some instances, shrimp allergy can be set off by partly cooked shrimp, but not by shrimp that is fully boiled or fried.

(Periodical References and Additional Reading: *New York Times* 12-29-90; *New York Times* 1-31-91; *Harvard Health Letter* 5-91, p 5; *Harvard Health Letter* 6-91, p 1; *Harvard Health Letter* 12-92, p 5; *New York Times* 5-4-93, p C3; *Scientific American* 8-93, p 62; *Scientific American* 9-93, pp 52, 64, 72, 80, 106, and 116; *Scientific American* 12-93, p 78; *Nature* 12-2-93, p 421; *New York Times* 12-28-93, p C3; *New York Times* 1-4-94, p C1; *Scientific American* 5-94, p 68)

INFLAMMATION AND ARTHRITIS

The immune system works in part by causing inflammation. Immune-system cells such as mast cells, basophils, and eosinophils secrete chemicals such as histamine, which brings more blood (and therefore more immune system cells) to the point of attack, causing the site to redden and swell. The nerves react to the process by transmitting pain signals to the brain.

While inflammation is painful, it is generally temporary and worth the trouble in dealing with a foreign invader. But some cases, for reasons that are poorly understood, the immune system provokes inflammation when there is no invader. Such inflammation experiences over a long period of time are recognized as a chronic disease. The archetype of such autoimmune diseases is rheumatoid arthritis.

Oral Tolerization

David Trentham and his coworkers of Harvard Medical School in Boston reported in the September 24, 1993 *Science* that they had significantly reduced symptoms of rheumatoid arthritis by a technique intended to selectively stop the immune reaction. The method, called "oral tolerization," has also been used against other autoimmune diseases, but the arthritis study produced the most hopeful results so far. The concept behind oral tolerization is to have the person under attack by the immune system to ingest regular amounts of the body substance being attacked, or something very much like it. Experiments with animals have shown that the substance used to change the immune attack need not be exactly the same as the one that provokes the initial attack by immune-system antibodies.

For the rheumatoid arthritis study, 59 patients with rheumatoid arthritis were fed either a chemical called type II collagen, which is a constituent of cartilage, or a placebo. The collagen was extracted in liquid form from chicken breastbones. After other drugs were withdrawn, half the patients drank collagen in their morning orange juice, while the others got juice flavored with vinegar.

Patients who got only vinegared juice tended to get worse for the most part (although a few improved on the placebo and no other medication). But statistically, the collagen treatment was effective, with most of the patients showing a reduction in swelling and joint pain from 25 to 50 percent. Four patients became symptom-free during the trial.

Background

Arthritis comes in many forms and has many causes. Indeed, *arthritis* by itself is only a vague term, and must be modified by another word to designate a specific disease.

A form of arthritis now thought to be caused by an autoimmune reaction is termed *rheumatoid*. Although the main symptom of the disease is inflammation of the membrane surrounding a joint (the *sinovium*), other nearby tissues are often involved, including the bone itself. Similar inflammation in other tissues, nowhere near the joints, can also be labeled as rheumatoid arthritis in clinical practice. Some patients also feel tired or just vaguely ill.

One theory is that rheumatoid arthritis is initiated by a virus in persons with a hereditary predisposition toward the disease. The condition most often begins in early middle age, between 35 and 50, with women about two or three times more likely than men to develop the disease. Severity of symptoms and frequency of periods when the condition is acting up both vary greatly from patient to patient. About one time out of seven the symptoms simply vanish, never to return. In severe cases, however, the joint damage can be considerable and permanent.

The main treatment for rheumatoid arthritis has been to use aspirin or steroids to reduce inflammation. But since rheumatoid arthritis is an autoimmune disease, it can be attacked more directly through the immune system. Patients with severe arthritis that is not helped by other means may use an immune-suppressing drug. These drugs, however, suppress a wide range of immune reactions, leaving the patient open to various diseases. Furthermore, immune-suppressors (and aspirin and steroids) have other serious side effects in many patients.

A Different Diet Connection

Foods definitely affect symptoms of rheumatoid arthritis. Most patients with rheumatoid arthritis experience symptomatic relief while fasting. One possible explanation is that certain foods produce an allergic response by themselves; but with the immune system already attacking tissues, the general higher level of chemicals and white blood cells caused by the food allergy also makes the arthritis symptoms worse. There is a second theory that proposes that a food alters the way that the allergic system operates. The relief during fasting, for example, could be caused when the body has fewer fatty acids (since none are being eaten) with which to make cell membranes. In any case, when the fasting is over, the symptoms begin again.

If the first theory is true, however, fasting works only because certain foods are missing from the diet, not food in general. Studies have shown that a few patients develop their arthritic symptoms from such foods as shrimp even in double-blind tests using capsules, but most patients react the same to placebos as to food capsules. Studies have also shown that mast cells are reduced in number when some patients avoid foods to which they might be allergic. But the number of rheumatoid patients for whom such specific food responses has been found is small—perhaps one in 20.

The second theory revolves primarily around different dietary fats. Research suggests, for example, that the famous omega-3 fatty acids, found in fatty fish such as salmon and sardines, may reduce symptoms of rheumatoid arthritis. A 1990 study showed that adding omega-3 supplements to the diet reduces joint symptoms. Another research trial in 1993 showed that a different fatty acid, gammalinolenic acid, which is not normally in food but which can be extracted from the seeds of the evening primrose or of the herb borage, also relieves arthritic symptoms. Another study put arthritic patients on a vegetarian diet, which contains a different fat profile from a diet that includes meat, poultry, and fish. The vegetarian arthritics also experienced reduced symptoms.

The Pregnancy Connection

In 1938 Philip Hench of the Mayo Clinic in Rochester, Minnesota, reported that pregnancy often causes symptoms of arthritis to abate. Experiments with this intriguing observation tried to connect the relief to the change in hormones that women experience during pregnancy, but to no avail. Finally in the April 12, 1993 the *New England Journal of Medicine* a group of researchers led by J. Lee Nelson of the Fred Hutchinson Cancer Research Center in Seattle, Washington, reported on research that suggests an entirely different mechanism hinting at an explanation to the mystery.

The Seattle team was eventually able over a period of nearly ten years to obtain useful data from 46 women who became pregnant after the onset of rheumatoid arthritis. Nearly 70 percent of the women found considerable loss of symptoms during the pregnancy—but that means that more than 30 percent did not. Knowing that rheumatoid arthritis is caused by the immune system, Nelson and her coworkers studied the problem from that point of view.

Physicians used to believe that the fetus and mother were protected from each other by barriers between the separate blood supplies, but now they know that some fetal cells wind up in the mother's bloodstream anyway (*see* "Fetal Diagnosis," p 108). It is not known what protects these cells from destruction by the immune system, but it is clear that they are protected. Of course, in some instances the fetus shares enough key genes with the mother to mitigate any immune response, but this would be expected to happen less often—about a quarter of the time in fact—than the opposite situation, in which the father's genes or repressed maternal genes are expressed on fetal cells.

Nelson and her coworkers found that the immune-system gene profiles were quite different between mother and fetus in the cases where remission occurred during pregnancy. When the fetal cells were genetically similar to maternal cells in their immune profile, there was no symptomatic relief. In two instances, when the same rheumatic mother had two pregnancies, relief was obtained for the pregnancy in which the fetal genes resembled the father and not when the genes were like the mother's. This suggests that whatever mechanism in pregnancy reduces the immune attack on fetal cells is initiated in some way by the reaction to the fetal cells. Furthermore this mechanism also protects cells being attacked by the immune system in the mother.

(Periodical References and Additional Reading: *Harvard Health Letter* 7-93, p 4; *Science* 9-24-93, pp 1669, 1727; *Science News* 9-25-93, p 198; *Science News* 10-23-93, p 266; *Harvard Health Letter* 3-94, p 1)

DIABETES

Estimates are that 14 to 15 million Americans have diabetes-mellitus, about six percent of the U.S. population—making it among the most common chronic diseases. But only one in ten of these people have Type I diabetes, which has been identified as an autoimmune disease. The large majority have Type II diabetes (also known as Non-insulin-dependent diabetes mellitus, or NIDDM), which may not have an autoimmune component at all.

Type II diabetes is associated with middle-age and excess weight, so it is somewhat surprising the Type II affects five percent of the population of the world, most of which is not middle-aged or older and most of which is not overweight. The increase in Type II diabetes around the world has been linked to a change to a Western diet and lifestyle. On the island of Nauru, for example, where mineral riches led the population to become sedentary and obese, incidence of Type II diabetes rose from zero percent at the end of World War II to 28 percent of the population at its peak. Since then, natural selection has taken its toll on the genetically susceptible portion of the population, so diabetes has begun to decline on Nauru, despite the continuing Western lifestyle.

New Thoughts on the Cause of Diabetes

Recognition of Type I diabetes as an autoimmune disease provides little help in determining the cause of the disease. As with asthma and rheumatoid arthritis, genes are suspected. After the discovery of bacteria, physicians looked for bacteria as the root cause of most disease, and likewise physicians today suspect genes are behind any disease for which the etiology is poorly understood.

Genes are thought to contribute about 40 to 50 percent of the reason Type I diabetes occurs, with the rest coming from an unknown cause. If Type I were caused by just the genes, as in a pure hereditary disease, 100 percent of people with those genes would develop the disease; instead, only about half of them develop diabetes. One theory, supported by experimental studies, is that the genes must be activated by a protein in cow's milk (see "Milk, Mothers, and Formula," p 126). The protein is bovine serum albumin, which has a small region that is almost exactly the same as a similar-sized region on the insulin-producing beta cells of the pancreas. A large-scale study is ongoing to determine if children who avoid that protein will develop fewer cases of Type I diabetes than matched controls who have an unrestricted diet.

Near the end of 1993, two studies reported that animal trials had shown that the enzyme glutamate decarboxylase (GAD) also contains a region that is about the same size and shape as one on the beta cells and also of a region of a virus linked with Type I diabetes. GAD is mostly found in the brain, where it synthesizes the neurotransmitter GABA, but it also is used as a cytokine by cells of the pancreas. Although a normal component of "self," GAD sometimes provokes the "non-self" reactions of the immune system. This was first observed in the autoimmune disease known as "stiff-man syndrome," a rare disorder in which the nerves signal muscles to tighten, producing painful spasms. It was observed that Type I diabetes is common in people with "stiff-man syndrome," suggesting the link that was later observed. Apparently the "non-self" reactions to GAD can cascade and engulf the beta cells of the pancreas, producing diabetes. GAD is not necessarily the start of the process or even the main actor, so there are plenty of roles left for genes, viruses, and milk. For example, the Coxsackie virus also has a region resembling a region in GAD.

In specially bred mice, injection with GAD can prevent the development of a disease similar to Type I diabetes in humans. This suggests that this line of research may lead to a way to prevent Type I diabetes in humans by similar methods.

By 1991, some researchers claimed that they had located the gene for one family's hereditary Type II diabetes on the long arm of chromosome 20, though the actual gene had not been spotted. Other researchers in the early 1990s found mutations of the genes for insulin, for the insulin receptor, and for a transfer-RNA in small groups of diabetics.

In 1992 a group of French researchers found that in 16 French families whose members experience Type II diabetes at an unusually young age, a gene on chromosome 7 was the common link. The following year Simon Pilkis of the State University of New York at Stony Brook reported that he and coworkers had found 23 different mutations in that gene, which is for an enzyme known as glucokinase, any one of which could initiate type II diabetes. Glucokinase starts the reaction that causes the pancreas to secrete insulin. If even one gene in the pair of glucokinase is defective, the patients in the study developed Type II diabetes as adolescents; this is much earlier than the normal pattern for Type II, which typically starts in middle age.

But three 1991 studies showed that middle-aged men, middle-aged nurses, and physicians who exercise regularly cut their risk of Type II diabetes in half, Thus genes cannot be the whole story. Another link was forged at the start of 1993 when a report in *Science* showed that obese rats overproduce a hormone that in turn depresses the output of the gene for the protein glut4. The function of glut4 is to combine forces with insulin to get glucose out of the blood and into cells by passing it through cell membranes. One form of Type II diabetes features an inability of insulin to accomplish the task of getting glucose into cells. Thus for mice at least, the connection between obesity, genes, and Type II diabetes became clearer. A month later, an Australian study linked dietary fat to insulin resistance in humans as well.

Late in 1993 Christine Reynet and C. Ronald Kahn of Harvard Medical Center in Boston, Massachusetts, announced that they had discovered that a member of the Ras family of proteins (*see also* "Molecular Biology Against Cancer," p 419) is over-expressed in the voluntary muscles of people with Type II diabetes. This suggests that the genetic component of this disease might be related to the protein, which they christened Rad (for Ras associated with diabetes).

Results of the Diabetes Control and Complications Trial

The *Harvard Health Letter,* a relatively conservative newsletter on advances in health, is aimed primarily at interested members of the nonmedical public. It relies a lot on the faculty at Harvard Medical School to help make its choices of topics to treat and to aid in tough calls on recommendations for healthful living or medical treatment. Each year the faculty advisors pick the top ten health advances for the past year. In 1993 the advisors chose for number one a treatment that is not especially new and that evidence suggests is being ignored by the people who could most benefit from it. The treatment is variously termed "intensive," "closely monitored," or just plain "tight" control of diabetes.

Intensive care for diabetes means monitoring blood glucose levels several times as day with a sensitive blood test (not just once a day with a urine indicator), adjusting insulin dosage to fit the levels, and injecting proper amounts of insulin four to seven times a day to keep the glucose level at optimum levels all the time.

Although this method of treatment goes back to the invention of home blood monitors in the late 1970s, it was not clear in 1983 whether or not all the trouble was worth it. Furthermore, the tight monitoring could cause problems by too fine an adjustment, often resulting in low blood sugar with attendant temporary loss of mental faculties. About half again as many cases of severe hypoglycemia requiring hospitalization occur with tight controls as do with conventional care.

Nevertheless, animal studies and anecdotal evidence suggested that tight control could prevent the complications of diabetes, complications that may result in three times as many deaths as diabetes itself causes directly and that additionally include several harmful conditions that are not life threatening.

The National Institute of Diabetes and Digestive and Kidney Diseases mounted a large-scale study of intensive care that began in 1983, called the Diabetes Control and Complications Trial. Almost 1500 persons (1441) with Type I diabetes agreed to be assigned randomly to either an intensive or a conventional care group. The average age of the subjects was 27 and none had complications from the disease when the trial began.

After almost ten years—but a year before the study was scheduled to end—the doctors, led by David M. Nathan of Massachusetts General Hospital in Boston, stopped the test and offered intensive care to everyone. The evidence was clear and direct: some of the worst complications of diabetes were greatly reduced in the intensive care group. The study showed that the complications were a direct result of glucose levels—the control group on conventional therapy had blood glucose levels nearly half again as high as the group in tight care.

Eye disease: Among those with no eye disease when they entered the study, the risk was 76 percent less of developing it in the tight care group. Even in those who already had the beginning of eye disease, the progression to greater severity was much faster among those receiving conventional therapy.

Kidney disease: Kidney disease with clinical effects often takes a long time to develop but damage to the kidneys can be detected much earlier from levels of certain chemicals in the blood. Based on these markers, damage to kidneys was reduced by 40 to 50 percent as a result of tight care.

Nerve disease: Painful or numbing nerve ailments were found in about 60 percent fewer patients using intensive treatment.

As a result of the success of the trials, they were stopped early in June 1993 and all the patients in the study moved into intensive care. Results of the study were published in the September 30, 1993 *New England Journal of Medicine.*

Manufacturers of devices and chemicals used in tight control all felt that the report on Type I diabetes would send sales of their products booming. But despite the great improvement in preventing deadly or undesirable complications, patients with diabetes did not rush to embrace tight controls. Children under 13 cannot manage the disease for themselves, and some older persons are too ill or too prone to hypoglycemia to take up intensive control of glucose levels. Cost can be off-putting as well, since the tight controls typically cost more than twice as much for monitoring and physician's visits.

No tests of tight control have yet been run on Type II patients, who constitute the large majority of people with the diabetes. Doctors conducting the Diabetes Control and Complications Trial believe that the results also apply to Type II, however, since the complications are similar.

Various groups have been trying for a decade to develop an "artificial pancreas," an implantable device that would produce insulin in relation to glucose needs. When developed, this would eliminate the need for careful monitoring. The first devices were only able to handle the needs of diabetic mice, but by 1993 versions were available that could be successfully implanted in diabetic dogs. The key to these devices is to use natural islets of Langerhans, the site of the beta cells that produce insulin in the pancreas. One group used islets from pigs in the device for dogs, protecting the islets from the immune system with a semipermeable membrane. The immune-suppressing drug cyclosporine is also used.

Human trials are under way using islets from humans, but the patients getting the implants still need cyclosporine. Therefore, the first trials are being conducted on people who already take cyclosporine for other reasons—essentially because they have had kidney transplants. These will be Phase 1 safety trials, with several years to go before Phase 2 effectiveness trials.

Other Advances

Other research on diabetes has been aimed at improving insulin delivery in more conventional ways, alleviating complications of diabetes, and preventing the disease from developing in the first place.

Insulin in use today, whether more traditional insulin from animal sources or human insulin produced by genetic engineering, has to be injected, not taken as a pill. Insulin is a protein and is digested when taken orally, converted into its amino acids. Injection is one of the main burdens of the diabetic who is keeping the condition under control. For decades, one alternative to injection that has been explored is administering insulin as a nasal spray, so that it could pass through thin membranes directly into the bloodstream without injection. Danish scientists announced in 1991 that they thought they had solved problems in dosage, transport across membranes, and irritation of nasal passages, and were beginning large-scale trials of their spray.

Scientists at the Weismann Institute of Science in Israel developed a sort of vaccine for Type I diabetes in mice. The part of the immune system that destroys beta cells in the pancreas is mainly the T cells. The Israeli group used an approach not unlike the one successfully developed by Pasteur as his first vaccine. They removed T cells from the mice, taking care to obtain the type that can attack beta cells. Then the scientists weakened the T cells *in vitro*. When the T cells were reinjected into the mice, the

Background

Diabetes mellitus ("sugar diabetes") is what the word *diabetes* by itself means to most people. The other diabetes, diabetes insipidus, is a different disease entirely. What they have in common is that both diseases are disorders caused by defects in manufacture or delivery of a hormone insulin for mellitus, antidiuretic hormone for insipidus. Among the symptoms of each is excessive urination; the word *diabetes* comes from Latin and Greek words for "passing" as in "passing water"; *mellitus* means "honey-sweet," used because glucose is in the urine; *insipidus* means "tasteless." For diabetes insipidus, the urine production is almost all there is to the disease, although it can have several causes, some of which can be serious in themselves.

As with many other chronic disorders, "diabetes" is more of a collection of symptoms than an actual disease. For example, persons with measles may show different symptoms, but they all suffer from a disease caused by the invasion of a recognizable organism. When the organism is routed and effectively disappears from the body, the measles disease is also gone. There is no such neat cause and effect in diabetes.

First of all, there are two main varieties of diabetes mellitus. In what is now called Type I diabetes, the body fails completely or nearly so to produce the hormone insulin. Insulin has many actions throughout the body, mostly connected to metabolism and particularly associated with utilization of glucose, the main circulating energy source for cells. In general, the failure in insulin-production for Type I diabetics comes from the immune system attacking the insulin-producing cells in the pancreas.

In Type II diabetes the mechanism is entirely different. Cells throughout the body for one reason or another lose some or most of their ability to use insulin, or the body just needs more insulin than a normal pancreas produces for some other reason. One suggestion is that Type II diabetes is more a disease resulting in free fatty acids in the blood than it is initially of insulin and glucose metabolism.

For Type I diabetes there is no effective treatment except injection of insulin to make up for the lack of production. Type II diabetes can be controlled in some cases with diet and exercise, but more severe cases may require oral medication. In many cases, Type II diabetes is also treated with insulin injections, providing the body with so much insulin that even poor uptake by cells will capture enough of it.

Some diabetes appears to be inherited, partly at least. Some diabetes is a secondary result of recognizable diseases of the hormone system. An infection may trigger the immune reaction of Type I diabetes. Overweight and over-eating combined can require too much insulin from the pancreas.

Diabetes mellitus is officially the seventh leading cause of death in the U.S. (after heart disease, cancer, strokes, accidents, emphysema, and infectious lung disease), but for the purpose of national mortality statistics, every death is attributed to one underlying condition. The immediate cause of death may be removed from the ultimate cause; a heart attack that causes an automobile accident that kills the driver of the other car results in one more accidental death, not one more death from heart disease. Almost no one dies of AIDS; people with compromised immune systems are killed most often by infectious disease or by cancer. Similarly, more people are killed as a result of complication of diabetes than the about 50,000 whose deaths are directly attributed to the disease in the official statistics. An informed calculation used in the *Harvard Health Letter* is that 160,000 persons in the U.S. die as a result of diabetes each year, making it the fourth leading cause of death instead of the seventh.

Death from diabetes may come in many ways. Among the most direct is coma from one source or another. Unable to utilize glucose because of a lack of insulin, a person with type I diabetes may go directly to fat for energy, which can cause the person to lose consciousness and perhaps to die. More likely as a cause of death is kidney disease, which strikes 35 to 45 percent of persons with Type I diabetes and 20 percent of those with Type II. For unknown reasons, people with either form of diabetes, but especially those with Type II, are more likely than most people to die from heart attacks or strokes.

Other complications of diabetes are less frequently fatal, but most people with Type I diabetes who live long enough become blind. A combination of loss of feeling (or unexplained pain) in the peripheral nerves with poor blood circulation often results in damage to tissues that leads to amputation of limbs. Treatment of diabetes can lead to hypoglycemia, or low blood sugar, which can produce confusion or a different kind of coma from the previously described *diabetic coma* caused by burning fat instead of glucose.

cells were no longer recognized by the immune system and were attacked. Other T cells of the same type were also attacked. With that population of T cells removed, the mice could not develop Type I diabetes.

Some work has been done in relieving diabetes with transplants of fetal pancreatic tissue (*see* "Cell Transplantation: Fetal Tissue and More," p 511).

In the early 1990s, because of the recognition that Type I diabetes is an autoimmune disease, experiments in injecting small amounts of insulin into children who were at high risk for diabetes were conducted. It is believed that these injections delayed the development of diabetes and in some cases may have prevented the disease from developing. The concept behind this treatment is about the same as the one used by many allergy specialists to induce tolerance to specific foods or other substances.

Of the many complications of diabetes, one of the ones that is most life-threatening is kidney failure. Half of the people with Type I diabetes eventually develop kidney failure by the time they are in their 30s or early 40s. Kidney failure also develops eventually in Type II diabetes, but the patients are typically much older and many die of other complications first. As a result of both forms of diabetes, however, a third of all 200,000 Americans with kidney failure are diabetics.

Experiments with mice in the late 1980s suggested that kidney failure could be avoided through use of a drug called an ACE inhibitor, specifically captopril (trade-named Capoten) which has been used to treat high blood pressure since 1970 (*see* "High Blood Pressure UPDATE," p 407). A three-year double-blind study with 409 humans with Type I diabetes demonstrated in 1993 that use of captopril reduced risk of kidney disease by 50 percent. Reduction of high blood pressure had not caused this improvement, as even the placebo-using controls had their blood-pressure stabilized with other drugs if necessary. While some physicians are waiting for further tests, others have immediately begun prescribing captopril to their diabetic patients.

(Periodical References and Additional Reading: *New York Times* 2-5-91; *New York Times* 2-15-91, p A17; *New York Times* 7-18-91; *Harvard Health Letter* 3-92, p 4; *Nature* 3-12-92, p 162; *Nature* 6-4-92, p 362; *New York Times* 7-30-92, pp A10 & A12; *Science* 10-30-92, p 766; *Harvard Health Letter* 11-92, p 6; *Science* 1-1-93, p 87; *Science News* 1-2-93, p 7; *Science News* 1-30-93, p 68; *New York Times* 3-1-93, p A13; *Scientific American* 6-93, p 18; *New York Times* 6-14-93, p A1; *New York Times* 6-15-93, p D4; *Science News* 6-19-93, p 388; *Scientific American* 9-93, p 107; *Nature* 11-4-93, pp 15, 69, & 72; *New York Times* 11-4-93, p A15; *Science News* 11-6-93, p 292; *New York Times* 11-11-93, p A1; 11-26-93, p 1441; *Harvard Health Letter* 1-94, p 4; *Harvard Health Letter* 3-94, p 1)

MULTIPLE SCLEROSIS

Multiple sclerosis, or MS, affects about 2.6 million people worldwide. Since 1982 it has been well established that MS is an autoimmune disease. For reasons unknown, a person's immune system begins to attack the myelin sheaths that cover and insulate many nerve cells. The attack replaces the sheaths with scar tissue, which impedes any messages transmitted by the nerve cells. These cells, called neurons, no longer function properly, whether they are in the brain or give instructions to muscles. Consequently, MS can have a wide range of symptoms that depend largely upon which nerve cells are affected.

Because the problem behind the symptoms is an attack on the neurons by cells of the immune system, recent attempts to treat the disease have involved attempts to suppress the immune system. Total suppression is not desirable, however. Most of the immune system is still needed for its regular purpose of fending off undesirables. The goal is to suppress just enough or to suppress just the very specific cells of the system that are causing the problem. It is agreed that these cells are T cells, but whether they are just a few specific T cells or a wide class of them is not a subject on which experts agree.

Treatment

In theory, a way of blocking a specific immune reaction could be based on the mechanism which to some degree protects the body from immune reactions caused by certain foods. Although some people have some specific reactions to foods, such as hives from undercooked shrimp, nearly all foreign proteins are tolerated by the digestive system. It seems that ingestion of a protein produces some kind of immune tolerance.

In 1993 this concept of oral tolerization was tried as a treatment for MS (and some other diseases as well; *see* "Inflammation and Arthritis," p 435 and "Autoimmune UPDATE," p 447) with uncertain results. Previous experiments with animals who had autoimmune diseases, including an animal model for MS, showed improvement. The study on humans involved 30 persons all with early-stage MS. Half were fed myelin obtained from cattle brains, purified, and screened for bacteria and viruses. The other half got a placebo of dried milk.

Although fewer of the experimental patients had major attacks than the controls did, any result in such a small sample could be the result of pure chance—the course

MS MYSTERIES

Multiple sclerosis offers many clues regarding its origins, but no definite answers.

- Three out of five persons with MS are female.
- Women respond differently to treatment than men do.
- A high proportion of people with MS have lived in a warm climate during adolescence.
- If one of two identical twins has MS, the chances are between one in five and one in three that the other has it also. This fact might point to genetic basis, but that does not seem to be quite the case.
- Five studies that have tried to identify the T-cell receptor associated with MS have located five different receptors.
- In some patients, the disease ebbs and flows for a quarter of a century, and most of these patients die from other causes.
- In some patients, the disease progresses rapidly and causes death within a year.
- Almost no one gets multiple sclerosis past the age of 60.
- At one time or another about 130 different remedies have been proposed for MS, but have failed more careful tests. A current folk favorite, bee venom, has not yet been tested in controlled studies, however.

of MS is so unpredictable. Furthermore, and somewhat mysteriously, none of the women in the study seemed to be helped at all by eating bovine myelin. This is particularly troubling since three out of five MS patients are women. Not only did the men who ate myelin have fewer attacks than the controls, but also they showed reductions in the number of immune-system cells that attacked myelin *in vitro*. Since no harmful side effects were observed, the study is now expected to be repeated with a larger sample.

The investigators were Howard L. Weiner, Glenn A. Mackin, Makoto Matsui, Samia J. Khoury, David M. Sawson, and David A. Hafler of Brigham and Women's Hospital in Boston and E. John Orvav of the Harvard School of Public Health, and the report of their study was in the February 26, 1993, issue of *Science*.

Much bigger news regarding MS was made the following month when a new genetically engineered MS-treatment drug was recommended for approval by a panel advising the U.S. Food and Drug Administration (FDA). After the FDA approved the drug, tradenamed Betaseron, in July 1993, however, it became apparent that production of the drug did not match the demand. Consequently, a lottery was organized to determine who would get the drug. Four out of five persons who wanted Betaseron were unable to obtain the drug when it went on the market in October 1993. About 100,000 persons in the U.S. have the form of MS for which Betaseron is recommended. The manufacturer estimated that there would not be enough Betaseron to treat everyone who wants it until 1996.

Betaseron is a genetically engineered version of beta interferon, one of a class of immune-system chemicals that were first recognized for their virus-fighting ability, but which are now known to have varied functions (*see* "Allergies and Asthma," p 431). Beta interferon has two functions that make it useful in treating MS. It calls forth the production of additional suppressor T cells, cells that tend to dampen the attack of the immune system on foreign tissues by reducing the quantity of antibodies produced.

And beta interferon inhibits the production of gamma interferon by T cells. Although once gamma interferon was used as a treatment for MS, when the patients became worse instead of better, the true role of gamma interferon in calling forth T cells and activating phagocytes was discovered.

Thus, the combined actions of beta interferon are good for people with MS whose nerve-cell coverings are being destroyed by the antibodies and by the attack cells called forth by gamma interferon. Destruction of myelin in MS begins when a T cell that is sensitized to a specific antigen in the sheath encounters the antigen, which has been picked up by a macrophage and is being presented on the cell surface of the macrophage. The T cell reacts by releasing a barrage of cytokines, including tumor necrosis factor (which kills cells) and gamma interferon, which summons more T cells to the vicinity. The gamma interferon stimulates macrophages as well; in response to gamma interferon, the macrophages attack by releasing more tumor necrosis factor and also by directly consuming the dead cells. In the brain, cells called glial cells can also initiate the process by presenting the antigen to a T cell.

In the principal test of Betaseron, the number of severe attacks among people with the intermittent, or "relapsing, remitting," MS was cut by a third with injections of Betaseron. Furthermore, damage to the brain, which increased nearly 20 percent for the controls, *decreased* over four percent among the persons receiving beta interferon. Like all interferons, Betaseron tends also to produce flu-like symptoms and inflammation as side effects, but these are easily tolerated.

Although Betaseron provides somewhat more than symptomatic relief, it is nevertheless not a cure for MS. A company called Neurocrine Biosciences has what it hopes will be a cure, although phase 1 safety tests are not to begin on its drug until the end of 1994. In fact, the drug does not even have a publicly announced name yet. The Neurocrine drug is a short chain of amino acids that blocks the action of T cells that attack myelin, and that ignores the rest of the immune system. Because it is a short chain, or peptide, the drug can be manufactured by chemical processes instead of the genetic engineering that produces Betaseron. Thus, if actually effective, the Neurocrine drug should be neither as scarce nor as expensive as Betaseron.

There are also genetically engineered antibodies that have also been designed to block the action of T cells. While this approach seems successful in lowering the level of MS symptoms, it also drastically reduces the number of cytotoxic cells, which also happens in AIDS.

(Periodical References and Additional Reading: *New York Times* 10-17-91, p A23; *Science* 2-26-93, pp 1263, 1321; *New York Times* 3-2-93, p C11; *New York Times* 3-20-93, p 1; *Scientific American* 5-93, p 128; *Nature* 7-15-93, pp 187 & 243; *New York Times* 7-24-93, p I-7; *New York Times* 9-8-93, p C12; *New York Times* 9-2-93, p A15; *Harvard Health Letter* 3-94, p 1)

Autoimmune UPDATE

In the 1950s the word *autoimmunity* meant something entirely different from its meaning today; at that time, it designated immunity acquired without apparent exposure to an antigen. The advent of organ transplantation, when rejection of foreign tissue became an immediate issue, made physicians and researchers realize that the immune system could attack more than just viruses, bacteria, and parasites. The theoretical basis for understanding transplant rejection was Peter Medawar's 1949 definition of "self" and "nonself" and his explanation how the body learns to distinguish between the two. During the 1960s, researchers led by Jean Dausset of the University of Paris discovered histocompatibility regions of white blood cells, which directly determine the self-nonself distinction. By the late 1960s *autoimmune* had come to be an adjective describing conditions in which the immune system mistakes parts of self for nonself and consequently mounts an attack. Systemic lupus erythematosus (SLE) and rheumatoid arthritis were among the early diseases identified with the new concept of autoimmunity. At a major conference on rheumatoid arthritis in 1967, a few investigators noted that the chemicals attacking the lining of joints in rheumatoid arthritis seemed to be similar to antibodies, for instance. By then the concept of autoimmune disease was gradually becoming a part of mainstream thinking.

Today it is believed that about one adult in 20 suffers from an autoimmune disease, at least in industrialized nations where parasites other than viruses and bacteria are minor problems. The reason for noting the absence of significant parasite infestations is that the same mechanisms that attack parasites are implicated in autoimmune diseases. When all known autoimmune diseases are considered, about twice as many women as men are affected, probably because estrogen enhances immune system production of the cytokine gamma interferon, which promotes immune system activity of the type associated with autoimmune diseases. For some diseases, notably SLE, the ratio of women to men affected is especially high.

Causes of Autoimmunity

It is not quite clear what causes autoimmune diseases. It is easy to show, for example, that the autoimmune disease myasthenia gravis occurs because antibodies begin to attack a key neurotransmitter receptor used by nerves to direct the activity of muscles. In this case, it is known that the thymus, where most T cells "learn" their immune-system roles, is involved in misdirecting a population of T cells to attack the acetylcholine receptor. If a person with myasthenia gravis is young enough, removal of the thymus may stop the disease (at a small risk to the immune system as a whole). But the missing link for myasthenia gravis and for all autoimmune diseases is what starts the process on the wrong path.

Viruses appear to have a role in initiating the immune error, perhaps because they have evolved to do so to evade immune attack. Thus, a virus that resembles antigenically the tissues of the human body may be better equipped to escape the human immune system. One known example is the virus known as adenovirus 2, one of the many common cold viruses. Adenovirus 2 has amino acid sequences that are remarkably like those of proteins in the myelin sheaths that cover nerves. Thus, it may be no coincidence that those sheaths are sometimes attacked by the immune system, producing the autoimmune disease multiple sclerosis.

Some bacteria may also have evolved to resemble the amino-acid sequences of human proteins. The damage to the heart caused by rheumatic fever is thought to result from an autoimmune attack promoted by the immune system's fight against strep bacteria, an attack in which "friendly fire" hits the myosin (the most common protein in muscle) of the heart.

Some persons are genetically more susceptible to a specific autoimmune attack than others, although this statement can increasingly be made for all sorts of diseases. The key to genetic susceptibility is in the type of human lymphocyte antigen (HLA) inherited. The HLA is a molecule presented on the surface of a cell that tells the immune system that the cell is self and not nonself. There are many different HLA types inherited—comparison of these types is the essence of tissue typing for organ transplants. One type of HLA is associated with rheumatoid arthritis, a different one with multiple sclerosis, and two different types with Type I diabetes. Conversely, some HLA types are associated with low incidence of a particular disease; for example in Japan, where the common HLA type is not liable to Type I diabetes, the disease occurs at a rate about 5 percent of the rate in the U.S.

Stress probably does not initiate autoimmune reactions, but it may partly account for the episodic incidence of many. Stress probably prompts the hypothalamus and pituitary gland to release hormones that promote inflammation, a useful response in many traumatic situations but damaging in the case of autoimmunity. Nerves themselves may also release neurotransmitters that add to the problem. Chemicals released by nerves during anxiety are thought to be a factor in psoriasis, a disease primarily of the skin in which cells proliferate and often become inflamed (it may also attack joints). Consequently, anxiety can worsen psoriasis. Similarly, anxiety has been linked to release of a hormone-like substance called corticotropin-releasing factor, which in turn has been shown to be present in excess in tissues affected by rheumatoid arthritis.

Systemic Lupus Erythematosus

Perhaps the archetypical autoimmune disease is systemic lupus erythematosus, usually known as SLE, or lupus. In this disease the immune system begins to manufacture antibodies aimed at various organs throughout the body, not just one specific tissue, such as the myelin sheath tissue attacked in multiple sclerosis. The pervasiveness of the attack in SLE is explained by the fact that the antibodies are components of the cell nuclei, including DNA. Almost all autoimmune diseases are more common in women than in men, but lupus attacks nine women for every man. No one knows what causes SLE, but the usual suspects include genetic predisposition and viral triggers. Some drugs or other chemicals seem to produce symptoms of lupus during exposure, but symptoms disappear after exposure ceases. Nevertheless, no one has been able to demonstrate that SLE is simply an allergic reaction.

The name "lupus," which means "wolf" in Latin, comes from the "sign of the wolf," a butterfly-shaped red rash on the bridge of the nose and upper cheeks, one of the most common symptoms of the disease. In its most serious form, the disease can affect almost every organ in the body.

Blood Both red and white blood cells, and even the small cell-like platelets, can be attacked by antibodies. Lowered platelet counts can lead to internal bleeding. Blood vessels can be blocked by inflammation and by damaged cells.

Brain About three-quarters of people with SLE have some cognitive problems, ranging from headaches to psychosis, although most impairments are mild and temporary. Depression and anxiety may be symptoms of lupus but more likely are emotional responses to a devastating disease.

Eyes Also subject to various types of damage.

Heart Pericarditis, or inflammation of the membrane around the heart, occurs in one-fourth of all patients, and rhythm disturbances in two-fifths. Treatment of SLE can also cause coronary artery disease for unknown reasons.

Kidneys Clogging and inflammation of the kidneys is among the most serious problems, and occurs in about half of the cases. The condition is caused by complexes of antibodies and antigens, which are carried to the kidneys in the blood and become trapped in the small passageways of the kidneys. This can lead to kidney failure in about one person in 20.

Lungs Inflammation of the membrane surrounding the lungs, or pleurisy, is common, as is difficulty in breathing caused by muscle damage in the rib cage.

Mouth Ulcers are common.

SLE is difficult to diagnose because it mimics so many other diseases. The best indication is antibodies to DNA, but only three-quarters of the persons thought to have the disease show such antibodies. Other antibody tests can also be used, although they are even less reliable. Possibly, as is often the case, SLE is really a collection of varied autoimmune diseases. On the other hand, research in the 1990s suggests that mice with a similar disease have a genetic defect that causes T cells and B cells to avoid programmed self-destruction, which results in a proliferation of older immune-system cells.

In the past, treatment of SLE has consisted of high doses of steroids to relieve inflammation, but more recently physicians have felt that the cost in side effects is too high. Physicians use small amounts of steroids to prevent acute damage; they do not use steroids just to relieve painful symptoms. The rest of the time such anti-inflammatory agents as aspirin and ibuprofen are used. Very serious attacks, especially on the kidneys, can be halted with immune-system suppressing drugs. This combination approach has stretched the lifetime of most SLE patients by years, even decades.

More on Oral Tolerization

Several different experiments in treating serious autoimmune disease have been based on a principle that seems to be as old as the practice of medicine: if a disease is troubling you, a bit more of the same thing might cure you, as the hangover victim reasons to justify a drink the following morning. With diseases that affect the immune system, this "hair-of-the-dog" approach is often effective, for reasons that are not entirely clear. Thus, some people with allergies are helped or even cured when the allergies are challenged by large doses of the allergen.

According to one theory, these challenges work because of oral tolerization. Foods almost always contain foreign proteins, but people and other animals eat most foods without an allergic reaction. Therefore, the body must be taking steps to suppress the immune reaction to certain proteins that enter the body through the digestive system. Thus, when a person ingests a protein that should cause an immune reaction, a mechanism mysteriously reduces or blocks the reaction.

Howard Weiner of the Harvard Medical School and the School of Public Health in Cambridge, Massachusetts, experimented with feeding animals antigens in the 1980s and was encouraged by his findings. His animal studies led to the creation of the commercial company, Auto-Immune of Lexington, Massachusetts. By 1993 Auto-Immune and several research institutions had begun to report on experiments with human beings. The goals of these experiments, however, were not to remove ordinary allergies, but to stop autoimmune diseases in their tracks.

In any autoimmune disease, a person's immune system produces antibodies against the organism's own proteins that are necessary for important functions. The protein that stimulates the immune system is an antigen that is essentially identical to an internal allergen. Thus, a technique known somewhat informally as "antigen feeding" and more formally as "oral tolerization" consists of feeding a person suffering from an autoimmune disease quantities of the antigen, or something very similar to it, in hopes that the immune system will use its own mechanisms to block a particular antibody.

Several diseases have been thus treated, so far with mixed results (*See* "Inflammation and Arthritis," p 435 and "Multiple Sclerosis," p 444). The treatment is difficult to evaluate, partly because most autoimmune diseases go into periods of remission from time to time for reasons that are poorly understood. Thus, for example, if (A) a multiple sclerosis patient consumes myelin from cattle to prevent the patient's immune system from attacking myelin and (B) the patient's multiple sclerosis goes into remission, there is no sure way to say that A caused B.

Further trials of the technique, which should also be applied to other autoimmune diseases, such as uveitis, or eye inflammation, will ascertain whether this method is effective or not. If it works, it will be a major breakthrough, since the treatment is simple and easily tolerated by patients. Furthermore, oral tolerization may have an impact beyond autoimmune diseases, possibly preventing transplant rejection.

KNOWN OR SUSPECTED AUTOIMMUNE DISEASES

Disease	Organs Affected	Classification
Addison's disease	adrenal glands	known
Alzheimer's disease	brain	suspected
amyotrophic lateral sclerosis	spinal cord and motor nerves	hinted at
atherosclerosis	arteries	possible factor
autoimmune heolytic anemia	red-blood-cell membrane proteins	known
Chron's disease	lower intestine	known

Disease	Organs Affected	Classification
diabetes mellitus type I	beta cells in pancreas	known
Duchenne muscular dystrophy	muscles	possible factor
Goodpasture's syndrome	kidneys and lungs	known
Grave's disease	thyroid	known
Hashimoto's thyroiditis	thyroid	known
idiopathic thrombocytopenic purpura	blood platelets	known
infertility, spontaneous	sperm	known
irritable bowel syndrome	colon	possible
multiple sclerosis	brain and spinal cord	known
myasthenia gravis	synapses between nerves and muscles	known
phemphigius vulgaris	skin	known
pernicious anemia	gastric parietal cells	known
poststreptococcal glomerulonephritis	kidneys	known
psoriasis	skin and joints	known
rheumatoid arthritis	connective tissue and joints	known
scleroderma	skin, heart, lungs, intestines, and kidneys	known
Sjögren's syndrome	liver, kidneys, brain, thyroid, and salivary glands	known
systematic lupus erythematosus	DNA, platelets, other tissues	known
uveitis	eyes	suspected

(Periodical References and Additional Reading: *Science* 2-26-93, pp 1263, 1321; *Science* 12-24-93, pp 1669, 1727; *Harvard Health Letter* 3-94, p 1)

OTHER CHRONIC DISEASES

The Senses UPDATE

Some conditions that affect the senses are considered diseases, while others are thought of more often as "handicaps," a word that has largely disappeared from politically correct usage (except when referring to golf). Inability to see, for example, can come from various causes—several different diseases, conditions such as untreated cataracts, accident, injury to the brain from any cause, genetic or birth disorders, or even psychological conditions. It is convenient to lump most of these causes and the treatments for them into one article under the rubric "chronic diseases," even though some of the actual diseases of eyes are infectious and not chronic in any sense.

To a lesser degree, the same can be said for hearing as for vision. Hearing loss comes from many possible sources, and may result from damage to mechanical parts of the system, to transmission facilities in the inner ear, or from defects in the brain.

Because sight and hearing are the two main ways humans communicate with the world, damage to either of these senses is viewed as much more serious than damage the senses of smell, taste, and touch. Loss of the sense of smell, for example, is usually temporary or harmless, although it can indicate a brain tumor—so it is a good idea to have such a loss of a sense checked by a physician.

A few serious conditions, although not life-threatening, involve the less obvious senses. Loss of "the sense of balance" is one of the most common. In Meniere's disease (cause not clear) and labyrinthitis (caused by infection, usually by a virus), loss of balance can lead to extreme nausea and vomiting.

Sight

Some vision problems are considered in other articles in this book: *See* "Testing the Senses," p 124 and "Vitamin UPDATE," p 160.

Glaucoma   Glaucoma is discovered in thousands of people in the U.S. annually. If untreated, glaucoma can lead first to loss of peripheral vision and later to blindness. The immediate cause is poor drainage inside the eye, causing a pressure build-up that apparently damages the optic nerve. Recent treatment has consisted of using eye drops twice a day to lower the pressure or surgery to open drainage channels.

It is not known exactly why the drainage of fluids is blocked. In older people, who have a higher incidence of glaucoma, poor drainage results from changes in the aging body. In the early 1990s, investigation of a family in Illinois resulted in the discovery of a gene, on chromosome 1, for a form of glaucoma that strikes earlier in life. Thus, it could be said that glaucoma sometimes has a genetic cause. Finding the actual glaucoma gene and determining the protein it makes should make the hereditary situation clearer and may also suggest a new treatment for the disease.

In the meantime, at least one new treatment has proven quite successful in a very small human trial (and earlier in animal trials). Four men and a women with severe and

DIFFERENT WAYS OF SEEING

Focusing problems for the eyes are among the most common disorders—so common in fact that they are not thought to be much of a disadvantage for most purposes. Until recently the more formal names have been *myopia* for nearsightedness, which comes from the Greek word "myops," indicating the squinting of a nearsighted person, and *presbyopia* for farsightedness, a Greek derivation indicating an old person's eyesight. But while nearsightedness is still myopia, the alternative names for farsightedness, hyperopia ("too much eyesight") or hypermetropia ("over-measuring eyes"), seem today to be more appropriate than presbyopia. For one thing, almost as many young people become hyperopic as become myopic. Today the name *presbyopia* is generally restricted to farsightedness that develops after the age of 40 or so.

The main purpose of many of the mechanisms in the eye, and especially of the lens, is to focus light on the retina, which provides a direct line to the brain. It is now known that nearsightedness often can be detected in very young children. One possible reason is that small lenses tend to focus light more, missing the retina by forming the image somewhere within the eye. As these children grow older, such early myopia tends to disappear (although recent research suggests that it may return in adolescence). Most children, however, are born with hyperopia because of the overall small size of the eyeballs. A normal lens focuses behind the retina in a small eye. Unlike myopia, this farsightedness does not typically return when the children grow to be teenagers. Presbyopia develops much later, when the ability of the eye to focus is lost to a degree, so that the focus is behind the retina. This can happen to a person whose eyesight had been myopic before, although at some point vision may be fairly normal in the myopic turning presbyopic. More typically, myopics who develop presbyopia end up wearing trifocal glasses, with three different corrections.

About one in four Americans is myopic. Because a great many people develop presbyopia as they age, the total number of farsighted people at any given time is about the same as the total number of myopics.

---

sudden (acute) glaucoma were injected with a drug that is normally used to promote urination. In all five, pressure in the eye dropped to safe levels almost immediately, as was reported in the May 1992 *American Journal of Ophthalmology*. The hitch was that the injections of ethacrynic acid were made directly into the eye, which many people would find difficult to accept. Acute glaucoma may be accompanied by pain and considerable loss of vision, both starting suddenly, so those suffering from such an attack may feel more willing to receive eye injections than people with chronic glaucoma, who may have no noticeable symptoms except a gradual loss of peripheral vision.

Although glaucoma is a condition of *increased* pressure within the eye, the ophthalmologist Sohan Singh Hayreh of the University of Iowa in Iowa City has found a connection between glaucoma and *decreased* pressure in the blood during sleep. He recommends, consequently, that physicians avoid telling patients with high blood pressure as well as glaucoma to take pills for their condition at bedtime. Hayreh also finds that a stroke affecting the optic nerve is connected to low nighttime blood pressure.

Misshapen eyeballs The two common eye defects that are the occasion for wearing glasses or contact lenses are commonly called nearsightedness—meaning that it is difficult to focus on objects more than a foot or two away—and far-sightedness—meaning that objects some distance away are clearer than those near at hand. Recent research confirms what many have long suspected: myopia (nearsight-edness) has a strong genetic component. But other recent studies show that a popular belief long rejected by most physicians is actually correct: excessive reading early in life does contribute to myopia. Close observation, whether of toys or the printed page, for long periods each day may interfere with the poorly understood mechanism that coordinates the growth of the eyeballs with the muscular focus of the lenses. Experiments with chickens have suggested that presenting signals more strongly to the growing eye may improve such coordination. This hypothesis is now being tested on children by giving them stronger patterns when they learn to read.

Eyeglasses correct the focus for either nearsightedness or farsightedness. Contact lenses, applied directly to the surface of the eye, accomplish the same thing. But because of their direct application on the eyes, contact lenses that become dirty in any way can injure or infect the eyes. Various forms of contact lens have been developed—soft lenses, lenses for long wear, and so forth—to solve some of the problems of the lens touching the eye. In 1993 Johnson & Johnson began to test market the first completely disposable contact lenses—to be worn for one day and then thrown away. The maker says that its studies have shown that the new lenses are more comfortable and outperform other types in correcting vision. And it is easy to keep the lenses clean and sterile before inserting the lenses in the eyes.

Hearing

For the individuals involved and their families, handling deafness is one of the most controversial health issues. People who do not hear sounds often feel they have their own language and culture, and no real need for medical intervention that may result in limited hearing. People who do hear often think that everyone should be able to hear to the extent that is medically possible, even if hearing is distorted. A middle ground is hard to find.

This disagreement in many ways affects many parts of the life of deaf. In an effort to reach a solution, researchers have focused on electronic devices called cochlear implants.

Cochlear implants About one in five persons who receives such an implant becomes able to hear well enough to understand speech in person and over the telephone. The same ratio of one in five gets no benefit at all. This leaves 60 percent of implant recipients with some hearing but not enough for most purposes. Nearly always, however, it is enough to warn of the kinds of danger preceded by sound—a truck backing up, a horn being honked, an alarm going off. Parents often cite that ability and the somewhat safer life it promises as an argument for an implant in a child.

Background

Translation of sound waves, which begin as coordinated movements of molecules of air, into electrochemical nerve signals takes place in a spiral-shaped part of the inner ear called the cochlea (from the Latin for *snail* or *snail-shell*, because of its shape), which is lined with about 25,000 tiny hairs and filled with fluid. The hairs are often called *hair cells*. The motion of air molecules is mechanically transmitted to the liquid in the cochlea. Within the cochlea in hearing individuals the motion of the liquid affects the hairs, which then produce nerve signals that are perceived as sounds. For such a Rube Goldberg device, largely constructed by evolution out of the jawbones of reptiles, the sensitivity is remarkable. Most humans hear sounds from 20 to 20,000 cycles per second, a range of three orders of magnitude.

The first crude cochlear implants were built by William E. House in 1961. Since then about 8000 have been used in deaf persons. Implants receive sound with a battery-powered microphone attached like a hearing aid to the outer ear. The microphone turns sound into electrical impulses. One or more wires carry the electric signals through holes bored in the mastoid bone to the inner ear and the cochlea, where the electric signal directly stimulates nerve endings, bypassing the tiny hair cells that normally do the job. One or more electrodes are used, although there are 30,000 nerve endings in the cochlea. Research in 1993 showed that use of more than one channel for the electric signals improves ability to recognize some words to somewhat over 60 percent, or three out of five.

Since 1991 the U.S. Food and Drug Administration has permitted cochlear implants in children.

Biological fixes for hearing problems   Cochlear implants are most useful when the cause of deafness is a mechanical problem with the hair cells. Loud sounds, some antibiotics, and various illnesses can literally knock the hairs off the nerves, for example. Birds can generate new hair cells in their somewhat different ears, if some are lost, but until March 1993, it was thought that mammals had no such ability. Two reports in the March 12, 1993 *Science*, by Andrew Forge and co-workers from University College in London, England, and Mark E. Warchol and co-workers from the University of Virginia in Charlottesville demonstrated that guinea pigs can regenerate lost hair cells that were deliberately removed by antibiotics. The scientists also demonstrated that in the test tube the linings of human cochleas as well as those from guinea pigs could also regenerate hair cells. Six weeks later a Belgian group of scientists showed that retinoic acid, a vitamin A relative, could improve such regeneration. So far, similar experiments on humans are about a decade away, according to some researchers, but it is reasonable to expect good results.

Damage to hair cells is only one cause of deafness. Genes involved in hearing development can also be inherited in alleles that either fail to ensure proper development or that somehow initiate the process of hearing loss later in life. (Many people lose hearing as they age, predominantly due to loss or inactivation of hair cells from trauma.) In 1991 one hereditary cause of deafness was located in a gene mapped to chromosome 5. People with a dominant allele of this gene, which the subjects studied inherited from a mutation that took place in Costa Rica in the eighteenth century, become profoundly deaf by about the age of 30. It is hoped that knowledge of such genes and their products will provide yet another way to treat deafness.

Another way to hear   From time to time someone will claim that he or she can perceive images although he or she blindfolded—but these claims have usually been invalidated or rejected. However, in the July 5, 1991, issue of *Science* researchers reported a similar "second way of hearing" experienced during an attempt to save endangered sea turtles. Martin L. Lenhardt of the Medical College of Virginia found that he could hear the ultrasound signals being used in an attempt to keep the sea turtles from laying eggs on a beach where the eggs or hatchlings might be lost. Experiments back in the laboratory demonstrated to Lenhardt that he and his co-workers were all able to hear sounds and even distinguish words if a device producing the ultrasound signals was in direct contact with the skull. The effect did not seem to use the normal pathways of hearing, which in humans are not effective for such high pitches. Trials with profoundly deaf subjects demonstrated that they could also use ultrasound transmitted directly to the skull to hear, and in about half of the instances they could recognize words.

Scientists hope to develop a small transducer that would take normal speech and other sounds and raise the frequency. The ultrasound version of the normal sounds would be conveyed to the skull of a person who is unable to hear normal sounds because of an ineffective cochlea.

(Periodical References and Additional Reading: *New York Times* 9-5-91; *Science News* 10-19-91, p 253; *Science News* 1-30-93, p 69; *Science* 3-12-93, pp 1616, 1619; *New York Times* 3-23-93, p C6; *Science News* 5-8-93, p 302; *New York Times* 5-18-93, p C3: *Science News* 6-12-93, p 376; *New York Times* 6-16-93, p D4; *Scientific American* 7-93, p 26; *Scientific American* 8-93, p 14)

ALZHEIMER'S DISEASE

Despite evidence of many people who continue into old age with their mental faculties intact, popular and even medical myth has long associated aging with inevitable loss of memory and cognitive faculties. The word *senile,* which means "old," became a short way of saying senile dementia, defined as a deterioration of mind and emotion associated with aging.

Reporting, in 1906, on an investigation begun five years earlier, the German neurologist Alois Alzheimer described "premature" senile dementia, noting characteristic brain damage. Later pathologists found that many persons who had died with this condition, defined loosely as having the symptoms of senile dementia before the age of 65, also had similar characteristic physical defects in the brain. Thus, Alzheimer's disease was first associated with what we would now call "early-onset" Alzheimer's disease. In the nine decades since Alzheimer's work, it has become clear that the same brain defects also occur with considerable regularity among people over 65 (estimates range from one out of 20 to one out of ten in this age group, although in many of these instances the patients are considerably older than 65).

Alzheimer's disease was largely unknown to the general public before 1980. In the early 1980s, however, as the demographic profiles of the population, especially in industrial societies, started clearly reflecting the growing percentage of the elderly, the concept of Alzheimer's as a major disease gained currency. Realizing the likelihood of living well beyond the biblical "three score and ten," people started worrying about senile dementia. Articles reported to this concerned audience that most senile dementia could be accounted for by alcoholism, prescription drugs, clinical depression (see "Depression UPDATE," p 299), multiple small strokes, chronic syphilis, brain tumors, head injury, kidney disease, thyroid hormone deficiency, vitamin B_{12} deficiency, infection, or brain fluid accumulation—a list of theoretically correctable, relatively rare, or even self-imposed conditions. But it was recognized that even when all these problems were subtracted, a pool of ten to 20 percent of the instances of senile dementia still could not be explained. Therefore, these particular conditions were attributed to Alzheimer's disease. Brain autopsies eventually confirmed that the unexplained physical condition Alzheimer discovered among younger individuals was the true cause of most of the unexplained senile dementia.

Diagnosing Alzheimer's Disease

Because Alzheimer's disease can only be reliably diagnosed by a direct examination of brain tissue—a process too dangerous to undertake for a condition that cannot be

Background

Alzheimer's disease is diagnosed by two specific abnormalities that can be seen in a microscopic examination of brain tissue. Nerve endings are damaged and link together in what are called neuritic plaques. And within nerve cells, new structures appear that are called neurofibrillary tangles. Furthermore, some nerve cells in the base of the brain simply die. These cells are producers of the neurotransmitter acetylcholine (see "The Ubiquity of NO in Life," p 305). Furthermore, a normal brain protein called beta amyloid, which also was discovered in other parts of the body in 1992, accumulates and acts as if it were toxic, possibly because it has transmuted into a sort of infectious protein called a prion (see "Prions Revisited," p 339). Another defect identified is that potassium channels in the brain close up.

Because these changes are normally only observed in autopsies, the diagnosis of Alzheimer's is generally based on various clues. First, all other causes of apparent dementia are eliminated if possible. About one potential case in ten is removed by such screening and the underlying cause treated. The remaining nine individuals are diagnosed on the bases of persistent memory deficit; emotional instability, including both depression and agitation; and loss of attention span and orientation in relation to time, place, and self-identity.

Ultimately, the disease, as it progresses, causes brain deterioration, and death. The more severe the early symptoms, the faster the progression. Survival after diagnosis has been reported in studies as from two to 16 years. According to some statistics, Alzheimer's disease, believed to affect as many as two to four million Americans, is the fourth leading cause of death—although other accounts regard accidents or diabetes as the fourth leading cause. Some studies find 100,000 deaths annually from Alzheimer's in the U.S., which would put it ahead of accidental death, but still far behind diabetes.

effectively treated even after diagnosis—considerable effort has gone into finding a method of definitely recognizing the disease by some reliable chemical test, such as a blood test. In the absence of effective treatment methods, the main point of such clear-cut diagnosis would be to show that Alzheimer's is *not* the cause of dementia. Then a more extensive search could be conducted to find the actual cause, which might well be treatable.

One expensive option tried in 1992 was use of magnetic resonance imaging (MRI) to look into the brain without surgery. Advanced MRI facilities at Massachusetts General Hospital in Boston were thought to be correct 95 percent of the time.

In the December 15, 1992, issue of the *Proceedings of the National Academy of Sciences,* Boyd Haley and Debra Gunnersen of the University of Kentucky found that all of the patients later determined by brain examination to have had Alzheimer's disease also had unusually high levels of the enzyme glutamine synthetase, a protein that acts on glutamate and ammonia. Both glutamate and ammonia are toxic to brain cells in large amounts, but necessary in small amounts for proper brain functioning. Release of glutamate in high amounts is the cause of much of the damage in strokes. Only one patient in a control group without Alzheimer's disease had high levels of the glutamine synthetase.

Another test, announced by Daniel L. Alkon of the U.S. National Institute of Neurological Disorders and Stroke in the September 1, 1993, issue of the *Proceedings of the National Academy of Sciences,* was based on the closure of potassium channels in cell membranes as a result of Alzheimer's disease. Alkon also claims that potassium channels are part of the memory process. Alkon and coworkers reasoned that if such channels were closed in the brain, they might also be shut off in other tissues. Cultured skin cells can easily be tested for open or closed channels with an electrical probe and with a dye that fluoresces when the channels are open and fails to glow when they are closed. Blind tests on 50 skin samples were used to identify correctly the 20 patients whose Alzheimer's had been diagnosed by other means, and also to identify correctly the individuals without the disease or with other brain diseases. Still, Alkon claims only the ability to identify 70 percent of Alzheimer's patients by this method.

A simpler approach, although hardly definitive, has been to determine the sense of smell. Research has shown that among the very early symptoms of Alzheimer's is a loss of smell and a loss of the memory of smells. Once again, the potassium channels are involved.

Alzheimer's Genetics

Alzheimer's disease would be easier to diagnose and to treat if scientists could identify a single cause for the condition. During the early 1990s, there was a proliferation of hypotheses concerning a possible cause.

At the beginning of this period, most scientists believed that the protein beta amyloid by itself caused the disease. In 1991 a researcher even demonstrated that injecting beta amyloid into the brains of mice caused them to forget tasks they had learned. But in 1992 four different groups of scientists discovered that beta amyloid is a normal protein found throughout the body. So, beta amyloid by itself could not be the cause.

Few diseases in the 1990s lacked a genetic explanation of either cause or susceptibility. Alzheimer's is no exception. As early as 1987 James Gusella of Massachusetts General Hospital in Boston, famed for his work on Huntington's Disease (*see* "Three-base Repeats: Fragile X, Huntington's Disease, and More," p 50), theorized that Alzheimer's could be caused by a gene on chromosome 21. A clue for this etiology comes from Down's Syndrome, caused by an extra copy of chromosome 21, whose victims develop symptoms of Alzheimer's disease if they live long enough. Furthermore, the gene for the precursor protein to the beta amyloid implicated in Alzheimer's is on chromosome 21. Even though the protein is found in various parts of the body, there might be an allele that did not harm most cells but was poisonous to some brain cells. Actually, this has been shown to be the case for Huntington's disease. Thus, the assumption that Alzheimer's was linked to the gene for the amyloid precursor protein on chromosome 21 made sense.

It was therefore something of a surprise when a study of a family with early-onset Alzheimer's (conducted by Margaret A. Pericak-Vance of Duke University in Durham North Carolina) found that the cause was apparently a gene on chromosome 19. Soon, however, a different family was found with a defect in the amyloid precursor gene on chromosome 21, a defect that also led to early-onset Alzheimer's. Yet another group determined that a gene on chromosome 14 caused early-onset Alzheimer's. But other families were investigated, and those families developed early-onset Alzheimer's in the pattern of a hereditary disease, but did not have the defective alleles on chromosomes 14, 19, or 21. Thus, by early 1991, it was known that at least three or four different genes might be implicated in early-onset Alzheimer's disease.

In any case, all of the genes identified were for the early-onset version of Alzheimer's disease. Other chronic disorders, however, may have a well-defined genetic version that often strikes early and that is uncommon, whereas the common version has a different cause, often unknown. In 1993, researchers from Duke University—led by Allen D. Roses, and including Pericak-Vance, Ann M. Saunders, and others—located the gene that predisposes people for late-onset Alzheimer's in about four cases out of five. It is the ApoE4 version of the gene for the protein apolipoprotein E, the protein that aids cholesterol in traveling through the bloodstream from the liver to where it is needed. The same ApoE4 allele also predisposes people to heart disease, which was previously known, but it apparently predisposes carriers to Alzheimer's to an even greater degree. People with two copies of the ApoE4 gene have eight times the chance of developing Alzheimer's; in addition, the presence of two copies of the gene leads to an onset of the disease at a significantly lower the age.

Very few people in the general population have two copies of the ApoE4 gene, perhaps as many as one person out of three has a single copy of the gene, which may double or triple the risk of developing the disease and also leads to an early onset, though not as early as in a carrier of two copies.

Within a few months, 20 different studies had confirmed the statistical connection between ApoE4 and Alzheimer's. Before the end of 1993 there was even a theory about an actual link between ApoE4 and the disease, though the theory received scant support. Allen D. Roses and Warren Strittmatter, also of Duke, conducted *in vitro*

studies that showed that the most common allele of the gene for the protein apolipoprotein, which is known as ApoE3, and also another uncommon allele, ApoE2, bind to a protein in brain cells that Roses and Strittmatter named "tau." In binding to "tau," the ApoE3 and ApoE2 protect the cells from disruption. But ApoE4 fails to bind to the tau protein, so cells become disrupted and die. In this theory, amyloid has nothing to do with the cause of Alzheimer's, but is simply a side effect. But other studies continued to find beta amyloid as one of the principal factors in Alzheimer's, possibly linked with ApoE4 or perhaps with another gene on chromosome 19 that is close to the one for the ApoE series. Furthermore, many critics faulted Roses and Strittmatter for using very high concentrations of proteins in their test-tube experiments, much higher than are found in nature.

Further help in understanding a genetic basis for Alzheimer's may come if genetic engineering efforts to create a mouse that will develop the disease are successful. The amyloid precursor gene on chromosome 21 was first introduced into mice in 1993 by two different groups of researchers. So far none of the mice has developed Alzheimer's, but if current efforts fail, a different allele of the gene may work.

Neurotransmitters and Cytokines

The neurotransmitter acetylcholine has long been known to be at abnormally low levels in Alzheimer's disease. In the October 9, 1993, issue of *Science*, researchers from the Massachusetts Institute of Technology in Cambridge reported that low levels of acetylcholine actually promote the formation of neuritic plaque in the brain—one of the principal concomitants of Alzheimer's. However, the scientists engineered the process with genetically altered cells *in vitro*, without proving that the experiment replicated the actual process in the brain.

In *in vitro* experiments, researchers from the University of California—Los Angeles identified a nerve-cell messenger called nerve growth factor (NGF) that is needed to keep alive the particular brain cells that die during Alzheimer's disease. This nerve-cell messenger attaches itself to a protein called p75, which is an NGF receptor on the surface of cells. The scientists' results, published in the July 16, 1993, issue of *Science*, suggest that if a way could be found to raise the levels of NGF in the brain, cell death, the major concomitant of Alzheimer's disease, might be stopped. This is not easy to do, however, since NGF, being a protein that cannot pass the blood brain barrier, will have no effect if introduced into the bloodstream. Scientists in Sweden are currently testing the possibility of administering NGF directly to the brain through an opening in the skull.

The Aluminum Connection

In 1965 it was discovered that rabbits developed seizures and neurofibrillary tangles similar to those found in Alzheimer's when they were injected with aluminum salts. Kidney dialysis patients also developed dementia and neurofibrillary tangles if aluminum was used in the dialysis machine. When Alzheimer's studies became more widespread investigators looked for aluminum in the brains of people who had died from Alzheimer's, and they found it. Other studies also linked aluminum—a toxic metal (to a certain degree) that is nevertheless excreted easily—to Alzheimer's. For example, the disease seemed more prevalent in places with high levels of aluminum in the drinking water. Some people stopped using aluminum cookware.

By 1992, however, the aluminum connection seemed rather dubious. This connection was dealt another blow in the November 5, 1992, issue of *Nature,* when a new microscopic technique demonstrated that if there was any extra aluminum in the brain, it is not in the neuritic plaques. The jury is still out on the presence of aluminum in the neurofibrillary tangles.

Hormones and Alzheimer's

In the fall of 1993 Victor Henderson of the University of Southern California in Los Angeles announced that his analysis of the death records of 2418 post-menopausal women revealed a 40 percent decrease in the incidence of Alzheimer's disease among the women on estrogen-replacement therapy. An earlier and smaller analysis of 253 women over several years had uncovered the same result with about the same decline in Alzheimer's among the women on estrogen-replacement therapy. Because of the small number of women in the study who developed the syndrome, results of the study were not considered to establish a link between estrogen and protection against Alzheimer's, but Henderson is initiating a larger study in an effort to establish a link.

Although estrogen is thought of largely in connection with its roles in initiating pregnancy and in development of bone, the hormone has powerful effects throughout the body and is thought by some to be more active in the brain than anywhere else. Animal studies have shown that estrogen interacts with nerve growth factor and indirectly with the neurotransmitter acetylcholine. As a result, estrogen helps maintain the network of cell interconnections in the brain. Some evidence with humans also supports the idea that estrogen replacement can improve scores on memory tests of information processed by reading, one of the many forms of memory that degrades in Alzheimer's.

There is a lot of evidence suggesting that estrogen may provide protection from Alzheimer's. More postmenopausal women than men of the same age develop the disease, possibly because most men continue to produce testosterone into later years, and testosterone can be converted to estrogen in the brain as needed. Postmenopausal women who are very thin make the least amount of estrogen and are also more susceptible to Alzheimer's than counterparts with more body fat.

Other hormones were also linked to Alzheimer's in a 1993 study by Michael Meaney of McGill University in Montreal. He and his co-workers found that the stress hormones cortisol and the glucocorticoids are negatively correlated with scores on cognitive tests—that is, high levels of these hormones are associated with low scores. Older people with low levels of the hormones have scores that resemble those of considerably younger people. Meaney believes that the stress hormones have an adverse, and cumulative, effect on the hippocampus in the brain, a center for memory and thinking.

Treatment

Efforts to diagnose and understand Alzheimer's disease have been frustrating because it is so difficult to devise appropriate treatment. However, in 1986 scientists started testing a 50-year-old drug for Alzheimer's. The drug is called tacrine (TACK-rin, short for tetrahydroaminoacridine), and some studies in the late 1980s showed that it caused slight improvement in memory. Its action is to slow the breakdown of the neurotransmitter acetylcholine, which has been shown to be in short supply in the brains of people with Alzheimer's. Unfortunately, tacrine also caused liver damage in three out of four subjects of the studies.

When tacrine reached the U.S. Food and Drug Administration (FDA) panel on March 15, 1991, the drug was turned down after a long, stormy session. A week later the FDA proposed a method of expanding clinical tests by a procedure that allowed about 4000 patients to use the drug. After a year, however, the story was the same: the results of a controlled trial, announced in November 1992, showed insufficient memory improvement and too many side effects. Nevertheless, many researchers were impressed that a careful study had shown any memory improvement at all. As a matter of fact, British and European research had shown more benefits than the U.S. trials. Results of a second U.S. study, reported in January 1993, indicated that higher doses of tacrine caused further memory improvement. Meanwhile, careful monitoring of patients' liver enzymes during the first few weeks of treatment could be used to determine which patients should either stop taking the drug or switch to a lower dosage. Patients who only had nausea, vomiting, diarrhea, and rash could continue taking the drug if they so desired.

As a result of a more favorable perception of tacrine in the scientific community, a second FDA advisory panel recommended in March 1993 that the drug be marketed. Even so, it was not approved until September 1993, after which it began to be marketed under the tradename Cognex. It was expected to provide help in mild and moderate cases, but, based on the clinical trials, only about 12 percent of the patients taking the drug would be helped at all.

In 1993 there were at least 15 other drugs, some with actions similar to that of tacrine and some with different approaches, being tested against Alzheimer's. Some of these were already available treatments for other diseases, such as the calcium-channel blockers used to treat high blood pressure. One of the drugs with an action similar to tacrine is a Chinese tea brewed from the club moss *Huperzia serrata*, which the Chinese have drunk for years to bolster memory.

Meanwhile another treatment strategy has been developing separately. Tacrine and similar drugs are used to increase acetylcholine levels in Alzheimer's patients, which, scientists hope, would improve memory. A decrease in acetylcholine is thought to be a concomitant of cell death. A drug that would prevent cell death by increasing the level of acetylcholine would get at the root of the disease. In the late 1980s several lines of reasoning and a few clever retrospective studies suggested that Alzheimer's might be an autoimmune disease, like rheumatoid arthritis. Consequently, scientists theorized that, if in Alzheimer's the immune system killed inflamed cells, an anti-inflammatory drug might provide symptomatic relief, just as aspirin and steroids can be used to relieve arthritis. But steroids were out of the question, mainly because of their toxic effect on nerve cells, the very cells this therapy is trying to preserve.

The first small clinical test of this theory used a non-steroidal anti-inflammatory drug (NSAID) called indomethacin, which acts like aspirin and ibuprofen in regard to inflammation. The trial started with 44 patients, half on indomethacin and half on placebos. While gastrointestinal side effects of indomethacin reduced the experimental population to 14, untreated Alzheimer's disease over the six-month trial also reduced the number of controls by 20 percent. The controls had emotional problems with the test, their reactions probably triggered by their progressing illness. However, the 14 experimental patients were generally stable throughout the trial. A larger trial was also launched, and results should be available sometime in 1994.

(Periodical References and Additional Reading: *Harvard Health Letter* 10-90, p 1; *New York Times* 2-16-91, p 1; *New York Times* 4-16-91; *New York Times* 2-26-91, p C1; *New York Times* 3-17-91; *New York Times* 3-23-91; *Harvard Health Letter* 4-91, p 8; *Harvard Health Letter* 7-91, p 8; *Harvard Health Letter* 7-92, p 3; *New York Times* 9-24-92, p A26; *New York Times* 10-9-92, p A19; *Science* 10-9-92, p 304; *New York Times* 10-29-92, p A20; *Nature* 11-5-92, p 65; *New York Times* 11-10-92, p C2; *New York Times* 11-11-92, p D20; *New York Times* 12-15-92, p C3; *Harvard Health Letter* 2-93, p 1; *New York Times* 3-19-93, p A18; *Science News* 5-8-93, p 300; *Science* 6-18-93, p 1719; *Science* 7-16-93, p 345; *New York Times* 7-20-93, p C3; *New York Times* 8-13-93, p A1; *Science* 8-13-93, pp 828 & 921; *Science News* 8-14-93, p 108; *New York Times* 9-1-93, p A16; *Science News* 9-4-93, p 153; *New York Times* 9-10-93, p A19; *Science* 9-17-93, p 1520; *Scientific American* 11-93, p 28; *New York Times* 11-9-93, p C3; *Science* 11-19-93, p 1210; *Discover* 12-93, p 26; *New York Times* 3-9-94, p C3)

PARKINSON'S PROGRESS

Parkinson's disease is a mysterious ailment that mostly strikes older people, especially Europeans. In the U.S. there may be as many as one million persons with the disease. Furthermore, there is a whole set of Parkinson symptoms that are caused by known factors and that are often called *parkinsonism*. Parkinsonism results from brain damage of various sorts, including that caused by drugs, viral diseases, toxic chemicals, and boxing. Guam disease, which also resembles amyotrophic lateral sclerosis, has strong parkinsonian features; this mysterious ailment was discovered on the island of Guam in 1947 and since then seems to be gradually disappearing.

Although it is not clear what causes Parkinson's disease, it is known that loss of cells that manufacture the neurotransmitter dopamine produces most of the symptoms. One approach to treating the disease has been simply to replace those cells with cells from an aborted fetus (*see* "Cell Transplantation: Fetal Tissue and More," p 511) or with dopamine-producing cells from another source. This approach has been successful with people who have drug-induced parkinsonism, but only slightly so for Parkinson's disease patients. Researchers in the area of treatment are seeking a better source of dopamine-producing cells, such as genetically engineered skin cells (being developed at the University of California at San Diego). There are some researchers, however, who believe that the ineffectiveness of fetal-cell transplants on people suffering from the disease should not be attributed to the dopamine produced by the cells but to various known or unknown nerve growth factors that the cells also manufacture.

Background

A key discovery concerning Parkinson's disease occurred during 1982, when an underground drug manufacturer accidentally created a drug now known as MPTP. Addicts injected this drug thinking it was a cheap heroin substitute; instead it caused them to develop the symptoms of advanced Parkinson's disease. Researchers found that MPTP killed the cells in a part of the brain called the substantia nigra, a part that uses dopamine to communicate with other parts of the brain. Animal models for Parkinson's disease have been developed using MPTP to destroy that part of the brain.

The symptoms of parkinsonism begin when the dopamine supply is reduced in regions in the brain known as the caudate and putamen in the striatum. When these areas fail to get dopamine, from the substantia nigra or from another source, they start sending incorrect messages to muscles and other parts of the body.

Instead of replacing the dopamine-producing cells, some treatments replace just the dopamine. A version of L-dopa, re-engineered so it so can cross the blood-brain barrier and enter the brain, works because L-dopa is converted into dopamine in the brain. While this drug is almost always successful in reducing symptoms, its effectiveness quickly decreases. Consequently, physicians try to reduce symptoms with any other means as long as possible before turning to L-dopa. The most useful drug for this purpose since 1981 has been selegiline, which postpones the need for L-dopa and permits a lower L-dopa dosage when the two are used together. Selegiline is a monoamine oxidase inhibitor and stops the reaction that clears dopamine after use. But selegiline is very similar to powerful antipsychotic drugs and has many of the side effects of those drugs. The dopamine agonist bromocriptine accomplishes the same task of increasing dopamine levels by a different route. Other drugs developed for other purposes, including amantadine, an antiviral, have also reduced the need for beginning L-dopa treatment.

Recently, a new treatment possibility emerged, although it is a long way from reaching the public. Frank Collins and co-workers at Synergen in Boulder, Colorado, reported in the May 21, 1993, issue of *Science* that they had discovered a protein similar to a growth factor, which they call "glial line-derived neurothrophic factor," or GDNF. Genetically engineered GDNF *in vitro* maintains cultures of certain types of neurons for three weeks; without the factor, most of the neurons die over this length of time. The crucial part of this story for Parkinson's disease is the fact that, thus far, it is the dopamine-producing neurons which respond to GDNF. GDNF seems to have no effect on other neurons, although not every possible neuron had been tested when the report was issued. The bad news is the usual problem; proteins such as GDNF cannot cross the blood-brain barrier, so some way would be needed to get GDNF to the brain.

Other researchers are heartened by the discovery of GDNF because they believe it demonstrates that new growth factors exist. Some of these other factors may turn out to be peptides small enough to cross from the blood-brain barrier. GDNF itself emerged from a program that began in 1987 when Hans Thoenen of the Max Planck

SYMPTOMS MAY VARY.

Parkinsonism and Parkinson's disease itself present an amazing array of symptoms, some quite odd. Some of the symptoms seem impossible to account for, although a few can be directly attributed to loss of the neurotransmitter dopamine (*see* "The Ubiquity of NO in Life," p 305) in the brain. Here is a brief glossary.

Blunted affect   Feeling and emotions that have been reduced in scope and intensity.

Bradykinesia   A general slowing down and reduction of movement, including gestures and facial movement. Not only do almost all activities slow down, but the decrease in energy also produces a kind of behavior that observers perceive as loss of personality.

Dementia   Possibly not a symptom of parkinsonism at all, although about ten to 20 percent of the people with Parkinson's disease have symptoms similar to those of Alzheimer's disease. The most likely explanation is that people exhibiting this symptom actually have Alzheimer's disease in addition to Parkinson's disease.

Festinating gait   Walking slightly stooped with small steps that do not raise far from the ground, leaning noticeably forward in the process.

Mask   Characteristic lack of expression and facial rigidity.

Micrographia   Handwriting becomes progressively smaller.

Monotone   Speech that is slow and soft, and maintains approximately the same pitch; lack of intonation.

Rigidity   Not the same as the rigid muscles symptomatic of some other diseases. Parkinson's rigidity is the replacement of continuous motion by discrete motion, often resulting in stop-and-go movements, like the gear of a old clock that is regulated by a cogwheel.

Tremor   Probably the parkinsonian symptom most associated in the public mind with Parkinson's disease, perhaps because it is so apparent. A famous example is the motion picture star Katherine Hepburn, who has continued to act and make public appearances despite her usually noticeable parkinsonian tremor.

Institute in Munich, Germany, ground up brains to look for growth factors. By 1991 various research groups that built on his work had located growth factors for dopamine-producing neurons, but GDNF is the first to be produced in significant quantities by genetic engineering.

(Periodical References and Additional Reading: *New York Times* 3-21-91; *New York Times* 11-12-91, p C3; *New York Times* 5-24-92, p I-1; *Harvard Health Letter* 5-93, p 1; *Science* 5-21-93, pp 1072 & 1130; *Harvard Health Letter* 6-93, p 3)

ALS—NOT JUST LOU GEHRIG'S DISEASE

Because amyotrophic lateral sclerosis (ALS) is so associated in the public mind with one famous victim of the disease—New York Yankee Lou Gehrig—it is often thought of as much rarer than other chronic diseases, with the exception of heart disease and cancer. It is comparatively rare—about 5000 cases a year in the U.S.—but because it is always fatal within three to five years, it has a disproportionate impact on society. In addition to Lou Gehrig, it has claimed other well-known Americans, notably musician Charles Mingus and New York Senator Jacob Javits.

The main symptom of ALS is that nerve cells that connect the brain and spinal cord to muscles gradually cease functioning. Patients gradually lose the ability to walk, swallow, or breathe, and eventually suffocate to death.

Causes and Treatment

One form of ALS is hereditary, and the gene that causes this form has been identified (*see* "Other Genetic Diseases," p 62). In this rare form of ALS, the gene allele produces an ineffective form of a protein that normally counteracts free oxygen radicals. Untamed, the free radical destroy neurons in the brain and the spinal cord. Between five and 10 percent of ALS is hereditary, but the other instances lack a satisfactory explanation.

One of the most promising leads, described in the May 28, 1992, issue of the *New*

GUAM DISEASE

Shortly after World War II, U.S. physicians stationed on the Pacific island of Guam noticed that the native Chamorros were dying from what appeared to be ALS at a rate 50 times that of the U.S. Further study showed that Guam disease was not exactly ALS—in many patients symptoms of parkinsonism also developed. The official name of the newly recognized disease became Guam ALS-PDC (for Guam amyotrophic lateral sclerosis—parkinsonism dementia complex), although many just call it Guam disease.

Guam ALS-PDC was thought to provide major clues to various illnesses that entailed similar brain deterioration, even diseases with mostly different symptoms, such as Alzheimer's, although both diseases are characterized in part by neurofibrillary tangles in brain cells. In the 1960s it was thought that high levels of aluminum in the soil cause Guam disease, suggesting a role for aluminum in other brain disorders.

But the aluminum is still in the Guam environment, while the disease is dying out. The most severe cases occurred during the 1940s and 1950s and resembled ALS the most. Gradually parkinsonian symptoms crept in. Later, the ALS symptoms began to vanish, leaving only parkinsonism. A new, symptomless, variant of the disease is also vanishing. There were about 40 cases annually the 1950s, and fewer than five new cases each year so far in the 1990s. Because of this change, investigators are looking for something that Chamorros ate or did in the 1940s that they no longer eat or do today as their society becomes increasingly westernized. Attention recently has focused on plants called cycads that contain potent toxins, but what seemed to be good leads have all been eliminated. Researchers are now rushing to understand Guam disease before it completely disappears.

England Journal of Medicine, has been the discovery that the neurotransmitter glutamate (*see* "The Ubiquity of NO in Life," p 305) in excess opens up calcium channels—the sudden influx of calcium kills neurons. Evidence has suggested glutamate as a possible factor in Guam disease, since glutamate is high in cycads, plants whose consumption is one possible cause of Guam disease. Following this lead, Jeffrey Rothstein of Johns Hopkins University in Baltimore, Maryland, and co-workers studied brain tissue of people who had died from ALS. They found that the brain tissue was lacking in the molecules that normally absorb glutamate. They also looked at the cerebrospinal fluid of living ALS patients, and found three to four times as much glutamate as normal. There was some hope that drugs could be developed that would block this overproduction of glutamate.

In December 1992, the *New England Journal of Medicine* contained a report linking antibodies against nerve cells to ALS. The antibodies appeared to attack the calcium channels, pores that also are affected by glutamate. If the antibodies cause the disease, which is still uncertain, then ALS is similar in that respect to multiple sclerosis.

One promising line of treatment, which seemed effective in experimental animals with a disease similar to ALS, has been to use a nerve growth factor of one kind or another to slow down the course of the disease. Large-scale clinical trials of this idea were being put in place at the end of 1993.

(Periodical References and Additional Reading: *New York Times* 5-28-92, p B10; *New York Times* 12-15-92, p C8; *Science News* 1-2-93, p 5; *Science News* 3-6-93, p 148; *Science* 7-23-93, p 424; *New York Times* 8-20-93, p A16; *Science News* 8-21-93, p 116)

New Tools in Medicine

NEW TOOLS: THE STATE OF MEDICAL DIAGNOSIS

Physicians tend to believe that diagnosis is more of an art than a science. Even today the basis of good diagnosis has remained patient history; visual, aural, and tactile examination; and a few simple tests using simple equipment. From early times until the present the examination of body wastes has also been important. Ancient Egyptian physicians also paid attention to such factors as expression, color of skin, swellings (if present), stiffness and ability to move, breathing, and sweat. The early Indians timed intervals between bouts of fever and examined samples of blood. Chinese physicians took stock in listening to the pulse and examination of the tongue. In Greek and Roman times and right on through the Renaissance, counting the pulse was one of the main areas of technological advance, as better clocks were developed.

The nineteenth century brought new tools, beginning at the stethoscope and ending with X rays. X rays were just the beginning of the many ways to observe the interior of the body without opening it. The twentieth century has seen a steady advance in imaging techniques (see "Imaging UPDATE," p 485).

Some of the old techniques have been updated with new technology as well. Ancient Egyptian physicians would smell a patient's breath as part of their diagnosis and physicians still do today when they suspect certain conditions. But in the early 1990s, the Battelle Memorial Institute of Columbus, Ohio, developed a mechanical sniffer that can provide instant readings of breath using mass spectroscopy. Not only are the results useful in detecting the hallmarks of specific diseases, but it can also detect toxic chemicals that have been ingested. The main problem with the device is that it is as big as a refrigerator and costs $400,000.

At the same time, old-fashioned observation of the patient's exterior continues, although sometimes with a new twist. The February 2, 1993 *Journal of the American Medical Association* reported that male baldness, especially the bald spot in the back of the head or the bald pate surrounded by hair, is positively correlated with the risk of heart attack. But there was no such connection to a receding hairline. For the most severe baldness at the top of the head, the risk of heart attack was more than three times the risk for the man with a full head of hair. Most of the 1437 patients studied were males of European descent under the age of 55, and the baldness pattern may be different for older men of different races. This was not the first recognition of the connection between heart attacks and baldness, but it was the first to try to quantify it and compare the different types of baldness.

Finding a Hidden Disease

While a few conditions produce signals that almost anyone can recognize—chicken pox, for example, has a distinctive rash—many diseases are difficult to diagnose. Typically, several different diagnostic tools used by physicians are brought into play.

What follows is a description of a diagnosis for a woman who comes to see a physician who complains of pelvic discomfort and abdominal bloating.

- A pelvic examination may or may not reveal the cause. While women from their teenage years throughout the rest of their lives should have such examinations often, there are often cases where such an examination fails to identify the cause of the specific symptoms.
- A patient history often points to diagnosis. For example, ovarian cancer is more likely to occur in a woman from a family from which other women also have ovarian cancer. One close relative, such as a mother, sister, or daughter, with cancer means five times the risk; two such close relatives mean fifty times the risk. Thus the physician asks about members of the family.
- Patient history can also reveal lifestyle factors, such as smoking or diet. For ovarian cancer some of the lifestyle factors are very specific, such as use of talcum powder which raises the risk, as does taking drugs to promote fertility. On the other hand, being pregnant, taking oral contraceptives, nursing, and tubal sterilization are among the lifestyle factors that reduce the risk of ovarian cancer.
- Increasingly, biochemical techniques are being developed for specific conditions. Cancer cells make larger amounts of certain proteins than normal cells do (see below). A blood test can reveal whether certain proteins are elevated. If so, cancer is a greater possibility. But cancer cannot be definitely identified by blood tests nor can most blood tests separate cancers from benign tumors. Like patient history and a physical examination, the best that can be expected from a blood test is partial elimination of a possibility or increased probability that a condition exists.
- For many conditions, imaging can aid in diagnosis (see also "Imaging UPDATE," p 485). An imaging system specifically developed for pelvic examination of women is called transvaginal color-flow Doppler ultrasonography. This technique makes blood flow in the ovary visible; since most cancers require higher than normal supply of blood, imaging in this way can often detect small tumors that are missed by other methods.

The good news is that an observant and knowledgeable physician who uses all the means outlined above can generally recognize early ovarian cancer, which can be cured if caught soon enough. The bad news is that the symptoms that can be noticed by the patient, which might start the whole process, do not occur until the cancer has progressed, when it may be too late for a cure. Furthermore, since ovarian cancer strikes only one woman in 70, it may be viewed as too expensive for every woman in the U.S. over 45 (the age when risks rise) to have annual blood tests or ultrasound— estimated in 1993 at a total cost of $14 billion for the tests. The cost would also be increased well beyond this figure because in tens of thousands of cases false positives would lead to unnecessary surgery.

Molecular Biology and Diagnosis

Before World War II there was very little in the way of understanding or even recognizing specific proteins, though some such as insulin and thyroid hormone were beginning to be used for diagnosis. The work of Linus Pauling, Frederick Sanger, and others shortly after the war contributed greatly to understanding individual proteins. Chemists also began to use on a regular basis various methods of separating a mixture of organic chemicals into its distinct components (*see also* "Synthetic Antibodies, Glowing Germs," p 478). The structure of DNA and the genetic code were unraveled. Most recently, methods have been developed (1) to take a small sample of DNA and amplify it as much as needed for any purpose and (2) to coax a gene into making the protein it normally produces.

Here is an example of the new methods. Many different cancers have as a common thread defects in a gene called *p53* (*see* "Genes for Cancer," p 54). Formerly the only way to tell which alleles of *p53* a person carried would be to sequence DNA from each chromosome one base at a time. At the end of 1992, however, a much quicker, though still tedious test, was developed. First a probe is used to locate and extract the gene from a patient's blood. Then the gene is made in quantity by the polymerase chain reaction (PCR). With plenty of copies available, the *p53* gene is inserted into animal cells that have been bred or engineered to lack *p53* entirely. The animal cells then cause *p53* to make its protein product. If that product is effective, it triggers another enzyme in the cells that causes the cells to change color. Circuitous as this procedure seems, the method reduces laboratory time for testing for defective *p53* from a few days to a few hours. Even so, such a test is a long way from becoming routine.

All of these advances have worked together to increase vastly the array of information that can be learned from a blood test or urinalysis.

PSA testing   A case in point is the blood test now routinely used to aid in diagnosis of prostate cancer (*see* "Prostate Problems," p 230). Prostate cells produce a protein that keeps semen liquid. The protein seems to have no other function, so the process that produces it is expressed only in prostate cells. A test was developed in the 1980s that can identify that protein, which is generally called PSA (prostate-specific antigen). In 1986 the U.S. Food and Drug Administration (FDA) approved the test for monitoring people diagnosed with prostate cancer, and the test became readily available by 1989. The main danger of prostate cancer comes when the cancer has metastasized and cancerous cells begin to grow in other organs, usually bone. With PSA testing, if the prostate gland has been removed, but PSA is still being found in the blood, there must be prostate cells elsewhere in the body—hence, the cancer has metastasized and additional therapy might be attempted.

Soon physicians reasoned that any increase in PSA in a man might indicate that the number of prostate cells was also increasing, which might very well mean cancer. Since PSA testing was available, this concept was tried out. Manufacturers of the test and of pharmaceuticals used in treating prostate cancer soon took a number of steps to promote further PSA testing. In many instances, observation of high levels of PSA led to detection of observable enlargement of the prostate gland. Furthermore, with or without such enlargement, random biopsies very often found cancer cells in the prostate. By the early 1990s, many physicians considered the PSA blood level to be a routine part of a general physical examination for men. The manufacturer of the test and the U.S. government financed a study of more than ten thousand men, published in the August 25, 1993 *Journal of the American Medical Association*, that showed that PSA was twice as effective in finding cancer as a physical examination. By then the PSA test was already approved for routine screening by the American Cancer Society and by the American Urological Association.

But by the end of 1993 the FDA had not approved PSA testing for what had become its most common use. Furthermore, other government and semi-governmental agencies in the U.S. also failed to endorse PSA screening of apparently healthy men.

Why is there this apparent discrepancy between the effectiveness of PSA testing in locating the second most common cause of death by cancer among men (after lung cancer) and the official attitude of the U.S. government? First of all, the test is unreliable in two ways. It has a rate of about 20 to 80 percent of false positives and of about 25 to 40 percent of false negatives, depending on which expert's data on false results you take. Second, the test costs only from $15 to $50 to perform but follow-up tests such as ultrasound and biopsies raise the actual costs considerably. The most common estimate is that, if all men over the age of 50 were routinely screened, the U.S. total cost would be about $28 million a year. And third, there is no evidence collected so far to show that routine PSA testing lowers the death rate from prostate cancer. A federal study to determine the long-term effect of PSA screening is underway—hampered in part because about 92 percent of all routine physicals for men over the age of 50 already include PSA testing—but results are not expected until about 2100.

PSA testing poses additional problems because a positive result so often leads to surgery or radiation therapy. For older patients, who are the ones most likely to have prostate cancer in any case, the risk for death from surgery is about one percent between 65 and 75 and double that afterward. Surgery and radiation at any age can lead to impotence (25 percent), incontinence (three to six percent), restricted urine flow (eight to 18 percent) and rectal injury (one to three percent), all destructive to the quality of life in an otherwise healthy man. Some 60 to 90 percent of men on Medicare are reported as impotent and 63 percent as incontinent if the prostate is removed. For older men, life with a small prostate cancer is often a safer option than treatment.

Other protein tests   Although PSA screening has received most of the publicity, the ability to detect specific proteins easily is leading to more and more blood or urine tests, simple tests that often lead to complicated decisions by physicians and patients.

The bone cancer that results from metastasis, whether from prostate or another cancer, is generally incurable, but perhaps the odds would be better if a test could detect it. Chemists from Metra Biosystems and Ciba-Geigy Corporation thought they had the answer when they found that the breakdown of collagen, which surrounds bone cells, produces measurable amounts of the proteins pyridinoline and deoxypyridinoline in urine. In May 1992 they told the American Society of Clinical

Oncology that the levels of these proteins rise when cancer metastasizes to bone. However, the chemicals also rise in cancer patients for whom no metastasis has taken place. The researchers optimistically suggested that in those cases, the newly developed test might predict that collagen degradation *preceding* metastasis might be occurring.

A different collagen test has been used in conjunction with measurement of enzymes produced by the liver to determine whether or not alcoholism has led to cirrhosis, which is scarring of the liver that in many cases leads to death. British researchers demonstrated that combining a standard screening method for collagen turnover in the liver with a standard battery used to measure various liver enzymes enabled them to detect cirrhosis without the need for expensive and invasive biopsy. The tests themselves typically cost about $2 each.

Protein tests are almost always indirect ways of measuring a problem, which is why they produce many false positives and negatives. For example, a test for colon cancer measures a carbohydrate-protein complex called carcinoembryonic antigen (CEA). The test is relatively expensive (over $50) and is used primarily for detection of reappearance of cancer after surgery (*see also* "Examining the Colon," p 482). A study released in the August 25, 1993 *Journal of the American Medical Association* demonstrated that while the test produced what exploratory surgery suggests were more false positive than correct results, it still led to detection of cancer recurrence in about five percent of the more than 1000 patients studied. However, follow-up studies showed that there was no statistical improvement in lifespan among those whose cancer recurrence was detected by CEA testing. As with many of the newer protein-based tests, it is far from clear whether or not CEA testing produces benefits commensurate with its costs. Of course, the few persons whose lives were saved by CEA testing do not think it is too expensive, nor do the people close to them.

Are Diagnostic Tests Reliable?

Analyses of the medical and social problems associated with protein-based tests are all based on the assumption that the laboratories performing the tests know what they are doing. One of the most common tests is the Pap test for cervical cancer that has been in use since 1928. When in 1993 a prominent woman in Newport, Rhode Island, died of cervical cancer after four Pap tests from the same lab were reported as negative for cancer or precancerous conditions, an investigation ensued. The Pap test uses slides with smears of cells that are examined under a microscope. Since the slides are preserved, the ones from this particular laboratory were available for re-examination by another laboratory and by federal investigators. Early results showed 17 tests that should have been reported as positive, but had not been, although re-study of the 19,000 samples covering the five years between 1988 and 1993 will not be completed until sometime in 1994. Poorly trained staff and sloppy procedures were blamed, and four technicians either resigned or were dismissed.

Testing blood and urine is a big business and highly competitive. One laboratory, for example, had revenues of nearly $200 million annually—but it was discovered in 1992 that some of that revenue came from overcharging the federal government for tests that physicians did not actually order. The question of how much should be spent on testing is a major issue for health-care legislation around the world, but it is further complicated by both cutting corners in laboratories and providing more tests than are actually needed to suggest ways that would improve a patient's health.

(Periodical References and Additional Reading: *New York Times* 7-19-92, p III-9; *New York Times* 8-4-92, p C3; *New York Times* 9-20-92, p I-1; *New York Times* 12-21-92, p D12; *New York Times* 12-22-92, p C6; *New York Times* 2-24-93, p A1; *New York Times* 6-2-93, p C12; *New York Times* 6-17-93, p A1; *New York Times* 8-25-93, p C10; *New York Times* 9-27-93, p A12; *New York Times* 9-29-93, p C12; *New York Times* 10-12-93, p C5; *New York Times* 10-27-93, p D3)

TIMETABLE OF MEDICAL DIAGNOSIS TO 1990

300 BC	At about this time, Herophilus studies the pulse, describing it in terms of size, strength, and rhythm, as well as attempting to measure its rate with a water clock.
170	Greek physician and anatomist Galen of Pergamum [born Pergamum (now Turkey), circa 130; died Sicily?, circa 200] becomes the first to use the pulse as a diagnostic aid.
1603	Sanctorius Sanctorius [born Justinopolis, March 29, 1561; died Venice, March 6, 1636] describes his device that uses a pendulum for counting pulse beats.
1707	*The Physician's Pulse Watch* by John Floyer [born Hintess, England, 1649; died Litchfield, England, February 1, 1734] introduces pulse-rate counting in medical practice and puts forth a special watch for it.
1747	*Primae lineae physiologiae* by Albrecht von Haller [born Berne, Switzerland, October 16, 1708; died Berne, December 17, 1777] is the first textbook on physiology.
1761	Giovanni Morgagni [born Forli (in what is now Italy), February 25, 1682; died Padua, Italy, December 5, 1771] writes *De sedibus et causis morborum per anatomen indagatis* (On the Causes of Diseases), the first important work in pathological anatomy.
	Leopold Auenbrugger [born Graz, Austria, November 19, 1722; died Vienna, Austria, May 18, 1809] uses his musical knowledge to develop the technique of percussion for diagnosis of chest disorders and publishes his findings in *Inventum novum*.
1816	Théophile René Laënnec [born Quimper, France, February 17, 1781; died Brittany, August 13, 1826] invents the stethoscope.
1819	*Traité de l'auscultation médiate* (On Listening to Organ Sounds with the Aid of an Instrument) by physician René Laënnec treats the use of the stethoscope for investigating the lungs, heart, and liver.
1822	William Beaumont [born Lebanon, Connecticut, November 21, 1785; died St. Louis, Missouri, April 25, 1853] starts his experimental study of digestion in the exposed stomach of a wounded man.
1826	René Laënnec writes *De l'auscultation médiate et des maladies des poumons et du coeur* (On Using Sound to Diagnose Maladies of Lungs and Heart), an extension of his work on the use of the stethoscope.
1827	Charles-Eduard-Ernest Delezenne [born Lille, France, October 4, 1776; died

August 26, 1866] develops his technique of "just noticeable differences" to study hearing.

1838   William Beaumont's *Experiments and Observations on the Gastric Juice and the Physiology of Digestion* relates his study of digestion *in vivo* and *in vitro* in a wounded man whose stomach remained partially accessible through a healed hole in the abdomen.

1847   Karl Friedrich Wilhelm Ludwig [born Witzenhausen (in what is now Germany), December 29, 1816; died Leipzig, April 27, 1895] develops a device that continuously records blood pressure, which he uses to show that the circulation of the blood is purely mechanical; no mysterious vital processes outside of ordinary physics needs to be invoked.

         Charles Babbage [born Teignmouth, United Kingdom, December 25, 1792; died London, England, October 18, 1871] invents an ophthalmoscope.

1850   Physician Carl Reinhold Wunderlich [born Sulz, Germany, August 4, 1815; died Leipzig, Germany, September 25 1877] about this time introduces the practice of taking accurate temperatures of patients with a thermometer as a regular part of diagnosis.

1851   Hermann von Helmholtz [born Potsdam, Prussia, August 31, 1821; died Berlin, September 8, 1894] reinvents the ophthalmoscope independently of Charles Babbage.

1852   Karl Vierodt makes the first accurate count of red blood cells, a technique that later becomes an important tool for diagnosing anemia.

1863   Physiologist Etienne-Jules Marey [born Beaune, France, March 5, 1830; died Paris, May 15, 1904] invents the sphygmograph, the predecessor of the sphygmometer used to measure blood pressure today.

1866   Physician Sir Thomas Clifford Allbutt [born Dewsbury, England, July 20, 1836; died Cambridge, England, February 22, 1925] develops the clinical thermometer; previously thermometers used in medicine were very long and it took about 20 minutes to determine temperature.

1895   Wilhelm Konrad Roentgen [born Lennep, Germany, March 27, 1845; died Munich, Germany, February 10, 1923] discovers X rays on November 8; he discovers that these rays pass through matter, a property that immediately leads to their application in diagnostic medicine.

1896   Michael I. Pupin [born Idvor, Austria-Hungary, October 4, 1858; died New York, March 12, 1935] of Columbia University takes the first diagnostic X-ray photograph in the United States; Eddie McCarthy of Dartmouth, New Hampshire, has a broken arm set with the new diagnostic aid less than three months after the discovery of X rays by Roentgen.

1897   Walter B. Cannon discovers that a bismuth compound can be used to make intestines visible to X rays.

1898   Herta Ayrton [born Portsea, England, April 25, 1854; died August 26, 1923], who invented a sphygmograph (an instrument for monitoring the human pulse), becomes the first woman to be elected to Britain's Institution of Electrical Engineers.

1903   Dutch physiologist Willem Einthoven [born Semarang, Java, May 22, 1860; died Leiden, Netherlands, September 29, 1927] develops in the Netherlands the string galvanometer, the forerunner of the electrocardiograph, used to measure tiny electrical currents produced by the heart.

1908   The tuberculin test, a skin test for tuberculosis based on an immune reaction to an antigen discovered by Robert Koch in 1890, is introduced by Charles Mantoux [born 1877; died 1947].

1911   American physiologist Walter Bradford Cannon [born Prairie du Chien, Wisconsin, October 19, 1871; died Franklin, New Hampshire, October 1, 1945] in *Mechanical Factors of Digestion* describes his use of bismuth compounds to make soft internal organs visible with X rays.

London doctor William Hill develops the first gastroscope, a tube that can be swallowed by a patient so that the doctor may look at the inside of the patient's stomach through the tube.

1913   Bela Schick [born Boglar, Hungary, July 16, 1877; died New York, December 6, 1967] introduces the Schick test for diphtheria.

1924   Willem Einthoven of the Netherlands wins the Nobel Prize for Physiology or Medicine for his invention of the electrocardiograph.

1927   Antonio Moniz obtains X-ray pictures of the arteries of the brain by injecting a contrast medium into the blood vessels.

1928   Dutch radiologist Ziedes de Plantes develops a method using a moving X-ray source that can keep a single plane of the patient's body in focus; this is a predecessor of what comes to be known as computerized axial tomography (CAT or later CT scan)

1928   Greek-American George Papanicolau [born Coumi, Greece, May 13, 1893; died February 19, 1962] develops the Pap test for diagnosing uterine cancers.

1929   German psychiatrist Hans Berger [born Neuses, Bavaria, May 21, 1873; died Jena, Germany, June 1, 1941] develops the electroencephalogram (EEG).

1932   Armand Quick [born Theresa, Wisconsin, July 18, 1894; died January 26, 1978] introduces the Quick test to measure the clotting ability of blood.

1949   X rays from a synchrotron are used for the first time in medical diagnosis and treatment.

1951   Rueben Kahn [born Kovno, Lithuania, July 26, 1887] introduces a "universal reaction" blood test for detecting several disorders at an early stage.

1956   Werner Forssmann [born Berlin, August 29, 1904; died Schopfheim, West Germany, June 1, 1979] Dickinson Richards [born Orange, New Jersey, October 30, 1895] and French-American physiologist André F. Cournand [born Paris, September 4, 1895] win the Nobel Prize for Physiology or Medicine for their use of the catheter for study of the interior of the heart and circulatory system.

1957   Allan Cormack [born Johannesburg, South Africa, February 23, 1924], then at the University of Capetown in South Africa, begins independent development of the CT scan; no one at the time seems interested.

1958   Ian Donald of Scotland is the first to use ultrasound to examine unborn children.

1959   Norman J. Holter [born Helena, Montana, February 1, 1914] introduces a portable electrocardiograph for continuous recording of an electrocardiogram to study heart patients.

1960	The U.S. physician H. Anger invents the "Gamma camera," a detector that allows the imaging of internal organs that are labeled with a radioactive element.
	William H. Oldendorf [born Schenectady, New York, March 27, 1925; died Los Angeles, December 14, 1992] begins work about this time on his version of the CT scan; working independently of researchers in South Africa and Great Britain at the University of California in Los Angeles, Oldendorf writes medical papers and obtains patents in the field, but fails to attract enough interest for development. In 1975 he (along with Godfrey N. Hounsfield, who did succeed in obtaining development support) receives the Albert and Mary Lasker Award, the main recognition for Oldendorf's contributions.
1967	Mammography for detecting breast cancer is introduced.
1967	Godfrey N. Hounsfield [born United Kingdom, 1919] uses medical X rays to reconstruct a three-dimensional image, the essential development of the CT scan, a method previously discovered by Allan Cormack and William H. Oldendorf; unlike Cormack and Oldendorf, however, Hounsfield finds medical personnel interested in pursuing the new method.
1971	Raymond V. Damadian [born New York, March 16, 1936] applies for a patent on using magnetic resonance imaging (MRI, also known as NMR) to detect tumors
	The first CT scanning X-ray machine is installed for testing at Atkinson Morley's Hospital in Wimbledon, United Kingdom; it takes 4.5 minutes to gather data followed by 20 minutes of computer time to construct an image.
1972	At Wimbledon in the United Kingdom, the first experimental CT scan imager for medical purposes at Atkinson Morley's Hospital detects a brain tumor in a living patient on October 4.
1973	John Malland at Aberdeen University in Scotland introduces nuclear magnetic resonance scanning (NMR or, more recently, MRI for "magnetic resonance imaging") for medical diagnosis.
1977	Raymond V. Damadian builds his first medical magnetic resonance imager (MRI), based on nuclear magnetic resonance spectroscopy techniques, and tests it successfully on July 7.
1979	Allan McLeod Cormack of South Africa and the United States and Godfrey N. Hounsfield of England win the Nobel Prize for Physiology or Medicine for their invention of computed axial tomography.
1986	Testing for prostate cancer by use of a simple blood test (for a glycoprotein called PSA, for prostate-specific antigen) is approved for use in the U.S.

SURPRISE: NORMAL TEMPERATURE ISN'T NORMAL

In September 1992, Philip Mackowiak of the University of Maryland School of Medicine revealed that re-measuring human body temperature showed that it is seldom 98.6° F or 37° C, even in normal people. Although Mackowiak found in 148 healthy volunteers an average temperature of 98.2° F, the main point of his report was that temperature measured under the tongue, as is the most common method, varies from about 96.0° F in the morning to about 99.9° F in the evening.

Although 98.6° is usually reported as normal temperature, there are numerous anomalies. The Becton Dickinson clinical thermometer for home use notes in accompanying literature that normal temperature under the tongue is 98.6° F, but the thermometers themselves appear to have an arrow, presumed to indicate normal temperature, at 98.5°, which the material on use of the thermometer fails to explain.

One has to wonder how the common "normal" temperature of 98.6° F came to be. In the nineteenth century, physicians began to use temperature as an aid in diagnosis on a regular basis. One of the main advocates of the practice was Carl Wunderlich, who is claimed to have averaged the temperatures of 25,000 people in the middle of the nineteenth century. Some evidence suggests Wunderlich, who reported on the normal armpit temperature in 1868, used a thermometer that was calibrated too high by modern standards. One has to expect also that Wunderlich may have used the nearest whole number in the Celsius scale (37° C) instead of an apparently more accurate measurement to tenths in the Fahrenheit scale. The report that he found the top of the normal range as 100.4° F might also be a translation, since 100.4° F is exactly 38° C, just as 98.6° F is exactly 37° C.

The situation is further complicated by Wunderlich's use of the armpit temperature, which the American Medical Association in its *Family Medical Guide* notes to be either 1° F or 0.5° C higher than temperature under the tongue which Mackowiak measured. In that case, one might have expected Wunderlich to have found (if Mackowiak is right) that normal temperature is 99.2° F or 37.3° C.

When Daniel Fahrenheit made the first of the mercury-glass thermometers that are still commonly used, he reported normal body temperature as 96° F but that low number is thought to have resulted from using a uniform bore in the thermometer. If there is no adjustment in the bore, a thermometer that registers 32° at the melting point of ice and 212° at the boiling point of water would be expected to be a degree or two short around the middle of that range. Thus, an early Fahrenheit thermometer could have reported body temperature lower than a more careful measurement would have shown.

Skin temperature, measured by hand when a child is suspected to be ill, is only about 86° F (30° C). Rectal temperatures, often used in hospital situations, are generally thought to range around 99.6° F or 37.5° C, although there has been no definitive report in the literature.

(Periodical References and Additional Reading: *Discover* 1-93, p 52)

SYNTHETIC ANTIBODIES, GLOWING GERMS

New diagnostic tests are often called by acronyms that end in "A," such as the PSA test for prostate cancer and the CEA test for colon cancer. In those cases the "A" is for *antigen,* a clue that the test actually works by binding a protein or glycoprotein (a common carbohydrate-protein combination on the surfaces of cells) with an antibody specific to that particular chemical. Furthermore, the antibody must be a *monoclonal* antibody, a chemical that binds to a particular antigen with exquisite specificity.

Although monoclonal antibodies have come to play an important part in diagnostic

Background

One of the most easily accessible parts of the immune system is a group of chemicals called antibodies that circulate in the bloodstream. Antibodies are the key to the success of vaccination, for example. Injection of a vaccine stimulates a B-cell lymphocyte to produce antibodies against proteins in the vaccine. Such antibodies home in on specific foreign proteins so that they can be destroyed. Vaccination confers long-lasting immunity because the B cells that have been stimulated to produce the antibodies reproduce and the line remains in the bloodstream, prepared to produce antibodies against a reinvasion of the specific protein.

Antibodies are usually called "proteins," although each one is actually a combination of four protein chains linked together. Proteins and their parts are often identified by "weight," a rough measure of the number of amino acids linked together to form a chain. The more amino acids, the heavier the chain. All antibodies consist of two identical heavy chains and two identical light chains. Each type chain is specified by a separate gene. The chains link together to form a Y-shaped molecule, with the arms of the Y being the active sites that link to an antigen.

In 1975 César Milstein and George Köhler developed in England a method of producing large amounts of specific antibodies by a cloning technique. Antigens from human cancer cells are injected into a mouse. The B cells in the mouse start producing antibodies that attack the antigens. These B cells are removed and fused with cancerous mouse B cells, forming hybrid cells called *hybridomas* that live and reproduce, continuing to produce large amounts of antibodies. Probes are used to pick out a hybridoma that produces a specific desired antibody, and this cell is then reproduced in large quantities. Antibodies from such a cell line are called *monoclonal* because they are produced from the clones of a single hybridoma.

The original mouse-produced antibodies have sometimes caused undesired immune reactions when used in human bodies. More recently, scientists have used human cells to make the hybridomas, reducing unwanted reactions. But the easier-to-produce mouse antibodies are sufficient for applications that take place outside of human bodies. Just like natural antibodies, monoclonal antibodies react with proteins or other chemicals with exquisite specificity. Thus, they can be used in diagnosis, one of the first applications of this technology.

testing, their manufacture is based on slow biological processes instead of chemical reactions, and tests based on biology often take some time to prepare and read. Preparation of monoclonal antibodies is beginning to bypass biological processes.

Also, new techniques based on getting cells or free-living creatures to glow under specified circumstances have proven a popular way to obtain a quick reading of biological tests.

Beyond Monoclonal Antibodies

In 1989 Richard Lerner of the Scripps Clinic in La Jolla, California, and coworkers proposed a new way to create monoclonal antibodies, a method that bypasses mammal cells entirely. The method using mammal cells often takes months and results in few clonal lines that have the specific reactions desired.

In the new method, which is sometimes called "antibodies from libraries," the starting point is the genes that specify heavy and light protein chains that will be eventually assembled to make the finished antibody. The "library" of the method is a repertoire of gene clones for the heavy and light chains of mouse antibodies.

The procedure that follows seems complex but is largely what has come to be routine genetic engineering. Heavy and light chain gene segments are checked out of the library and inserted into a phage—a virus that infects a bacterium. The phage is used to infect *E. coli* bacteria, which then has the capacity to manufacture large numbers of combinations of heavy and light chains—in effect, a wide variety of antibody-like fragments, though they are antibodies to no particular antigen. Using rapid screening methods, scientists can screen as many as a million of these antibody fragments in a day. If they find a few dozen fragments that react to the antigen used in screening, these fragments can then be compared with each other for activity. The best can then be produced in quantity by the same method. Furthermore, deliberate mutations can be introduced to improve binding if needed. This method was hailed as one of the great medical advances of 1989.

But in 1992 there was continuing controversy about antibodies from libraries. The main objection was a theoretical one, namely that the probability of obtaining the same antibodies as produced in nature was low. A laboratory study of one antibody-antigen reaction showed that the artificial library antibody fragments to that antigen were not the same as antibodies derived from mammal cells. This difference suggests caution in using library antibody fragments in applications inside human bodies, but should be no deterrent to diagnostic applications based on blood or urine samples.

In 1993 chemists developed a way to produce another kind of artificial antibody, one that required no mice, human cell lines, phages, or bacteria. Klaus Mosbach, George Vlatakis, Lars I. Andersson, and Ralf Müller of the University of Lund in Sweden developed a way to make what amount to plastic antibodies.

They chose to demonstrate their method by making plastic antibodies to the "antigens" theophylline (a common asthma medication marketed under many brand names) and diazepam (best known as Valium). The principle is essentially the same as recording a body part in the sidewalk outside the Chinese Theater in Hollywood, but using a molecule instead of a hand or foot and a polymer combination instead of concrete. The theory behind this approach states that the main way that an antibody sticks to its antigen is mechanical. The "lock and key" metaphor is more than just an analogy, although there is some reason to believe that electrical forces play some part in actual antibody-antigen reactions. In any case, after the shape of the molecule of theophylline or of diazepam has been copied in relief by the plastic, the model molecules are freed and the plastic antibodies left to float in an organic solvent.

Tests were conducted with doctored blood (antigen-free blood in which a known amount of either theophylline or diazepam had been added) and with real blood from people using and not using the drugs. The plastic antibodies did as well as biological counterparts in binding to the antigens, making a few mistakes with similar chemicals (just as the biologicals do), but correctly identifying all the instances of the real chemicals. Because the plastic used in the artificial antibodies had been tagged with radioactive atoms, the assay was easy to complete. A measurement of the level of radioactivity after the plastic antibodies have been separated from the samples being tested translates directly into a measure of the amount of antigen.

The main disadvantage of the radioactive plastic antibodies is that the versions developed so far need organic solvents in which to work. Biological antibodies can be used in water. The chief advantages are that the plastic versions are inexpensive compared to their biological counterparts, can be easily stored or transported, and are even reusable after chemically removing the antigens that cling to them.

Glowing Health

In 1984 Keith Wood of the University of California at San Diego and coworkers isolated the gene for the protein that causes the firefly to glow and glimmer, an enzyme known as luciferase. By 1989 the gene and the genes for four other luciferases with slightly different colors, taken from the kittyboo beetle, were being installed in various bacteria and other single cells or even in viruses. In a cellular environment, luciferase works with the cellular energy source adenosine triphosphate (ATP) to produce a characteristic glow, just like the firefly's "fire." By 1991, the luciferase gene had been installed in artery cells of living dogs, showing that it was possible to use genetic engineering to change the gene structure of cells *in vivo*. At that point, putting a luciferase gene into a cell was just a test for an engineering technique. But a couple of years later, the same idea was being used in a new kind of diagnostic test.

It is important to diagnose drug-resistant tuberculosis (*see* "The Return of Tuberculosis," p 363) as soon as possible because treatment for the drug-resistant strain is different from that for "wild" tuberculosis. Furthermore, knowing exactly which drugs the strain is resistant to suggests which ones to avoid in treatment. Use of luciferase to make the bacteria glow reduces the time needed to identify a particular drug-resistant strain by weeks. Without the test, the bacterium takes three to five weeks to grow into quantities great enough to analyze; another five or more weeks are needed to test the samples against various tuberculosis treatment drugs to find which ones kill the bacteria or prevent them from multiplying. It is this second period, the one for testing drug resistance, that is reduced from weeks to days by use of the technique developed by William Jacobs and Barry Bloom from the Albert Einstein College of Medicine with Graham Hatfull of the University of Pittsburgh and described in the May 7, 1993 *Science*.

The cultured bacteria are first given a dose of an anti-tuberculosis medicine and then infected with a genetically engineered phage that carries the gene for luciferase, the same technique used for making artificial antibody fragments with bacteria. Then the phage carries the gene into living bacteria, where the energy source ATP interacts with the luciferase to cause the bacteria to emit light within two hours of infection. If the drug has killed most or all of the bacteria or weakened them so that they are not very energetic, the glow is nonexistent or weak. Drug-resistant bacteria, however, shine brightly. Thus it is easy to tell a few hours after the phage begins to infect the bacteria whether or not they are resistant to the particular drug being used.

The same test is also being used with new drugs or new drug combinations. This not only enables a quick assay of possible benefit, but it means that drugs that might break down over the course of several weeks can be tested before any such break-down occurs.

The same method is available for use with all sorts of bacteria, including staph and strep, although the primary use so far has been for tuberculosis.

(Periodical References and Additional Reading: *Discover* 11-89, p 12; *Science* 12-8-89, pp 1250 & 1275; *Science* 12-22-89, p 1544; *Science News* 6-22-91, p 391; *Nature* 5-21-92, p 201; *Nature* 10-29-92, p 782; *Science News* 2-6-93, p 90; *Nature* 2-18-93, p 645; *Science News* 2-27-93, p 132; *Science* 5-7-93, pp 750 & 819; *New York Times* 5-7-93, p A17; *Harvard Health Letter* 8-93, p 1)

EXAMINING THE COLON

Among cancers common in the United States cancer of the lower bowel or of the rectum is second only to lung cancer as a killer among the cancers common in the U.S. It is estimated that 57,000 Americans died from colorectal cancer during 1993. This death rate is more than a third of the incidence rate, meaning that somewhat more than one out of three persons who develops colorectal cancer in the U.S. will die from the disease.

The major research development in fighting colorectal cancer has been the location of genes involved in such cancers (*see* "Genes for Cancer," p 54), but it will be some time before routine DNA analysis will be a part of the annual checkup for people over 50. In the meantime, experts believe that majority of colorectal cancer deaths could be prevented by better use of the tests now available. Of particular concern are growths called adenomatous polyps, which can be detected by some of the following tests and which often are precursors to cancer.

The primary lines of defense are a test of a sample of fecal material and visual examination of the interior of the colon. Both have been involved in some controversy during the early 1990s.

Fecal occult blood screening   The idea behind fecal screening is that a diseased colon often bleeds slightly. If the blood is not obvious in fecal waste, it is called *occult,* which in this context simply means "hidden." Detection of occult blood is accomplished by chemicals that reveal hemoglobin. Among the problems with this test is the long list of other situations or substances that can be mistaken for cancer by the chemical analysis of the fecal samples: this includes blood from rare meat, bleeding caused by aspirin, hemorrhoids, ulcers, or diverticulitis. Furthermore, raw broccoli, turnips, horseradish, cauliflower, red radishes, parsnips, cantaloupe, or even vitamin C supplements can cause false-positive results.

The actual collection of fecal samples is left to the patient. Various methods have been used and recent ones involving special wipes are not difficult to use at all, although some people refuse to take samples out of misplaced fastidiousness.

On May 13, 1993, the *New England Journal of Medicine* published the results of a study of 46,551 Minnesota residents over a period of 13 years that showed that those in the experimental group, who took the fecal occult blood test, had a third fewer deaths from colorectal cancer. The problem with this result is that about one person

GUT TALK

One minor problem people have when dealing with matters intestinal is a lack of clarity about which part is which. Even today, some people find language referring to the lower part of the digestive system a bit too plain for ordinary discourse. The whole length under discussion, presented alphabetically below, is about 30 feet. Many of the traditional divisions assigned by anatomists are somewhat arbitrary, as one part flows into the other. Also defined are the three different instruments used by physicians to examine the colon and rectum.

Alimentary canal The tube of the digestive system from the lips and teeth through the esophagus, stomach, intestines, rectum, and anus; also called the digestive tract.

Anus The end of the line—the opening at the base of the rectum.

Appendix A thin projection from the cecum, about the size and shape of a pencil when healthy.

Bowels Both intestines taken together—hence, the "large bowel," often used for the large intestine.

Cecum Also known as the "blind gut," the cecum is a large pouch that forms the upper part of the large intestine—above the colon. The small intestine joins the large near the end, but not at the end, forming a T juncture. One branch of the T is the cecum, while the other is the colon. If this were a maze, the colon would be the way out.

Colon The main part of the large intestine—technically, the part from the cecum to the rectum, a distance of about six feet. Names are based on the direction that wastes travel when passing through: the colon is divided into an ascending colon, above the cecum; a transverse colon, across the midsection; and a descending colon, heading toward the rectum. The last part between the descending colon and the rectum is an S-shape; anything shaped like an S curve is *sigmoid,* so this part is the sigmoid colon (sometimes called the sigmoid flexure, which just means "S-shaped bend").

Colonoscope A long (about five feet) flexible-tube periscope, often using fiber optics, that can view the entire colon as well as the rectum. It is equipped with a mechanism for removing and retrieving small parts of the wall of the colon under the direction of the physician performing the test, who watches the progress of the lighted tip on a monitor.

Colorectal The inclusive term for the colon and rectum.

Gut A term with different meanings depending on the speaker, but most often representing the same as *bowel* or *intestine,* although sometimes indicating the whole alimentary canal.

Intestine A general word used for the whole apparatus extending from the stomach to the anus.

Proctoscope A foot-long rigid tube used as a periscope for examining the rectum and lower colon. The prefix *procto-* comes from the Greek words for anus and for rectum. Seldom used anymore.

Rectum The last section of the alimentary canal, where fecal matter is stored before evacuation through the anus. The name *rectum* refers to its straightness. It is usually about eight inches long.

Sigmoidoscope   A flexible periscope 18 inches long, which can provide a view of the lower third of the colon as well as of the rectum.
Small intestine   Consisting of three labeled sections from the stomach to the large intestine, (1) the first foot or so is the duodenum, best known as a site of some peptic ulcers; (2) the next eight or nine feet is the jejunum, about which little is heard; and (3) the last nine feet or so is the ileum, which sometimes becomes inflamed, a condition called ileitis. Don't confuse the ileum with an ileus, which is a failure of the intestines to perform properly.

---

in ten has a positive (blood detected) fecal occult blood test for each test performed, but only one person in 30 has precancerous conditions or colorectal cancer. Most of these have precancerous polyps. The only good way to be certain which persons with positive results have cancer is to administer expensive colonoscopic examinations to everyone with a positive result. Only 2.2 percent of those with a positive fecal blood test, which amounted to 38 percent of the persons screened when taken over the whole 13-year period, were found to have cancer when further examined with a colonoscope.

Some cancers do not produce blood, even occult blood. Approximately eight percent of colorectal cancers are thought to fall into this group, and thus show up as false negatives on the fecal occult blood test. Combining this information with the large number of false positives, a study in the March 10, 1993 *Journal of the American Medical Association* concluded that there was no definitive proof that fecal occult blood screening by itself saves lives. Because there are so many false positives that are followed up with colonoscopy, however, the follow-up examinations do save lives, which would account for the results of the Minnesota study announced later in 1993.

Tumor Associated Antigen (TAA) screening   A test more controversial than the fecal occult blood test is one for a protein produced in greater abundance by cancers (*see also* "New Tools: The State of Medical Diagnosis," p 469 and "Synthetic Antibodies, Glowing Germs," p 478). The TAA test is only about 40 percent accurate and is used primarily by insurance companies to screen for cancer. While a positive result may mean nothing more than a turn down on an insurance application, improvements might someday make it an additional tool in screening for colorectal cancers (or other cancers), especially when combined with fecal occult blood screening.

Sigmoidoscopic examinations   The American Cancer Society recommends that everyone over the age of 50 should have fecal occult blood screening annually combined with sigmoidoscopic examinations every three to five years. A review of two large studies published in the March 10, 1993 *Journal of the American Medical Association* concluded that regular sigmoidoscope examinations on the whole population over the age of 50 could reduce deaths from colorectal cancers by 60 to 70 percent. Despite this, sigmoidoscopy can only detect half of all colon cancers. (The figures make sense when you recall that only somewhat more than a third of persons with colon cancer die as a result of the disease.)

Double-contrast barium-enema X rays   Since 1897, physicians have used heavy elements that stop X rays to observe soft parts inside the human body. A barium enema provides a strong X-ray picture of the interior of the colon and can in some cases detect cancers there. The American Cancer Society recommends that people whose family history suggests a high risk of colon cancer have either a barium X ray or a colonoscopic examination every five years after the age of 35 or 40. But if anything suspicious shows up on the X ray, the patient will then have to have a colonoscopic examination to verify and quantify the cause, so many physicians believe that it is more effective simply to bypass the X ray and proceed directly to colonoscopy.

Colonoscopy   In theory—and perhaps even in actual practice—all colorectal cancers can be detected by colonoscopy, so a few experts in the field have proposed that all the other tests be abandoned. Just give everyone a colonoscopic examination every year they say.

Not only can a colonoscope view the entire length of the colon, but also it can remove suspicious growths. If they are small enough, the colonoscope can remove them entirely. If they are larger, the colonoscope can remove a sample for examination for cancer (a *biopsy*).

The problem is that colonoscopy is too expensive to use in mass screening. Furthermore, since it is quite invasive and requires some sedation, colonoscopy entails a slight risk, which is not true of fecal occult blood testing or of TAA testing (and extremely remote for other tests as well).

(Periodical References and Additional Reading: *Harvard Health Letter* 3-91, p 4; *New York Times* 3-10-93, p C12; *New York Times* 4-24-93, p 36; *New York Times* 5-13-93, p A1; *Harvard Health Letter* 10-93, p 8)

Imaging UPDATE

In 1896, Wilhelm Konrad Roentgen demonstrated in public that the bones inside his hand could be observed without removing the flesh covering them. Doctors within days began to use Roentgen's X rays to aid in setting bones. This was the beginning of routine imaging inside living humans—although William Beaumont in a famous instance had previously been able to observer the interior of a man's stomach through an opening caused by a healed wound.

New Developments in Imaging the Circulatory System

For many heart attack victims, the first symptom is death. Thus imaging the heart before the attack, and taking steps to forestall the attack, is an important part of medical practice.

A straightforward X ray of the heart can show whether or not it is enlarged, but not much else. Putting dyes that are opaque in the heart and exposing it to X rays, however, shows much more. The dyes make the coronary arteries show up and make any blockage of them visible on the film. The dyes are injected directly into the arteries that supply the heart with blood. This technique is called a coronary angiogram. About a million such angiograms are done each year in the U.S. One study reported in the November 11, 1992 *Journal of the American Medical Association* found that half the coronary angiograms performed were unnecessary, but many physicians disputed the claim, which was based on an analysis of 171 patients in the 1980s, mostly men and with an average age of 60.

Although the angiogram is an invasive procedure, and thus has some risk to the patient, the main objection to excess angiograms is the cost, ranging from $1500 to $5000 each.

A cheaper, noninvasive procedure was developed by a company called Imatron, founded by scientists from the University of California at San Francisco. The method uses an ultrafast CT scan, taken by X rays that are electronically rotated around the body (in conventional CT scans, the X ray emitter is rotated mechanically). The ultrafast scan takes images so fast that it captures the heart mid-beat. Also, it can pick up sharp images of any calcification of arteries. It is believed that calcification has a one-to-one correlation with atherosclerosis, the deposits of plaque that clog up arteries and cause heart failure or heart attacks (see "Heart Disease and Strokes UPDATE," p 400). While the new machine is expensive, most hospitals charge less than a third of the cost of a coronary angiogram for the ultrafast CT scan of the heart. Experts believe that the absence of calcium is a sure sign that there is no coronary heart disease, but that there has been too little experience so far with the new scans to be sure what the presence of calcium means for treatment, such as angioplasty or bypass operations.

Another new technique is little used so far because of its expense. Intravascular ultrasound consists of threading a tiny sound-producing and detecting device through the arteries and into the heart. Echoes inside the blood vessels can be used to detect plaque and to determine its consistency. While this method can detect conditions too subtle to show up on an angiogram, its main purpose is to determine whether or not balloon angioplasty will work or whether another method, such as laser angioplasty or a bypass operation, would be more successful.

Blood clots are dangerous in places other than just in the heart. When a blood clot is suspected in a vein, the traditional way to look for it is to use a venogram, essentially the same technique as a coronary angiogram—except that the dye is injected into a leg vein instead of a heart artery. Although reliable, the venogram is invasive and sometimes causes difficulties, including allergic reactions to the dye used. Late in the 1980s, the technique of ultrasound scanning was shown to be a good noninvasive alternative.

New Developments in Imaging the Fetus

Although ultrasound has other uses, such as inspecting the coronary arteries or veins in the leg, most people automatically think of fetal sonograms when they think of the method. Sonography is routine in some European countries and with many physicians in the U.S. But a study reported in the September 16, 1993 New England Journal of Medicine concluded that routine ultrasound scanning was of no value. After following 15,530 low-risk pregnancies (no bleeding, diabetes, high blood pressure, kidney abnormalities, or mother's age below 17) over a six-year period, the researchers found that the same rates of fetal defects occurred at birth whether or not ultrasound was used. There is thought to be virtually no damage caused as a result of ultrasound scanning—although there could be a slight risk from elevated temperatures caused by acoustic heating—so the principal concern here is the cost of making the procedure routine.

Early in the 1990s an invasive, but highly useful, alternative or supplement to ultrasound began to be used by a couple of physicians in the U.S. and one in France. The technique, called embryoscopy, uses a version of a device developed for examining the insides of coronary arteries. It can be inserted through the wall of the mother's abdomen and into the amniotic sac just as the needle used in amniocentesis is, making about the same sized hole and with about the same degree of risk. Among its advantages over ultrasound is that it can detect fetal malformations much earlier in pregnancy. Furthermore, it seems likely that the equipment can be adapted for use in fetal surgery.

New Developments in Magnetic Resonance Imaging

The result of a stroke when brain cells are being destroyed by a blood clot (about 85 percent of the instances) or a burst blood vessel (in the remaining 15 percent of strokes) can be observed by conventional MRI scanning. By then, however, it is too late to institute treatment that might limit the damage caused by the stroke. What is detected in such conventional magnetic resonance scanning is an image of water molecules that have leaked from the blood into the damaged areas of the brain—but it takes hours for enough water to leak to make the shape of the damaged area visible on an MRI scan. A new method, called diffusion-weighted MRI scanning, works on somewhat the same principle that Doppler radar uses to detect thundershowers. In diffusion-weighted MRI the movement of water molecules is tracked, not just their position. For unknown reasons, the speed at which water diffuses through the brain is slowed by a stroke, so slow moving molecules indicate where brain cells are dying. Instead of hours, results can be obtained in 15 or 20 minutes after a stroke.

An even better MRI version, called echo planar MRI scanning, uses brief pulses of magnetism to obtain images much faster than any previous equipment. This method can observe an entire brain, section by section, within a few seconds. A stroke can be observed while the damage is in the earliest stages. Medication exists that can limit damage of strokes provided the physician knows what the stage and location of the stroke is, so this information has therapeutic value as well as enabling physicians to understand strokes better.

In March 1993, a collaborating group of U.S. and British scientists announced in *Lancet* a new way to modify computer programs and frequencies used in MRI to image individual nerve cells within the body. The technique can screen out all the other tissue in which the nerves are embedded, even the sheaths around individual fibers in a bundle. One use of the new technique is expected to be locating pinched nerves, a major cause of pain that is hard to diagnose and also difficult to treat. Because the modifications of standard equipment are simple and cheap, this procedure should spread quickly.

Improving imaging is not the only concern for operators of MRI equipment. Because a person's whole body is put into a tube rather like a torpedo launcher on a submarine, where one is subjected from half of a hour to two hours to loud, strange noises from the operation of the magnets, the patient is frequently terrified during an

Background

Nearly all imaging methods depend on observation of electromagnetic radiation, which stretches from the long radio waves used in magnetic-resonance imaging to the short gamma rays involved in radioactive tracers and PET scans.

Ordinary X rays   Initially, bone was the only obvious tissue observed on X-ray photographs, although keen-eyed surgeons soon learned to obtain more information from the subtle shades of gray, finding tumors and spots on the lungs. Soon every small town across the U.S. and other industrialized nations had X-ray machines installed in shoe stores so that children and their parents could make sure that new shoes were not squeezing young bones. Dentists learned to find the details of previously hidden cavities.

In addition to being too penetrating to reveal soft tissues, the problem with X rays is that they cause much more damage than early scientists expected. X rays can induce cancer. When it became clear that X rays were damaging, the shoe store machines were withdrawn, and doctors and dentists learned to leave the room while an X ray was being taken.

X rays combined with opaque fluids   X rays were miraculous, but only fairly hard tissue showed up even as a different shade of gray. Within the first year of use for the new rays, clever doctors found fluids that are opaque to radiation, fluids that could be swallowed or injected or otherwise inserted into a desired region of the body. Stomach ulcers and colon cancers would be observed after a glass of chalky bismuth or barium solution or a barium enema. Dyes were injected into the circulatory system to reveal the interior of the heart (angiograms) or brain.

X rays combined with computers   Although the comic book hero Superman could focus his X-ray vision on details, medical X rays originally involved no discrimination whatsoever. Radiation passed through the body and collected on a flat piece of film or fluoroscope screen. Images from different planes within the body were merged into a single plane.

As early as 1917, however, mathematicians had shown that images from several different angles can be combined to give three-dimensional views. An early effort to accomplish something like this was made by Dutch radiologist Ziedes de Plantes. He used a moving X-ray source to obtain a single "slice" of the target. The mathematical method for building an image uses a large number of such slices to reconstruct the target object.

After World War II, the invention of powerful computers made mathematical reconstruction feasible. Several attempts to accomplish this were made in England, South Africa, and the U.S. Today this three-dimensional method, known as computed tomography (CT) scanning, has become a common diagnostic tool.

Radioactive tracers   Radioactivity was discovered in 1896 shortly after X rays. From the beginning, scientists knew that radioactivity also could be used to make photographs through opaque substances; indeed, that is how Antoine-Henri Becquerel discovered radioactivity. It was not until the 1930s, however, that doctors found ways to use radioactivity to see inside the body. Accelerators used for studying subatomic particles by then were producing radioactive versions of various familiar elements. The radioactive "tracer" was ingested or injected, and its progress through the body could be determined by measuring radioactivity through body tissues, even using the radioactive element to produce photographs.

Radioactive iodine has been used since the 1940s to observe the thyroid, which concentrates iodine. Some experiments in the 1940s and 1950s in using radioactive elements in living humans became controversial during the early 1990s when it was widely reported that many of the subjects of the first experiments were poorly informed or mentally unable to grasp the meaning of the experiments in which they were the subjects. Furthermore, a few experiments used extremely dangerous plutonium to find out what would happen to people who were exposed to the element.

Like X rays, radioactivity damages tissue. Both are frequently used to treat tumors as well as in diagnosis. As a treatment, they are focused on or placed in tumors to kill cancerous cells.

Thermography Instead of using high-frequency X rays or gamma rays, thermography uses low-frequency infrared radiation to observe the interior of the body. Generally the infrared radiation is produced from heated portions of the body itself. For example, blood is warmer than bone, so blood circulation can be observed to some degree with thermography. Images are fuzzy, however, because of the longer wavelengths involved. A frequent use for thermography is to locate a tumor by the extra blood that tumors often attract. Similarly, inflamed regions of the body, caused by immune reactions, are warmer than regions around them and can be detected by thermography.

Magnetic resonance imaging The CT scan produces better images than conventional X rays, but still uses damaging radiation. Another approach solved that problem and achieved more as well. Chemists found a way to make specific atoms or parts of molecules produce characteristic radio waves on demand. Weak radio waves and strong magnetic fields, used to induce the radio waves, are not generally thought to be harmful.

The essence of the method is to use powerful electromagnets to cause the nuclei of atoms to line up, somewhat the way that iron filings can be aligned by an ordinary horseshoe magnet. When the field is removed, the nuclei return to their normal disarray, in the process emitting radio waves at frequencies that vary depending on the particular nucleus and its state in a molecule.

In the early 1970s several inventors, notably Raymond Damadian, created machinery that could use this effect on whole human bodies. The result, now known as magnetic resonance imaging (MRI), reveals soft tissue that would not be otherwise observable. Medical doctors renamed the technique, known as nuclear magnetic resonance to chemists, out of fear that patients would think it had something to do with nuclear fission or fusion. Instead of involving such dangers, MRI provides the safest way to look inside the body.

MRI is especially favored for examining brain tissue for tumors, strokes, or changes caused by such diseases as multiple sclerosis or AIDS. It can also be used for images of softer tissues in any part of the body.

PET scans Some radioactive elements emit positrons, the antiparticles of the electron. When an electron and a positron combine, they vanish in a cloud of high-energy electromagnetism, similar to X rays but at a higher frequency (equivalently, at a shorter wavelength). Such electromagnetic waves are gamma rays. For a PET (Positron-Emission Tomography) scan, the positron-emitting radioactive element is put into a molecule of interest, such as glucose, which then can be traced as it moves through or concentrates in the body as the attendant gamma rays are being observed from outside the body. Such scans have been particularly helpful in imaging brain metabolism, suggesting which regions of the brain are active at a given moment.

Ultrasound Sonography is a method of obtaining images (called *sonograms*) that does not depend on electromagnetic radiation passing through the body. This technique based on high-frequency sound waves ("ultrasound") is thought to be remarkably safe and, unlike MRI, also inexpensive enough to be used routinely in a physician's office. The imaging devices emit high-frequency sounds because the higher the frequency, the sharper the image—which is true of all forms of imaging dependent on waves. Instead of reading waves that pass through the body, however, ultrasound devices usually use echoes from body parts. The most common use in the U.S. is for fetal examination. Nearly all pregnant women who are cared for by an obstetrician or gynecologist, or even who visit a clinic, have the position, progress, and even the sex of the fetus diagnosed by this method.

Each scan involves moving the sound emitter and receiver across the region to be observed. A series of scans may be used and analyzed in two-dimensional images by a computer, although the newest development combines scans in a computer to produce the kind of 3-D images more familiar from CT scanning.

MRI. Studies in 1993 showed that 35 percent of people being tested undergo panic attacks to some degree, while in one case out of ten the anxiety level is high enough for the exam to be postponed or dropped.

Among the ways physicians can cope with patient anxiety is to provide music chosen by the patient and directly piped into earphones; to provide special prism glasses that enable the patient to observe something outside the MRI tube or even to watch movies during the scan; and to use somewhat lower-quality open scanners for which the patient does not have to be inside a reasonable facsimile of a coffin.

And although MRI has been touted as the safest form of imaging, there are a few people who believe that this safety is illusory. The problem is not thought to be with the present generation of MRI scanners, but with new machines that are more powerful and that scan more rapidly. Higher magnetic fields improve the resolution of the images, while faster scanning has many benefits. Nevertheless, some patients claim to feel the effects of rapid switching of powerful magnetic fields, and some physicians think that these small effects could signal deeper trouble. Although the last scientific session on MRI safety was in 1991, before the new machines began to be used, the U.S. Food and Drug Administration has announced that it believes the new devices are safe.

New Ideas

A part of the electromagnetic spectrum that has been difficult to use for scanning inside the body is the part we are most familiar with, i.e., visible light. In 1991 scientists found a way to combine several ideas from lasers, holography, and interferometry so that visible light could reveal details beneath skin and muscle. The trick is to use a second beam that is adjusted to cause the scattered light of the first beam to be canceled. Unscattered light will pass through the skin and muscles to show what is underneath.

Although the question of who should obtain routine mammograms has been controversial (*see* "Breast Cancer," p 216), there is no doubt that many mammograms are needed and that the number is rising. Radiologists, who may screen a hundred mammograms before finding something suspicious, may miss the subtle clues. Philip Kegelmeyer has developed a computer program that uses digitized mammograms to point out areas that may need special attention. Early tests showed that it increased the ability of radiologists to locate breast cancers in mammograms by about ten percent.

(Periodical References and Additional Reading: *Harvard Health Letter* 1-90, p 2; *New York Times* 6-4-91; *New York Times* 8-16-92, p III-1; *New York Times* 8-23-92, p III-8; *New York Times* 11-11-92, p A16; *Science News* 1-9-93, p 28; *New York Times* 3-16-93, p C3; *New York Times* 4-6-93, p C1; *New York Times* 7-6-93, p C3; *Scientific American* 10-93, p 106; *New York Times* 11-3-93, p C16)

Diagnostic Tests

Regular medical check-ups are often recommended, especially for persons over the ages of 40 or 50. If you take the advice and get the check-up, here are some of the ways your doctor will examine you for disease and some of the things the doctor will be watching for. Also included are a few tests that are not part of a normal physical check-up, but which may be needed if certain diseases are detected. A few tests are specific to men or to women.

Name of Test	Test Procedure	What Can Be Learned
Ausculation	Physician listens to chest sounds with a stethoscope.	Physician can hear blood flowing through heart valves as well as heart beat; also, sounds of breathing can be used to observe fluid in lungs or other problems.
Biopsy	Tissue is removed with a needle or a punch or cut out of a suspicious growth anywhere on or in the body.	Examination of the tissue through a microscope can, with near perfect accuracy, detect the difference between a malignancy (cancer) and tissue that is abnormal for some other reason (a benign growth).
Blood Chemistry	Several cubic centimeters of blood are taken from a vein on the inside of your elbow.	The blood sample is separated and many different tests are run on the samples, of which for a healthy person the most important is to measure cholesterol in the blood; most of the common blood tests are described briefly below along with tests of chemicals found in urine.
Body Temperature	A thermometer is placed in the mouth, rectum, or under the arm for a minute or two.	Normal body temperature varies for several reasons (*see* "Surprise: Normal Temperature Isn't Normal," p 477); although patients most often connect high body temperature to infection, it can result from any process in which normal metabolism is speeded; a slight increase around ovulation is used in determining a fertile period in women.

Name of Test	Test Procedure	What Can Be Learned
Breast Examination	Doctor presses breasts between fingers (women).	Search for lumps that can be cancer; according to one large study, physician is able to identify nearly half the tumors present by this method alone, and almost 90 percent of lumps at least a centimeter in diameter; the American Cancer Society recommends that women over 40 have this done once every three years.
Chest X ray	Patient leans chest onto flat plate, while nurse or physician leaves room briefly.	Primary purpose is to observe any signs of lung damage from cancer or tuberculosis, but can also be used to spot enlarged heart or bone conditions.
CT (or CAT) Scan (for Computed Tomography or Computerized Axial Tomography)	Patient lies still on table while machine scans body or head.	Brain abnormalities or various abnormalities in the body are detected in 3-dimensional X-ray views.
Dilatation and Curettage (D&C)	Woman is anesthetized and scrapings are removed from her uterus.	Used to diagnose any of a number of gynecological problems, including cancer; also used sometimes as a method of abortion in early pregnancy.
Electrocardiogram (ECG or EKG)	Patient has several receptors placed on wrists, ankles, and chest that lead to machine.	Measures electrical activity in the heart; sometimes patient is also asked to exercise (Stress Test); many common heart defects can be recognized from this test, especially from changes in activity from year to year.
Electroencephalogram (EEG)	Patient has a couple of dozen sharp electrodes attached to scalp and by wires to a machine.	Measures several kinds of brain waves; abnormalities can signify epilepsy or other brain conditions such as trauma or tumors.
Fecal Occult Blood	Patient takes samples of stool at home over several days.	Stool samples are tested chemically for any small traces of blood; a positive test (indicating the presence of blood) can be caused by cancer of the colon or rectum; there are, however, many false positives caused by other sources of blood or by chemicals in some foods; a positive test only means that a direct examination of the colon with a colonoscope is called for; about 90 percent of the time, direct examination shows cancer is not present; furthermore, a negative test does not rule out cancer; despite such problems, the American College of Physicians (ACP) and the American Cancer Society (ACS) recommend such tests annually for persons over 50.
Fundoscopy	Physician shines a bright light into eyes and looks through lenses.	The region observed is the only place in the body where tiny blood vessels and a part of the brain (the optic disc) can be directly observed; especially useful in detecting diseases that affect the circulatory system, including diabetes and consequences of high blood pressure, as well as pressure on the brain.

Name of Test	Test Procedure	What Can Be Learned
Interview	Physician uses a checklist of possible changes to ask patient about symptoms.	Sometimes called the most important part of the examination because it reveals symptoms not obvious all the time and also informs physician of what to watch for during remainder of physical examination.
Mammography	Breasts are squeezed to nearly uniform thickness and X rays are taken of them (women).	Although sometimes painful, this test is not dangerous and reveals changes in breasts too small to be found by direct examination; there is good evidence that annual mammography for women over 50 reduces mortality, but evidence of benefits for younger women is controversial.
Palpation	Physician presses hand against abdomen below ribs and above pelvic bone; palpation of chest is to detect heart disease.	Physician can detect unusual lumps, size of organs such as liver, and hardness or softness; a painful reaction by the patient can indicate such diseases as peritonitis.
Pap Smear	Sample taken from cervix during pelvic examination (women).	Slides of cells are examined for abnormalities that can be cancerous or precursors of cancer.
Pelvic Examination	Patient lies on table with legs in stirrups; vagina is held open with a speculum (women).	Physician is feeling for abnormalities of the uterus or ovaries; light is used to look at cervix and vaginal walls.
Percussing	Two fingers are placed on chest and tapped with fingers of other hand.	Hollow sounds may indicate emphysema; location of heart and heart beat also checked by tapping chest.
Sigmoidoscopy	Patient lies on examining table while physician inserts an instrument through the anus and into the rectum; some air is pumped into the intestines during this procedure.	A lighted tube allows the doctor to examine the lower part of the rectum and colon for cancer or other conditions; although the test is expensive and somewhat uncomfortable, studies have shown that such a screening even as seldom as once a decade in persons over 50 can substantially reduce death from cancer of the colon or rectum; both the ACP and ACS suggest this test every three to five years for persons over 50.
Sphygmomanometry	Cuff pumped up around arm.	How well your heart is working by measuring your blood pressure, which is expressed as two numbers given in the same order (verbally expressed as "over" although they are not parts of a fraction). A pressure of 120 over 80 is about right for most people. Higher numbers, especially above 160 or 95, can signal heart attack or stroke risk, kidney disease, or damage to the eyes. Very low blood pressure is mostly a sign of danger in the event of other illnesses, such as accidental injury or massive infections.

Name of Test	Test Procedure	What Can Be Learned
Spinal Tap (Also known as Spinal Puncture or Lumbar Puncture)	Needle is inserted into lumbar region of back and spinal fluid removed.	Fluid reveals damage to brain or spinal cord caused by disease or trauma.
Urinalysis	Patient urinates into a cup.	Like the blood, urine is separated into several samples that are tested chemically; the urine and blood tests are outlined below.

CHEMICAL TESTS (BLOOD AND URINE)

Substance tested	Expected levels	Comments
Albumin	3.70 to 4.70 gm/dL	Protein that, along with gamma globulins, forms blood plasma.
Albumin/globulins ratio	1.10 to 2.00	Ratio of albumin to globulins can be too low in liver disease.
Alk. phosphatase	35.0 to 145 units/L	Enzyme that, when levels are elevated, can indicate any of several different conditions, though higher levels are often a side effect of medication.
Bilirubin (direct)	0.00 to 0.20 mg/dL	Waste product from normal breakdown of red blood cells; the direct form results from action by the liver and may be detected in either blood or urine.
Bilirubin (total)	0.30 to 1.40 mg/dL	Total bilirubin and direct bilirubin both increase as a result of liver disease or gallstones, as well as a side effect of several drugs; the yellow color of bilirubin results in the symptom known as yellow jaundice (when skin and whites of the eyes develop a yellow cast).
BUN	9.00 to 26.0 mg/dL	Stands for "Blood Urea Nitrogen"; a high BUN may indicate kidney disease.
Calcium	8.70 to 10.0 mg/dL	Both low and high levels can indicate any of a number of conditions, ranging from osteoporosis (high) to inactive parathyroid glands (low).
Chloride	95.0 to 107 mmol/L	Electrolyte
Cholesterol	150 to 249 mg/dL	Many physicians believe that levels between 150 to 200 protect against heart disease.
Cholesterol rank	1.00 to 75.0 percentile	A rank of 40 means that 40 percent of the population has a lower cholesterol level than you do.
Creatinine	0.80 to 1.40 mg/dL	A measure of kidney function; can also be measured in urine; high blood levels and low urine levels indicate poor kidney performance.
Globulin	2.20 to 3.50 gm/dL	Proteins in the blood other than albumin; of four types, gamma globulin is best known, since it consists of antibodies to infection.

Substance tested	Expected levels	Comments
Glucose	65.0 to 115 mg/dL	Carbohydrates are converted into glucose, so test measures ability of body to metabolize carbohydrates; a high level may indicate diabetes or other hormonal diseases, while a low level can be called hypoglycemia.
HCT (Hemocrit)	39.0 to 52.0 percent	Percent of blood volume occupied by cells (mostly red blood cells); low levels indicate anemia.
HDL cholesterol	39.0 to 79.0 mg/dL	HDL means "high-density lipoprotein"; HDL cholesterol is nicknamed "good cholesterol" since it is necessary for health and prevents, rather than causes, heart disease. A ratio of HDL cholesterol to low-density (LDL) cholesterol higher than four is considered beneficial even when total cholesterol is high.
HGB (Hemoglobin)	13.2 to 17.7 gm/dL	Low levels indicate anemia.
Iron	50.0 to 160 mcg/dL	Low levels mean anemia; high levels may be involved in heart disease.
LDH (Lactic dehydrogenase)	104 to 250 IU/L or 200-600 IU/L	High levels often indicate that a heart attack has taken place or that there has been other tissue or cell damage; different expected levels represent different types of measurement used from lab to lab.
Lymphocytes	1049 to 3581 mm^3	About a fourth of the white blood cells are lymphocytes, classed into B cells and T cells; a subclass of T cells is killed by the HIV virus that causes AIDS.
Magnesium	1.40 to 2.10 meq/L	Low levels may indicate a hormone deficiency, while high levels may occur after a heart attack.
MCH (mean corpuscular hemoglobin)	27.0 to 33.0 PG	A red-blood-cell index used in diagnosing anemia.
MCHC (mean corpuscular hemoglobin concentration)	31.0 to 37.0 percent	A red-blood-cell index used in diagnosing anemia.
MCV (mean corpuscular volume)	84 to 105 fl	A red-blood-cell index used in diagnosing anemia.
Phosphate	2.20 to 4.20 mg/dL	Used to measure phosphorus in blood; high levels occur in kidney disease or vitamin D deficiency as well as in rarer conditions.
Platelets	140 to 440 1000/mm^3	Platelets are small bodies in the blood that are important in forming clots.
Potassium	3.50 to 5.30 mmol/L	Electrolyte; high levels in blood may indicate kidney or liver disease (usually accompanied by low levels in urine).

Substance tested	Expected levels	Comments
Prostate specific antigen (PSA)	0.50 to 4.00 mcg/L	High levels suggest the need for additional testing for the possibility of prostate cancer.
Prostatic acid Phos.	0.00 to 2.50 mcg/L	High levels suggest the need for additional testing for the possibility of prostate cancer.
Protein (in blood)	6.30 to 7.90 gm/dL	
Red blood cells	4.30 to 5.80 $1,000,000/mm^3$	High values may indicate kidney diseases or lung problems, while low values are the main indicator of anemia; low values also occur during malaria.
Sodium	134 to 144 mmol/L	Electrolyte; high values may suggest endocrine disorders, while low values are associated with diabetes.
Transferrin Sat.	15.0 to 50 percent	A measure of iron-binding, it can be useful in identifying iron-deficiency anemia.
TR4 as thyroxine	4.50 to 12.5 mcg/dL	High and low levels indicate thyroid function.
Triglycerides	50.0 to 200 mg/dL	Triglycerides are the main way that dietary fat is carried in the blood, so high levels may contribute to heart disease and possibly to some forms of cancer.
Uric acid	3.40 to 8.70 mg/dL	High levels indicate gout.
White blood cells	4.00 to 10.9 $1000/mm^3$	Important in determining the presence of an infection and its severity.

NEW TOOLS:
THE STATE OF SURGERY

Surgery has to one degree or another been separate from internal medicine throughout most of human history, even when practiced by the same individuals. In the middle ages in Europe, surgeons were held in low regard, whether they were barber-surgeons or surgeon-apothecaries. In recent times, however, surgery has been viewed as the apex of the medical profession, requiring more training and skill than most other specialties. At some point in the post-World War II period, the situation changed from "They have to operate—he must be at death's door" to "They think they can operate, so he has a chance." In other words, it came to be felt that surgery was a safe and effective way of producing a cure, while internal medicine and other forms of treatment (radiation, for example) were merely adjuncts to surgery. Patients too sick for heart transplants or removal of a lung or intervention in the brain or a coronary bypass would be expected to die from their disease, while patients undergoing surgery were given a good chance of survival.

Surgery is perhaps not quite as exalted as its reputation, but nevertheless surgeons have made great strides in recent years and continue to do so.

New Devices and Materials

The invention of devices such as the obstetrical forceps (a closely guarded secret for years) and development of materials such as sutures that are eventually absorbed by the body are ways that surgery has progressed over the last few centuries. Here are some of the surgical improvements of the early 1990s:

Artificial bone grafts The Collagraft Bone Graft Substitute is intended to be used as a scaffolding between parts of a fracture so that bone cells will have something on which to grow. It is a mixture of a ceramic that is slowly dissolved by the body and collagen, a natural protein found in bone.

Carpal tunnel-plasty The carpal tunnel syndrome is a repetitive stress injury in the wrist and hand that causes ligaments to thicken, which then press on the nerve and tendons running into the palm through a passage known as the carpal tunnel. Surgery involves cutting the ligament and perhaps cleaning out the tunnel to make more room. J. Lee Berger of St. Joseph's Hospital and Medical Center in Patterson, New Jersey, has developed a device that inserts a small balloon under the ligament. When the balloon is inflated, it raises and stretches the ligament, relieving the pressure on the nerves and tendons. Unlike traditional surgery, this procedure can be repeated if needed—or the ligament can then be cut.

Cataract knife sheath About 1.35 million cataract operations are performed in the U.S. each year, and cataract surgery is the most common operation for persons over the age of 65. In 1991 surgeons discovered that by using a small tunnel to get to the lens, it was possible to do cataract surgery without stitches. Fluid pressure from within the eye would seal the tunnel, so long as the opening was well shaped and not nicked. But this happens only 30 percent of the time; the rest of the time a slip of the knife as it passes through the tunnel destroys the sealing ability. Self-sealing, stitchless cataract surgery is highly desirable since healing takes place within ten days instead of taking four to six weeks. In 1993 Alexander Eaton of Fort Myers, Florida, developed a plastic sheath that goes around the knife while it is in the tunnel, making it almost impossible for the knife to cut into the tunnel wall.

Cryogenic surgery   Dermatologists have long used the extreme cold of liquid nitrogen to destroy warts or even skin cancers. Since July, 1992 a device has been available commercially that can be used to attack cancers and other conditions deep in the body with freezing cold, a technique called cryosurgery. In the February 1991 *Cell*, Gary M. Onik of Allegheny General Hospital in Pittsburgh, Pennsylvania, reported that he had used an experimental version of the device to operate on liver cancers that had been deemed inoperable by conventional methods. Of the first 18 patients, five lived for more than two years after cryosurgery and appeared to be in complete remission, while all of the others lived a year or so longer than had been expected without the surgery. Soon the cryosurgery device was being applied to prostate cancer and on enlarged prostate, cutting costs in half, shortening hospital stays, and protecting nearby organs from damage (with warm catheters). Ultrasound is used to position the freezing tip of the device, which is called an Accuprobe. Experiments have begun on using Accuprobe freezing on other cancers, including lung and brain cancer.

Glues   Sewing even a small patch of skin onto a visible part of the body, such as the face, can lead to unwelcome scars. In 1990 some surgeons began to glue patches of skin in place instead of sewing it. The key is that the glue used is made from the patient's blood. The glue is called fibrin, and is made from fibrinogen taken from the blood and combined with two other proteins. After five or six days, the blood supply to the skin patch is restored by the body and the glue is carried away in the blood. There are no scars.

A different organic glue, a green dye mixed with proteins and sugars, acts like Krazy Glue in repairing parts of the eye or even in brain surgery. Among its advantages is that instead of causing bleeding as conventional surgery does, gluing temporarily seals off blood vessels. The glue is dried on the spot with a laser (which is why the glue is dyed green, to absorb the wavelength of laser light used). As the wound heals, the organic proteins and sugars are absorbed by the body.

Modular knee caps and joints   Modular knee replacements, made from titanium alloy, cobalt alloy, or polyethylene, are now available in six sizes, which can be mixed or matched to replace any damaged knee. The three main parts are a femoral component to replace the end of the large single bone in the upper leg; a tibial component to connect the new knee to the lower leg; and the patella, or kneecap. There are also various small parts that are used in putting the whole gadget together.

Robot surgeons   Several firms around the world have produced either passive robotic arms (used for positioning instruments for human surgeons) or full robotic surgical arms. The robots are used mainly for finely controlled work in brain surgery or for procedures that require such mechanical operations as drilling in bone. Thus far, robots are largely an adjunct to human surgery, however.

Scar prevention   British surgeons have demonstrated in animals that scar tissue can be prevented by counteracting a cytokine called transforming growth factor beta, types 1 and 2, substances that affect collagen. Too much of the growth factors, a condition that typically occurs in adults as a response to injury, promotes the formation of permanent scars. A third cytokine, transforming growth factor beta, type 3, works to prevent scarring. The first two types can be neutralized with monoclonal antibodies against them, while a genetically engineered or synthetic version of type 3 is injected into the wound. The trick has yet to be tried on humans, but it is quite effective on mice.

Stomach staples   In 1991 a panel of the U.S. National Institutes of Health endorsed procedures for stapling up the wall of the stomach in obese patients. The reduced stomach volume was shown to be a significant aid in lowering weight. The operation even suppresses the patient's appetite before eating, although why this happens is not known. Although the truly obese seldom reach an "ideal" weight from the procedure, they do lose enough to escape the worst medical consequences of obesity (*see* "Weight and Health," p 144).

Virtual bodies   Surgeons often have difficulty finding subjects upon whom to practice before developing surgical skills. Some work is done with cadavers. Surgery on animals such as pigs or dogs is sometimes used. Watching other surgeons is important, but does not do the trick. Now several organizations have developed computer-assisted virtual reality in which surgeons can practice and even make mistakes without harm. This technique has been used most often with laparoscopy, in which the surgeon regularly works by watching a monitor and not by looking directly at the body.

New Trends: The Laparoscopic Revolution

Real laparoscopy is fast becoming the norm for certain kinds of operations. But in most cases, long-term studies have not been conducted on patient survival and other measures of effectiveness for all the applications of laparoscopy. Laparoscopic surgery is conducted through at least two small incisions through the skin and usually through the wall of the abdomen or chest. One or more incisions permit long narrow tools to be inserted, the tools that actually cut, staple, and remove. Another incision is for the laparoscope itself, a combined light and camera on a stick. The laparoscope both lights the scene and conveys an image of what is going on to the monitor, which the surgeon watches to guide the instruments. In general, laparoscopic surgery produces less pain and faster healing, both as a result of the smallness of the incisions (often called "postage-stamp" incisions). It is more expensive than conventional surgery, however.

Laparoscopy began as a technique in gynecology. In the late 1980s it was adapted to gall-bladder surgery and went into a boom phase. In the April 18, 1991 *New England Journal of Medicine* a detailed analysis showed that the rate of complications was less for laparoscopic surgery than for traditional gall-bladder surgery. Today 80 to 90 percent of gall-bladder operations in the U.S. are performed using laparoscopic techniques.

As surgeons learned the technique they came to apply it to different types of operations. Laparoscopic hernia repairs and appendectomies soon became common. Although some physicians now perform almost all surgical procedures using laparoscopic techniques, others await the outcome of controlled, long-term studies on results. It is not clear, for example, whether or not there is much or any advantage to a laparoscopic appendectomy, which produces about the same amount of scarring as conventional surgery for this operation, may not reduce pain or length of hospital stay, and costs much more than traditional methods.

New Trends: Outpatient Surgery

In the 1970s almost 90 percent of all surgical procedures were conducted in hospitals and involved a stay of at least one night ("inpatient" operations). Throughout the 1980s and into the 1990s, there has been a steady increase in the number of surgical procedures that are performed on patients who then go home ("outpatient" operations) instead of staying overnight or longer in hospital. In 1990 for the first time the number of outpatient surgical procedures in community hospitals in the U.S. exceeded the number of inpatient operations. At the rate of growth in the early 1990s, perhaps as much as 70 percent of all surgical procedures will be handled on an outpatient basis by the beginning of the twenty-first century. Among the procedures often performed on an outpatient basis in the early 1990s were breast biopsies, tonsillectomies, knee surgery, hernia repair, gall-bladder removal, cosmetic surgery, vasectomies and tubal ligations, and hemorrhoid and cataract removal. It is no coincidence that some of these procedures are the very ones for which the incidence of laparoscopic surgery is rising. Costs of hospital stays have also been a factor in the rise of outpatient surgery. Because of the new emphasis, hospitals are building special wings solely devoted to outpatient surgery.

A study in the September 22, 1993 *Journal of the American Medical Association* of outpatient surgery at the Mayo Clinic in Rochester, Minnesota, showed that possibly fatal complications were very low—0.000007 percent of the 45,090 operations included in the study. About a third of all postoperative complications occurred well after the patient had returned home, however. Careful home monitoring of symptoms and a quick return to the surgeon for additional care is essential. It is considered necessary that a person other than the patient be present for the first night after surgery. Surgeons at the Mayo Clinic may be better trained than those at many small hospitals, so results are not necessarily comparable.

New Trends in Heart Surgery

Heart surgery for all practical purposes was nonexistent before the mid-1930s, when pioneering work by John Gibbon and Alexis Carrel produced the necessary tools and procedures. After World War II the heart surgeon became (along with the brain surgeon) one of the elite practioners of medicine. By the 1970s the coronary artery bypass grafting operation (often just called bypass surgery) entered widespread use. Today heart surgery is one of the most common procedures in the U.S., with perhaps 400,000 coronary bypass operations annually as well as valve replacements, installation of pacemakers, removal of arrhythmic circuits, balloon or laser angioplasty, and surgery connected with angiograms (*see* "Imaging UPDATE," p 485), not to mention heart transplants (*see* "Organ Transplant Proliferation and Problems," p 505).

For a time, it appeared that the future of heart surgery was in the artificial heart, but in 1990 the U.S. Food and Drug Administration banned the common variety of artificial heart then in use because of mechanical problems. (It could still be used in emergencies, although that did not happen.) In any case, the main virtue of the artificial heart of any type thus far developed seems to be in keeping a patient alive until an organ transplant is possible. The first such use of an artificial heart was in 1985, and the patient, after nine days on the artificial heart, got a transplant and lived for four and a half years. After 1990 it was not until 1993 that a patient had an artificial heart implanted, and the goal was once again to keep the patient alive until an organ transplant could be arranged. The artificial heart, made by the CardioWest corporation, was based on the same technology as the Jarvik heart that had been banned in 1990.

After a false start, a device similar to the well-known Roto-Rooter was approved for use in human leg veins (at the end of 1992) and in coronary-artery angioplasty (in June 1993). The Rotoblater system uses a diamond-coated burr that spins at 190,000 rpm inside a vein or artery, removing plaque instead of merely shoving it aside as is done in balloon angioplasty.

One problem with balloon angioplasty (and to a lesser degree with other forms of angioplasty) is that the arteries reclose after the operation about 40 percent of the time. In the early 1990s the U.S. Food and Drug Administration approved the use of small metal coils to keep the arteries open. These coils are called "stents." Studies released in November 1993 found that the stents prevent such reclosure about a third of the time, reducing the overall rate of closing up after balloon angioplasty to about 13 percent. The main problem with the stents so far has been bleeding associated with blood thinners that need to be used during application. In 1994, studies began using stents that were coated with blood thinner before application in the hopes that this will be safer.

Animal tests have suggested that another approach, using a polymer to form a sort of internal cast in the artery, is also effective. Furthermore, after the artery has recovered from the angioplasty, the polymer cast gradually dissolves and disappears.

Clogging of arteries after bypass surgery is also a problem, though it may take years for it to develop. One study, completed in 1992, showed that after about 20 years there was no difference in death rate between heart patients who had bypass surgery and those who were treated with drugs, although the bypass patients all did better in the first years after the operation than did the drug-treated patients.

(Periodical References and Additional Reading: *New York Times* 12-4-90; *New York Times* 1-29-91, p D1; *New York Times* 3-28-91, p B12; *New York Times* 4-10-91, p D9; *Harvard Health Letter* 3-92, p 1; *New York Times* 7-1-92, p C12; *New York Times* 7-19-92, p III-9; *New York Times* 11-22-92, p III-9; *New York Times* 1-13-92, p A14; *Harvard Health Letter* 2-93, p 8; *New York Times* 2-26-93, p A15; *New York Times* 6-3-93, p D10; *New York Times* 6-7-93, p D2; *New York Times* 6-14-93, p D2; *New York Times* 9-14-93, p C3; *New York Times* 10-25-93, p D2; *New York Times* 11-12-93, p A24; *New York Times* 12-14-93, p C3)

TIMETABLE OF SURGERY TO 1990

2500 BC	Egyptian carvings from this time show a surgical operation in progress.
1550 BC	The Edwin Smith Surgical Papyrus is written, although it appears to be a copy of a manuscript written about 2500 BC; the papyrus is a scientific treatise on surgery.
100	Surgery is used to remove breast cancer in Alexandria about this time.
1050	Albacasis, a Muslim living in Spain, writes the only known Arabic discussion of

surgery from this period; in Latin translation the book is influential on Europe in the Middle Ages.

1240   A decree of the Holy Roman Empire permits the dissection of human cadavers.

1275   William of Saliceto writes a comprehensive surgical text, reviving the use of the scalpel and describing case histories of patients in Bologna, where he taught.

1319   The first recorded case of body snatching (procurement of buried bodies for medical dissection) is prosecuted.

1320   Henri de Mondeville's *Chirurgia* (Surgery) advocates sutures and cleansing of wounds.

1460   Heinrich von Pfolspeundt writes *Bündt-Ertzney*, the first book on surgery to be published in Germany.

1490   An "anatomical theater" is opened in Padua by A. Benedetti da Legnano for demonstrating the dissection of corpses.

1505   The Royal College of Surgeons of Edinburgh is chartered.

1540   English barbers and surgeons are united as the "Commonality of the Barbers and Surgeons."

1549   An anatomical theater is established in Padua (Italy).

1584   Walter Raleigh introduces curare to England from South America.

1655   Johann Shultes' *Armamentarium chirugicum* (The Hardware of the Surgeon) describes a procedure for removing a female breast.

1666   Richard Lower [born Cornwall, England, circa 1631; died London, January 17, 1691] demonstrates the direct transfusion of blood between two dogs.

1697   Jacques de Beaulieu, known as Frère Jacques, develops a new method for removing bladder stones that, with various refinements, becomes the main technique used in the West during the 18th century.

1728   Giovanni Lancisi's posthumously published *De motu cordis et aneurysmatibus* discusses heart dilatation.

1731   The Royal Academy of Surgery is founded in Paris, France.

1736   Claudius Aymand performs the first successful operation for appendicitis.

1788   French surgeon Pierre-Joseph Desault [born Magny-Vernois, France, February 6, 1744; died Paris, June 1, 1795] is appointed surgeon-major to the Hôtel Dieu, where he becomes famous for teaching improved surgical techniques and for improvements in instruments used in surgery.

1793   John Hunter is the first to ligate the femoral artery for treatment of aneurysm.

1800   Humphry Davy [born Penzance, England, December 17, 1778; died Geneva, Switzerland, May 29, 1829] discovers nitrous oxide ("laughing gas") on April 9 and suggests its use as an anesthetic.

In England the Royal College of Surgeons is founded in London.

1822   The first successful hysterectomy is performed.

1824   Henry Hickman [born England, 1800; died 1830] uses carbon dioxide on an animal as a general anesthetic.

1825   Pierre Bretonneau [born St. Georges-sur-Cher, France, April 3, 1778; died Passy, France, February 18, 1862] successfully performs the first tracheotomy to restore breathing to a child suffering from croup.

1830	Physiologist Marshall Hall [born Basford, England, February 18, 1790; died Brighton, England, August 11, 1857] denounces bloodletting as a treatment for disease.
1831	Chemist and physician Samuel Guthrie [born Brimfield, Massachusetts, 1782; died Sackets Harbor, New York, October 19, 1848] discovers chloroform.
1832	Codeine is discovered.
	The Warburton Anatomy Act legalizes the sale of bodies for dissection in England, ending the practice of body snatching and sometimes murder to provide bodies.
1841	Charles Thomas Jackson [born Plymouth, Massachusetts, June 21, 1805; died Somerville, Massachusetts, August 28, 1880] discovers that ether is an anesthetic.
1842	The first use of ether in surgery is by Crawford Williamson Long [born Danielsville, Georgia, November 1, 1815; died Athens, Georgia, June 16, 1878] on March 30, but lack of publication allows credit for the discovery to go to William Morton in 1846; Long publishes his own results in 1849.
1844	Charles Thomas Jackson suggests to dentist William Thomas Green Morton the use of ether to deaden pain.
	Horace Wells [born Hartford, Connecticut, January 21, 1815; died New York, January 24, 1848] is the first to use nitrous oxide as an anesthetic in dentistry.
1846	William Thomas Morton [born Charlton City, Massachusetts, August 9, 1819; died New York, April 2, 1872] uses ether as an anesthetic during operations as advised by Charles Jackson, who discovered that ether is an anesthetic.
	Sir James Simpson [born Bathgate, Scotland, June 7, 1811; died London, May 6, 1870] discovers that chloroform is a better anesthetic than ether or nitrous oxide; he starts the use of chloroform in childbirth. In 1847 his *Account of a New Anesthetic Agent* describes his discovery.
1856	Karl Friedrich Wilhelm Ludwig is the first to keep animal organs alive outside the body, which he does by pumping blood through them.
1859	German chemist Albert Niemann isolates cocaine from the leaves of *Erythroxylon coca*; the stimulant properties of cocaine had long been known to natives of South America, and Europeans had learned of them after their conquest of the Inca empire.
1881	Alexander Graham Bell invents two types of metal detectors for locating bullets in the human body; one type, the induction balance, is used on President Garfield when he is assassinated.
1884	Czech-American surgeon Carl Koller [born Schüttenhofen, Bohemia (now Czech Republic), December 3, 1857; New York, died March 21, 1944] uses cocaine as a local anesthetic.
1885	Swiss surgeon Emil Theodor Kocher [born August 25, 1841; died July 27, 1917] develops surgical removal of the thyroid as a cure for goiter.
1890	Surgeons at Johns Hopkins Hospital in Baltimore, Maryland, begin using rubber gloves during surgery.
1893	American surgeon Daniel Williams [born Holidaysburg, Pennsylvania, January 28, 1858; died August 4, 1931] performs the first open-heart surgery on a patient injured by a knife wound.

1896	Johannes von Mikulisz-Radecki invents the gauze mask to be worn by surgeons when performing surgery.
1904	Albert Einhorn synthesizes procaine, also known as Novocaine, a local anesthetic that is the first usable substitute for the use of cocaine in medicine.
1905	The first modern instance of the transplant of an animal organ into a human takes place, without success.
	Alexis Carrel [born Lyon, France, June 28, 1873; died Paris November 5, 1944], working at the Rockefeller Institute in New York City, develops techniques for rejoining severed blood vessels, paving the way for organ transplantation.
1905	George Washington Crile [born Chile, Ohio, November 11, 1864; died January 7, 1943] performed the first direct blood transfusion.
1913	German surgeon A. Salomen develops mammography for diagnosing breast cancer.
1914	Alexis Carrel performs the first successful heart surgery on a dog.
1917	The natural anticoagulant heparin is discovered.
1921	C. O. Nylen and G. Holmgren introduce microsurgery using the operating microscope they invented.
1924	Acetylene is used as an anesthetic.
1935	John Gibbon [born Philadelphia, Pennsylvania, September 29, 1903] and his wife develop the first prototype of the heart-lung machine.
1936	Alexis Carrel, working with Charles A. Lindbergh, develops a form of artificial heart that was used during cardiac surgery.
	Ernest H. Volwiler and Donalee L. Tabern formulate sodium pentothal, used for inducing hypnotic sleep as a preparation for full anesthesia for surgery and also known as "truth serum" because of the state of suggestibility it induces.
1938	English surgeon Philip Wiles develops the first total artificial hip replacement, using stainless steel.
1944	Alfred Blalock [born Culloden, Georgia, April 5, 1899; died Baltimore, Maryland, September 15, 1964] and Helen Brooke Taussig [born Cambridge, Massachusetts, May 24, 1898; died May 20, 1986] perform the first "blue baby" operation, correcting blood supply to the lungs of a female infant.
1951	American surgeon John H. Gibbon, Jr., develops the heart-lung machine.
1952	The world's first sex-change operation is performed on George Jorgenson, who becomes known to the world by the post-change name of Christine.
1953	Surgeon John H. Gibbon, Jr., uses his heart-lung machine to keep Cecelia Bavoleck alive while he repairs a leak in her heart.
	The first kidney transplant is performed in Paris; the graft fails after 21 days because of rejection.
	In one of the first successful organ transplants and the first uses of near-fetal tissue, Julian Sterling of Philadelphia, Pennsylvania, successfully transplants the thyroid and parathyroid glands from a newborn, but doomed, baby into a 29-year-old woman; because the tissue came from a newborn whose immune system had not developed, this operation was the first such to succeed.
1960	John Charnley implants a two-part joint replacement made of plastic and cobalt-chrome.

1962	Lasers are used in eye surgery for the first time.
1963	A man has the kidney of a chimpanzee transplanted into him in an operation at Tulane Medical School in New Orleans, Louisiana; he survives for nine months.
1963	James Daniel Hardy performs the first lung transplant.
	Thomas Starzl [born Le Mans, Iowa, March 11, 1926] and Francis Moore [born Evanston, Illinois, August 17, 1913] perform the first liver transplant.
1967	Surgeon Christiaan Neething Barnard [born Beaufort, South Africa, November 8, 1922] performs the first partially successful human heart transplant December 3; the recipient of the new heart is Louis Washkansky, who lives for 18 days.
1967	Cleveland surgeon Rene Favaloro develops the coronary bypass operation.
1968	Christiaan Neething Barnard performs a second human heart transplant; this time the patient, Philip Blaiberg, lives 74 days with his new heart.
1969	In Texas, Denton Cooley [born Houston, Texas, August 22, 1920] and Domingo Liotta replace the diseased heart of Haskell Karp with the first artificial heart to be used in a human being; Karp lives for nearly three days.
1971	In the United Kingdom, the diamond-bladed scalpel is introduced.
1976	The basic law regulating surgical implants in the U.S. is passed; it allows equipment makers to sell products without lengthy government testing or reviews, provided that the implants are substantially similar to devices already in use. One result is that surgical implants are inserted into humans with very little testing for long-term safety.
1977	Andreas R. Gruentzig [born Dresden, Germany, June 25, 1939; died October 27, 1985] invents balloon angioplasty, a method for unclogging diseased arteries.
1978	Alden H. Harken, Mark E. Josephson, and Leonard H. Horowitz devise a surgical procedure that successfully treats cardiac arrhythmia.
1982	A team of doctors led by William DeVries [born Brooklyn, New York, December 19, 1943] implants the first Jarvik 7 artificial heart on December 2; the patient, Barney Clark, lives 112 days. Patrick Walsh devises a new operation for prostate cancer that is generally successful in avoiding impotence, a common side effect of previous surgical treatments for the disease.
1983	The immunosuppressant cyclosporine is approved by the United States Food and Drug Administration, making transplants of organs much safer than they had been previously.
1985	Lasers are used in the United States for the first time to clean out clogged arteries.

ORGAN TRANSPLANT PROLIFERATION AND PROBLEMS

The modern history of organ transplantation begins in 1953, although regular and confirmed successes were not easily obtained until 30 years later when the immune suppressor cyclosporine became available.

Kidney transplants were a popular first choice. People have two kidneys and only need one, but people *really* need at least one kidney. If the second one fails, it means either an unsatisfactory and moderately unhealthy life on dialysis, a kidney transplant, or death.

A lot can go wrong with a kidney, but it seldom happens suddenly, so there is time to plan for a transplant. Furthermore, a living relative can donate a kidney, providing a better immune match and a healthier kidney than can usually be obtained from a cadaver (by about ten percent, according to one estimate). Kidney transplants even from cadavers are still the most successful transplant operations, with over 90 percent of patients surviving more than a year after the transplant. As a result, kidney transplants accounted for over seven-tenths of all organ transplants in the early 1990s.

Many of the remaining three-tenths of transplants involve the heart. Heart transplants are no longer front-page news, mainly because they are now predominantly successful. In the late 1960s the first two heart transplant recipients survived fewer than 100 days each after the operation. Today the one-year survival rate for heart transplants is about 90 percent. In 1994 one transplant survivor, Dirk van Zyl, died at the age of 68, from an unrelated stroke. He had lived 23 years since becoming the sixth transplant patient of Christiaan Barnard, the South African pioneer surgeon. There are about 3500 heart transplants annually around the world, with most of them performed in the U.S.

Other organs have become additional transplant success stories, including the pancreas, the liver, and lungs. Sometimes two organs are easier to transplant than one — hearts and lungs go together, for example. In 1988, a combined liver-small intestine transplant was the first successful small-intestine transplant. By 1991 the first successful series transplants of the small intestine were announced by the University of Pittsburgh. All five recipients in the series had shortened small intestines, although the causes for the "short-gut syndrome" varied. The first operation in the series, in May 1990, produced the first instance of a transplant of a small intestine by itself. The Pittsburgh team credited the successful series to the then experimental immune suppressor FK506.

The chances of a one-year survival after an organ transplant were calculated by the United Network for Organ Sharing based on data from the late 1980s. Except for kidneys, the source of the organ was not indicated.

SURVIVAL RATE AFTER ORGAN TRANSPLANTS

Organ	Survival of recipient (one year or more)	Survival of organ (one year or more)
Kidneys (from live donors)	97%	91%
Kidneys (from cadavers)	92%	81%
Pancreas	89%	71%
Heart	83%	82%
Liver	76%	69%
Lung*	48%	57%
Heart-lung combination*	57%	48%

* Based on a very small number of donors.

The survival figures were much higher than for earlier periods (in the 1970s only 30 percent of liver transplant recipients survived a year, for example). Thus it can be presumed that there was additional improvement for these percentages in the early 1990s. About 16,000 U.S. transplants take place each year; because of multiple organ donations, there are only about 4500 donors.

A Shortage of Organs

In 1993 there were about 20,000 people in the U.S. who hoped to obtain kidney transplants. Kidneys from cadavers become available at a rate of about 7500 a year, not enough to catch up, as new potential recipients are also added to the list each year. Some of the gap is made up by living relatives of potential recipients. In the early 1990s, these relatives donated about 2300 kidneys each year. In a few cases, friends offer to donate their kidneys.

In India, Egypt, and other developing countries, the shortage of kidneys and the ability of a healthy person to give up one kidney and live has led to an aggressive trade in kidneys for donation. In India in 1992 a kidney could bring $1000 or more to the selling donor, a large sum in a poor country. The ethics of the spare organ trade bother many people, and most nations have tried to suppress the sale of kidneys. For the most part, however, suppression merely moves kidney sales onto the black market and raises prices all along the line.

Another approach to improving organ supply is being tried by the Regional Organ Bank of the University of Illinois. When a person with a healthy kidney dies suddenly, the Illinois Organ Bank perfuses the abdomen with a preserving fluid. After a few hours or a day or two, the family is asked whether or not they would like their now dead relative to donate the kidneys. The first transplants from this procedure were scheduled for late in 1993.

Kidneys are not the only organs in short supply—another 10,000 potential recipients await other organs. About 4000 persons in the U.S. are on the waiting list for new hearts at any one time, but only about 2000 hearts suitable for transplant are expected to become available each year. And living friends are not the only altruists, although they are the most dramatic. People who have some healthy organs, but who know they are dying, can also donate organs to be removed as soon as their hearts stop beating—at least at the University of Pittsburgh Medical Center. If dying individuals do not make such a provision, the requirement in most states is that they be brain dead, which may be much later. A brain-dead patient (whose brain shows no functioning at all) can be maintained for a time on a device called a ventilator so that organs stay healthy enough for transplanting.

In the U.S. as a whole, there are about 10,000 to 12,000 patients declared brain dead each year, far short of demand; and most of those, in any case, are not suitable donors—they might be too old, have died from a transmissible disease, most often AIDS, or have damaged organs.

For the most part, organ receipt policies are set by the United Organ Sharing Network, which not only keeps the waiting lists of potential recipients and is a clearing house for donors, but also tries to set ethical policies. Preference is normally given to the potential recipient who has waited the longest, though some physicians argue that the healthiest patients for whom a transplant is required should be the first recipients. Organ recipients who have waited a long time are usually in poor condition and may not have as good a chance of surviving the operation or of returning to normal life as recipients who are comparatively healthy before the operation. Also, there is some evidence suggesting that the patients with the most aggressive physicians often shove ahead in the line.

Trans-Species Transplants

One solution to the shortage of organs would be to find a way to use organs from common domestic animals which can be bred in almost any amount imaginable if there is a reason to do so. But the kidney of a pig or even of a baboon is even more foreign to the immune system than an organ from a totally unrelated human. Early efforts to give humans animal organs, some of which preceded the first known transplants between humans, all failed.

With the ability to use drugs to suppress the immune system, transplants between unrelated humans has become possible, though not so easy as between close blood relatives. Given the organ shortage, some physicians have tried a combination of transplant between species along with massive immune suppression.

The most famous of these recent attempts took place in the U.S. in 1992 and 1993. On June 28, 1992, physicians from the University of Pittsburgh, headed by transplant pioneer Thomas E. Starzl, implanted the liver from a baboon in a man dying from complications of hepatitis B (*see* "Through the Alphabet with Hepatitis," p 345). Patients with active hepatitis B are prohibited from human-to-human liver transplants because the virus invariably infects the new liver and causes it to fail also. Baboons are thought to be immune to or at least to resist hepatitis B.

The Pittsburgh team had shown some success with interspecific transplants or transplants between two different species. The surgeons had shown that with the proper combination of immune suppressors and anti-inflammatory drugs, they could transplant hamster hearts and livers into rats. The evolutionary distance between hamsters and rats is thought to be about the same as that between baboons and humans. Hamsters and rats are in adjacent but different families of rodents, just as humans and baboons are in adjacent but different families of primates.

The Pittsburgh patient who received the baboon liver on June 28, 1992 died on September 7, 1992, just 70 days after the operation, but the cause was not transplant rejection. Death came from a mixture of causes unrelated to the transplant, most prominently a stroke caused by a fungus blocking arteries in the brain. The several infections and cause of death started rumors that the patient had succumbed to AIDS, which is transmitted by the same pathways as hepatitis B. The hospital issued an equivocal denial of the rumors, and later Starzl said the patient was infected with HIV, but that the infection had not yet caused AIDS.

On January 10, 1993, the same team tried again with a second man whose liver had been destroyed by hepatitis B. He lived 26 days before succumbing to an infection probably caused by a leaky suture from the transplant operation. The liver appeared to be healthy.

Pigs, although not closely related to humans, are for many reasons a logical choice

BABOON BUSINESS

Since 1905 at least 35 different attempts have been made to transplant an organ from a nonhuman animal into a human being, including transplanting seven baboon kidneys, two baboon hearts, and two baboon livers. One person survived 98 days with a baboon kidney. Baboons are considerably smaller than humans and they are not our closest animal relative. Furthermore, they are not exactly domestic animals. When a surgeon wants to practice on an animal, he usually chooses a pig, which is about the same size as a human, organized in much the same way, is an omnivore (so its digestive organs are similar to those of humans), and is raised by the millions every year.

Baboons are, of course, primates in the group known as Old World monkeys. Humans are also primates, in a small group that includes two or three species of chimpanzee and the gorilla—orangutans and gibbons are now thought to be in a separate group by most evolutionists. The two groups of primates have been separate for about 20 to 30 million years.

Why not use organs from a chimpanzee or a gorilla, our closest relatives from whom we have been separated by about seven to nine million years? To begin with, chimpanzees and gorillas are endangered species. Furthermore, they are expensive and in short supply in captivity. But perhaps a more compelling reason is that they are too closely related; many people believe that killing a chimpanzee or gorilla is uncomfortably close to murder. On the other hand, a few experiments with chimpanzee organs have been tried anyway. The longest survivor of an interspecific transplant into a human received a chimpanzee kidney in 1963 and lived for nine months.

Baboons are smaller than humans, but that makes them more suitable for organ transplants into human babies or young children. In 1984 the transplant recipient known as Baby Fae lived 20 days with a baboon's heart. Although an adult baboon's liver is about the same size as that of a 13-year-old male human, a successfully transplanted organ grows to adult human size, which happened with the first baboon liver transplant in just 70 days.

---

for many medical procedures (much the same can be said for sheep—although sheep, but not pigs, are subject to the transmissible brain disease scrapie). In the future, pigs may be genetically engineered to be more closely related to humans than they are now (see "Pigs and Other Animals Become More Human," p 47), but for now the farmyard variety has to suffice.

On October 12, 1993 a young woman received a pig liver to replace her own, which had malfunctioned with autoimmune hepatitis since childhood. The pig liver was intended as a holding action, so the defective human liver was also kept in place, giving the woman two less than satisfactory livers until a suitable donor could be found. Time was of the essence, as the woman was dying from liver malfunction when the operation began. Either the pig liver was too late or the interspecific gap was too great, as the woman died from brain swelling induced most likely by acute liver failure a few hours after the operation. The brain swelling had begun two hours before the operation, suggesting that the attempt was too late. Physicians at Cedars-Sinai Medical Center in Los Angeles, California, where the operation took place, might try the same tactic again—but sooner—if confronted with similar circumstances.

Fighting the Immune System

The human immune system did not evolve rejection mechanisms with the idea of rejecting organ transplants. The parts of the immune system that cause organ rejection appear to be designed by evolution to deter parasites, such as worms and protists (see "The State of the War Against Parasites," p 378). An unwanted complication, from the standpoint of modern medicine, is that to one degree or another cells from a different human are viewed as unfamiliar parasites, so the immune response is to search out and destroy the foreign cells. Unlike real parasites, however, transplanted organs have evolved no defenses against the immune system, so that without outside aid of some kind, the immune system wins and the organ is rejected.

In recent transplant history, the main outside assistance has come from drugs that suppress the immune system, primarily cyclosporine and FK506, although sometimes monoclonal antibodies have been used. Scientists from Wyeth-Ayerst in Princeton, New Jersey, announced in 1993 that they had synthesized rapamycin, soon expected to join the short list of immune-suppressor chemicals. Like cyclosporine, rapamycin was originally obtained from a fungus. The existing version breaks down too fast in the body for effective use, but it is hoped that the synthesized version can be modified to avoid this defect.

The chemical approach can be successful, but it is very dangerous as it exposes the body to attack by real parasites of one kind or another. Furthermore, most drug-suppression of the immune response knocks out more of the system than would be desired for simple transplant protection.

Some new approaches to fighting this battle have been developed in animal studies. The immune system is much better understood today, so researchers have found ways to interfere with specific parts that are causing trouble while leaving the rest of the system intact. Transplants are attacked by killer T cells (see "Allergies and Asthma," p 431) in response to chemicals that signal the T cell to attack and to summon help, a process called graft rejection. As in many organic processes, graft rejection has a cascade effect as one chemical stimulates another, which may then stimulate others or may inhibit others; such cascades enable specific, modulated responses. The killer T cells must be stimulated by helper T cells. For the helper T cells, the four chemical signals (cytokines—messengers—and receptors) involved in transplant rejection are the molecule B7, the receptor CD28, a protein called MHC that picks up an antigen from the graft, and a receptor called the T-cell receptor. The T cells also contain a different receptor called CTLA4 that normally is not involved in graft rejection. For a graft rejection cascade to begin, a different immune cell introduces the graft (i.e. transplant) to the helper T cell by presenting the MHC with an antigen from the graft. At the same time, it presents B7. The T-cell receptor locks onto the presented MHC, while one of its CD28 receptors grabs the B7. This double connection is what provokes the graft response to begin. It is also the way that an autoimmune reaction is started (*see* "Autoimmune UPDATE," p 447).

In 1992, Peter Linsley, of Bristol-Myers Squibb Pharmaceuticals, and coworkers revealed that they discovered in 1991 that the CTLA4 molecule would connect to B7 even tighter than CD28, preventing CD28 from attaching to the presenting white blood cell. They reasoned that if the region contained loose CTLA4 molecules, graft rejection would not be initiated and that autoimmune reactions might be suppressed—both without turning down the whole immune response. To make this work, CTLA4 needs to be in the blood, which was accomplished by combining the molecule with the protein immunoglobin, normally present in blood, a combination named CTLA4Ig. Linsley's group tested CTLA4Ig against the autoimmune response in 1993 and reported a successful test in mice in the August 7, 1992 *Science.*

The same issue of *Science* contained a positive report on the use of CTLA4Ig in preventing transplant rejection. Jeffrey Bluestone and Deborah Lenschow of the University of Chicago Medical Center in Illinois demonstrated that CTLA4Ig allowed diabetic mice to accept foreign pancreatic tissue. Furthermore, it altered the immune response so that additional cells from the same donor could be accepted. Yet a third study showed that CTLA4Ig would prevent graft rejection in rats with heart transplants. The catch is that unlike immune-suppressing chemicals like cyclosporine or FK506, the molecules of CTLA4Ig need to be continually supplied to the rats to prevent graft rejection. This knocks out a part of the immune system needed for various other purposes. Still, it may be possible with experience to use CTLA4Ig to remove just the T-cell population involved in a specific graft rejection, leaving the remaining T cells as well as the immune system intact.

(Periodical References and Additional Reading: *New York Times* 1-29-91; *New York Times* 6-1-91, p A1; *New York Times* 6-29-92, p A1; *New York Times* 6-30-92, p C3; *New York Times* 7-2-92, p A17; *New York Times* 7-5-92, p I-18; *New York Times* 8-7-92, p A12; *Science* 8-7-92, pp 751, 789, & 792; *New York Times* 8-17-92, p A20; *New York Times* 9-2-93, p D18; *New York Times* 9-8-92, p D14; *New York Times* 9-9-92, p A13; *New York Times* 10-13-92, p C6; *New York Times* 10-14-92, p A16; *New York Times* 1-11-93, p A12; *New York Times* 1-20-93, p C14; *New York Times* 2-6-93, p 6; *New York Times* 6-2-93, p A15; *Science News* 6-5-93, p 358; *New York Times* 6-30-93, p C14; *New York Times* 7-7-94, p D19; *Scientific American* 8-93, p 62)

CELL TRANSPLANTATION: FETAL TISSUE AND MORE

On one level there is no significant difference between transplanting a liver and transplanting a fetal brain cell. In both cases a primary motive is to produce within the transplant recipient's body a chemical or group of chemicals that would otherwise either have to be supplied continually from some outside source or done without. In either case the transplant, if successful, integrates itself into the part of the body. Livers grow by multiplying cells; conceivably fetal brain cells might also reproduce (although adult brain cells in humans no longer duplicate themselves).

Looked at from a different point of view, however, fetal transplants present so many different ethical issues, different techniques, and additional possibilities that they are generally classed in a different group from the organ transplants.

Other cell transplants also pose different problems. The most common cell transplant operations in the U.S. are bone-marrow transplants, used to treat perhaps as many as 10,000 patients with blood-cell malignancies in the U.S. each year. Bone-marrow transplants are controversial largely because of insurance-company resistance to paying for the expensive and somewhat experimental operations. What bone-marrow transplants have in common with fetal cell transplants is that cells are expected to reproduce and to add something lacking to the body. The difference is that the lack is not a chemical *per se,* but is instead whole groups of red and white blood cells along with platelets.

Often the reason for a bone-marrow transplant is not because the recipient's bone marrow has anything wrong with it. Instead, the occasion of the transplant is to allow a procedure that involves whole-body radiation to suppress tumors. The bone marrow is removed and replaced after the radiation treatments to keep it from harm. In other instances, where the problem is a disease such as leukemia that has its origin in defective bone marrow, the marrow has been removed and treated in some way and then replaced. When the donor and the donee are the same person, there are few ethical issues, though there are as noted above, financial issues.

Most cell transplants in which the donor is a different person from the recipient involve the same kind of immune rejection problems as organ transplants do. But sometimes the cell transplants can be handled in a different way. On May 8, 1993, a Type I diabetic human received insulin-producing pancreas cells from donors, for example (*see* "Diabetes," p 438). He was not the first diabetic for whom this had been tried, but it had failed in the past because the same autoimmune reaction that destroyed the original pancreatic cells also destroyed the new ones. But in this case, the pancreas cells were protected from antibodies by a seaweed gel covering each. The gel keeps antibodies out but allows insulin to escape. The technique had been successful previously on dogs for periods as long as seven months to two years. Even if the gel eventually fails, the operation itself is minor (it takes a half hour and involves only local anesthesia) and could be repeated for another period of months or years with reduced insulin shots or none at all.

Another approach has been to transplant insulin-producing cells into Type I diabetics who, because of organ transplants, already have their immune systems suppressed chemically. Because kidney impairment is a common complication of diabetes, this strategy is not so bizarre as it might at first seem. In some patients this approach has produced enough insulin within the pancreas itself to arrest the diabetes.

Tissue Transplants

Whole groups of cells, such as bone marrow, are technically *tissue,* since more than one type of cell can be involved. In addition to bone marrow, bone, skin, cartilage, ligaments, and tendons for grafts and blood vessels for bypass operations are commonly transplanted from one part of a body to another or from one person to another. Corneal tissue for eye treatment and heart valves are also transplanted, mostly from cadavers. All in all, there are thought to be about 400,000 tissue grafts from one person to another, coming from about 10,000 dead or living donors—about 25 times as many tissue grafts as organ transplants. These figures do not include self-grafts, which although uncounted probably occur more often than grafts from one person to another.

The number of grafts far exceeds the number of donors. One cadaver is known to have supplied 61 separate organ or tissue transplants. In this particular case, the cadaver was the body of a man from Virginia who died (in a shooting in 1985) carrying an undetected infection with HIV, and seven of the recipients developed AIDS as an unwanted consequence of their transplants. As a result of this case, when the HIV infection somehow slipped through the tests that should have caught it, the U.S. Centers for Disease Control and Prevention (CDC) began revising its tissue-transplant guidelines, a process that started in December 1991 and was not complete late in 1993. Congress has also begun steps to regulate tissue transplants, although none has so far reached the status of law.

In 1992 a man dying of AIDS received a bone-marrow transplant from a baboon. Baboons are thought not to be subject to such human viral diseases as AIDS or hepatitis B. The baboon cells failed to take, and the man died. Baboon bone marrow was also given to the second recipient of a baboon liver (*see* "Organ Transplantation: Proliferation and Problems," p 505) in the hope of creating a combined baboon-human immune system that would accept the liver. Further baboon bone-marrow experiments are planned.

A series of transplants using human identical twins has shown that transplanting bone marrow from a twin not infected with HIV to one that is can be helpful. Although the first experiments, which began in the early 1980s, did not save the lives of the infected twins, results have been steadily improving with practice. Most of the 36 recipients since 1986 were still alive in 1994.

Many types of tissue are kept in "banks" from which specific matches can be selected and withdrawn as needed. There are about a hundred each of banks that specialize in eye tissue and bone tissue, while there are smaller numbers of clinics specializing in other human transplant materials. All are modeled on the well-known blood banks that have made blood transfusion accessible to almost everyone who needs it.

Fetal Cell Transplants

There are several virtues for the use of cells from an aborted human fetus in cell transplants. The first, cited mostly by proponents, is that the fetus has not developed a full set of antigens, so fetal cells do not provoke the same immune response as cells from adults. The second, cited mostly by opponents, is that fetal tissue can be found in considerable supply as a result of natural or induced abortions. A third possible virtue is that fetal cells may continue division in their new home, while adult cells from many parts of the body have long ago stopped reproducing themselves.

Fetal nerve cells are particularly useful. Brain cells taken from a fetus will survive in a laboratory dish for as long as a week, but adult cells succumb within ten minutes of removal from the brain. This makes fetal cells the cells of choice for brain tissue even though the immune system does not affect brain transplants as much as it does other parts of the body. Also, scientists hope that fetal brain cells can produce cytokines that will cause new connections to grow between the transplant and the old brain, which adult cells are not expected to do. A lot of the theory behind these operations is a bit fuzzy, however.

The administrations of U.S. presidents Ronald Reagan and George Bush opposed fetal-cell research and even banned government support of it, mainly, people believe, because of fears that success with fetal cells might lead to additional abortions, although the Bush administration did propose developing a fetal-tissue bank from natural miscarriages. The bank failed to come to pass. In the meantime, some patients paid out of their own pockets as much as $50,000 to become subjects of fetal-tissue transplants.

The succeeding administration of U.S. President Bill Clinton ended the ban on fetal-tissue research, but fetal-tissue research in the U.S. in 1993 was just getting restarted after its ban. In other countries, however, fetal-tissue research was well along. Some nations had already established fetal-tissue banks to collect and preserve cells from abortions.

One possible alternative to fetal cells for nerve cell or brain cell transplants is the nerve cells of the nose. These nerve cells, unlike others in the body, continue to divide and grow in adult humans.

Diabetes   In Russia and its neighboring former-Soviet states, physicians had accomplished more than 3000 transplants of fetal insulin-producing cells into patients with Type I diabetes by the early 1990s. In no case has this procedure provided a complete cure, but dependence on injected insulin has been reduced by as much as 90 percent. Presumably, the steady supply of insulin from the transplanted cells will also help prevent the complications from diabetes. In 1993 researchers in the U.S. planned to import fetal tissue from the Russian tissue banks that had already been established.

Parkinson's disease   The most dramatic cure from fetal brain cell implants has come in the case of two persons with drug-induced artificial parkinsonism (*see* "Parkinson's Progress," p 463). The patients, who developed their condition simultaneously in 1982 from a chemical called MPTP (sold to them as a cheap substitute for heroin), were each largely cured by a massive dose of fetal brain cells taken from as many as seven different donors. The transplants took place in Sweden, where fetal-tissue research began on animals in the 1979 and has since been in advance of most of the rest of the world. Results of the operation, conducted by Hakan Widner, of the University of Lund, and coworkers were announced in the November 26, 1992 *New England Journal of Medicine.*

Parkinsonism is not exactly the same as Parkinson's disease, however, and much milder improvements have been noted so far in dozens of experiments with the disease in which it arose from natural causes. The first human cell transplants for Parkinson's disease were attempted in 1987 with controversial results. Nevertheless, hundreds of patients since then have received the transplants. Typically cells are obtained from fetuses that are six to 11 weeks past the date of implantation in the uterus. The fetal cells are placed in a liquid suspension and then injected into the part of the brain where they are needed.

Huntington's disease   In 1990 the first attempt to cure Huntington's disease with a fetal-cell transplant was undertaken by Ignacio Madrazo of the La Raza Medical Clinic in Mexico City (*see* "Three-Base Repeats: Fragile X, Huntington's Disease, and More," p 50). Although preliminary results were somewhat promising, experts generally felt that Huntington's was not sufficiently well understood for this approach to be successful. Animal research, however, suggests that the cells involved in Huntington's disease can be replaced by fetal transplants.

Other attempts   Fetal cells have been tried in cases of liver failure, muscular dystrophy, and even as a way to handle severe pain.

(Periodical References and Additional Reading: *Harvard Health Letter* 5-92, p 1; *New York Times* 5-24-92, p I-1; *New York Times* 7-27-92, p A1; *New York Times* 4-11-93, p I-19; *Science News* 4-24-93, p 263; *New York Times* 5-16-94, p I-24; *New York Times* 8-15-93, p I-28; *New York Times* 7-19-94, p C3)

NEW TOOLS:
THE STATE OF DRUGS AND
MEDICAL DEVICES

Use of medicinal herbs may antedate humans. Many insist that chimpanzees, monkeys, and other mammals or even birds have used specific plants to improve health under a variety of circumstances. The old folk belief that dogs eat grass to cure themselves of worms resembles a theory that monkeys seek the leaves of certain tree species to rid themselves of a parasite.

Biologically derived medicines still make up the bulk of drugs used by humans today, although modern chemistry often synthesizes copies of the natural substance or even makes improvements on its basic molecule. Inorganic compounds for the most part came later than the biologicals, although consumption of kaolin—clay eating—to relieve stomach problems may well be prehistoric. The general practice of using inorganics, however, is thought to have originated in the sixteenth century, and inorganics have always lagged behind the biologicals. Nature had millions of years to find the complex chemicals plants use in fighting their parasites and predators, which are the biologicals of most use in human medicine as well.

Medical devices also must have been used in prehistoric times, provided one counts bandages and splints.

Whatever drugs or devices physicians prescribe, they work better than they might for chemical or normal biological reasons, especially when they are new to a patient and highly touted. No matter what the illness—asthma, duodenal ulcer, herpes—a new drug or procedure administered by a convincing and convinced physician helps about 70 percent of the patients, even when the drug itself is worthless. At least that was the result of a retrospective study of nearly 7000 patients, 40 percent of whom were helped a lot by the useless treatment, while another 30 reported that the results of the treatment were only good, not excellent. The results of this study, directed by Alan H. Roberts of the Scripps Clinic and Research Foundation in La Jolla, California, were published in the August 1993 *Clinical Psychology Review.*

Earlier research in the 1950s (by Henry Beecher) had shown that a third of patients improve when given placebos—supposedly neutral medicines—if the patients think they will work. In controlled studies, however, patients know that they have a fixed chance of getting a placebo instead of the drug, and improvement would be expected to be less. Research on double-blind studies, however, has shown that a different factor interferes with the placebo effect; because of side effects or real improvement or perhaps some other factor, 78 percent of patients and 87 percent of physicians (according to one study) can tell whether they are getting the drug or the placebo.

Despite the complexities introduced by the placebo effect and lack of blindness in supposedly blind studies, many new drugs and devices work very well. These are detailed in separate articles later in this chapter. The remainder of this article deals with problems that have been encountered in drug development and in the financial burden of pharmaceuticals in the U.S. and other nations.

Drugs That Don't Work

Perhaps the spate of nonworking cures in the early 1990s was the inevitable result of increased competition for sales, but perhaps it was just hubris. Knowledge of how the body functions at a genetic and molecular level increased so much in the 40 years from 1953 to 1992 that scientists and drug companies began to think that they actually knew how the body works and could correct any small errors in design that had been made by previous planners. In any case, here is a brief recounting of some of what went wrong.

June 1992   The antibiotic Omniflox, approved in the U.S. in January, was withdrawn from the market on June 5, 1992, after the drug was implicated in three deaths as well as many adverse reactions.

September 1992   Studies in Europe and Canada showed that the drug Arasin, marketed by Genesia Pharmaceuticals, Inc., to prevent heart attacks and reduce damage during bypass surgery, did not do so for most patients. Before the drug was marketed, clinical tests in the U.S. had found the drug effective.

October 1992   A drug called Proscar, produced by Merck & Company, was found to be less effective than surgery for its intended use in treating enlarged prostates.

January 1993   A much-touted drug, Centoxin, a monoclonal antibody also known as HA-1A, intended to cure the fatal bacterial infection known as sepsis was found to work on gram-negative bacteria, but physicians could not tell in advance which sepsis was caused by such germs. Furthermore, a different group of patients were harmed rather than helped by Centoxin. As a result, the difference in mortality between those in trials treated with the drug and those receiving a placebo was not statistically significant, and the trial was halted on January 28, 1993. The drug was also withdrawn from overseas markets at that time.

A similar drug known as E5 failed to win approval from the U.S. Food and Drug Administration (FDA) on two occasions because of apparent lack of effectiveness, but its manufacturer quietly gave up that drug after saying that it would try again. In 1994 two other attempts to develop a drug to treat sepsis were also abandoned, but the pharmaceutical companies involved planned to continue working with other approaches to the problem.

April 1993   A drug being sold as a treatment for congestive heart failure, Manoplax, was found to stop working after three months; after that, it makes the heart fail more rapidly. The manufacturer, Boots Company, could not estimate how many deaths the drug might have caused because most patients who took the drug were near death even before starting medication.

Also in April, the asthma treatment tipredan, a steroid, failed to work in several trials in different countries and was dropped by its British developer.

Lorenzo's Oil   A widely seen movie in 1993 told the story of how two parents of a son with a genetic disease found, with limited help from the medical community, a treatment for their son's condition. The treatment for adrenoleukodystrophy, which has symptoms similar to multiple sclerosis but is even more devastating, consisted of a blend of two natural oils, known as erucic and oleic acids. In the movie, the treatment worked. In scientific studies, it did not. Discovery of the gene and therefore the protein involved in the disease soon after the motion picture may lead to a more effective treatment.

Drugs That Induce Illness

Sometimes drugs do more than simply fail to work, perhaps allowing a few people who are already at the point of death to die. Some drugs cause new illnesses that are much worse than the ones being treated. Others result in dramatic deaths in people who are merely ill (*see* "The Calamity of a Viral Medicine," p 335). In addition to drugs that cause problems because of their inherent nature, some medicines are contaminated with viruses, bacteria, or toxic compounds accidentally.

OTC Drugs   Because they are over-the-counter (OTC) instead of prescribed drugs, people in the U.S. tend to think of simple painkillers such as aspirin, ibuprofen (Advil and others), and acetaminophen (Tylenol and others) as safe and effective in all situations, in all doses, and all the time. But this is not the case (*see also* "New Uses for Aspirin," p 527).

A 20-year study in Switzerland of the drug phenacetin (which was taken off the OTC market in the U.S. by the FDA in 1980) showed that women who used the drug regularly had a death rate more than twice that of those using aspirin or no painkiller at all. High blood pressure and kidney disease were the main causes of death. Phenacetin is converted into acetaminophen in the body. A separate study in 1990 found that regular users of phenacetin had five times the risk of kidney disease, while regular users of acetaminophen had three times the risk. The phrases "regular use" and "regular users" apply to people who take several doses daily.

Another problem with painkillers surfaced in 1993, although the basic ideas were well known earlier. An FDA advisory panel on June 29, 1993 recommended that people be warned not to drink alcohol and take acetaminophen because of the risk of serious liver damage. The reaction can occur when people take more than the four grams a day (eight Extra-Strength Tylenol tablets) that is the recommended maximum dose, provided that they normally have at least two alcoholic drinks daily. On September 8, 1993, two different advisory panels also recommended that warning labels for drinkers be added to aspirin and ibuprofen. Liver damage was not the issue; stomach bleeding was. To some degree this seemed to be an attempt among the makers of OTC painkillers to point accusing fingers at each other. None of the warning labels discussed here have actually been added to the drugs.

Quinine is not only sold over drugstore counters, but is also available in quinine water and similar products. A report of two cases of kidney failure in the July 31, 1993 *Annals of Internal Medicine* reminded physicians that quinine could in rare cases lead to blood-sugar deficiencies. The report called for warning labels on tonic water as well as on quinine sold in tablet form for malaria prevention or to relieve muscle cramps.

Contamination   In France in July 1993, four health officials were given jail sentences as a result of 1200 hemophiliacs becoming infected with the HIV virus that leads to AIDS as a result of virus-infected blood factors. Two French physicians were charged with producing human growth hormone that infected 25 children with invariably fatal Creutzfeldt-Jakob disease (*see* "Prions Revisited," p 339). The hormone was harvested from cadavers, although genetically engineered growth hormone has been available since 1985.

In the United States it may sometimes seem that all a pharmacist does these days is to count pills from one bottle to another, but there are still preparations that pharmacists mix in the store. Batches of one of these, Indocin eye drops, manufactured by a pharmacist in Pittsburgh, Pennsylvania, somehow became contaminated with the bacterium *Pseudomonas*. Although the pharmacist regularly sterilized his materials and equipment, some of the 2000 bottles of Indocin eye drops he made in 1990 were not sterile. Two women lost the sight of one eye, and other users had severe eye infections from the bacterium, which invaded small cuts made during cataract surgery.

Interactions   Two drugs, each of which may be perfectly safe by themselves, can interact to create a life-threatening situation. Antibiotics are often one of the interacting drugs, especially erythromycin. Added to the list of drugs not to be taken with erythromycin in 1992 (which previously included the antiseizure medication phenytoin and the bronchodilator theophylline; patients with liver disease should also avoid erythromycin) were the antihistamines terfenadine (Seldane) and astemizole (Hismanal). This interaction has been known to lead to cardiac arrest and death. Terfenadine also interacts with oral ketoconazole (Nizoral), which is an antifungal agent, to produce potentially fatal cardiac arrhythmias.

The Conservative U.S. Food and Drug Administration

In the U.S., drug problems are often less severe and more quickly contained than they are in other industrialized nations. Largely this has been because the FDA has a conservative tradition, though it can be duped. For example, in the 1980s a concentrated anesthetic, Versed, made by F. Hoffmann-La Roche, caused a number of serious comas and deaths because even the slightest amount beyond the effective dose could result in an overdose. This happened in Europe, where Versed had been licensed several years before the FDA accepted the drug. In this case, however, the manufacturer suppressed information about the problems in its filing with the FDA, and the FDA did approve the concentrated form in 1985. In the next 18 months, 46 or more deaths occurred as a result. Around the same time as the FDA approval, Hoffmann-La Roche reformulated the drug for British use in a less concentrated form but failed to notify the FDA of this either. With normal notification, the FDA would not have approved Versed in the concentrated form. For similar reasons, many other drugs have what amounts to a public trial in other countries before the FDA allows use in the U.S.

Because of problems like the Versed situation, the FDA on June 1, 1993 called for greater reporting of any adverse reactions to drugs or medical devices. It said that it would set up new mechanisms to make that possible. A couple of weeks later it also announced that it planned to have pharmaceutical companies disclose financial ties to physicians who conduct drug tests. Many pharmaceutical companies at present pay physicians to perform tests, and the FDA indicated that it thought that it was possible that financial concerns might affect results of drug trials.

OTC products are also in the domain of the FDA. The FDA in the early 1990s made "sweeps" of OTC products about once a year. In 1990 it found 223 ingredients commonly used in OTC preparations that the FDA thought were ineffective for the conditions the medicines were intended to treat. In 1991 it banned 111 products altogether. In 1992 it called for hundreds of OTC manufacturers to take false claims off labels. In 1993 it found that Warner-Lambert had improperly trained lab technicians, changed drug formulas without FDA approval, and let drugs that failed quality checks be marketed. As a result, a federal court ordered a halt in all Warner-Lambert OTC drugs and stopped the sale of all but 13 Warner-Lambert prescription drugs. (The 13 were exempted because of medical necessity.)

In general, during the early 1990s, the FDA moved in the direction of greater conservatism as to what drugs and policies it would accept, although activists for particular causes (notably AIDS) pushed for policies that would admit more drugs earlier in the process. AIDS activists have often banded together in "clubs" to import drugs not approved by the FDA or that are sold at lower prices in other countries. In an acknowledgment of the problem, the FDA offered in May 1993 guidelines to clubs so that they could continue their activities without violating laws.

At the same time, the FDA was less conservative in the sense that it attacked misleading claims vigorously. For example, the FDA openly endorsed a report that found that 30 percent of the statistics used in medical advertisements directed at physicians come from inconclusive, dissimilar, or poorly designed studies but were not presented that way in the ads; that 19 percent of the advertisements mentioning side-effects in headlines were misleading; and that nine percent of the graphs used misrepresented the studies they depicted. In fact, the FDA division of drug marketing claimed that half the ads in the study violated FDA guidelines.

A different U.S. agency was a bit too conservative. The Drug Enforcement Administration (DEA) delayed approval of a request to manufacture more Ritalin to meet the needs of an increasing population of attention-deficit disorder afflicted children and adults. As a result of the DEA inaction, supplies of the drug were extremely low during the fall of 1993. The DEA sets manufacturing policy because Ritalin is considered in the same class as cocaine and morphine, although there are no known cases of the use of Ritalin as a recreational drug.

The High Price of Medicine

First of all, pharmaceutical companies are not all bad, despite high drug prices. Merck & Company, for example, has donated millions of doses of the drug Mectizan worldwide to treat the parasitic infection that causes river blindness (see "The State of the War on Parasites," p 378).

But on the other hand, a constant refrain through most of the early 1990s was that drug prices are too high and pharmaceutical companies make too much money—to wit, about ten percent of total U.S. health-care costs, or (in 1990) $70 billion. After prescription drug prices rose at a rate nearly three times as high as other prices in 1991, 73 percent of people polled said that the federal government should set the prices for all prescription drugs and a number of congresspersons announced that they would look into the problem. The following year drug prices in the U.S. increased four times as much as other products.

A study by the U.S. General Accounting Office in 1992 found that in Canada, where the government has more control over drug prices, selected prescription medicines averaged 32 percent lower than the same drugs in the U.S. Congressional hearings were held early in 1993 by the U.S. House Small Business Subcommittee on Regulation and Business Opportunities. The concern expressed was that high prices were being charged for drugs that had been developed largely with U.S. government funding, such as Taxol, which was supported by the U.S. National Cancer Institute. A month later on February 25, 1993, the U.S. Office of Technology Assessment, another congressional agency, reported that drug-company profits were two or three percentage points higher than those of other high-risk, high-development-cost industries, resulting in about $2 billion in "excess" profits each year. Actually, drug profits were about five times as high as the rest of U.S. industries on a percentage basis.

The pharmaceutical industry began to fight these charges in 1993. On March 8 industry representatives informally asked the Clinton administration for an antitrust exemption so that they could work together to lower drug prices. A few days later, the industry took a different approach and formally agreed to keep drug prices at the national inflation rate as a voluntary move. Ten large manufacturers as well as the trade association announced the policy. Later in 1993 there was considerable evidence of actual price competition between drug manufacturers; SmithKline Beecham, Upjohn, and Schering-Plough used cash rebates to consumers in hopes of increasing business, while Proctor & Gamble offered a money-back guarantee if their prescription drugs for treating urinary-tract infections failed to please.

(Periodical References and Additional Reading: *New York Times* 12-9-90, p I-39; *New York Times* 1-17-91; *New York Times* 6-9-92, p D2; *New York Times* 8-27-92, p A21; *New York Times* 9-23-92, p D4; *New York Times* 9-25-92, p D3; *New York Times* 10-21-92, p D4; *New York Times* 10-22-92, p D1; *New York Times* 10-30-92, p D4; *Harvard Health Letter* 11-92, p 3; *New York Times* 1-26-93, p C6; *New York Times* 2-9-93, p C1; *New York Times* 2-12-93, p A1; *New York Times* 2-26-93, p D1; *New York Times* 3-2-93. (C5; *New York Times* 3-10-93, p A16; *New York Times* 3-16-93, p D4; *Harvard Health Letter* 4-93, p 4; *Science News* 4-3-93, p 220; *New York Times* 4-7-93, p D4; *New York Times* 5-26-93, p A18; *New York Times* 6-2-93, p A17; *New York Times* 6-16-93, p A19; *New York Times* 7-20-93, p C3; *New York Times* 7-22-93, p A9; *Scientific American* 8-93, p 115; *New York Times* 8-1-93, p I-33; *Nature* 8-5-93, p 476; *New York Times* 8-17-93, pp C3 & D3; *New York Times* 9-9-93, p A18; *New York Times* 11-14-93; *New York Times* 7-19-94, p D1)

TIMETABLE OF MEDICAL TECHNOLOGY TO 1990

2100 BC	The oldest medical text that has been preserved in its original form is a cuneiform tablet from about this time that lists a sequence of recipes for various external poultices and plasters.
1550 BC	The Papyrus Ebers gives a description of 700 medications; it also shows that physicians prescribe diets or fasts and massage, and that some practice hypnosis.
10	Thaddeus of Florence describes the medical use of alcohol in *De virtutibus aquae vitae* (On the Virtues of Alcohol).
40	*De materia medica* by Greek physician Pedanius Dioscorides of Anazarbus, Turkey [born circa 20 A.D.] deals with the medical properties of about 600 plants and nearly a thousand drugs.
900	Arab chemists and physicians prepare alcohol by distilling wine.
1286	Allesandro della Spina is said to make use of the invention of a friend, Salvino degli Armati; the invention is eyeglasses made with convex lenses to correct nearsightedness. Later, in 1306, Friar Giordano of Pisa claims to have known

the person who invented eyeglasses 20 years earlier—although it is not clear that Friar Giordano's reference is to Armati.

1300   Eyeglasses become common, being produced in the glassmaking center of Italy, Venice; but lenses often are made from inferior glass that refracts light unevenly.

1345   The first English apothecary shop is opened in London.

1398   The Florentine *Receptario* is the first official pharmacopoeia.

1410   Benedetto Rinio's *Liber de simplicibus* describes and illustrates 440 plants that have medicinal uses.

1426   The herbal of Celsus [born circa 14 A.D.; died circa 37 A.D.] called *De re medicina* (On Medicine) is rediscovered and when the printing press is invented, it becomes one of the first medical books to be printed.

1450   Nicholas Krebs, known as Nicholas of Cusa [born Kues, Germany, 1401], constructs spectacles for the nearsighted.

1490   About this time the Chinese invent the modern form of toothbrush with pig bristles at a right angle to the handle.

1493   Christopher Columbus on his second voyage finds that American natives use tobacco as a medicine.

1520   Physician and alchemist Philippus Aureolus Paracelsus, or Theophrastus Bombast von Hohenheim [born Schwyz, Switzerland, May 1, 1493; died Salzburg, Austria, September 24, 1541] introduces tincture of opium, which he names laudanum, into medicine about this time.

1530   Paracelsus's *Paragranum* argues that medicine should be based on nature and its physical laws and is the first to suggest the use of chemical substances, such as compounds of mercury and antimony, as remedies.

1535   *Dispensatorium* by Valerius Cordus [born Germany, 1515; died 1544], one of the first books to describe most known drugs, chemicals, and medical preparations, is published.

1543   English apothecaries are legalized by an Act of Parliament.

1579   The first glass eyes are probably made about this time.

1596   The *Pen-ts'ao kang mu* compiled by Li Shih-Chen [born China, 1518; died 1593] includes a description of over 2000 drugs from the animal, vegetable, and mineral kingdoms, as well as detailed prescriptions and references to other texts.

1617   The Guild of the Apothecaries of the City of London is founded.

1618   The first edition of the *London pharmacopoeia* is published.

1714   Dominique Anel [born Toulouse, France, 1679; died 1730] invents the fine-point syringe, still known by his name, for use in treating *fistula lacrymalis*.

1775   William Withering [born Wellington, England, March 1741; died Birmingham, England, October 6, 1799] introduces digitalis to cure the dropsy associated with heart disease.

1778   William Brown publishes the first U.S. pharmacopoeia.

1784   Benjamin Franklin invents bifocal eyeglasses, mounting half lenses for near and for distant vision in the same frames.

1785	William Withering's *Account of the Foxglove* reports on his discovery of the use of digitalis in treatment of heart disease.
1811	Samuel Hahnemann publishes a catalog of homeopathic drugs.
1818	Jean-Baptiste Dumas [born Alais, France, July 14, 1800; died Cannes, France, April 1884] treats goiter with iodine.
1829	The first edition of the *U. S. Pharmacopoeia* is published.
1845	The hypodermic syringe is introduced.
1862	Alexander Pagenstecher introduces the use of yellow mercury oxide salve as an ophthalmological ointment.
1876	Lydia E. Pinkham [born Lynn, Massachusetts, February 9, 1819; died Lynn, May 17, 1883] starts advertising her patent medicine for female reproductive disorders, the main active ingredient of which was alcohol.
1878	On May 2, George Francis of Adelaide, Australia, observes that a common pond scum of the genus *Nodularia* was poisonous to mammals, the first observation of a toxin produced by cyanobacteria (also known as algae).
1883	Sydney Ringer [born Norwich, England, 1835; died Lastingham, Yorkshire, October 14, 1910] discovers that an isolated frog heart kept in a saline solution will beat longer if calcium and potassium are added to the solution; the combination is known today as Ringer's solution. Ringer also finds that other activities of cells require calcium.
	Antipyrene, a powder used to reduce fever and relieve pain, is synthesized.
1887	A German glass-blower, F. A. Muller, develops the first form of contact lens, which covers the whites of the eye as well as the cornea.
1890	Benzocaine is developed in Germany; it is a local anesthetic that is given the trade name Anesthesin.
1891	George Redmayne Murray treats myxedema (the common form of hypothyroidism) with a hormone extracted from the thyroid gland.
1893	Felix Hoffman, working for the Aldolf von Bäyer firm in Elberfeld, Germany, synthesizes aspirin (acetyl salicylate).
1902	Millar Hutchinson in New York invents the first electrical hearing aid.
1903	Niels Ryberg Finsen of Denmark wins the Nobel Prize for Physiology or Medicine for his treatment of skin disease with light.
1904	Procaine, a local anesthetic, is discovered.
	Dr. William Scholl [born La Porte, Indiana, June 22, 1882; died March 29, 1968] sells the first one of his newly patented arch supports, now known as the Foot-Eazer.
1907	Ross G. Harrison [born Germantown, Pennsylvania, January 13, 1870; died New Haven, Connecticut, September 30, 1959] demonstrates the *in vitro* growth of living animal tissue.
1908	Physician Allvar Gullstrand [born Landskrona, Sweden, June 5, 1862; died Uppsala, Sweden, July 21, 1930] publishes *Die optische Abbildung in heterogenen Medien und die Dioptrik der Kristallinse des Menschen* (The Optical Imaging in Heterogenous Media and the Dioptrics of the Lens of the Eye of Man); he also develops eyeglasses to correct astigmatism and for use after lenses have been removed in cataract operations.

| 1913 | John Jacob Abel [born Cleveland, Ohio, May 19, 1857; died Baltimore, Maryland, May 26, 1938] develops the first artificial kidney. |

1913   John Jacob Abel [born Cleveland, Ohio, May 19, 1857; died Baltimore, Maryland, May 26, 1938] develops the first artificial kidney.

1914   Roger Adams [born Boston, Massachusetts, January 2, 1889] synthesizes Adamsite (phenarsazine chloride), a substance that causes sneezing.

1921   Frederick Grant Banting [born Alliston, Ontario, Canada, November 14, 1891; died Musgrave Harbour, February 21, 1941], Charles Best [born West Pembroke, Maine, February 27, 1899; died Toronto, Ontario, March 31, 1978] John McLeod, and James Collip extract insulin from the human pancreas and start experiments on dogs in an effort to develop a treatment for diabetes.

1922   Frederick Banting and Charles Best's *Internal Secretions of the Pancreas* is published.

1923   Sir Frederick Banting of Canada and John J. R. Macleod win the Nobel Prize for Physiology or Medicine for the discovery of insulin.

1927   Philip Drinker and Louis Shaw [born September 25, 1886; died August 27, 1940] develop the iron lung, a device for mechanical artificial respiration.

Julius Wagner von Jauregg [born Wels, Austria, March 7, 1857; died Vienna, Austria, September 27, 1940] win the Nobel Prize for Physiology or Medicine for the treatment of syphilis of the brain by using malaria inoculation to induce fever, which kills the bacteria in the brain.

1930   Ernest H. Volwiler [born Hamilton, Ohio, 1893; died Lake Forest, Illinois, October 3, 1992] and Donalee L. Tabern [born United States, 1900; died 1974] formulate Nembutal (pentobarbital sodium), a barbituate used for inducing hypnotic sleep.

1932   German chemist Gerhard Domagk [born Lagow (in Poland), October 30, 1895; died Burberg, Germany, April 24, 1964] discovers the first sulfa drug, Prontosil; he finds it kills streptococci and is very effective against blood poisoning.

1934   Quinacrine (also known as mepacrine, Atabrine, or Atebrin) is introduced as an effective treatment for malaria.

1935   Gerhard Domagk uses the first sulfa drug, Prontosil, on his youngest daughter to prevent her death from a streptococcal infection; this is the first use on a human being. Its success in this and other instances make Prontosil famous worldwide as the first "wonder drug."

Edward C. Kendall isolates cortisone, a substance present in the cortex of the adrenal gland.

1936   Daniele Bovet [born Neuchâtel, Switzerland, March 23, 1907], Leonard Colebro, and coworkers discover that the wonder drug Prontosil breaks down in the body and that the part that kills streptococci is a known chemical, sulfanilamide; they show that sulfanilamide is as effective as Prontosil.

Ernest H. Volwiler and Donalee L. Tabern formulate sodium pentathol, used for inducing hypnotic sleep as a preparation for full anesthesia for surgery and also known as a "truth serum" because of the state of suggestibility it induces.

1937   Based on the model of the successful drug sulfanilamide, scientists create sulfapyridine, the second sulfa drug.

A version of the antibacterial drug sulfanilamide called elixir of sulfanilamide that has been contaminated with poisonous diethylene glycol (antifreeze) is administered, resulting in 107 deaths; concern over this disaster contributes to the passage of the U.S. Food, Drug and Cosmetic Act of 1938, which establishes the U.S. Food and Drug Administration.

Pharmacologist Daniele Bovet, working at the Pasteur Institute in France, develops the first antihistamine.

1939   Scientists create sulfathiazole, the third sulfa drug.

Gerhard Domagk of Germany wins the Nobel Prize for Physiology or Medicine for discovery of the first sulfa drug, Prontosil.

1940   Herbert M. Evans [born September 23, 1882, Modesto, California] uses radioactive iodine to prove that iodine is used by the thyroid gland.

1941   Canadian-American surgeon Charles Branton Huggins [born Halifax, Nova Scotia, September 22, 1901] shows that administration of female sex hormones can be used to control prostate cancer; this is considered the first use of chemotherapy as a treatment for cancer.

1942   Georg Keble Hirst [born Eau Claire, Wisconsin, 1910(?); died Palo Alto, California, January 22, 1994] develops the first test for a viral infection, the hemagglutination assay; influenza viruses cause red blood cells to clump and allow researchers to determine how much influenza antibody there is in the blood.

1943   Dutch doctor Wilhelm Kolff [born Leiden, Netherlands, February 14, 1911] develops the first kidney dialysis machine; it is a machine that cleanses the blood outside the body and is used for patients with nonfunctional kidneys.

1948   American optician Kevin Touhy develops the modern corneal contact lens when he accidentally breaks off the corneal part while making a lens of the older type, which also covered the whites of the eye.

1950   Robert Wallace Wilkins [born Chattanooga, Tennessee, December 4, 1906] introduces the treatment of high blood pressure with reserpine, following the practice of using the drug in the form of snakeroot in India.

1951   Antabuse, a drug that prevents alcoholics from drinking, is introduced.

1952   The drug isoniazid, the first effective treatment for tuberculosis, is introduced.

Radiation therapy for cancer using cobalt 60 as a source of radioactivity is introduced.

1953   Frederick Sanger [born Rendcombe, England, August 13, 1918] becomes the first to determine the molecule-by-molecule structure of a protein, insulin.

1956   The kidney dialysis machine, developed by Wilhelm Kolff in 1943 comes into use in the United States.

Frederick Charles Novello introduces the diuretic drug chlorothiazide.

1958   Bifocal contact lenses are introduced.

Clarence Walton Lillehei [born Minneapolis, Minnesota, October 23, 1918] introduces the external pacemaker for controlling heart action.

1959   Ake Senning implants a pacemaker (heart stimulator).

1962   The drug MER-29 (Triparanol), intended to lower blood cholesterol, is found to cause cataracts in some users and is withdrawn from the market.

After reports became public that the use of the medicine thalidomide to control morning sickness had resulted in the birth of from seven to fourteen thousand children with deformed limbs, mostly in England and Germany (the drug was never approved for the U.S. market, although 2.5 million tablets were distributed in the U.S. for experimental use by 1200 doctors), the U.S. Congress in October establishes new and stricter guidelines for introduction of new drugs. Although thalidomide had been tested in animals, it had not been found to cause the birth defects in those tests, so it was introduced commercially in Europe in 1959 and used until 1962.

1964   Home kidney dialysis is introduced in the United Kingdom and the United States.

1965   Soft contact lenses are invented.

1975   César Milstein and George J. F. Köhler announce in the United Kingdom their discovery of how to produce a single line of identical antibodies, which are termed "monoclonal antibodies"; because they all represent the same lineage or clone of antibodies, each binds with the same chosen protein or antigen. In years to come, monoclonal antibodies will find a variety of uses in identifying specific molecules.

Miguel A. Ondetti, David W. Cushman, and coworkers at the Squibb Institute for Medical Research attack the problem of blocking human angiotensin-converting enzyme (ACE) and succeed in producing the first ACE inhibitor, an effective agent against high blood pressure known as captopril.

1976   Erwin Neher and Bert Sakmann develop the patch-clamping technique to study the traffic of ions across cell membranes; by tightly sealing a very thin glass pipette against a cell membrane, one can isolate a small patch of it and study the ion channels it contains.

1980   Dornier Medical Systems of Munich, West Germany, develop the lithotripter, a machine that uses sound waves to break up kidney stones while the stones are still in the kidney.

1982   On August 5, health authorities in Britain recall the drug known as Oraflex or Opren (generic name benoxaprofen) because it is blamed for 61 deaths and about 3500 other adverse reactions; in the U.S., the manufacturer voluntarily stops marketing the drug, only three months after its approval by the U.S. Food and Drug Administration.

1983   The U.S. Orphan Drug Act is passed, granting manufacturers of drugs designed to treat diseases with fewer than 200,000 victims an exclusive seven-year marketing period and other incentives to produce such drugs.

1984   César Milstein of Britain, Georges J. F. Köhler of West Germany, and Niels K. Jerne of Denmark share the Nobel Prize for Physiology or Medicine—Milstein and Köhler for their research on monoclonal antibodies and Jerne for his studies of the immune system.

1986   The U.S. Food and Drug Administration approves OKT3, the first monoclonal antibody to be approved for therapeutic use in humans; it aids in organ transplants.

Tony Hodges patents a split computer keyboard (the two halves can be adjusted to different angles of attack for each hand) to prevent such repetitive stress injuries as carpal tunnel syndrome.

1987   The U.S. Food and Drug Administration approves the drug AZT (generic name zidovudine), marketed as Retrovir, for treatment of persons with AIDS; AZT is the first approved treatment for the syndrome.

1988   Drug Delivery Systems develops the electric skin patch; it contains a battery that passes a tiny current through the skin under the patch, reducing its resistance to the absorption of drugs.

Disposable contact lenses go on sale; these can be worn one to seven days without removal or cleaning.

Elias J. Corey [born Methuen, Massachusetts, July 12, 1928] Myung-Choi Kang, Manoj C. Desai, Arun K. Ghosh, Ioannis N. Houpis, and Wei-Guo Su announce the synthesis of ginkgolide B, the chemical thought to be the active ingredient in many herbal remedies based on ginkgo leaves; ginkgolide B fights asthma and other allergies by suppressing the immune system.

The American geneticist Philip Leder [born Washington, DC, November 19, 1934] receives a patent for a mouse genetically engineered to be highly susceptible to cancer; the first patented animal in the world (although bacteria had been previously patented) is used in cancer research.

NEW USES FOR ASPIRIN

Since ancient times, practitioners of traditional medicine (formerly known as "witch doctors" among other appellations) have used infusions of willow bark as medicine. Legend has it that the concept was brought to the attention of science when Edmund Stone, an eighteenth-century Anglican clergyman in England, discovered that he obtained headache relief by chewing on the bark of the white willow tree. Recent research has shown that the active ingredient in willow bark, salicylic acid, is manufactured by plants to protect against viral infections. This ingredient of the willow-bark infusion has come to be known, as *asprin*, from its original trade name.

Until recent times, which have seen the rise of acetaminophen and ibuprofen as competition, aspirin has been the sovereign home remedy for headaches and muscle pains. Americans still take about 30 billion aspirin each year, mainly to relieve headaches or muscle or joint pain. Increasingly, however, millions of people take aspirin in small doses daily or every other day as a preventive measure against other illnesses.

In October 1993, partly in response to the increased use of aspirin as a preventive, the U.S. Food and Drug Administration (FDA) began to seek public opinion on a proposal for labeling products containing aspirin with a warning to consult a physician before beginning long-term use. FDA policy at the time was to label aspirin-containing products prescribed by physicians with information that the drug might be useful in preventing certain classes of heart-related conditions in men (no mention of women) after particular conditions (e.g. stroke precursors, heart attacks, or some forms of chest pain), but to eschew similar labeling on over-the-counter medications. A spokesperson for the FDA said that the risk of excessive bleeding from aspirin use was well documented but the benefits for heart disease were still controversial.

Over-the-counter aspirin in 1993 already contained a number of warnings. The most dramatic on the bottle itself—"it is especially important not to use aspirin during the last three months of pregnancy unless specifically directed to do so by a doctor because it may cause problems in the unborn child or complications during delivery" — is given in capital letters and was added in 1991. In ordinary type on the bottle, children and teenagers were warned not to take aspirin for flu or chicken pox because it could lead to Reye's syndrome, a rare but frequently fatal transformation of a viral disease into brain and liver damage, leading to seizures that may progress into coma or even death.

Indeed, aspirin definitely causes bleeding in the stomach and other parts of the digestive tract, making it a danger to persons with ulcers in that region. It can also cause bleeding in the brain, which is one form of stroke. And aspirin can cause allergic reactions in some people, leading in extreme cases to shock and death. Minor side effects include stomach pain, heartburn, or nausea.

In short, aspirin is a powerful drug. Like most powerful drugs, it can be utilized in many ways. A surprising number of new uses turned up in the early 1990s, and during this period further confirmation came for aspirin's benefits to the circulatory system. The earlier benefits had been discovered in the course of about 300 different studies of aspirin around the world.

Aspirin is even being tested for effectiveness against AIDS, in a study that started in August 1993 and is directed by Donald Kotler of St. Luke's-Roosevelt Hospital Center in New York City.

Heart Attacks and Strokes

The first fame for a new use for aspirin came in 1988 when the Physicians' Health Study revealed that male doctors who took an aspirin every other day had fewer heart attacks or strokes. In 1991 a similar, but less definitive, study of 87,678 female nurses showed that women also have fewer heart attacks if they take small amounts of aspirin. The difference in the studies was that the men deliberately took aspirin to prevent circulatory problems, while the women were grouped into those who took aspirin for headaches or other conditions and those who did not regularly take aspirin. The women showed a 30 percent drop in first heart attacks, as opposed to the 50 percent reduction for men. Other studies showed that patients with stable angina — chest pain caused by the heart when stressed which is relieved by standard medications or by rest — are also less likely to suffer heart attacks. The same does not seem to be true for unstable angina.

The protective effect of aspirin for heart attacks and stroke apparently comes from the ability of aspirin to reduce prostaglandins, which cause platelets in the blood to stick together. Thus blood clots formed by aggregation of platelets do not occur. Such clots when lodged in the heart are a major cause of the death of heart muscle cells and the heart attacks that follow; when lodged in the brain, clots similarly result in the loss of brain cells that is the direct damage from a stroke.

Platelets exposed to aspirin can no longer produce an enzyme that causes clotting. Once this happens to an individual platelet, it never recovers the ability to produce the enzyme. About ten percent of the platelet supply is replaced daily, so the effect of aspirin lingers. Thus, many persons taking aspirin to prevent clotting take only one dose every other day.

Furthermore, low doses of aspirin block the action of a chemical (thromboxane) that promotes clotting but fail to block another chemical (prostacylin) that reduces clotting. Higher doses inhibit both chemicals and thus cancel each other out. For blocking clotting, the most effective dose seems to be half of a baby aspirin or even a little less.

Continued research has confirmed the usefulness of aspirin taken or introduced in various ways as a treatment for heart attack and stroke as well as a preventive measure. Given soon after a heart attack, for example, aspirin reduces deaths to 75 percent of what they otherwise would be. Continued use of small daily doses of aspirin cuts the risk of a second heart attack to nearly half of what nonusers experience. The chance of a stroke following a heart attack is also reduced when aspirin is administered. There is less danger of clots during or after balloon angioplasty. It seems that whenever clotting is a problem, aspirin helps.

One common problem involves blood clots in persons who have had artificial valves implanted in their hearts. A small study by Alexander G. G. Turple of the Hamilton Civic Hospital Research Center and McMaster University in Hamilton, Ontario, reported in the August 19, 1993 *New England Journal of Medicine,* showed a 77-percent reduction in the number of serious clots among the patients taking aspirin as compared to those using a placebo. Furthermore, there was only a slight risk of excess bleeding in the aspirin patients, who were taking 100 milligrams of aspirin daily in time-release doses.

Preeclampsia

Somewhat confusingly, preeclampsia ("before eclampsia") is a serious condition in pregnant mothers that by itself primarily affects the baby by causing premature birth, while eclampsia is an acute problem that affects both the mother and the child and can be deadly. A high percentage of premature deliveries, variously estimated from one in four to one in three, result from preeclampsia. The condition also results in a lower birth weight among babies with preeclampsic mothers whose pregnancies come to term. About one in 20 women develop preeclampsia during their first pregnancy, but the condition is much less common in second or later pregnancies. The main symptoms are elevated blood pressure and fluid retention, while protein in the urine (which can be caused by high blood pressure) indicates that the mother is at a greater risk for the convulsions of eclampsia. (An older name for preeclampsia and eclampsia is *toxemia.*)

The most likely cause of preeclampsia is insufficient blood supply to the placenta, which then sends out chemical signals that affect the mother's blood vessels. As blood flow is reduced, the problem becomes self-perpetuating through feedback. If the original blood-flow problem is prevented, however, the feedback mechanism has no chance to get started. Aspirin was tried as a preventive measure with this in mind.

Results of a number of studies released since 1989 have shown consistent aid in prevention among mothers at higher risk for the disease or in whom the very beginning of the preeclampsia cycle can be detected. Thomas F. Imperiale and Alice Stollenwerk Petrulis of the Case Western Reserve University School of Medicine reported on July 10, 1991 in *Journal of the American Medical Association* that women at high risk for preeclampsia developed the condition 65 percent as often if they took low doses of aspirin. The aspirin also improved birth weights of newborns.

On the other hand, a large-scale study of 3135 first-time pregnancies conducted by Baha M. Sibai of the University of Tennessee, Robert C. Cefalo of the University of North Carolina at Chapel Hill, and coworkers, and reported in the October 21, 1993 *New England Journal of Medicine* showed that low doses of aspirin failed to make any difference unless the mother already showed moderate high blood pressure (systolic above 120) before the aspirin regime began.

Low doses of aspirin (on the order of 60 to 80 milligrams in most studies with pregnant women) are more effective than high doses and also safer. High doses of aspirin can result in excessive bleeding, for example. Even low doses were found to put mothers and the fetus at risk from a life-threatening condition called *abruptio placentae,* in which the placenta and uterus separate.

Migraines

The Harvard study on aspirin and heart attacks showed that the incidence of migraine attacks was reduced by 22 percent among men who took aspirin daily and were migraine sufferers. The exact cause of this relief is not known, but there seems to be a connection between platelets and migraines, which might account for the effect of aspirin.

Migraine cries out for relief, and a great many medicines have been found to provide it—at least some of the time to some people. Although aspirin is a standard headache remedy, it is not particularly effective *during* a migraine attack (the reduction found in the Harvard study was in the *incidence* of attacks). Since 1894, derivatives of a fungus found on rye (ergot) have been successful in providing relief during a migraine attack, although with severe side effects in some cases. Several high blood pressure medications, included both beta and calcium-channel blockers, provide relief for many migraine suffers and may reduce incidence. A folk remedy, the herb feverfew, has been found helpful in controlled studies in reducing incidence migraines. The exact role of any of these drugs in preventing migraines is even less well understood than the role of aspirin.

Cancer

In March 1993, the American Cancer Society released a study by Michael J. Thun that reported lower death rates for four different types of cancer among people who take aspirin daily, thereby building on a December 5, 1991 study that found lower death rates for one of the types, colon cancer. Both studies came from a retrospective look at a population of 635,000 persons living in the U.S. between 1982 and 1988.

One puzzle is that the four cancers in the study—involving the stomach, esophagus, and rectum as well as the colon—are considered different enough that one chemical would not be expected to affect all of them. Although all are cancers of the digestive tract, there is a considerable difference from one to another in the environmental factors that affect the four cancers.

Colon cancer has been reduced in laboratory animals with drugs similar to aspirin. A controlled study with sulindac, which acts like aspirin, found that the drug reduced polyps in people with a hereditary predisposition toward precancerous polyps. Other

SQUEEZING DATA FROM A MILLION PEOPLE

In 1982 more than a million Americans agreed to take part in a research effort known as the American Cancer Society's Cancer Prevention Study II. Since then, every two years the study participants update information about their occupation, living habits (including diet, smoking, alcohol consumption, exercise, drugs taken, and so forth), and any other potentially useful information that might relate to cancer. Statistics are also collected on causes of death, with special attention, of course, to cancer. Data is available covering 1982 through 1988.

With that kind of information, the study has been a boon to any researchers who want to examine the effects of lifestyle on health. The two studies by Michael Thun each involved about 635,000 people that provided suitable data concerning their aspirin use. Researchers from the University of Michigan were able to use data from about 900,000 people who described their smoking or nonsmoking habits in analyzing lung cancer risks.

---

studies with humans also have suggested that aspirin could help prevent colon cancer, which led to Thun's original look at colon cancer. In that study, people who took aspirin or a related drug (such as ibuprofen) on an average of at least every other day were shown to have a 40 percent lower risk of dying from colon cancer. The 1993 look at the same data base showed a similar 40 percent reduction in the other digestive-tract cancers among people who take aspirin regularly.

The mechanism by which aspirin might prevent cancer of any type is not known. Aspirin is thought to stimulate production of gamma interferon and interleukin-2, immune-system chemicals that are known to fight cancer (*see* "Allergies and Asthma," p 431).

Further study of the relationship between aspirin use and cancer, including controlled studies, will be conducted.

Pain

Although the public normally thinks of aspirin in terms of pain relief first, people also recognize that for acute or major pain, aspirin is not as effective as such opiates as morphine or as various synthetic pain blockers. In blind tests, however, aspirin fares much better than might be expected when matched against other pain relievers.

Aspirin's pain suppression is in part a result of its influence on transmission of nerve impulses and in part a result of its suppression of the inflammation that is causing the pain. In both cases scientists thought, until recently, that aspirin's effects were only local—affecting pain transmission from the wound itself and inflammation of the wound, for instance.

A study by Tony L. Yaksh and A. B. Malmberg of the University of California at San Diego (published in the August 28, 1992 *Science*) showed that the effect of aspirin (and its sister drug, ibuprofen) on pain is more general and less related to anti-inflammatory properties than previously believed. In their study, the scientists stimulated pain in mice and then injected aspirin or ibuprofen directly into the spinal column. They found that even though there was no aspirin near the pain stimulus, the longer-lasting pain that persists after a stimulus was reduced more than when the drug was taken by mouth and carried by the bloodstream to the site of the injury. Indeed, the pain-reducing potency was 100 to 500 times as great when directly injected into the spinal cord. Thus aspirin acts in part by reducing transmission of pain throughout the system. This work may lead to new ways to administer aspirin and comparable drugs, ways that would be both more effective and have fewer side effects.

TIMETABLE OF ASPIRIN

circa 400 BC   The school of Hippocrates recommends chewing willow bark as a cure for a variety of illnesses.

1763   In England, a description is published of the success Reverend E. Stone is having in reducing fever through the use of dried willow bark.

1838   Italian chemist R. Piria is the first to isolate salicylic acid, which he obtains from willow bark; this step was an important precursor of aspirin.

1853   Charles Frédéric Gerhardt obtains acetyl salicylic acid, a closer precursor of aspirin, from the bark of the silver birch.

1859   Hermann Kolbe synthesizes salicylic acid, the active principle of aspirin, from inorganic chemicals; although effective in reducing pain and fever, the new chemical is poorly tolerated by the stomach.

1893   Felix Hoffman, working for the Adolf von Bäyer firm in Elberfeld, Germany, synthesizes aspirin (acetyl salicylate); in its production, he uses a variant of the method introduced earlier by Hermann Kolbe to produce salicylic acid, but aspirin is not as unfriendly to the stomach lining as is salicylic acid; Hoffman's motivation is to develop a treatment for his father's rheumatoid arthritis. In 1899 aspirin is first taken for arthritis treatment, though it was previously administered for fever and pain reduction in other diseases; aspirin is still among the most effective treatments for arthritis.

1899   The Adolf von Bäyer company begins to market aspirin.

1950   Lawrence L. Craven [born United States, 1883; died Glendale, California, 1957] publishes the first of several articles based on the effects of regular aspirin use to prevent heart attacks and strokes, based on his research of 8000 patients; he continued to report on the preventive powers of aspirin in articles in obscure medical journals until 1956, but fails to convince others of his discovery.

1971   British scientist John R. Vane, while working with prostaglandins, discovers that aspirin helps keep platelets in blood from clotting, which brings him a share of the Nobel Prize for Physiology or Medicine in 1982.

1981   Studies about this time link aspirin taken for flulike symptoms or chicken pox with Reye's syndrome, a sometimes fatal transformation of a viral disease into seizures connected with brain and liver damage and coma; in November the U.S. Centers for Disease Control proposes warning labels.

1982   Regulations proposing warning labels for Reye's syndrome on aspirin products are drawn up by the U.S. Department of Health and Human Services, but not enacted.

1983	Babette B. Weksler and coworkers at Cornell University Medical Center in New York City discover that high doses of aspirin fail to prevent coronary artery disease, but speculate that lower doses will be effective.
1985	U.S. Secretary of Health, Education, and Welfare Margaret Heckler asks aspirin manufacturers to put warning labels against Reye's syndrome on bottles of aspirin; many comply.
1986	Warning labels against Reye's syndrome on aspirin products becomes mandatory in the U.S.
1988	In January, results of a study of more than 22,000 male physicians between the ages of 40 and 84 with no previous history of heart disease or stroke are announced; the data show that taking one buffered aspirin every other day reduces the risk of heart attack. The study is halted years before it had been scheduled to complete so news of the benefits can be released.
1989	On March 22, the Stroke Prevention in Atrial Fibrillation Study announces that regular aspirin use prevents mild strokes caused by abnormalities of heart rhythm in persons younger than 75.
	A team led by Eyal Schiff at Chaim Sheba Medical Center in Israel announced that pregnant women treated with 100 milligrams of aspirin daily are less likely to develop high blood pressure or the related complications grouped together as preeclampsia.

NEW USES FOR OTHER OLD DRUGS

Drug	Old use	New use
ACE inhibitors (e.g. Captopril)	Control high blood pressure	Retards progression of kidney disease in people with Type I (insulin-dependent diabetes).
Testosterone gel	Hormone replacement	Lowered risk of heart attack in men in a Swedish study reported in August 1993.
Thiazide diuretics	Lower levels of water and salt in high blood pressure	Study in January 1991 showed increase in bone density, reducing osteoporosis.
Valium (diazepam)	Tranquilizer	Six-year study released in July 1993 showed reduction in risk of convulsions caused by fevers (febrile seizures) in infants and young children.

(Periodical References and Additional Reading: *Harvard Medical School Health Letter* 5-90, p 1; *Harvard Health Letter* 12-90, p 4; *Harvard Health Letter* 1-91, pp 7 & 8; *New York Times* 3-16-91; *New York Times* 7-9-91, p C3; *New York Times* 7-14-91, p I-15; *New York Times* 10-31-91, p A24; *New York Times* 12-5-91, p A30; *Harvard Health Letter* 3-92, p 3; *Science* 8-28-92, p 1276; *New York Times* 9-1-92, p C3; *New York Times* 10-23-92, p A12; *Harvard Health Letter* 12-92, p 4; *New York Times* 3-21-93, p I:32; *Science* 7-23-03, p 422; *Science* 8-6-93, p 754; SN 8-7-93, p 85; *New York Times* 8-19-93, p A18; *New York Times* 8-31-93, p C5; *Science News* 11-6-93, p 302; *Science News* 11-13-93, p 311; *New York Times* 12-7-93, p C7; *Scientific American* 1-94, p 24; *New York Times* 1-7-94, p A20; *New York Times* 2-23-94, p C12; *Readers Digest* 4-94, p 85)

SYMMETRY AND DRUGS

Simple ideas are sometimes extremely powerful. Among the simplest ideas of mathematics is that of symmetry, which can be viewed most easily as any operation that produces an identical copy of the original. Sometimes, however, the identical copy is not truly identical in a basic way. The mirror image of a person or other object appears to be the same as the original, but right and left are reversed. This is most easily seen for writing, for which reversal of right and left makes many letters almost unreadable. Such mirror images can be constructed in three dimensions as well. They are also present in drugs.

You may read or hear from a friend that you should buy "D Vitamin E", or that "Dl Vitamin E" is a waste of money. What's the difference? Essentially, the difference is the same as the one between the L-Dopa used to treat Parkinson's disease and the D-Dopa that no one ever mentions. Like most organic compounds with biological activity, a molecule of alpha tocopheryl acetate (commonly used as vitamin E) or a molecule of dopa can come in two different forms, called chiral forms. These forms are like the two gloves in a pair—the same in all respects except that each fits only one hand. The right-handed form is called, depending on the author, D (for *dextro-*) or R (for *right*), while the left-handed form is called L (for *levo-*) or S (for *sinister*). A mixture of the two ought to be DL or RS, but drug manufacturers prefer Dl in the apparent hope that no one will notice the lower-case letter l.

For most compounds that come in left- and right-handed versions, only one form is biologically active. In the case of dopa, it is the L form, while for vitamin E, it is the D

Background

Although the first realization of the difference between the D and L forms goes back to Louis Pasteur's work of 1848, the full realization of the implications for medicine were a long time coming. It was not until the 1880s that Emil Fischer developed a system to classify organic chemicals into the D and L forms and not until 1955 that Fischer's system was proved to be correct. The study of the shapes of organic chemicals has since come to be called stereochemistry (three-dimensional chemistry), the two different forms are known as enantiomers (opposite shaped), and the chemicals that occur in both D and L forms as chiral (handed) compounds.

The essential molecules for life are chiral. Proteins are made from 20-odd chiral chemical units called amino acids. In living creatures only the L enantiomers of the amino acids are utilized. When these are combined into proteins, the resulting chain of L forms always is a three-dimensional spiral, or helix. The combination of left-handed subunits produces a helix that curls the other way, so the protein itself is right-handed. Similarly, the bases (or nucleotides) that make up RNA and DNA are left-handed, producing the single right-handed helix of RNA and the famous right-handed double helix of DNA. The right-handed helices of DNA, RNA, and proteins are the master chemicals of the body, ultimately controlling all other chemical reactions. Thus it is not surprising that the body deals with different enantiomers of chiral compounds in different ways.

form. Often the other form is simply inert and therefore biologically useless, as is believed to be the case for the L form of vitamin E. In some cases, however, both forms are biologically active, but result in different effects. One form of naproxen is anti-inflammatory, while the other one is poison. It is believed that only one chiral form of thalidomide caused the severe birth defects of the 1960s, while the other form has the mild tranquilizing effect doctors sought when the medicine was prescribed to pregnant mothers to prevent morning sickness. Other medicines such as ethambutol and benoxaprofen can cause blindness or death in one form, but not in the other. On a more positive note, synthetic L-menthol has become a major flavoring, since it is the form that people taste as mint.

Sadly, methods of producing drugs chemically by ordinary means produce equal amounts of the D and L forms mixed together. When thalidomide was prescribed, therefore, the medicine was dispensed with both the slightly useful tranquilizer and the producer of birth defects combined in each dose. One survey of the pharmaceutical industry in 1985 found that more than three-quarters of all drugs that are active in only one chiral form were sold in mixtures of both forms. Thus, these drugs as sold consist of a half-and-half mixture of a drug with known useful properties and a similar drug that is at best useless. In May 1992, the U.S. Food and Drug Administration began to require that manufacturers reveal the presence of one or both chiral forms in drugs.

Manufacture of one of the two forms of an organic compound has been difficult. It is known, for example, that only the D form of common table sugar, or sucrose, is used by the body, although we taste the L form as sweet. From time to time companies announce that they will offer L-sucrose as a noncaloric sweetener that has all the other properties of sugar in cooking—which is not the case with common artificial sweeteners. So far, none of the proposed L-sucrose sweeteners have made it to the market. In addition to difficulty of manufacture, it remains to be proved that L-sucrose is completely neutral. On the other hand, the common sweetener aspartame is produced by a process that uses organic enzymes to insure that its molecules have the correct handedness. Table sugar is manufactured by sugar cane or beet plants, so it normally comes in a form with a single handedness. Although synthetic L-menthol has to be catalyzed, natural menthol from mint plants is already in the L form. A classic method of drug manufacture is to use the same idea—get an organism to produce the desired form of the drug. Bacteria are used to produce the proper form of vitamin C, while enzymes taken from microbes are also used to make the correct form of aspartame.

In the late 1980s and early 1990s, several new methods were developed that made production of molecules with controlled handedness easier. One approach relies on inorganic catalysts that can be adjusted to produce either right- or left-handed forms during chemical reactions. A New Jersey company, Advanced Separation Technologies, patented a method based on using a sugar called cyclodextrin, developed by chemist Daniel Armstrong, as a filter to separate the two forms of a compound.

Another method uses organic catalysts of a novel type—monoclonal antibodies. Kim D. Janda, Charles G. Shevlin, and Richard A. Lerner of the Scripps Research Institute in La Jolla, California, announced in the January 22, 1993 *Science* that they had developed monoclonal antibodies that could catalyze reactions so that specific handedness would occur. In the reaction they worked on, handedness was not the only issue, however. The chemical they wanted to produce normally appears in only one form in the particular reaction, but the antibodies change the energy at a crucial stage, resulting in a different form. A few months later another group of California chemists and biologists reported the production of a desired form of an organic compound using the monoclonal-antibody approach.

Both inorganic and organic catalysts interact with other molecules without the catalyst molecule itself changing, so the right catalyst can be used to produce thousands of chiral molecules for each molecule of catalyst.

Some promising new medicines violate nature's chirality by using both L-amino acids and D-amino acids to produce peptide chains not found in nature (peptides are similar to proteins, but with fewer amino acids). One drug made this way, nafarelin, is a promising treatment for endometriosis, produced by slightly altering the hormone luteinizing-hormone releasing hormone (LHRH). Other drugs based on this idea can be used to block receptors, having one part that fits the receptor and another that, because of incorrect chirality, fails to do anything biologically. Among the diseases being countered with this method is AIDS. Another idea is to strengthen enzymes with new twists so that they do not break down as quickly as the natural version.

Antisense Genetics

Screws and other threaded machine parts must be either right-handed or left-handed—also called clockwise and counterclockwise. The thread, taken by itself, is a kind of three-dimensional spiral called a helix. Until the 1953 discovery that DNA, the chemical of heredity and cell direction, was shaped as two linked helices, the helix was at most a mathematical concept. But now symmetry entered the worlds of biology and medicine in a new way.

Symmetrical considerations for the helices of DNA and RNA go beyond their shapes. Both nucleic acids are right-handed helices, but DNA also uses a symmetry of its four bases to link its two helices. Just as the mirror image of a right-handed person appears to be left-handed, each of the four bases that make up a strand of DNA has a "mirror image" base that always faces it, linking one DNA strand with its image strand. The four bases of DNA are usually known by their first letters as A, C, G, and T. The mirror image of A is T, while that of C is G. Thus if a very simple gene is coded as ACTCATGAGATTAG, its image on the matching strand of DNA is TGAGTACTCTAATC. DNA is matched with RNA by essentially the same system, although the T base of DNA is replaced with a base known as U. Thus, the RNA image, or transcription, of the simple gene ACTCATGAGATTAG would be UGAGUACUCUAAUC. An RNA transcription of the image of the gene would be like the original gene, but with T replaced by U—ACUCAUGAGAUUAG.

At each step of the process, the original is replaced with its "mirror image." Biologists have borrowed terminology from mathematics to discuss these changes. In mathematics replacing a figure with its mirror image is called changing the sense of the figure. So the original RNA is said to have one sense, while its image has the opposite sense. This is abbreviated by calling the opposite sensed RNA "antisense RNA."

A gene functions when RNA produces its antisense image of the gene and, in a several-step process, proceeds to manufacture a protein. Interfering with any of the steps can cause the gene to stop functioning.

At first thought, one might wish to have all the genes functioning, but this would be far from healthy. Life proceeds in a series of stages, with genes being turned on when needed and turned off when not. Cancer is caused when certain genes are turned on or off inappropriately. Other diseases are caused by genes that produce too much of a substance or that produce an incorrect version of the substance. Viruses are strands of DNA or RNA that act like genes and subvert the cells' production of proteins. Thus the ability to shut off genes selectively, completely, or partially can be a powerful tool for medicine.

When it was learned how genes worked, scientists quickly realized that one way to shut down the work would be to use the mirror symmetry of DNA or RNA. If a mirror image of the RNA was available, it would tie up the RNA so that it could not be used to transcribe the gene. Since the mirror image has the opposite sense of the original RNA, it is called antisense RNA. The trick is to make the antisense RNA bind tightly to the original RNA, blocking the next steps in the process. This is easier in theory than it was found to be in practice.

In 1993, however, Brian C. Froehler and other researchers from Gilead Sciences, Inc., a biotechnology company from Foster City, California, found a way to modify the link between two of the bases so that it is from ten to 100 times as strong. Thus once the mirror image attaches itself to its intended target of messenger RNA, it stays there much longer, making the drug more powerful.

Clinical trials of antisense drugs began in 1991, but results were not expected to be published until 1994. Prepublication leaks, especially about studies of drugs in animal models, suggest the possibility that some products based on symmetry would appear as early as 1995. Drugs known to be in development or about to be put into development in 1993 included antisense RNA to treat genital warts, the degenerative eye disease cytomegalovirus retinitis (which mostly affects AIDS patients), the bone-marrow cancer, myelogenous leukemia, lung cancer and inflammation in general. Tests of one of the antisense drug directed against RNA which has been used in treating myelogenous leukemia show that the antisense RNA is so much safer than conventional chemotherapy that patients can administer the drug to themselves at home. In the lung-cancer therapy, the idea is to use a viral vector to insert an antisense version of the *p53* gene into the cancerous cells (*see* "Genes for Cancer," p 54).

In laboratory tests, antisense approaches have been used to block the enzyme that cancer cells produce, the enzyme that pumps chemicals directed against the cancer out of the cells. If this approach works in the body, it would halt one major form of resistance that cancers develop to chemotherapy.

Right Keyhole, Wrong Key

Shape has been recognized in the twentieth century as one of the main ways that organic molecules function. This is the essential idea behind the symmetry of D and L forms of drugs and, in a less obvious form, behind the sense and antisense relationship of DNA and RNA. A third way that shape is essential is in the relationship between enzymes and other catalysts and the molecules on which they work, called the substrate molecules. Each enzyme causes chemical processes to proceed at a much greater rate by bringing parts of molecules that will interact with each other closer together. To do this, the enzyme has a part, often called the key, that fits into the substrate molecule like a key into a lock. When the key is in the lock, forces between parts of the key and parts of the lock cause the substrate molecule (or molecules if the key causes two molecules to interact faster) to change in a specific way. For example, some enzymes cause a molecule to break into two parts, while others cause two molecules to join together in a specific way. This key and lock mechanism accounts for the way that most reactions in living creatures occur.

Just as antisense RNA can be used to block the action of viruses or unwanted genes, fitting a wrong key into a substrate lock and leaving it there will prevent the correct key from even getting into the lock. This concept has become an important idea in manufactured drugs, but has long been a part of life. For example, many of the organic poisons used by venomous creatures or poison plants work by this principle, blocking some reaction essential for life by flooding the organism with wrong keys to the reaction.

One target for such wrong keys in medicine is the disease-causing virus. Each virus includes enzymes that act as keys to enable the virus to perform such essential tasks as entering and leaving cells or slipping into the DNA structure of the cell. To block such an enzyme, one can cause the virus to encounter a false lock for its key. In 1993, for example, researchers found two false locks for the enzyme that enables influenza viruses produced in cells to escape so that the viruses can infect other cells. One of the false locks, developed by Mark von Itzstein and coworkers at Monash University in Victoria, Australia, in conjunction with Glaxo of England, was shown to work in flu-infected ferrets, blocking the illness and its transmission.

(Periodical References and Additional Reading: *New York Times* 11-2-92, p D2; *Science* 1-22-93, pp 469, 490; *Science* 1-22-93, pp 479 & 490; *New York Times* 1-26-93, p C3; *Science* 4-16-93, p 337; *Science News* 5-29-93, p 348; *Science News* 6-5-93, p 366; *New York Times,* 6-6-93, p C3; *New York Times,* 6-8-93, p C3; *New York Times* 1-3-94, p C14)

PROMISING PILLS AND POTIONS

Everyone seems to feel better if they can take a pill or get an injection to solve whatever problem they have. The idea is often used as a metaphor for conditions far removed from medicine, such as a "bitter pill" indicating an unpleasant economic remedy. This is perhaps one reason that people dose themselves with, and that even physicians prescribe, antibiotics (only useful against bacteria) for diseases caused by viruses, such as the common cold.

Nostrums of various types proliferate in the age of new medical technology. These include various mirror-image approaches (*see* "Symmetry and Drugs," p 534), new biologicals taken from plants and animals, medicines from fungi, protists, or bacteria, drugs manufactured by genetic engineering, treatments based on monoclonal antibodies, more traditional synthetic organic compounds, and even inorganic chemicals that have biological effects. In the early 1990s, while living organisms provided most of the ideas, increasingly very specific chemistry located the drugs.

New Drugs from Animals, Plants, and Fungi

Many of humanity's oldest and most reliable remedies, as well as even more that are ineffective, derive from other living organisms, ranging from fungal fruiting bodies (toadstools) to the sex organs of such mammals as lions and tigers and bears. Periodically, as when digitalis is located in foxglove, antibiotics in molds, or aspirin in willow bark, an ancient herbal remedy becomes one of the wonder drugs of science.

Today one of the major arguments used by persons trying to defend species from extinction is that some untested species may become lost before we find that it contains a more potent cure for cancer (or AIDS or malaria or heart disease) than Taxol—a chemical found in the bark of an endangered yew. The search ranges from lowly cyanobacteria (formerly known as blue-green algae) to frogs, sharks, and other vertebrates. In the early 1990s, this informal program has led to several major new classes of drugs.

The U.S. National Institutes of Health (NIH), National Science Foundation, and Agency for International Development all recognized the promise of biological drugs and together set up an award program called the International Cooperative Biodiversity Groups Program that funds teams of U.S. and foreign scientists in searching for biologicals in endangered environments. The first five awards, amounting to $2.5 million in all and announced in December 1993, sponsored research in rain forests of Suriname, Costa Rica, Nigeria, and Cameroon as well as in arid and semiarid regions of Latin America.

Shark Antibiotic   Sharks are especially interesting to humans. Although we think of them as fish, it is clear that sharks and their relatives are a considerable evolutionary distance from trout or cod. In modern taxonomy, the cartilaginous sharks, rays, and ratfishes are given a separate class from the fish. The complete list of vertebrate classes consists of jawless fishes; sharks and relatives; bony fishes; amphibians; reptiles; birds; and mammals.

Legends abound about sharks. Among them is the legend that sharks never develop cancer. This is not true, but those who hold that it is claim that the cause is a chemical in the cartilage that sharks have instead of bone. As a result, there was in the early 1990s a flurry of commercial interest in selling shark cartilage extract to prevent cancer.

Another legend is that sharks do not develop infections, even after surgery and despite lifestyles that expose them to all sorts of bacteria and fungi. This legend, however, has considerable basis in fact. The story intrigued Michael Zasloff when he first heard of shark resistance to infection in July 1989. Zasloff had already founded a corporation to locate biological antibiotics after his discovery in August 1987 of a new family of potent antibiotics in the skin of the African clawed frog. Since the frog discovery, which was a group of chemicals named magainins, Zasloff has pursued antibiotics in less exotic places, such as pig intestines and cow tracheae. But his most potent discovery may have been in February 1993 when he and Karen S. Moore located an entirely new form of antibiotic in the stomach tissues of a shark called the spiny dogfish (*Squalus acanthias*), which they described in the *Proceedings of the National Academy of Sciences*.

Squalamine, as the chemical has been named, is a modified steroid that chemically pokes holes in the cell membranes of bacteria, protozoans, and fungi, but ignores the cell membranes of vertebrates. Chemically it is similar to cholesterol.

The key idea behind any antibiotic is to attack something that germs or classes of germs have and that humans lack. Penicillin and relatives, for example, act on an enzyme used in bacterial reproduction. Antibiotic resistance occurs when some germs that use a different pathway to achieve the same end proliferate in the absence of those destroyed by the antibiotic. It is thought that it will be more difficult for microbes to develop resistance to squalamine since it is not likely that a microbe exists with a totally different type of cell membrane.

Squalamine should be especially useful in treating fungal diseases, which are not affected by antibiotics aimed directly at bacteria. Although fungal diseases are often limited by human immune systems (think of athlete's foot), they are hard to eliminate and when the immune system is suppressed, as in AIDS or after organ or cell transplants or during other forms of modern therapy, fungal diseases become much more serious.

Since squalamine is a steroid, a class of drugs whose chemistry is now well known, it has rapidly been synthesized. Zasloff and his colleagues at Magainin Pharmaceuticals in Plymouth Meeting Pennsylvania continue to explore its chemistry in hopes of making it even more effective.

Ghana Traditional Healer's Herb   The plant *Desmodium adscendens* is used by traditional healers in Ghana for asthma and a variety of other conditions, all of which biologists recognize as involving constrictions of smooth muscles. Three different triterpene glycosides were isolated from the West African plant according to a report in 1993; they were shown to relax smooth muscles *in vitro*. Because of the long tradition of the plant's use, the scientists working on the chemicals expect the glycosides to be successful in humans as well.

Deerfly Blood Thinner   In the October 1, 1993 *Proceedings of the National Academy of Sciences,* researchers for Massachusetts General Hospital-East in Charleston, Massachusetts announced that they had extracted a chemical they named chrysoptin from the common deerflies found along the New England Coast. Chrysoptin keeps blood platelets from sticking together. The previous year the same team found a chemical with the same action in the tropical sandfly. Biting flies use the chemicals to keep wounds open while the flies feast. Similar chemicals from other sources, notably from viper venom, are already in use to stem clotting in heart attacks or strokes.

Poison Arrow Frog   The Ecuadorian frog *Epipedeobates tricolor* is known as the poison arrow frog, named for its main use by traditional South American natives. In 1992 John Daly and coworkers at the NIH discovered that, for mice at least, one of the chemicals in the glands of the poison arrow frog is a potent pain blocker; furthermore the chemical is of an entirely different family from the opiates.

A year later at least two teams had developed synthetic analogs to the chemical, which is named epibatridine. Although epibatridine as it now exists, natural or synthetic, is too toxic to use as a human painkiller, scientists believe that they can engineer the toxicity out and leave the painkilling in. Even if that fails, the chemical's action points to a previously unknown receptor.

Domestic Animal Sources   Because of easy access to animal organs from slaughterhouses, some drugs are extracted from cows, sheep, or pigs. For example, a new drug known as GM-1 ganglioside, which allows some patients to recover motion after an injury to the spinal cord, is extracted from the brains of cattle.

New Immune Suppressor   Since the discovery of the effectiveness of penicillin from molds in the middle of the twentieth century, the search for biological agents in other molds and fungi, soil bacteria, and even protists has increased in intensity. Some 120 different useful antibiotics have been obtained from soil microbes, including the first, found before penicillin was clinically available.

Although cyclosporine (from a fungus) has made organ transplants possible, it is not for everyone. It can cause hypertension, kidney problems, and liver damage, which may aggravate conditions that exist in those who most need the transplant. Twenty years ago another immunosuppressant was discovered in a different fungus and named rapamysin. Clinical trials are underway with rapamysin made by fermentation in large batches (the way penicillin was first manufactured), but in 1993 chemists were able to synthesize the drug. This may lead to production of new and improved versions, although synthesis at present seems unlikely to be cheaper or more efficient than fermentation.

A Bacterial Toxin   The poison produced by the anaerobic bacterium *Clostridium botulinum* is best known for causing paralysis or death when it is eaten in spoiled foods. It has long been considered among the most potent natural chemicals. The botulism toxin paralyzes by preventing nerves from releasing the neurotransmitters that cause muscles to contract. In 1990 the U.S. Food and Drug Administration (FDA) approved using the toxins to stop the uncontrollable winking known as blepharospasm and "crossed eyes," officially known as strabismus. Research continues on other ways to use the unique properties of the toxin.

Genetically Engineered Proteins

Genetic engineering has to a large degree lived up to the initial excitement over its medical possibilities. In most current genetic engineering, a bacterium, yeast, immortalized mammalian cell, or possibly some other cell (although much less likely than the types named) is given a bit of DNA that causes the cell to produce a desired protein. In some experimental instances, a mammal or plant expresses the protein in milk or some other way. Notice that genetic engineering is essentially a new way to make quantities of proteins.

Stimulating Cell Growth   In 1991 two new drugs for promoting cell growth became available through genetic engineering. These drugs may be the beginning of a broad class of treatments. Both are known as colony stimulating factors. Because they can have many uses, ranging from adjuncts to cancer treatment to attacking viruses and bacteria by stimulating the immune system, one scientist has called their introduction "of a similar magnitude to what the discovery of antibiotics represented." Granulyte colony stimulating factor (G-CSF) improves the immune-system response in people undergoing chemotherapy. Granulocyte macrophage colony stimulating factor (GM-CSF), marketed as Leukine, causes bone marrow to produce more white blood cells.

Clotting Factor   In 1992 the FDA approved genetically engineered clotting factor VIII, a blood protein missing in people who are born with hemophilia A. Although the artificial clotting factor is thought to be exactly the same chemically as the natural one, it cannot be contaminated with viruses as natural clotting factor has been in the past. (Modern techniques are believed to be efficient in preventing such contamination.) The genetically engineered version is 25 to 50 percent more expensive than clotting factor VIII made from human blood.

Bone Morphogenetic Protein   Since 1945 it have been observed that some chemical in bone can actually change muscle cells into bone cells. During the 1990s workers found nine such chemicals in bone, which generically are called bone morphogenetic protein (BMP). Although there is not much BMP in ground up bone cells, there was enough to develop genetically engineered forms of the various proteins in this class. Two separate sets of field trials using BMP with human subjects were approved by the FDA in 1993. The companies involved, Genetics Institute, Inc., of Cambridge, Massachusetts, and Creative Biomolecules of Hopkinton, Massachusetts, have each received various BMP-related patents, and it was not clear who would emerge as the winner from the patent fight. In the meantime, the field trials will establish whether or not there is something worth winning.

Synthetic Organic Compounds

Although nearly always based upon knowledge of chemicals produced by the body, synthetic organic drugs are produced by chemical reactions, not by natural or genetically engineered living organisms.

New Class of Neurotransmitter-Related Drugs   The new drug for migraine headaches, sumatriptan, became the first of a new class of drugs that resemble neurotransmitters. Previous effective treatments such as various psychoactive drugs and L-dopa act on neurotransmitter receptors or stimulate natural neurotransmitters.

Peptide Screening and Design   The first artificial version of a protein, produced in 1953, depended on the ability to combine amino acids in a correct sequence and shape. The ability to form short chains of amino acids, called peptides, proceeded rapidly and by the 1960s became an easy trick for organic chemists, instead of a Nobel Prize-winning feat. For the most part, however, no one had any idea of which peptides might be useful and which might be just random chains of amino acids. In the early 1990s, however, a number of methods were developed for screening peptides for biological activity. Among the results of random peptide manufacture and biological screening are promising new treatments for asthma and blood clots.

Other groups are working on the more traditional approach of developing specific peptides. Many of these peptides are intended to replace proteins that have to be made by genetically engineered bacteria, yeast, or mammalian cells. Such peptides, if found, would be more stable than proteins and probably produce fewer side effects.

RU 486   Although RU 486 was developed primarily as an abortion inducer or as a "morning-after" birth-control pill, it has various biological effects throughout the body. One of the first uses permitted for the drug in the U.S. was a special ruling by the FDA that permitted a brain cancer patient to use the drug as a treatment. The drug was also proposed as useful in treating endometriosis, depression, and cancers of the breast, ovaries, or prostate.

Cholesterol for Sepsis   A surprising drug for an old enemy is that relatively new enemy and even newer friend cholesterol. The old enemy is sepsis, often known as "blood poisoning." Sepsis is the overreaction in the immune system of bacterial poisons called endotoxins. Worldwide about 300,000 to 400,000 persons a year develop sepsis and about half of them die as a result.

Daniel M. Levine and coworkers of the Rogosin Institute at New York Hospital-Cornell Medical Center reported in the December 15, 1993 *Proceedings of the National Academy of Sciences* that sepsis is reduced by the kind of cholesterol known as HDL (high-density lipoprotein), also nicknamed "good cholesterol" because it helps reduce heart disease. The Rogosin scientists showed that mice genetically engineered to produce large amounts of HDL survive an injection of endotoxins that is about six times more than the amount needed to kill mice engineered to produce small amounts of HDL cholesterol. Furthermore, giving normal mice an injection of synthetic HDL also improved survival rates.

The researchers have patented the use of synthetic HDL for sepsis treatment. Testing on humans should begin late in 1994 or early 1995.

An Antiviral Drug   Drugs that work on viral diseases are in very short supply (*see* "The Calamity of a Viral Medicine," p 335). In 1993 Australian and British researchers found two new drugs that in animals at least seem to work against influenza. They were able to use computer simulations to locate chemicals that block an enzyme called a sialidase that is on the viral coat, and to model these chemicals to be directed solely at the form of the enzyme found on influenza viruses. Many other pathogens also have sialidases on their surfaces (and so do some mammal cells, including some in humans), so the hope is that blockers can be found that attack specific pathogens but not other cells.

Fat Blocker   The drug known as orlistat (chemically tetrahydrolipstatin) prevents fat from being absorbed by the walls of the intestines, so most of the fat in food is excreted. For people on a weight-loss diet, this doubles the amount of weight lost in a given period of time, although it does produce a fair amount of gastrointestinal problems, such as flatulence, diarrhea, and malodorous stools. In 1993 orlistat was still undergoing clinical trials with obese patients.

PNP Blocker   The enzyme purine nucleoside phosphorylase (PNP) recycles a part of DNA or RNA for reuse. It also interferes with the AIDS drug ddI, which is an artificial nucleoside. A collaborating group of scientists from Birmingham, Alabama, worked three years on finding a drug that would inhibit PNP, finding several. The apparent best of the lot, known as BCX-34, has also shown effectiveness in limited trials against psoriasis and cutaneous T cell lymphoma. Another even more potent inhibitor may be effective against arthritis. This is a tremendous payoff from the designer-drug approach to developing specific drugs for biochemical actions.

Cell Adhesion Molecules   In the 1980s it was realized that a number of molecules involved in cell adhesion had common active sites and that drugs might be made to mimic or block them. The first such drug, Telioderm, imitates the active site for cell adhesion in a gel that promotes wound healing in skin and is mainly aimed at curing bed sores. However, a large number of applications involving cell adhesion molecules are in the works—for strengthening bones weakened by osteoporosis, preventing blood clots, reducing inflammation, treating multiple sclerosis, stopping cancer metastasis, and even curing the common cold.

(Periodical References and Additional Reading: *New York Times* 12-15-90, p D1; *Harvard Health Letter* 2-91, p 7; *New York Times* 3-6-91, p D4; *New York Times* 6-27-91; *New York*

Times 10-9-91, p D22; *New York Times* 10-26-91, p 20; *New York Times* 7-30-92, pp A10 & A22; *New York Times* 10-6-92, p D1; *New York Times* 11-10-92, p C5; *New York Times* 12-11-92, p D5; *New York Times* 2-15-93, p A8; *Science News* 2-27-93, p 143; *New York Times* 3-22-93, p D2; *New York Times* 4-4-93, p III-2; *Science* 5-14-93, pp 906 & 910; *Nature* 6-3-93, pp 401 & 418; *Science News* 6-5-93, p 358; *New York Times* 6-8-93, p C3; *Nature* 7-22-93, p 285; *Science* 8-27-93, p 1117; *Scientific American* 10-93, p 24; *Science News* 10-9-93, p 235; *Scientific American* 12-93, p 92; *New York Times* 12-8-93, p A20; *Science News* 12-18/25-93, p 406; *Discover* 1-94, p 86; *Scientific American* 1-94, p 78)

TECHNICAL FIXES FOR OLD PROBLEMS

Although people tend to think first of drugs or surgery when considering medical treatment, there are many mechanical or electrical devices that have been developed for handling special conditions. The most common of these, such as hearing aids and eyeglasses, are treated elsewhere (*see* "The Senses UPDATE," p 452).

Like hearing aids and eyeglasses, many important medical devices replace or augment natural organs—artificial kidneys, livers, hearts, for example, as well as various "inert" implants. One way to group these replacement parts is by those that are permanently implanted in the body and those that are support devices outside the body.

MEDICAL DEVICES AND THEIR PURPOSES

Device	Intended Medical Purpose
Common permanently implanted devices in the patient's body	
Annuloplasty ring	Heart valve attachment
Aneurysm clip	Closes a bulging and weakened blood vessel
Breast prosthesis	Inflatable or gel breast replacement or enlarger
Cardiovascular intravascular filter	Filters outs blood clots
Central nervous system fluid shunt	Drains excess fluid from the brain
Chin prosthesis	Silicone used to reshape face
Defibrillator (internal)	Controls irregular heart rhythms
Diaphragmatic-phrenic nerve stimulator	Stimulates breathing
Heart valve	Replaces leaky or nonworking valve
Intercardiac patch	Used to patch a hole in the wall of the heart
Pacemaker	Electrically stimulates heart beat when needed
Penile implant	Silicone device used in maintaining erection
Spinal implants	Keeps spine straight and disks in place
Testicular prosthesis	Replaces missing testicle(s)
Vascular graft	Synthetic blood vessel wall
Ventricular bypass assistance	Temporary heart pump
Common support devices used outside the body	
Apnea monitor	Warns of halt in breathing during sleep

Device	Intended Medical Purpose
Defibrillator (external)	Controls irregular heart rhythms
Dialysis equipment	Replaces all or part of kidney function
Oxygen generator	Aids breathing
Tracheostomy tube and cuff	Used to permit breathing through neck
Ventilator	Maintains breathing

Other medical devices remove something (stones or pathogens or arterial plaque, for example) or add something (drug delivery systems).

Device Failure

Until 1976, the U.S. Food and Drug Administration (FDA) did not regulate medical devices. Today there are about 16,000 devices under FDA regulation. Even after regulation started, there were some notable failures—especially the Bjork-Shiley heart valve, which easily developed cracks and had to be removed from the market in 1986 (*see also* below).

In the early 1990s it sometimes appeared that there were even more problems with medical devices than with nonworking or dangerous drugs. About 53 persons a year were thought to die as a result of poorly working or badly designed medical devices. Another 1150 annually were seriously injured by devices. Silicone implants were among the most controversial products (*see* "Implants and the Immune System," p 223). Among the other devices under inspection by the FDA were various models of heart defibrillators, a device intended to help control urinary incontinence, and a laser angioplasty device.

The Bjork-Shiley valve   There were about 23,000 people in the U.S. and 55,000 to 86,000 worldwide (both figures are widely used) who had been fitted with the Bjork-Shiley heart-valve implant. By 1992 a total of 468 of the valves had failed and more than 300 people had died. Although some of the heart valve recipients have had the valves removed and others have died from other causes, most still live with the knowledge that their heart could fail at any time. There is about a one in 20 chance of dying from the valve-removal operation and the procedure costs about $35,000. No one knows exactly who received the valves, so it is possible that many of the recipients still do not know that anything is wrong with their heart repair.

In 1992 the manufacturer, a division of Pfizer, announced that a new X-ray method could detect cracks well before the breakage led to failure of the valve. Pfizer said that it would pay for anyone with the Bjork-Shiley valve (about 51,000 persons at that time) to have X rays taken twice a year with the special technique and for the valve to be removed if it appeared to be developing cracks.

Deadly radiation   In 1992, machines built by Omnitron International of Houston, Texas, failed to remove radioactive iridium-192 from two patients' bodies after a cancer treatment that was to take only a few minutes. Although this was a purely mechanical problem, the results could be devastating. In one instance, an alert technician noticed the error and solved the problem before any serious damage to the patient. In the other, despite radiation alarms, the iridium wire was not removed at all. After about 90 hours the wire fell out on its own (probably because of tissue destruction), was sent out in the trash, and got caught by the radiation detector at the waste hauler. The patient died the next day. One source noted at the time that at least 40 other people had also died from overdoses of medical radiation since 1975.

Baby monitors   Devices were developed to detect the breathing of infants, as sudden loss of breath might be the onset of Sudden Infant Death Syndrome (*see* "SIDS UPDATE," p 128). Although the devices were intended to work from transformers, it was possible to plug them into wall sockets. When this was done, however the surge of electricity killed the baby.

Defibrillator   According to the Public Citizen Health Research Group, a consumer activist organization, the FDA had received a thousand complaints of defects in the Physio-Control electric heart defibrillator, used by emergency medical services and hospitals, over a fifteen-month period in 1992-93, including reports of 322 deaths associated with device problems. According to the manufacturer, 150,000 of the defibrillators were in use on more than a million cases of cardiac arrest annually. The FDA had suspended sales of the defibrillator for ten months prior to May 18, 1993, while the company made design changes, but the FDA did not recall the existing models.

Improvements in Current Devices

Device failure is not typical of most medical machinery. A lot of it works just fine, and in the early 1990s some of those machines began to work better than ever.

Dialysis   Kidney dialysis, although still not perfect, has been one of the great medical success stories of the period since World War II. While dialysis solves the main problem caused by kidney failure, it does not replace all the important functions of the kidney. Medical engineers hope someday to produce a true "bionic kidney," an implantable device that will perform kidney functions such as waste removal and fluid control on a continuous basis with no monitoring by the patient. Work on development of such a device has been under way for many years, but the challenges in developing the bionic kidney are very great.

On the way to a bionic kidney, new miniaturized pumps and sensors can be used to reduce the size of the artificial kidney to as little as 60 pounds. Such a compact, lightweight unit can be used at home and even carried on trips, making the whole process of dialysis easier on the patient and more flexible. The same general principles as in today's artificial kidney are employed, but the difference is like that between a minicomputer of the 1970s and the desktop computers of today. Further development along this line could lead to the equivalent of a "laptop" dialyzer.

Another entirely different approach uses the body as part of the equipment. In peritoneal dialysis, the dialysis fluid is pumped or allowed by gravity to flow into the abdominal cavity, which is naturally lined by a thin film called the peritoneum. The same transfers of wastes as in hemodialysis take place between blood in tiny vessels in the peritoneum and the dialysis fluid. After several hours, the dialysis fluid, now increased in volume and containing the wastes, is pumped or allowed to flow out.

In 1990 inventor Dean Kamen became interested in peritoneal dialysis after a

Background

The kidneys are a pair of organs that remove waste products from the blood. They are vulnerable to injury and infection, which can cause either progressive loss of function or sudden catastrophic loss. Many sudden changes are reversible if the patient can be kept alive for a few days. Kidney failure that is not reversed or compensated for leads to poisoning by the body's own waste products. The patient dies after a short time.

Healthy kidneys control what is in a person's blood—how acid or how salty it is, for instance. Kidneys also determine how much of the blood is water. Additionally, kidneys help control blood pressure and release hormones that stimulate production of red blood cells and some steroids. Kidneys also help activate vitamin D and produce other substances useful to the body.

Chemicals that form as waste products of cells get carried to the kidneys by the blood. Most of these wastes are removed and discarded, although kidney cells recycle some into new chemicals that cells can use. Different parts of the kidney remove parts of the blood from or return useful chemicals through the walls of the capillaries.

Early in the twentieth century doctors realized that a technique for separating two kinds of chemicals can clean the wastes from blood just as natural kidneys do. Since the chemical process at the heart of the artificial kidney is called dialysis, the artificial kidney is usually called a dialysis machine. Because blood is the liquid involved, a more technical name for the process is hemodialysis (hemo means "blood").

Kidney failure can either be a slow, step-by-step process or it can happen very suddenly. The slow (or chronic) type is often caused by infections or by high blood pressure that has not been treated. If it is caught and treated with diet and perhaps vitamins and minerals, chronic kidney failure need not lead to dialysis. If not treated, however, it can result in kidney failure that can only be treated with dialysis or with a transplant.

The most common cause of sudden kidney failure is untreated chronic kidney disease. For unknown reasons diabetes can also cause kidney failure. Sometimes sudden kidney failure is a result of an acute infection, a drop in blood pressure from any cause (including bleeding), or anything that blocks release of urine. While the kidneys will recover when the cause is resolved, dialysis is often needed while recovery takes place, although changes in diet can control problems for many patients.

For nonrecovering kidney failure, life-long dialysis or a kidney transplant are the only long-term solutions. Today many patients use dialysis to stay healthy while a kidney suitable for transplanting is located.

Dialysis of blood can also be used in cases of acute poisoning, when it is too late for a stomach pump. Dialysis in some forms of liver failure can carry a patient through a crisis. This is because the dialysis process can remove many kinds of small molecules from a person's blood.

An artificial kidney pumps blood into a unit called a dialyzer, and there the blood enters a network of tubes running through a salt solution known as dialysis fluid or dialysate. The tubes are made from thin cellulose. Wastes pass from the blood into the dialysis fluid through the walls of the tubes.

If the supply of dialysis fluid were static, the process would remove only half the dangerous wastes from the blood. But the artificial kidney takes away used fluid and replaces it with new dialysis fluid that contains no wastes. Usually the machine mixes a powder with water to make fresh fluid as the dialysis process takes place.

Although this is a continuous process, you can picture it in terms of a number of passes. The first pass of the blood though the machine removes half the wastes, leaving half. With new fluid, the second pass removes half the remaining wastes, leaving a fourth of the original amount. Another pass would cause only an eighth to be left. After ten such passes, less than a thousandth of the original wastes would remain in the blood. The rest would be drained off into the dialysis fluid.

Although cleansing takes place in the dialyzer, most of the machine is involved in keeping blood pressure and temperature constant and in moving the blood and the dialysis solution through the dialyzer. In addition, a blood thinner such as heparin must be added and monitored to prevent clotting.

Small molecules, such as salts and acids, can pass through a thin membrane, such as cellophane. Large molecules, such as proteins and antibodies, cannot.

As blood and dialysis solution pass by each other, the small molecules gradually get into equilibrium. Dialysis solution contains minerals such as calcium in the same amount as there normally is in blood. Such minerals are already in equilibrium. Wastes, such as the chemicals creatine and uric acid, are not in dialysis fluid. To get into equilibrium, half of those chemicals must pass into the fluid from the blood. Some chemicals may also be in too great supply in the blood, but are also in the dialysis fluid so that the equilibrium position still leaves much of the chemical that was there originally in the blood.

manufacturer approached him to redesign a valve. Instead of a valve, he reinvented the whole process as a 22-pound computer-controlled pump and monitor. Manual controls were reduced from 37 operating keys to two. Furthermore, a physician can prescribe the way the flow of fluid is controlled, which was not possible on early peritoneal devices. Already approved in Canada, Europe, and Japan, the new home-dialysis device was awaiting FDA approval late in 1993.

TIMETABLE OF DIALYSIS

1861   British chemist Thomas Graham discovers and names the chemical process dialysis.

1913   In animal experiments, John Jacob Abel develops the first artificial kidney.

1943   Dutch physician Wilhelm Kolff develops the first practical kidney dialysis machine.

1960   Beldane H. Scribner and Wayne Quinton develop a permanent blood connector so that repeated hemodialysis becomes possible; the first patient to use the new connector lives on dialysis for another 11 years.

1964   The first systems for home kidney dialysis are introduced in the United States and United Kingdom.

1972   The U.S. Congress passes Public Law 92-603, enabling patients on Social

Security and under the age of 65 to be paid 80% of the cost of dialysis from federal funds.

1978   U.S. Food and Drug Administration approves peritoneal dialysis devices that can be worn continuously.

1992   About 150,000 patients in the U.S. and 500,000 worldwide rely on dialysis to lengthen their lives or as a bridge to a kidney transplant.

Blood Pressure Monitoring   Blood pressure has been measured since Stephen Hales took the blood pressure of a horse in 1726. The method Hales used was similar to the one used today in operating rooms and intensive-care wards, based on a catheter that directly measures pressure in an artery. Such an invasive technique is extremely accurate and provides continuous reporting, but it is hardly convenient and there is a risk of clotting or infections. The noninvasive pressure cuff used in many doctor's offices is not so accurate, but it is simple and causes no complications. Today many people stick their arm into a cuff when they visit the pharmacy and get a free or inexpensive quick checkup. A patient in a hospital may also use a variation of this technique that measures blood pressure every two and a half to five minutes.

Every couple of minutes is not really good enough for many patients, however. Continuous monitors are needed. Also, physicians would like to have continuous monitors that a patient could wear while going about routine activities, as that information would make it possible to monitor medications much better than the present practice, which may consist of asking the patient to use a pressure-cuff, digital-readout monitor once or twice a day. In the early 1990s, technology has made the goal of continuous, noninvasive accurate monitor possible — the new devices use crystals that emit electricity when pressure changes, for example, or that measure changes in electrical resistance that occur with pressure changes. The mid-1990s should see the first truly portable monitors that an ambulatory patient can wear all day.

High-Tech Hipbones   Replacement of joints has come a long way from Captain Ahab's ivory leg. Modern hipbone implants have been made from special cobalt-chromium alloy balls seated in polyethylene sockets, but the polyethylene tends to wear, producing small pieces that activate the immune system. Balls made of alumina or zirconia, although brittle, are so smooth that polyethylene wear is cut dramatically. In 1991, an even higher-tech approach was introduced: blasting the metal-type balls with nitrogen ions, which smooth and lubricate the surface.

Another innovation, this from 1992, has been adding a coating to the implant stem (the part attached to the leg bone) of hydroxylapatite, which is chemically so similar to bone that the bone tissue quickly bonds to it. Layers of tiny metal beads are also used by some manufacturers to get the implant stem to permit the bone to grow into it.

Catheters   Nothing could be more "low-tech" than a simple catheter, which is essentially a small flexible tube that can be inserted into veins, arteries, or other body tubes to withdraw fluids for analysis or excretion or to add fluids for nutrition or medication. Perhaps that is why catheter-related infections accounted for one out of six infections acquired in hospitals in 1991. Of the catheters, a type called the central venous catheter, inserted in veins near the heart for medication delivery or blood monitoring, is a particularly dangerous type. According to the U.S. Centers for Disease Control and Prevention, the central venous catheters cause 86 percent of bloodstream infections that begin in the bloodstream (not counting infections elsewhere that spread into the blood). These are extremely dangerous infections.

In 1991 a new form of central venous catheter was introduced by the Arrow International, although it was developed by the smaller Daltex Medical Sciences of Fairfield, New Jersey. The Arrow catheter is made from a polymer impregnated with an antibiotic, which according to a study results in an 80 percent decrease in the number of bacterial infections of the bloodstream. Daltex is developing a number of other polymer-based products similarly laced with antibiotics. The company also plans to develop polymer products, such as surgical gloves or condoms, that have an antiviral agent built into them. The advantage would be to reduce the chance of AIDS or hepatitis B, which is also one of the purposes of surgical gloves and condoms made from ordinary latex.

Implanted Artificial Heart Pump   A device used experimentally for the first time in 1991 is less than an artificial heart, but unlike the Jarvik artificial heart, the implanted left ventricular assist pump (or VAD, the general name for a ventricular assist device) uses an internal motor powered by an external belt battery pack. A VAD is usually implanted in the abdomen, since the heart is left in place. The first test of the implanted version of a VAD failed for reasons having nothing to do with the assist.

Previously a very similar left ventricular assist had been powered by an external air compressor, much like the Jarvik heart. Both external and internal assists are intended for use in keeping a patient alive until a heart transplant, which an external one has done for as long as a year. All told, more than 1300 externally powered artificial hearts or VADs (mostly the latter) have been used to keep patients alive while awaiting heart transplants.

Implanted Heart Defibrillbrators   Many lives have been saved since 1985 by implanted devices that recognize that a damaged heart has stopped working correctly and provide a sharp jolt of electricity to get it back on track. All told, more than 48,000 defibrillators had been implanted in the U.S. since FDA approval and in early 1993 some 35,000 of the implantees were still alive.

An improved version called the pacer-cardioverter-defibrillator also senses irregular heartbeats and if needed uses electrical pulses to restore normal heart rhythm. The advantage of the new type, approved by the FDA early in 1993, is that it begins with a low-level electric pulse. If that does not speed up a slow rhythm or start a stopped heart, a second pulse at a higher intensity is provided; a third level can also be used if the first two fail to do the task.

Ridding Arteries of Plaque   Plaque is a general term that physicians and dentists seem to prefer in describing any build-up of an undesirable substance. In the arteries, the substance contains lipoproteins and is called atherosclerosis or, if in heart arteries, coronary heart disease. By far the most common way to deal with arterial plaque without replacing an artery is balloon angioplasty, in which a balloon inserted into the artery at the end of a tube is pushed to where the plaque is and then inflated, pushing the plaque into the walls of the artery and unclogging the blood vessel.

Although this method is effective to a considerable degree, many inventions have been proposed to accomplish the same task in a way that would remove the plaque instead of just pushing it aside. The method called directional coronary atherectomy, which is a "Roto-Rooter" analog, was approved by the FDA in 1990. Studies since have shown, however, that removing plaque in this way is not any more effective than balloon angioplasty and is more dangerous. In 1993 researchers invented a method of directing with ultrasound the tiny high-speed drill on its journey through the artery. Perhaps it will improve the record of directional coronary atherectomy, although the ultrasound device may not be approved for use for several years.

Subsequent to directional coronary atherectomy, the FDA has approved a device that vacuums out plaque as well as a laser that evaporates it. The laser device has proved dangerous on occasion, however.

New Devices

Some new medical devices may arise because a visionary conceives of an entirely new solution to a problem or even discovers a new problem. More often, however, both the impairment to health and what might be done to correct it have been long recognized—but the technology for making the correction has been too difficult. In the early 1990s, technology began to catch up to some previously unsolvable problems.

The Artificial Liver Just as a dialysis machine is an artificial kidney and a heart-lung machine can replace those organs for a time, an artificial liver is a device outside the body through which blood can flow and be cleaned of toxins. While cleaning the blood is far from the only function of the liver, it is the one most likely to result in death in short order when the liver fails. Solve the toxin-cleaning problem and there may be time to deal with digestion or cholesterol manufacture or another liver function in some other way. If you fail to clean the blood, the patient dies. About 40,000 people each year suffer liver failure in the U.S., mostly as a result of poisoning, alcoholism, or infection.

Until recently, attempts to produce an artificial liver, none of which were very successful, relied on chemistry, including filters, enzymes, and absorbent activated charcoal. In 1993 an artificial liver based on biology became the first outside-the-body liver substitute to keep alive a patient who did not have a liver. The artificial liver was a 20-inch-long, 4-inch-wide cylinder filled with pig liver cells surrounded with cellulose fibers.

In 1992 the same model of artificial liver was used for the first time on humans on six different occasions, keeping all six alive until they were able to obtain transplants of human livers. In the first operation in 1993, that had been the plan as well. The patient's own liver, damaged beyond repair by an overdose of medicine, was producing toxins instead of cleaning them up, so it had to be removed. The patient lived 14 hours on the artificial pig-cell liver before she was able to get a satisfactory human-liver transplant. A different approach using pig-liver cells, but just treating plasma, has also been successfully used on more than eight humans as well.

Other artificial livers are in the works. One uses liver cells from rats and has been successful in animal tests with rabbits and dogs, with human trials expected sometime in 1994. Another uses a cell line derived from a human liver cancer (cancer cells often form "immortal" lines that can be kept alive much better than noncancerous cells).

Some experts are concerned that the cancer cells in this device might somehow escape during blood treatment. By the end of 1993, however, 11 humans had been treated with the cancer-derived artificial liver.

The best hope may be an artificial liver using normal human liver cells in a specially designed bioreactor that keeps the cells alive. First trials of this device on animals were scheduled for 1994.

In addition to technical problems with artificial livers, there is the question of how they will fit into the social problems connected with liver transplants. So far the main purpose of the artificial livers has been to keep patients alive for a short while until a liver with a good tissue type match was available for transplant, but in 1992 there were only 3,059 livers donated for the 15,000 people who needed them. Livers regenerate after some forms of damage, but the time involved for regeneration is great compared to the time the present generation of artificial livers are expected to be used on a given patient. One possible hope is to use pig livers genetically altered to express human antigens (*see* "Pigs and Other Animals Become More Human," p 47) as organs to transplant into humans.

The Artificial Pancreas   Transplants of insulin-producing cells into diabetics using animal cells have to be protected from the body's immune system just as the animal cells used in three out of five of the artificial livers. One way uses beads of cells enclosed in a seaweed gel and simply let loose in the abdomen (*see* "Cell Transplantation: Fetal Tissue and More," p 511), but most devices based on animal insulin-producing cells isolate the cells in plastic. The idea is much the same as the artificial liver, but since the pancreatic cells are intended to produce an additive to the blood (insulin) instead of removing substances from the blood (toxic wastes), there is no need to pump blood through them. Consequently, several pancreas substitutes based on animal cells are small devices that are implanted somewhere in the body. These can use plastic coatings with pores large enough for insulin molecules to pass through but small enough to keep out white blood cells and most immune-system chemicals. Some versions of a pancreas substitute based on this method do shunt blood past the cells, but most place the plastic-housed animal cells where the cells can be bathed with fluids (as in the peritoneal cavity). The main problem so far has been the immune system's attempt to wall off the foreign substance, depriving the animal cells of their nutrients and the blood of its insulin.

Blood-clot Remover   Just as a powerful hose can remove a caked-on piece of clay from a sidewalk, a device called the Angiojet flushes away blood clots from inside a blood vessel. Three powerful jets of saline solution are directed at the clot from one side, freeing it from the walls of the blood vessel. Another three jets push the clot from the other side, breaking it up and shoving it into a tube from which it flows out of the body. The entire task takes a couple of minutes. This product was just going to be tested in 1993 after several years of development.

Electric Drug Delivery   Skin patches, like the well-known patches used to deliver nitroglycerine or nicotine on a steady basis, have many advantages over oral medicines—and one big disadvantage: skin is designed by evolution to keep foreign molecules out. Small molecules can sometimes diffuse into the blood through the skin (*transdermal delivery*) without any special technology, but larger molecules need to be pushed. This has been done in the past hundred years in some instances with low voltage electricity. Over long periods of time, low-voltage current can drive a drug that has been engineered to carry an electric charge on each molecule through the skin. New devices of this type have recently been introduced, and they have their own power source built into the patch, delivering three to 12 volts of electricity to the skin along with the drug.

In the November 15, 1993 *Proceedings of the National Academy of Sciences*, Robert Langer and coworkers at the Massachusetts Institute of Technology in Cambridge suggest a different method to achieve transdermal delivery. They found that brief, higher-voltage pulses of current could temporarily rearrange the outer layers of skin, opening up pores through those layers. Still too new to be used for drug delivery, this approach appears to be a way to get drugs into the blood without breaking the skin. Also, the same idea might be used in reverse. Combined with a vacuum it could get blood out of the skin for blood tests—skipping that invasive and slightly painful needle in the arm. Early tests of the method have all used patches of human skin in the laboratory, but tests on living animals were scheduled for late 1993 or 1994.

Laser Replacement for Glasses Eye surgery was one of the first medical applications of the laser, that intense beam of coherent light that can transport energy to a specific designated area. In medical practice the energy is usually used in the form of heat, drilling holes or fusing cells (as in reattaching a detached retina). In 1992 the FDA approved using an existing medical laser system for treatment of glaucoma, an application based on the ability of lasers to drill holes in tissue without damaging surrounding tissue. New ducts in the eye created by the laser drain away excess fluid (*see* "The Senses UPDATE," p 452).

An experimental treatment for using lasers to cure myopia shows great promise and might be approved by the FDA as early as 1995. Trials using the lasers have produced excellent, 20-40 vision in more than 90 percent of the patients six months after the surgery. The laser treatment is based somewhat on the same idea as radial keratotomy, which uses scalpel surgery to reshape the eyeball. Some surgeons who have used both techniques prefer the laser version because it shaves the outside of the cornea instead of cutting into it, leaving the reshaped cornea stronger.

Heavy Cancer Treatment For nearly a hundred years, electromagnetic radiation of sufficient power has been known to kill cells, and for much of that time the electromagnetic radiation in the form of X rays or gamma rays has been directed at cancer cells (*see* "Report from the War on Cancer," p 412). Synchronotron radiation produced by particle accelerators has been used for this purpose intermittently since 1949 (and use is increasing in the early 1990s), but radiation from a synchronotron accelerator also consists of gamma rays, albeit more effective.

In the past 20 years, an entirely different form of "radiation" has been directed experimentally against cancer. Some particle accelerators use as particles atoms that have been stripped of some or all of their electrons. These particles are called ions, and the most useful ions come from heavy elements. The unofficial headquarters of experimental cancer treatment in the U.S. using heavy ions has been the Lawrence Berkeley Laboratory (LBL) in Berkeley, California, which treated about 400 patients over two decades. But the heavy-ion accelerator at LBL was closed in 1992 because it was outmoded for work in nuclear physics, its main mission. Japan, however, decided that the heavy-ion approach was successful with cancers that resisted electromagnetic radiation, and the Japanese have built a large particle accelerator just for medical use, the Heavy-Ion Medical Accelerator in Chiba (Himac). Chiba is a suburb of Tokyo. Himac began treating patients early in 1994.

Meanwhile, in the U.S. some cancer patients are being treated at Loma Linda Medical Center in California and Massachusetts General Hospital in Boston with very light ions—proton beams in fact. (A proton and a positive hydrogen ion are exactly the same entity.) Protons are not the best alternative to electromagnetic radiation, say experts, but they are a much less expensive option than heavy ions. Himac cost the Japanese about $300 million to build and will cost about $50 million annually to operate, though it only treats about a thousand patients a year.

(Periodical References and Additional Reading: *New York Times* 1-4-91, p A1; *New York Times* 5-26-91; *New York Times* 7-24-91, p A16; *New York Times* 3-29-92, p IV-2; *New York Times* 7-16-92, p D4; *New York Times* 8-20-92, p D4; *New York Times* 11-9-92, p A1; *New York Times* 11-29-92, p III-7; *New York Times* 12-17-92, p A24; *New York Times* 2-13-93, p 37; *New York Times* 2-24-93, p A1; *New York Times* 3-5-93, p A18; *New York Times* 3-21-93, p III-9; *New York Times* 3-25-93, p III-16; *New York Times* 5-13-93, pp D1 & D6; *Science* 5-14-93, p 912; *New York Times* 5-19-93, p C13; *Scientific American* 6-93, p 18; *New York Times* 7-14-93, p D5; *New York Times* 7-22-93, p A17; *New York Times* 7-26-93, p III-9; *New York Times* 8-27-93, p A20; *New York Times* 11-9-93, p D4; *Science News* 11-20-93, p 327; *New York Times* 11-21-93, p I-28; *Scientific American* 12-93, p 30; *New York Times* 12-21-93, p C3)

New Drug or Device Actions of U.S. Food and Drug Administration

About 5000 new drugs or medical devices come onto the market in the U.S. each year, so this is not the place to attempt a complete list. The most significant drug and device actions are included below, however.

Trade name(s)	Generic name	Intended use	Action
Accuprobe	liquid nitrogen delivery system	Treatment of liver and prostate cancer and for enlarged, noncancerous prostates (hypertrophy)	Approved 4-91
	alpha interferon	Treatment for hepatitis B	Approved 1992
Ambien		Sleeping pill	Approved 12-21-92
Arrow central venous catheter		Antibiotic tube to be inserted into veins near the heart for infusing and withdrawing fluids	Approved 1991
Betaseron	1B beta interferon	Treatment of multiple sclerosis	Approved 7-23-93
Biaxin	clarithromycin	Antibiotic used to treat mycobacterium avium complex (MAC) in AIDS patients	Approved 12-29-93
Centoxin	monoclonal antibody HA-1A	Treatment of septic shock after surgery or other trauma	Denied 4-92

Trade name(s)	Generic name	Intended use	Action
Ceredase*		Treatment of Gaucher's disease, a hereditary disorder that causes fat to accumulate in some organs	Approved 1991
	cladribine	Treatment of hairy-cell leukemia by killing white blood cells	Approved 1993
Claritin		Once-a-day antihistamine that lacks the potential cardiovascular side effects of other drugs for hay fever	Approved 4-14-93
	clotrimazole	Nonprescription treatment for vaginal yeast infections	Approved 12-3-90
Cognex	tacrine	To relieve symptoms of Alzheimer's disease	Approved 9-9-93
Contigen Bard Collagen Implant		An implant to relieve urinary incontinence; a collagen ring narrows the opening from the bladder to the urethra	Approved 10-18-90
Daypro		A one-a-day anti-inflammatory that is not a steroid; for treatment of osteoarthritis and rheumatoid arthritis	Approved 10-31-92
Depo-Provera	medroxyprogesterone acetate	Injected to prevent conception for three months at a time	Approved 10-3-92
ddC	zalcitabine	Treatment of advanced cases of AIDS	Approved 1992
ddI	2',3'-dideoxyinosine	Treatment of advanced cases of AIDS	Approved 1991
E-5	monoclonal antibodies	Treatment of septic shock after surgery or other trauma	Denied twice in 1992
Effexor		Antidepressant similar to Prozac, but affects norepinephrine as well as serotonin	Approved 12-93
Felbatol	felbamate	Controls partial epileptic seizures in adults and Lennox-Gastaut epilepsy in children	Approved 8-2-93
	gamma interferon	Used to combat the hereditary disease chronic granulomatous disease	Approved 1990
Halfan		Anti-malarial drug	Approved 1992
Imitrex	sumatriptan	Injected to control migraines	Approved 12-29-92
	interleukin-2	Treatment of kidney cancer	Approved 5-92
Kytril Injection		Antinausea drug for patients undergoing chemotherapy	Approved 12-30-93
Leukine; Prokine	genetically engineered granulocyte macrophage colony stimulating factor (GM-CSF)	Increase growth of macrophages (infection-fighting white blood cells) in cancer patients who have had bone-marrow transplants	Approved 3-6-91

Trade name(s)	Generic name	Intended use	Action
Lotensin		To treat high blood pressure	Approved 6-91
Lovenox	enoxaparin	To prevent blood clots after hip surgery	Approved 4-16-93
Manoplex		To treat congestive heart failure (withdrawn by manufacturer 7-20-93)	Advised MDs to halt use 4-93
Marogen	genetically engineered erythropoietin	To compete with Orphan Drug Epogen (essentially the same drug) approved in 1989	Denied 1-15-91
Mepron		To treat pneumocystis carinii pneumonia (PCP), which mainly affects AIDS patients	Approved 11-30-92
Naprosyn	nalproxen sodium	Analgesic and anti-inflammatory uses (similar to aspirin, ibuprofen, and acetaminophen) (used as a prescription drug since 1976)	Use in OTC market denied 6-2-93; approved for OTC use 1-11-94
Neupogen	granulocyte colony-stimulating factor (G-CFS)	Improve the immune system during chemotherapy	Approved 2-91
Norplant	levonorgestrel	Implanted to prevent conception for periods up to five years	Approved 11-90
Nutropin	genetically engineered human growth hormone	Treatment of growth failure in children with chronic renal insufficiency	Approved 11-17-93
Omniflox		Antibiotic used to treat infections of upper respiratory tract, urinary system, and skin	Approved 1-92, but withdrawn from market by manufacturer after three deaths and at least 50 adverse reactions
Oncoscint CR/OV		Imaging agent used in detection of colorectal or ovarian cancers	Approved 1992
Oralet	fentanyl in a lollipop	Calm children's nerves before surgery	Tentative approval 10-93
Paxil		Serotonin-enhancer, similar to Prozac	Approved 12-30-92
Proscar		Treatment for benign enlarged prostate glands	Approved 6-92
Pulmozyme	Dnase	Enzyme to break up mucus in lungs of cystic fibrosis patients	Approved 12-30-93
Stavudine (d4T)		Treatment of AIDS in patients who cannot take AZT or DDI	Approved for this use 10-5-92
Recombinate	genetically engineered blood factor VIII	To prevent symptoms in patients with hemophilia A (to replace Factor VIII derived from donated blood)	Approved 12-10-92

Trade name(s)	Generic name	Intended use	Action
rhDNase	recombinant human deoxyribonuclease	To break up mucus in patients with cystic fibrosis, who inhale the drug from an atomizer	Approved 1993
Rotoblator		Used for angioplasty; drills out plaque in arteries and veins	Reapproved: Leg veins, 12-92; coronary arteries, 6-2-93
Taxol	paclitaxel	Treatment of ovarian cancer	Approved 12-29-92
Tetranune		Combination DPT vaccine with vaccine against *Hemophilus influenzae* type B	
Trasylol Injection	aprotinin	Prevents excessive bleeding in heart-bypass surgery	Approved 12-30-93
Various drugs (Bantron, Cigarrest, Nikoban, Tabmint, etc.)		Intended to help smokers quit tobacco use	OTC use prohibited as of 12-1-93
Vasotec	enalapril	Already popular for treating hypertension, new use is to prevent heart failure	Approved for new use 11-15-93
Ventak	Pacer-cardioverter-defibrillator (PCD)	Implant that senses irregular heartbeats and if needed uses electrical pulses to restore normal heart rhythm	Approved 2-12-93
Videx (ddI)	didanozine	Treatment of AIDS as an alternative to AZT	Approved for this use 9-28-92
Zofran (injectable)		Anti-nausea drug	Approved 2-91
Zofran (oral)		Anti-nausea drug	Approved 1-4-93
Zoloft		Serotonin-enhancer, similar to Prozac	Approved 1992

* Ceredase is also known as the world's costliest drug; at $875,000 an ounce, costs of the drug alone range from nearly $88,000 a year to more than $380,000 a year, depending on weight of the patient and timetable of drug administration.

(Periodical References and Additional Reading: *New York Times* 12-15-90; *New York Times* 12-30-92, pp A10, D3; *New York Times* 6-5-92; *New York Times* 6-9-92, p D4; *New York Times* 10-30-92, p A1; *New York Times* 10-31-92, p 39; *New York Times* 11-22-92, p III-12; *New York Times* 1-11-93, p D2; *New York Times* 1-19-93, p D1; *New York Times* 1-30-93, p D5; *New York Times* 6-2-93, p A17; *New York Times* 6-3-93, p D1; *New York Times* 6-15-93; *New York Times* 1-9-94; *New York Times* 1-12-94, p A10; *Discover* 3-94, p 56; *Scientific American* 5-94, p 68)

Aging and Death

THE STATE OF GERONTOLOGY AND THANATOLOGY

The population of the earth is becoming older. In 1910 less than one percent of the population of the world was over the age of 65, traditionally considered the lower border of old age in the U.S. By 1992 that percentage had risen to 6.2 percent of the world's population. By 2050, estimates are that about 20 percent of the projected population of 12.5 billion will be over 65—one person in five.

The Shape of Populations to Come

At present the population structure of the world is described as a pyramid, which has a large base of young people and is capped with a tiny apex of old ones. By the year 2050, if present trends continue, in many currently developed nations the present population pyramid will be replaced by a rectangular form. That is, the numbers of young people, middle-aged people, and old people will all be about equal. In a perfect population rectangle, the number of people whose ages are in any similar interval— such as decades, as in ages 20-29 or 50-59—will be equal.

In a population pyramid, the average age of the population stays low because of the many young people forming the base of the pyramid. When the rectangular age structure is reached (which is not the case today anywhere in the world, although the age structure is close to rectangular in Sweden and Switzerland), the average age of the population is the midpoint of the rectangle. The average therefore depends on the age that the oldest people in the population will reach, not on how many young people there are in the total population.

Analysis of the kind of rectangular age structure expected by 2050 combined with reasonable expectations for longer lifespans show that after rectangularity has been reached, more than 90 percent of the people born in any given year will live to be over 65. Furthermore, the same analysis reveals that in a rectangular age profile, about two-thirds of the population will, at birth, be expected to live to the age of 85 or greater. Similar age structures are presently observed in laboratory mice or in other populations that live in protected environments. The same age distribution is largely true of Sweden and Switzerland, with their nearly rectangular population structures.

As Long as We Live

The age rectangle may be the final form. Only in science fiction could one expect an inverted pyramid, reflecting an immortal—barring accidental death—population. In such a mythical society, recruitment (that is, birth) would be kept low, thus maintaining an inverted pyramid form. But this is not an expected scenario.

The phrase "average life expectancy" refers to the expected age of death for the average person at the time the person is born if conditions stay the same. Only 100 years ago, the average life expectancy in the U.S. was less than 50 years. Many experts believe that the average life expectancy for humans in any society can never exceed 85 years of age. On the other hand, James Vaupel of Duke University in Durham, North Carolina, and Odense University in Denmark thinks that in some societies the average lifespan for men will reach 94 by 2080. Women, who live longer now, would perhaps reach an average life expectancy of 100. Of course, all bets are off in case of a major scientific breakthrough.

One such scientific breakthrough has already been confirmed for many types of laboratory animals, including mice, flies, fish, and nonhuman primates—and a few humans are experimenting with it. Given two populations of animals, the one that eats the least but still enough for survival will have an average life expectancy that is greater than the one that eats as much as it would like. Furthermore, the gain seems to come by postponing the changes recognized as old age, not by simply slowing down the whole process. After old age finally sets in, even the starved animals die at the normal rate. (*See also* "Slowing Aging, Delaying Death" p 568.)

But very few humans seem to be prepared to starve for extended youth, and it is not known for sure whether it would work in any case. As a result, the time spent with illnesses that disable the elderly increases. Today in the typical Western society, an average man lives to be 72 years old, but spends over 14 years in ill health; the average woman lives longer—about 79 years—but spends nearly 20 of those years disabled by illness. In general, as the population ages, disease patterns are different. Infectious diseases are less of a problem; nearly everyone will suffer from and eventually die from what are thought of as "degenerative" diseases.

Intimations of Mortality in the U.S.

Because the population profile of the U.S. is constantly changing as more people live longer, mortality tables need to be adjusted for age in order to be meaningful. With the adjustment, one observes a striking drop in mortality over the past 35 years. The age-adjusted death rate for men has dropped more than 27 percent since 1960, while that for women has fallen even faster, more than 32 percent. In 1991, the last year for which complete figures are available, the men's death rate was 645.9 per 100,000 and the longer-lived women had an age-adjusted rate of only 368.2 per 100,000.

One result is that in the U.S. today, one person out of eight is 65 or older. By the year 2050 it is expected that, depending on advances in medical care and lifestyle changes, one in five or even one in four persons will be age 65 or older.

Even with a higher benchmark to define old age, the growth of the senior population will be spectacular. The age of 85 is now viewed by many experts as the borderline between normal old age (from 65 to 84) and extended old age (from 85 on up). In the early 1990s there were about 4 million Americans in extended old age— 3.3 million people over the age of 85 in the 1990 census. The U.S. Census Bureau

AGING AND DEATH

Few subjects have inspired so many pithy sayings, startling discoveries, or simple theories as old age and death. Most of the theories and many of the "facts" are based on observation or extrapolation instead of scientific studies, however. Here are a handful of facts, factoids, and hypotheses:

- In all societies, the rich live longer (and are healthier) than the rest of the population.
- Most old people today are in China—71 million over the age of 65. This is largely because China has such a large population.
- Most old people in the year 2050 will still be in China, but by then the number will reach about 270 million. Not only will China continue to have the largest overall population of any nation, but also the population over 65 will go from about 6.4 percent today to about 20 percent over 65 in 2050.
- *Life expectancy* as used by demographers is the average number of years from a given age that people in a population will live if the death rate does not change during their lifetime. Therefore, when the death rate is undergoing reduction, the life expectancy figure cited at birth is always lower than it will become during a person's lifetime.
- Each human has a genetically determined maximum potential lifespan; for a large population of humans, these potentials form a rough normal distribution (the familiar bell-shaped curve) with a mean of 85 years and a standard deviation of seven years.
- The best way to insure a long life is to choose your parents carefully.
- The average number of years that people today enjoy good health is increasing at a slower rate than the average number of years that people live with major disabilities.
- Complete elimination of all deaths under the age of 50 in the U.S. would raise life expectancy at birth by less than four years.
- The oldest verified ages of living people in the early 1990s were about 120 years; no one was any older. Although some populations claimed older individuals, closer inspection found the presumed ages could not be confirmed and were, in fact, based on hearsay.
- Risk of death in every population doubles every eight years past the age of 30.
- If you live long enough, you will die either from heart disease or cancer.
- All men develop prostate troubles if they live long enough.
- The longer you live, the more likely you are to die; indeed, mortality rates increase exponentially with age (*see,* however, "Slowing Aging, Delaying Death," p 568, for a modified view of this commonplace).
- Death is nature's way of telling you to slow down.

Light will be shed on whether or not these adages and axioms are true in the articles that follow, though in many cases it is not possible to be certain whether the statement can be scientifically established.

predicts that the number will grow by the year 2080 to be 18.7 million, almost five times the present number. Others think that the Census Bureau is too conservative by far. Kenneth Manton of Duke University thinks that there will be 43 million over the age of 85 by the year 2040, even if there are no significant improvements in treating major diseases. The aforementioned James Vaupel, also of Duke University, thinks that the U.S. population over 85 could reach 72 million by 2080.

Disability in the elderly in the U.S. is less than had been expected just a few years ago. A study in 1993 found that although the U.S. population over 65 increased by 14.7 percent between 1982 and 1989, the chronically disabled population over 65 increased by only 9.2 percent during that same period. Another measure of disability, the number of elderly requiring personal assistance to get through the day, decreased by ten percent during the same period. Furthermore, the study found that the improvement in health came after the age of 75, not in the group between 65 and 74. Much of the improvement has come from better handling of vision problems, including cataracts, and from the use of artificial joints to replace natural ones that had worn out.

Lifestyles of the Old and Infirm

Many concerned people in the U.S. have banded together since the Great Depression of the 1930s (and before) to help feed the poor. In the early 1990s, many of the elderly were among the poor, but nutrition problems in senior citizens go well beyond lack of money, and charitable organizations, notably Meals on Wheels, are devoted to the problem of providing better food for old people who live outside of institutional settings. Other organizations have worked for better nutrition in nursing homes and in assisted-living facilities, where healthier persons prepare their own meals, but the less healthy eat communally.

On July 30, 1992, the U.S. General Accounting Office released a summary of studies on nutrition in the elderly whose title told it all: "Nutrition Information is Limited and Guidelines are Lacking." Indeed, some available studies showed that between 30 and 60 percent of old people do not get enough protein. The Tufts University Center on Hunger, Poverty and Nutrition Policy claimed that in 1990 about 10.5 percent of all Americans 65 and older experienced hunger, mostly because they failed to eat food that was available to them. The New York State Department of Aging estimated that about 86 percent of elderly people who need home-food delivery, such as Meals on Wheels, do not get it.

In 1993 a survey by the Nutrition Screening Initiative, a five-year project designed to promote better nutritional screening and care among the elderly by health-care providers, found that 25 percent of the persons 65 or older do not have healthy diets. This figure is heavily weighted upwards by survey results stating that doctors and nurses estimate that 40 percent of the elderly in nursing homes and 50 percent in hospitals are malnourished. The survey results were not the same as those reported by nursing-home and hospital administration staff, but even the administration staff reported on their survey forms that 25 percent of nursing-home residents and 34 percent of hospital patients eat the wrong food or else too little of the right food. Nutrition Screening officials say that poor nutrition leads to diabetes, heart disease, and cancer (*see also* "Slowing Aging, Delaying Death" p 568).

Medication and Old Age

Despite the obvious graying of the American population, the medical community does not seem to have fully grasped the implications of longer life. A study in the October 6, 1993 *Journal of the National Cancer Institute* found, for example, that older women are not treated aggressively for cancer, as they are referred to a specialist less often, given surgery less often, and, if operated upon, followed up with chemotherapy or radiation less often than younger women. Although this study was of women and cancer, there is no reason to think that the results would be different for men or for another disease.

Indeed, a study in France showed that surgery for colorectal cancer in patients over the age of 80 was as effective in preserving life for five years as it was in younger patients. In the July 1, 1992, issue of the *Journal of the American Medical Association,* researchers in the U.S. reported similar results for breast cancer in women 70 and older. And in the July 2, 1992, issue of the *New England Journal of Medicine,* a study reported that aggressive treatment of people 75 and older with clot-busting drugs produces better results than more conventional treatment that omits the drugs. Another study, in the June 26, 1991, issue of the *Journal of the American Medical Association,* reported that drug intervention in older people with age-related high blood pressure (a type that one in four Americans over the age of 80 develops) greatly lowered the risk of strokes. The therapy also improved heart function and reduced heart attacks in the elderly.

Early in the 1990s, concern for the differences in the way elderly people and their bodies deal with drugs began to surface. At that time, people over 65 represented only 12 percent of the U.S. population, but they consumed more than 30 percent of the prescription medicine (and more than 40 percent of the non-prescription drugs). Physicians realized that many older patients who live independently simply do not take the medications prescribed—sometimes not at all and sometimes in the wrong amounts or at incorrect times. Only about one in 20 patients over 65 takes his or her medicine in a supervised setting. Furthermore, the physicians themselves often failed to take into account how the physiological concomitants—changes in the body—of aging might affect the metabolism of drugs, perhaps because, in many cases, no one had ever studied the problem. In elderly patients side effects are often different from those in younger persons. In one famous case, unanticipated side effects were lethal: in 1982 the anti-arthritis drug Oraflex caused over 60 deaths among elderly patients before being withdrawn.

The U.S. Food and Drug Administration (FDA) in March 1990 asked the drug manufacturers to provide separate drug evaluation for the elderly. Later in the year the FDA took steps toward providing people over 65 with information about the specific effects a particular drug has on the elderly.

Another problem, especially in nursing homes and hospitals, has been the excessive use of certain medications for elderly patients, particularly sedatives, tranquilizers, and mood-altering drugs. One study reported in the July 16, 1992, issue of the *New England Journal of Medicine* found that nursing home patients were not disrupted by a 27-percent cut in sedatives and tranquilizers. While some patients who had been on tranquilizers became more depressed, others became less anxious on a reduced dose of tranquilizers.

(Periodical References and Additional Reading: *Science* 11-2-90, p 634; *New York Times* 12-1-90, p 50; *Science News* 1-4-92, p 4; *Harvard Health Letter* 3-92, p 8; *New York Times* 8-5-92, p C12; *New York Times* 10-10-92, p 1; *New York Times* 11-16-92, p A1; *Scientific American* 4-93, p 46; *New York Times* 4-7-93, p A1; *Science News* 10-8-93, p 229; *Statistical Bulletin* 4/6-94, p 10)

TIMETABLE OF GERONTOLOGY TO 1990

2600 BC   Egyptian embalmers take the first steps toward mummification of bodies by beginning the practice of removing the internal organs of dead pharaohs; these organs are preserved in jars in a salt solution, while resin-soaked linen replace them in the body.

1268   Roger Bacon discusses spectacles for the farsighted in *Opus majus*.

1825   Benjamin Gompertz proposes what comes to be known as "Gompertz's law": mortality rates increase exponentially with age in any species.

1858   Franciscus Cornelius Donders [born Tilburg, Netherlands, May 27, 1818; died Utrecht, March 24, 1889] discovers that farsightedness can be caused by eyeballs that are too shallow.

1905   John B. Murphy [born December 21, 1857, Appleton, Wisconsin; died 1916] develops the first artificial joints for use in the hip of an arthritic patient.

1935   Clyde McCay of Cornell University reports that white rats, which normally live two years in a laboratory setting, live for four years on a low-calorie diet that still provides good nutrition.

1957   George C. Williams of Michigan State University proposes that aging happens because genes that have survival value during reproductive years are preserved by evolution, but the same genes may have damaging effects later in life after reproduction ceases, when natural selection is no longer operative.

1978   Jean Bourgeois-Pichat of Paris calculates that the average human life expectancy will never exceed 77 years. Shortly after he publishes his findings, several nations publish statistics showing that their average life span already exceeds that limit.

1981   James F. Fries of Stanford University hypothesizes that the average biological limit of human life cannot rise above 85 years because better lifestyles only postpone the onset of major fatal diseases, compressing the period of morbidity.

1982   Richard Weindruch of the U.S. National Institute on Aging and Roy Walford of the University of California–Los Angeles show that adult mice one year old (corresponding in age to 35-year-old humans) who are put on a low-calorie, high-nutrition restricted diet live ten to 20 percent longer than mice fed their ordinary diet.

UNDERSTANDING AGING

People have always striven to elucidate the phenomenon of death. Aging, however, has apparently been a less thought-provoking subject: there are very few, if any, explanations of the necessity of aging. The mechanism of aging is known: cells in

Background

Aging happens after growing up; it is also called growing old. While technically some changes associated with aging begin at birth (ability to heal wounds is an example), for most of the decline that we think of as aging, a better start date would be after full growth, including development of muscular strength, takes place. Some specific age-related changes occur at later stages in life. The far-sightedness called presbyopia often begins around age 45, while menopause and many attendant changes for women may follow a few years after that. Because there is enormous variability from person to person, it is not possible to identify exactly when most of the changes associated with aging will begin.

CHANGES DURING AGING

Changes	Control
Balance sense becomes impaired	Learn to use available aids to keep steady
Basal metabolism falls about 12 percent	None
Bones become lighter, more brittle, and easier to break; bone mineral content decreases about 17 percent between ages 25 and 70	Diet, vitamins, and estrogen patches may help; a 1991 study showed that thiazide diuretics reduce bone thinning by 70 percent in elderly women
Bowel movements become hard to control; constipation more common than incontinence	Caused by underlying condition, usually treatable
Cataracts cover lenses of eyes in many people, with the process starting in the 50s and 60s	Avoiding sunlight all your life may forestall; cataracts can be removed
Cell solid constituents decrease by 37 percent between ages 25 and 70	None
Deafness often gradually increases	Cause uncertain; often can be corrected with hearing aid
Disease susceptibility increases	Vaccinations against diseases such as influenza help
Farsightedness very likely by 65	Glasses or contact lenses can correct
Fat in the body more than doubles between ages 25 and 70	Exercise and diet can prevent this increase
Fatigue strikes organs more easily	None
Growth hormone production begins slowing about age 50 and may stop completely	Injectable, genetically engineered hormone is being tested in various trials
Hair often thins on top of head, appears in nose and ears	Cosmetic changes can be made
Heart's efficiency decreases 30 percent	Exercise reduces decrease
Height diminishes	None
Itching may occur because of dry skin	Physician may prescribe treatment
Kidneys lose about 40 percent of efficiency	None
Liver's efficiency decreases by ten percent	None
Lungs lose about 40 percent of ability	Exercise reduces decrease

Changes	Control
Menstruation in women ceases as estrogen levels drop	Hormone replacement can help prevent heart disease or osteoporosis
Muscle cramps increase	Exercise may help
Prostate in men enlarges or develops cancer	Can be treated with surgery
Skin loses elastic tissues, causing wrinkles, sags, and thinner skin	None
Sleep patterns often change, with insomnia at night and sleepiness during day	Make sure you get enough rest; a nap is okay; a 1993 study found that a melatonin pill, replacing low levels of nighttime melatonin, improved night sleep in the elderly
Smelling and tasting ability decreases	None
Spots appear on skin	In 1992 it was discovered that tretinoin (Retin-A), a prescription drug, removes spots caused by age (liver spots)
Temperature changes cannot be sensed	Be sure to keep house properly heated
Testosterone levels decrease in men	Can be supplemented with patches or injections
Tooth loss causes increasing problems and may require implants, bridges, or dentures to fill in gaps where teeth are missing	Teeth may be lost at any age, but since they do not grow back, loss may be more of a problem in elderly
Urine discharge becomes hard to control	Caused by underlying condition, usually treatable
Vaginal lubrication slows in women	Creams can supplement
Water content of cells is reduced by about 13 percent between ages 25 and 70	None
Wounds heal more slowly, a slowing down that starts right after birth	None

Loss of sexual function, especially in men, that is often associated with aging is the subject of considerable debate. Many gerontologists believe that impairment only occurs as a result of an underlying functional disorder such as alcoholism or diabetes or from lack of a cooperating partner. Popular opinion remains that sexual function deteriorates in old age. Data from surveys conducted from 1988 through 1991 by various organizations when combined suggest that 27 percent of married couples over 60 make love once a week or more often, of which 16 percent are in the "more often" category. Where surveyed, however, there was a decline from those in their 60s to those in their 70s or older. One survey of healthy men and women found 81 percent of the women and 91 percent of the men were sexually active in their 60s, while only 65 percent of women and 79 percent of men were having sex in their 70s or beyond (see "Sexual Surveys," p 237, for a discussion of discrepancies between male and female respondents). Another survey found that 50 percent of the senior citizens in their 80s and 90s still wanted to maintain sexual activity, but often did not succeed in doing so. Also, drugs taken for other conditions common in old age, especially those for high blood pressure or heart disease, can decrease sexual functioning, often producing impotence in men.

humans fail to reproduce themselves very well in older people, even the cells that normally reproduce, such as skin cells or bone-marrow stem cells.

British author Anthony Smith calls aging the "perfect mechanism" since it always succeeds: "No one ever fails to die."

Theories of Aging

Although aging may be the "perfect mechanism" causing death, it is far from clear why aging has to occur. It would certainly be more pleasant if human beings were built like Oliver Wendell Holmes's "Wonderful One-Hoss Shay," a vehicle constructed in such an ingenious fashion that at the end of a hundred years of functioning perfectly, all the parts wore out simultaneously, and it suddenly collapsed into a pile of dust. Although it is not certain why our aging pattern is so different from that of the famous shay, theories abound.

All theories about humans seem to apply to other mammals, but often fail when applied to other kinds of organisms. Among the plants, for example, some, such as the peach tree, have short lives and age in a way similar to mammals, but it is not clear whether giant redwoods or desert Joshua trees age at all. Many fish do not seem to have a fixed size or lifespan; they just keep growing larger until some problem develops that kills them. Amoebas seem to be immortal, as do cancer cells from humans. Testing theories of human aging on creatures other than mammals generally shows considerable deficiencies. If the same theory is to hold for mammals and fish, for mayflies and redwoods, for brain cells and cancer cells, no hypothesis posed so far seems quite satisfactory.

Cells die and are not replaced   Certain cells die during growth and development by what is termed "programmed cell death." These cells die because they have done their part in development, and are no longer needed. But after an animal matures, cells continue to die for other, often unknown, reasons. Brain cells are notorious for dying without an apparent cause or owing to injuries from alcohol, drugs, radiation, and illness. Brain cells cannot be replaced. According to this theory, cell death accounts for aging.

But the theory does work even for the brain, which, among the organs, seems to provide the clearest validation of the cell death theory. Normal cell loss does not seem to impair brain function. Cell loss from injury is quite different, and alcoholism wards of hospitals are filled with people who no longer function as a result of irreparable brain-cell loss. But cell damage caused by injury is different from damage underlying the aging process.

Cells mutate as they divide   Over a lifetime, the hereditary material passed from cell to cell gets changed as a result of accident or injury. One theory of aging is that these mutations accumulate and cause poor organ function as well as cancer, often a disease of old age. One of many problems with this theory is the fact that many cells in the body stop dividing during the earliest phase of aging; the theory fails to account for the fact that most of the observable changes occur at a later stage in the aging process.

Chromosomes become shorter   Genes in humans are found on some 23 pairs of independent bodies called chromosomes, which can be identified only when a cell is dividing. When genes are literally missing (*see* "The State of Genetic Medicine," p 19), cell operations may or may not be impaired, since only a small number of genes are turned on in any particular cell at any one time. Nevertheless, recent work suggests that some changes associated with aging result from chromosome shortening. In June 1992, a team of biologists including Carol W. Greider from Cold Spring Harbor Laboratory in New York and Silvia Bachetti of McMaster University in Hamilton, Ontario, reported that immortalized cancer cells activate an enzyme for chromosome repair that is normally inactive in cells from adults (although found in youthful cells). The enzyme, telomerase, is always active in protists and yeasts, for example; those are single-celled creatures that do not age. These creatures reproduce by dividing forever so long as the environment remains friendly. Human cells, on the other hand, reproduce about 70 to 100 times and then stop. From lack of telomerase, human chromosomes become shortened by about 50 letters of the genetic code with each division. Toward the last few divisions the chromosomes become warped and sticky as well. Cancer cells, which produce telomerase, are as immortal as yeasts. This theory, which might explain aging in cells, does not seem to explain aging in whole individuals unless humans become old because their cells become old and cease dividing.

Toxic chemicals accumulate   An old theory about aging is that the body is gradually poisoned by the accumulation of wastes and other buildup of substances. This theory assumes that there is a reduced number of working cells because the buildup of substances interferes with their operation. Thus, this is a variation on the first theory above.

Free radicals accumulate   In a sense, this concept is just another toxic-cell theory, since free radicals are toxic versions of ordinary molecules that have an electron too few or too many. The difference is that free radicals do not come from outside the body, and are not wastes. Most are produced by normal background radiation. Various chemicals, notably certain vitamins, are thought to "mop up" the free radicals before they can cause damage. (*see* "Vitamin UPDATE," p 160).

(Periodical References and Additional Reading: *New York Times* 1-22-91; *Science News* 2-22-92, p 123; *Harvard Health Letter* 6-92, p 1; *New York Times* 6-9-92, p C1; *Harvard Health Letter* 10-92, p 8; *Harvard Health Letter* 11-92, p 1; *Harvard Health Letter* 4-93, p 1; *Science News* 5-29-93, p 343; *New York Times* 6-29-93, p C3)

SLOWING AGING, DELAYING DEATH

Two intertwined issues have long concerned humans: staying young and living forever. These are not necessarily the same.

It is possible to picture a population in which each person lives to be about 85, maintaining good health with few wrinkles, no muscle loss, clear vision, and a clear brain—and then dies quite suddenly from cancer or heart disease. Indeed, some researchers into aging think this possibility is quite likely.

It is also easy to imagine a population in which people age much as they do today—but medical science keeps them alive for much longer, postponing death to ages of 120, 150, or even beyond. The elderly would be the largest portion of the population, and society would have to be completely remade to their needs—which would be great, because of poor health. Cataracts would form, but be removed. Hearts would fail, but receive pump assists and electrical pacemakers. Other organs, such as kidneys and livers, would also be aided by implanted or external machines. All the old men would have no prostates, and the old women would have no breasts, since these cancer-prone organs would be removed when trouble started. Old age would last for 40 to 80 years or more, longer than most lifetimes in earlier days. Certain scientists think that this is the way that the world will be in the future.

Since we are just imagining, we can daydream about combining the two scenarios to obtain perpetual youth and longer life, but the combination is harder to come by. At least it is most likely that if both of the possible changes in aging or death can ever take place, one will happen first and the other much later. As Sir Adolphe Abrahams remarked, "Everybody wishes to live a long time. Nobody wishes to be old."

In the meantime, scientific evidence is piling up to suggest that the way people age and die is different from what we thought and is possibly amenable to change.

Chemical Cures for Aging

In 1990 a study reported that a dozen elderly men regained muscle strength after taking genetically engineered human growth hormone (hGH). Many people who learned of the study thought that at last science had found the way to prevent aging, and for only about $14,000 a year.

The original group consisted of men between the ages of 61 and 81 who gave themselves daily hGH injections for six months. During that time they developed 8.8 percent more lean body mass, 7.1 percent thicker skin, and lost 14.4 body fat. Daniel Rudman of the Medical College of Wisconsin, the researcher who reported these results, expanded his study to 26 men in 1991. This time he observed similar changes in body mass, fat, and skin, but also measured volume increases in the liver and spleen by eight and 23 percent respectively. Lean body mass goes with muscle, and the 1991 group showed an 11 percent increase in muscle volume as well. Some authorities, however, point out that similar results—at least for muscle and fat—could be obtained with regular exercise and no hGH injections. Also, it should be noted that the effects stopped after the injections were halted, and the men returned to their normal ratio of muscle to fat.

Growth hormone has many effects on the body, not all of them beneficial. The principal effect, for which it gets its name, is to ensure normal growth. In older men hGH produces swollen joints, enlarged breasts, and carpal tunnel syndrome in addition to its benefits.

Further studies, now ongoing, are testing hGH on women as well. One study in particular is aimed at seeing if hGH can reduce osteoporosis in older women, while other researchers are looking at effects in both men and women on strength.

If benefits from hGH are found that exceed side effects, hGH may become available in the U.S. for reducing the effects of aging some time after the end of the 1990s. Of course, as with any drug that has been approved by the U.S. Food and Drug Administration (FDA) for any purpose, physicians can prescribe hGH injections at their own discretion. The hormone is currently approved for use with children who for genetic reasons lack it entirely or do not have enough of it to grow properly.

On another front, a chemical called dehydroepiandrosterone (DHEA) has been said to retard aging. As its chemical name indicates, DHEA is one of those steroids based on male sex hormones. The body's production of DHEA diminishes as people age—this is also true of testosterone. One small study suggested a connection between low DHEA levels and certain effects of aging, such as decreased cognitive abilities, in older males; the study did not provide any conclusive findings on DHEA, however. Accounts of DHEA's ability to slow down the aging process may have stemmed from wishful interpretations of the above-mentioned study.

Aging occurs in cells being kept alive in a petri dish, as well as in whole organisms. After dividing 20 to 60 times, for example, human endothelial cells become old, stop dividing, and eventually die. According to a 1990 report, however, there is a way of significantly extending cell life, up to as many as 160 divisions. Inhibition of a single cytokine, interleukin alpha-1, did the trick. However, scientists do not know why.

The Diet Connection

Since 1935, dozens of studies have shown that laboratory animals fed calorie-restricted, but nutritionally sound diets live much longer than those fed an ordinary laboratory diet—sometimes twice as long. In 1991 the U.S. National Institute of Aging announced that a study it had funded showed that the occurrence and timing of 136 different tissue changes associated with aging—representing all organs—were nearly all retarded or reduced in mice fed a restricted diet, so the results are far more than skin deep.

It is not clear why this strategy works. One theory, based on studies of biochemical markers, is that the restricted diet somehow protects DNA from damage and facilitates DNA repair if that protection fails (this line of reasoning appeals to those who think that damage to DNA causes aging). A study, reported in 1992 by Linda D. Youngman of the University of Oxford, England, and Bruce N. Ames of the University of California–Berkeley, and co-workers, shows that restricted diets lead to less radiation-induced free-radical damage (a result appealing to those who think free radicals cause aging).

Youngman and Ames used a low-protein diet instead of a low-calorie diet. Erkki Ruoslahtin of the La Jolla Cancer Research Foundation in California showed in 1991 that low-protein diets reduce the amount of a hormone that induces the body to make structural material between cells. Other scientists also have observed that low-calorie or low-protein diets reduce various hormones. All of the studies just cited also demonstrated that the low-calorie or low-protein diets reduce tumor formation.

Dr. Roy L. Walford, a professor of pathology at the University of California, Los Angeles, School of Medicine, after studying aging for 30 years, has come to believe that a high-nutrition, low-calorie diet can cause humans to live to be from 110 to 150 years old and stay relatively healthy in their extended old age. Aside from himself—he is a thin, healthy 70 in 1994—and his family, his most extensive experiment with humans was Biosphere II, for which he developed a diet plan. The eight Biosphere voyagers averaged 1780 calories a day during the six-month-long experiment, which was described in the December 1992 *Proceedings of the National Academy of Sciences.* Only ten percent of the calories were from fat, meaning that the Biospherians consumed about 20 grams of fat a day. Most of the food was vegetarian, including six fruits, five grains, four legumes, two potatoes (sweet and white), and 19 other vegetables and greens, augmented by small amounts of goat-based dairy products, chicken and other meat, and eggs (*see* "Health Concerns and Common Foods," p 204). During the half-year of the study the subjects lost an average of 22 pounds, 35/15 millimeters on the blood-pressure scale, and 75 mg/dL of serum cholesterol. But it is not known whether this will translate into longer life.

It should be clear that a reduced calorie diet must also be highly nutritious to confer any benefits. Many studies show that poor nutrition, whether high or low in calories, reduces lifespan. Feeding older people a high-nutrition diet reduces symptoms of aging, calories or no calories, as reported in a study by Howard Fillit of Mt. Sinai Medical Center in New York City.

People exposed to Walford's diet say that the food is so bad that even the possible life-extending effects fail to provide a sufficient initiative stay on it.

Other Secrets of a Long Life

People who live to advanced ages are often asked how they managed when so many fail. Interviewees on the subject seem to attribute their success to odd causes in many cases, including habits such as drinking and smoking that for most people reduce lifespan. The baseball star Satchel Paige, who seemed to age more slowly than other humans, gave a list of secrets for longevity of which the most famous is: "Don't look back; something may be gaining on you."

More scientific studies have uncovered some of the general truths embedded in various stories about people who have successfully retarded the aging process. A Swedish study, released late in 1993, found that stress and isolation reduce lifespans. In the study, a random sample of 50-year-old male urban Swedes were surveyed to find out whether they thought they were stressed and whether they had close friends or good relations with an extensive family, among other social factors. Seven years later the same researchers examined the death record to see what had happened to their survey subjects. Only 3.3 of the men with little reported stress and lots of friends or family died during that time, but 11 percent of those with stress and few social contacts had died. Of course, this survey looked at men in their 50s, not the truly elderly. A similar study of two groups of Americans close in age was conducted in the late 1970s in California. During a nine-year period, there were twice as many deaths in the group consisting of individuals with few social ties as in the group whose members enjoyed close friends or family support.

That friendless people die early comes as no great surprise, but another study in late 1993 produced some apparently paradoxical results. A population was located that had been extensively studied from the early 1920s, when the average age of the population was 11, to the 1990s. The group consisted of children in California who scored above 135 on Lewis Terman's groundbreaking IQ test. These boys and girls were interviewed and tested every few years for the rest of their lives, first by Terman and then by other psychologists. Most of them had died by 1993. Howard S. Friedman of the University of California at Riverside gathered the accumulated data, grouped it into general psychological categories, and compared the categories with lifespans.

- Sociability and extroversion: no correlation with lifespan.
- Self-esteem and confidence: no correlation with lifespan.
- Conscientiousness and caution: traits connected with a longer lifespan.
- Cheerfulness and optimism: traits connected with a shorter lifespan.

The personality traits tended to stay the same throughout each person's life. The study was published in the October 1993 issue of the *Journal of Personality and Social Psychology.*

Scandinavian Studies

People have been known to lie about their age for one reason or another. After living many years, some people begin to add years to their true age. It is possible that some of those centenarians Willard Scott relentlessly salutes on the *Today Show* are only in their 90s. This factor has complicated the study of aging.

Scandinavian countries, particularly Sweden and Denmark, where records of all births and deaths are kept by the Lutheran church, have produced what are believed to be the most accurate death data available to science. James Vaupel of the University of Odense, Denmark, and recently also at Duke University in Durham, North Carolina, used Swedish data going back to 1750 to investigate extreme old age. He was particularly interested in looking at death rates for women and men aged 85, 90, 95, or 100. Since World War II, death rates for women at all of those ages have been reduced by more than a third and the rates for men have been reduced by about a sixth. These data conflict with the concept that there is a predestined lifespan. Vaupel thinks that the data imply that there is no set limit, or if there is, the limit must be much higher than 100 years old.

Vaupel then turned to death data from Denmark. He wanted to find out whether the concept of senescence makes sense. *Senescence* has been defined as an individual's deterioration with age leading to increased mortality. (According to Sir Peter Medawar, it "renders the individual progressively more likely to die from accidental causes of random incidence".) In other words, senescence is the "old age" implied when it is said that a person "died from old age." Vaupel and a collaborator, Niels Holm, used computer modeling to investigate the senescence factor in 55,000 Danish twins, both fraternal and identical. If there were genetic senescence, identical twins would be more likely to die at the same time than fraternal twins are, but the data did not reveal such a correlation. In fact, the study showed Vaupel and Holm that there was no senescence factor that they could locate below the age of 110; in other words, the mean age of death attributed to senescence was greater than 110.

A study of very old individuals by Finnish demographer Vaino Kannisto looked at data from 27 countries and observed that, as in Sweden, the very old have had increasing lifespans since 1950.

Really Old Fruit Flies

Data on the oldest population of humans, those over 85, are weak because the people in question are few in number, scattered about (until recently, at least), and not counted in most mortality tables (which typically cut off at 79 or at 85). Vaupel's Scandinavian data suggested that experiments with a large animal population might clarify the problems of senescence and life expectancy. Therefore, James R. Carey of the University of California at Davis and James W. Curtsinger of the University of Minnesota each decided to study a large population that would be easy to keep track of. Although fruit flies are not humans, they are born, live, age, and die in quick succession. The life expectancy for fruit flies is about a month. It is relatively easy to count dead flies every day to see when they die, and also to hatch large numbers of flies at once so that the age at death can be easily determined.

It was Carey's intention to examine a very large population of fruit flies and find out how long each one lived under both optimal and average conditions. He learned that in Mexico facilities had been set up to raise billions of male Mediterranean fruit flies (*Ceratitis capitata*) so that the flies could be sterilized and released in California to halt the fly population explosion in that state—a method that had been successful years before in controlling populations of other flies. Using the Mexican facilities, Carey and Mexican biologists (and Vaupel, who had inspired the study) examined two "small" populations of about 20,000 flies each under nearly optimal conditions and one very large population of 1.2 million flies under normal conditions. Because each population was studied until all the flies in it died, exact life expectancies at any given time could be calculated by working backward. These were still averages, but they were averages of real numbers for this population.

The two small populations had as a whole life expectancies of about 30 days. But in one of those optimal groups one fly lived to be 216 days old, while in the other, one fly lived to be 241 days old. Thus, the result tended to confirm Vaupel's idea that if there is senescent death, it can come to some individuals at a multiple several times the average life expectancy. If humans were fruit flies, the best cared for humans would live to seven or eight times the average life expectancy, or to as much as 560 years for men or 640 for women. But, of course, humans are not fruit flies.

The most interesting data came from the large population of flies. The likelihood of a fly dying in that population (which had a life expectancy at birth of only about 20 days) reached a peak between 40 and 60 days old. At that point each fly had about a 15 percent chance of dying on a given day. After that period, those flies that had survived had much lower probabilities of dying. Flies 100 or more days old had a chance of only four to six percent of dying on a given day. Out of 1.2 million flies at the beginning, only 62 were still alive at the end of 100 days. The half life of this population was 24 days—on day 125 there were only 31 flies left alive, but two had died on day 124. The half life of the original population was 20 days; thus, the super-old flies seemed to be healthier on the average than young flies.

One of the most likely ways to account for Carey's results would be if a small population were genetically superior to the other fruit flies. Curtsinger investigated this possibility with a different kind of fruit fly, *Drosophila melanogaster*, the mainstay of genetics research for most of the twentieth century. Because of that research, highly inbred lines of fruit flies were available. Curtsinger and coworkers at the University of Minnesota in Minneapolis, working with Vaupel, used four of these inbred lines and six first-generation hybrids between the four lines to investigate the effect of gene differences on lifespan. Although this team noted that different strains did have different lifespans, the important result was a confirmation of Carey's work. Within each group, individuals who lived past the age of maximum probability of death then had a lower probability of death and some of them lived many times the average life expectancy for the whole strain.

In a newspaper interview Carey said that if the fruit-fly results applied to humans at all, they might mean something like "a 60-year-old on average would live ten more years, but an 80-year-old would live 20 more years." Vaupel was more willing to make the transition between flies and folks: "We have a better and better chance to live into our 80s, and if we live into our 80s, there is a better chance that we will live into our 90s."

Long-Lived Worms

Although the work with fruit flies was exceptionally dramatic, this study was not the first to suggest that very old individuals have a lower mortality rate than that of merely old individuals. The same phenomenon had previously been observed in calorie-deprived rodents and in certain genetically manipulated strains of the nematode *Caenorhabditis elegans,* a tiny worm that has been so thoroughly studied that the development of every cell of its body is known. But these were thought to be unusual phenomena resulting from special circumstances.

The nematode *C. elegans* also figures in two other surprises connected with mortality. In the August 24, 1990, issue of *Science* Thomas E. Johnson of the University of Colorado in Boulder reported that nematodes with a defect in the gene *age-1* had a four-fold decrease in reproductive capacity along with a 65 percent increase in the mean lifespan and a 110 percent increase in the maximum lifespan. The lifespan increase resulted from a decrease in mortality rate for older worms. This was related to another increase in *C. elegans* lifespan announced by Wayne A. Van Voorhies of the University of Arizona in Tucson in the December 3, 1992, issue of *Nature*. Van Voorhies found that sperm production in hermaphrodites (the most common sex for the nematode) and in males decreases lifespan; this suggested that perhaps the effect described by Johnson was a result of decreased reproductive ability.

But in the December 2, 1993, issue of *Nature*, a team from the University of California–San Francisco, reported that the mutation of a single gene in *C. elegans* more than doubled its lifespan. The average lifespan in the worms with the mutated gene is 48 days, compared to 18 days for the wild type. This time the gene was not the one aptly (if accidentally) named *age-1*, but a developmental gene named *daf-2* whose normal role is to instigate a special kind of larval stage that conserves energy during bad environmental conditions, thus permitting the nematode to live longer in hopes of better times. The mutated *daf-2* fails to produce the special larval stage, but still ensures longevity. If a human could do the same, life expectancy would be about 150 or 160. While there is no obvious application of this result to humans, this discovery is a powerful example of how genetics affects length of life.

It also affects the aging process. Mutant worms appear healthier and more muscular at any adult age than their wild counterparts.

(Periodical References and Additional Reading: *Science* 8-24-90, p 908; *Science News* 9-29-90, p 198; *Science News* 10-5-91, p 215; *Science* 11-15-91, p 936; *Harvard Health Letter* 6-92, p 1; *New York Times* 10-10-92, p 1; *New York Times* 10-16-92, p A22; *Science* 10-16-92, pp 398, 457, & 461; *New York Times* 11-16-92, p A1; *Science News* 11-21-92, p 346; *Nature* 12-3-92, p 458; *Harvard Health Letter* 4-93, p 3; *New York Times* 11-9-93, p C3; *Nature* 12-2-93, pp 404 & 461; *Science News* 12-4-93, p 375; *New York Times* 12-7-93, pp C5 & C13; *New York Times* 7-20-94, p C1)

DEATH

ACCIDENTAL DEATH, HOMICIDE, AND SUICIDE

The number of accidental deaths in the U.S. has declined significantly in recent years. Indeed, we do not consider this surprising; we expect the death *rate* to be lower, especially since the rates in such countries as Japan (26.2 in 1990), the United Kingdom (24.4), and the Netherlands (24.3) are considerably lower than in the U.S. What is surprising, however, is that since 1988 the *total* number of accidental deaths has been declining by about five percent a year in recent years, even though the population continues to increase.

Year	Number of accidental deaths (U.S.)	Rate per hundred thousand
1992	84,000	32.9
1991	88,000	34.9
1990	93,500	37.5
1989	94,500	38.1
1988	96,000	39.1

Estimated rates were very high earlier in the century—82.7 per hundred thousand in 1910 (based on figures from about half the total population).

According to the U.S. National Safety Council, the 1992 total is the smallest in the U.S. since 1922. By 1923 the number of accidental deaths had climbed to 84,400. One high point was in 1941, when the total reached 101,513, after which rates declined until the early 1960s. By 1963, the total number had once again climbed above 100,000, to reach 116,000 in 1969—subsequently, accidental death began an irregular decline in the U.S. due to factors such as the Occupational Health and Safety Act of 1970, the imposition of the 55 mile-per-hour speed limit in the 1970s (still the limit in many states today), movements such as Mothers Against Drunk Driving, Students Against Drunk Driving, and greater public awareness of household hazards.

In June 1992, the U.S. Department of Health and Human Services recognized the importance of dealing with trauma and death from resulting from such events as unintentional poisonings, drowning, electrocution, and so forth. The department created the National Center for Injury Prevention and Control. Instead of being part of the National Health Institutes, the Injury Prevention group is part of the Centers for Disease Control and Prevention.

In May 1993, the Second World Conference on Injury Control took place in Atlanta, Georgia. At the conference, professionals from 50 nations decided not to use the words "accident" or "accidental" in any form, to emphasize that injury from causes other than disease is largely preventable. A typical statistic resulting from the conference was that bicycle helmets are 85 percent effective in preventing serious injuries from falls.

Motor-Vehicle Accidents

A big part of the U.S. decline in deaths from injury was in motor-vehicle accidents. The reduction resulted from a combination of several factors.

- Alcohol-related deaths: down to 45.8 percent of fatalities in 1992; accounted for 57.3 of fatalities in 1982.
- Seat-belt usage: up 59 percent in 1991, 62 percent in 1992, and 66 percent in 1993 according to Department of Transportation surveys; usage was just 12 percent in 1982, based on slightly different criteria.
- Air bags: installed on half the cars sold in 1993.
- Such safety features as anti-lock brakes and better tires, as well as autos designed with safety in mind, have saved more than 240,000 lives in the U.S. since 1967.

Consequently, the fewest number of people died in motor-vehicle accidents in 1992 of any year since 1962. Still, there were 39,235 fatalities in 1992, resulting from 6.2 million crashes. The number of deaths was expected to decrease as automobiles became safer, but it actually rose slightly in 1993, to 39,850, because people drove more.

The number of deaths per vehicle mile, however, has decreased steadily in recent years in the U.S.

Year	Deaths per vehicle mile
1993	1.7
1992	1.8
1991	1.9
1990	2.1
1989	2.2
1988	2.3

Guns Kill People, Too

A statistic concerning accidental death, surprising to many people, results from a sharp rise in the number of gunshot wounds combined with the steady decline in serious injuries from automobile accidents. The combination of these trends in six states and the District of Columbia has produced a situation by 1992 in which the number of deaths from shootings exceeds the number from automobile accidents. In New York that year, for example, 2345 died from gunshots and 1959 from gunshot wounds. The other five states with similar statistics were California, Louisiana, Nevada, Texas, and Virginia.

Although most people learning this have been mainly concerned with the rise in the number and use of guns, including automatic weapons, the decline in automobile deaths is the largest part of the story. Overall in the U.S. in 1991, the last year for which figures for causes of death were available at the start of 1994, gun-related deaths were 38,317 and motor-vehicles claimed nearly as many lives, 43,536; but, if the rate of automobile-accident deaths had been the same as it had been in the 1950s, the total for 1991 would have been nearer 60,000 instead of about 44,000. The year 1956 was the high point for motor-vehicle accidents in the U.S. on a per-person basis. The total that year was 39,628 deaths, but the U.S. population was much smaller. If that figure had grown directly with the population, by 1992 the number of motor-vehicle deaths would have reached 60,631.

By way of contrast, the gun-related deaths in 1956 were only 2,202. If that had grown directly with the population increase, it would have reached about 3369 by 1992 instead of being more than ten times that number.

Estimates by the U.S. Department of Health and Human Services early in 1994 are that the total number of gun-related deaths in the U.S. as a whole will exceed the total number of motor-vehicle deaths for the first time in 2003. The fall in motor-vehicle deaths has been so sharp in recent years that Garen Wintemute of the University of California at Davis calculated in the *Journal of the American Medical Association* that if rates did not change, gun-related deaths would exceed those from motor vehicles in the U.S. in 1994.

Even though the reduction in automobile deaths accounts in large part for the near reversal in order of importance, the rapid rise in gunshot fatalities is dramatic when looked at independently. Indeed, by 1992 the editors of the *Journal of the American Medical Association* had termed gun-related deaths a "public health epidemic."

While many view guns primarily as an external threat, firearms are also the leading mode of suicide among both men (65 percent in 1991) and women (40 percent). According to studies, family members are 43 times as likely as intruders to be hurt by guns kept in the home.

On June 9, 1992, the National Center for Health Statistics released their study of gun-related deaths in the late 1980s. The main victims of guns in the 79 U.S. metropolitan areas studied were black males aged 15 through 19; in the Washington D.C. area, with the highest rate in the study, the young black men were killed at an annual rate of 227.2 per 100,000 in the total population.

Homicide and Suicide Are Steady

Although the age-adjusted mortality rates for the U.S. have fallen dramatically for men and somewhat less significantly for women since 1960, primarily because of the reduction of heart disease and stroke, the portion of those deaths from suicide or homicide continues to increase. In 1991, the latest year for which there are complete data, suicide was the eighth leading cause of death in the U.S. and homicide the tenth (preliminary results for 1992 suggest that AIDS-related deaths had passed suicide by then, leaving suicide just ahead of homicide to fill the ninth and tenth positions). As a consequence, the U.S. leads the industrialized countries in deaths from homicide and legal intervention (a category that includes all deaths as a result of police activity, on or off duty, as well as executions). Violent acts cause nearly ten times as many injuries as deaths.

Figures like these contribute to a public perception that violence has become the major problem in American life. The statistics, however, do not tell the whole story and even a closer look at the statistics reveals a very different side to the problems of violence and suicide. First of all, it makes a considerable difference which year is chosen for comparison. If you go back to the end of the Eisenhower era—that is, to

1960—homicide rates for both men and women have more or less doubled, but suicide rates have stayed relatively constant. But if your point of departure is the end of the Vietnam War in 1975, the difference in homicide rates is very slight, up from 10.2 in 1975 to 10.8 in 1991, with slight annual rises or falls over the 16-year period. More than half of all homicides in 1991, or in earlier years, result from quarrels among family members or acquaintances, and 90 percent of the time both the victim and the perpetrator of the crime are of the same ethnic group. Homicide has a disproportionate effect on society because it is a problem chiefly of the young—almost 80 percent of all homicide victims are between the ages of 15 and 44. The victim rate for young men between the ages of 15 and 24 has risen amazingly since 1985, going from slightly less than 20 per 100,000 in that age group to over 35 per 100,000 and still rising steadily.

Suicide rates have remained fairly steady over a long stretch of time:

U.S. SUICIDE RATE

Year	Suicide rate in U.S.
1920	10.2 per 100,000
1925	12.1 per 100,000
1930	15.7 per 100,000
1935	14.3 per 100,000
1945	11.2 per 100,000
1950	11.4 per 100,000
1970	11.6 per 100,000
1979	12.1 per 100,000
1980	10.9 per 100,000
1986	12.8 per 100,000
1990	12.3 per 100,000
1991	12.0 per 100,000
1992	11.7 per 100,000 (provisional)

Clearly, the Great Depression of the 1930s affected suicide rates (which reached a high of 17.4 per 100,000 in 1932), but little else has made much of a change. It should also be noted that most experts believe that suicides are under-reported; survivors' evidence suggests that many automobile "accidents" or other apparent "accidents" were intended as suicides. The assumption is that with so many known near suicides, there must also be a large number of successful suicides buried in the accidental death statistics. If somewhere near a quarter of all "accidental" deaths could be classified as disguised suicides, the suicide rate would double.

(Periodical References and Additional Reading: *New York Times* 6-11-92, p B10; *New York Times* 1-17-93, p IV-6; *New York Times* 5-13-93, p A14; *New York Times* 5-26-93, p C11; *Scientific American* 11-93, p 14: *New York Times* 11-9-93, p C1; *New York Times* 12-19-93, p I-44; *New York Times* 1-28-94, p A12; *New York Times* 4-3-94, p I-15; *Statistical Bulletin* 4/6-94, p 10)

TIMETABLE OF TRAUMA TREATMENT TO 1990

1360	*Chirurgia magna* by Guy de Chauliac [born circa 1300; died circa 1368] describes fracture and hernia treatment.
1497	Hieronymus Brunschwygk [born circa 1452; died 1512] publishes the first known book on the surgical treatment of gunshot wounds.
1545	A book on surgery by Ambroise Paré [born Mayenne, France, 1510; died Paris, December 20, 1590] advocates abandoning the practice of treating wounds with boiling oil and using soothing ointments instead.
1667	In an experiment demonstrated before the Royal Society, Robert Boyle [born Ireland, January 25, 1627; died London, December 30, 1691] shows that an animal can be kept alive by artificial respiration.
1691	Clopton Havers [born Stambourne, England, circa 1655; died Willingale, England, April 1702] publishes the first complete textbook on the bones of the human body.
1746	The compressive bandage to stop bleeding from wounds is introduced.
1869	German surgeon J. Friedrich A. von Esmarch [born 1823; died 1908] demonstrates the use of a prepared first-aid bandage on the battlefield.
1877	J. Friedrich A. von Esmarch introduces the antiseptic bandage.
1920	Johnson & Johnson introduces the Band-Aid, a sterile-packaged individual bandage using tape to hold an absorbent pad in place over a minor cut.
1971	In the United States, it is shown that electric currents can speed the healing of fractures.
1987	A team led by Hari Reddi at the National Institutes of Health extracts and identifies bone morphogenetic protein (B.M.P.), a substance predicted first by Marshall Urist in the 1960s; B.M.P promotes new bone growth and is expected to help cure fractures that otherwise are resistant to healing, as well as to speed healing in more ordinary fractures and bone damage caused by surgery.

OPTIONS FOR DEATH, DYING, AND AFTERWARD

Death is inevitable, although it can sometimes be postponed or made easier. In some cases, people have decided that for their own incurable illness, a quick death is better than a long agony. In other cases, those with an incurable illness choose to live as comfortably as they can for as long as they can.

For hundreds of thousands of Americans in the early 1990s, the option taken for living out the last months or years of an incurable illness is different from what it used to be. For most of history, people died at home, cared for by relatives or servants or perhaps not cared for at all. A recent survey found that 86 percent of Americans asked would prefer it to be that way still, although Americans increasingly die in hospitals. But the same people, when asked to speculate how they would feel if they only had six months to live, also thought that they would like to spend it in a homelike setting with good medical care—a description of what a hospice is supposed to be (and what most hospices actually are). The hospice idea is still new to many people, but in 1991 about 210,000 patients were in these terminal care facilities on a full or part-time basis instead of in a regular hospital or nursing home.

The basic criterion for entry into a hospice program is one that people would not care to qualify for—a life expectation of less than six months. The actual time spent in the hospice, however, generally ranges from a few days to over a year, although the average stay is two months.

Euthanasia and Assisted Suicide

Does the name Dr. Jack Kevorkian mean anything to you? In the U.S., the "death doctor" has enjoyed the fame of a great celebrity whose name is instantly recognized by people. In part, his fame is due to a plethora of jokes by comedians on television and in clubs. The Michigan-based retired physician gained that fame by assisting terminally ill women and men in dying, usually by supplying them with carbon monoxide gas from a device of his own invention, recently in the back of a van known to the comedians as Kevorkian's deathmobile. He has worked mostly in Michigan because that state's laws—at least when Kevorkian started—were lenient toward death assistance. So far Kevorkian has survived a number of legal challenges, although his activities have become more limited by changes in laws covering assisted suicides even as his fame grows.

Suicide is legal in every state in the U.S., but assisting suicide is generally illegal, which can create problems not only for a Dr. Kevorkian, but also for any physician or nurse or family member who accedes to a dying patient's request to accelerate the process of dying. Helping an elderly or infirm patient to die is generally known as euthanasia (a derivation from the Greek for "good death").

Around the world, views on euthanasia vary considerably. In the West, the least restrictive policy has long been found in the Netherlands, and laws there became even less restrictive in 1993. But even in the Netherlands, where the prosecutors and courts have generally protected doctors who assist in suicides, such assistance is technically illegal, even when the patient is terminally ill. However, under a provision adopted in 1993, a physician who reports that he or she had assisted in the death of patient at that patient's request and provides the courts with an account of the process will not be prosecuted.

Death by Dehydration

In 1994 an 85-year-old physician's widow and physician's mother demonstrated that unassisted suicide can be relatively graceful. According to a report by her son published in the July 19, 1994, issue of the *Journal of the American Medical Association,* Virginia Eddy chose a slice of birthday cake, prepared to celebrate her 85th birthday, as her last life-sustaining meal. For most of her 85 years she had been healthy, but in the last year she endured two major surgical operations and pneumonia; and her health-related problems included failing eyesight, incontinence, and serious pain. After that birthday cake, Eddy ceased eating and, more importantly, ceased drinking any fluids. Her only input was morphine that she used for the pain, prescribed by her physician.

The dehydration that eventually killed Virginia Eddy—in only six days—did not add to her suffering, according to her personal physician Timothy Cope. Instead, it seemed to bring relief. She died in her sleep. She had told her family that she wanted to die, but wanted to do so "without hoarding pills, without making [her physician son] a criminal, without putting a bag over her head, and without huddling in the back of a van with a carbon monoxide machine." Courts in the U.S. have generally ruled that a competent person cannot be forced to eat or drink anything that he or she does not want.

A couple of years before Eddy's death, a committee of Roman Catholic bishops had denounced suicide by fluid deprivation, calling it a widespread practice. But their concern was somewhat different, focusing on patients thought to be in irreversible comas and who, therefore, were kept alive by nutrients—including fluids—that were supplied through tubes. The bishops' aim was to prevent physicians, nurses, or family members from obtaining court orders to have the feeding tubes removed. In the U.S., state laws vary on whether nutrition and fluids can be withheld, but since 1991 federal law has required hospitals and nursing homes to tell patients whether they are allowed by their state laws to refuse treatment that would prolong their lives. Such a refusal is most often reported in a document curiously known as a "living will," signed by the patient before entering treatment (such as a risky operation) that might leave the patient in a coma or otherwise incapable of making wishes known.

Keep Frozen until the Cure is Found

For a long time science-fiction writers have described the preservation of dead or dying humans by flash freezing so that they can be revived when the disease from which they are suffering or which killed them can be cured or reversed. Also, fictional accounts suggest preserving humans by freezing for the most boring parts of space missions, as in the motion picture *2001: A Space Odyssey*. In real life, there has been a small, but apparently thriving, business in freezing cadavers in liquid nitrogen, awaiting the development of new technology.

The wait may be a long one, but there are new developments that warrant some hope. Embryos of placental mammals, including mice, cattle, sheep, and humans, are routinely frozen and then successfully implanted in mothers who nurture the embryos through to normal birth and normal life. Such embryos are most likely to survive at the earliest possible stage of life, when there are only a few cells, typically eight. Nematode larvae with hundreds of cells are also routinely frozen and revived. These feats are a far cry from freezing and reviving a whole adult animal. (Fish and frogs are adapted to occasional light freezing, which they may encounter in nature; while they can be revived after a few months in normal winter ice, they cannot be deep frozen and revived years later.)

The closest to success for longer-term deep freezing of developed animals has been the successful freezing and revival of later-stage embryos (with guts, muscles, a nervous system, and a head) of fruit flies, as reported in the December 18, 1992, issue of *Science* by Peter Mazur of Oak Ridge National Laboratory and co-workers.

The motive for this research is that fruit flies are one of the standard laboratory animals, with about 15,000 different genetic lines being expensively kept at laboratories around the world. It is much easier to preserve a purebred strain in the freezer than to continually breed and feed its adult members.

The method used with the fruit flies is both simple and complex. Viewed simply, the process removes a membrane with household bleach, dissolves a waxy coating with gasoline, and adds ordinary antifreeze before putting the embryos in the deep freeze. In practice, each stage is delicate, with concentrations of chemicals carefully monitored and with very fast freezing and warming required. The method is not so delicate, however, that it could not be immediately duplicated by another laboratory with similar equipment.

Freezing fruit-fly embryos is still a long way from the ideals of science fiction. For one thing, the success rate of developing adult fruit flies from the process is only 40 percent. While this is sufficient for large fruit-fly stocks, the odds are not so good for any one individual.

(Periodical References and Additional Reading: *New York Times* 12-8-90; *New York Times* 4-3-92, p A10; *Science* 12-18-92, pp 1896 & 1932; *New York Times* 2-9-93, p A1; *Harvard Health Letter* 4-93, p 9; *New York Times* 12-22-93, p C2; *New York Times* 7-20-94, p C10)

TEN TOP CAUSES OF DEATH IN THE U.S.

A number of striking changes have occurred in the leading causes of death in the past 20 years. By far the most important has been the reduction in death from heart disease, but the most dramatic has been the swift rise of AIDS up the list. It is also noticeable that in 1970 none of the ten leading causes had a death rate per 100,000 that was less than 15, but in the 1990s there are three causes of death in the top ten with rates less than that.

Some scientists believe that as death from heart disease goes down, the rate for cancer will rise. Underlying this belief is the assumption that people who survive heart disease will eventually confront cancer. That has certainly happened, but a cause-and-effect relationship does not seem obvious.

	Rate per 100,000
1992 **TOTAL DEATHS**	**853.3**
1. Heart disease	282.5
2. Cancer	204.3
3. Stroke (Cerebrovascular accidents)	56.3
4. Breathing disorders (Chronic obstructive pulmonary disease, including bronchitis, asthma, and emphysema)	35.2
5. Accidents	33.8
6. Pneumonia and influenza	29.8
7. Diabetes mellitus	19.7
8. AIDS	13.2
9. Suicide	11.7
10. Homicide and legal intervention	10.4

	Rate per 100,000
1991 TOTAL DEATHS	**854.0**
1. Heart disease	283.3
2. Cancer	202.9
3. Stroke (Cerebrovascular accidents)	56.8
4. Accidents	36.2
5. Breathing disorders (Chronic obstructive pulmonary disease, including bronchitis, asthma, and emphysema)	35.2
6. Pneumonia and influenza	29.6
7. Diabetes mellitus	19.7
8. Suicide	11.9
9. AIDS	11.8
10. Homicide and legal intervention	10.8
1990 TOTAL DEATHS	**851.9**
1. Heart disease	289.0
2. Cancer	201.7
3. Stroke (Cerebrovascular accidents)	57.9
4. Accidents	37.3
5. Breathing disorders (Chronic obstructive pulmonary disease, including bronchitis, asthma, and emphysema)	35.5
6. Pneumonia and influenza	31.3
7. Diabetes mellitus	19.5
8. Suicide	12.3
9. Homicide and death from law enforcement	10.2
10. Liver disease (including cirrhosis)	10.2
1980 TOTAL DEATHS	**878.3**
1. Heart disease	336.0
2. Cancer	183.9
3. Stroke (Cerebrovascular accidents)	75.1
4. Accidents	46.7
5. Breathing disorders (Chronic obstructive pulmonary disease, including bronchitis, asthma, and emphysema)	24.7
6. Pneumonia and influenza	24.1
7. Diabetes mellitus	15.4
8. Liver disease (including cirrhosis)	13.5
9. Atherosclerosis	13.0
10. Suicide	11.9

	Rate per 100,000
1970 **TOTAL DEATHS**	**945.3**
1. Heart disease	362.0
2. Cancer	162.8
3. Stroke (Cerebrovascular accidents)	101.9
4. Accidents	56.4
5. Pneumonia and influenza	30.9
6. Pregnancy and childbirth (Perinatal-related conditions)	21.3
7. Diabetes mellitus	18.9
8. Atherosclerosis	15.6
9. Liver disease (including cirrhosis)	15.5
10. Breathing disorders (Chronic obstructive pulmonary disease, including bronchitis, asthma, and emphysema)	15.2

(Periodical References and Additional Reading: *New York Times* 9-16-93, p A16)

LIFE EXPECTANCY IN THE UNITED STATES

Life expectancy is not so simple as it seems at first thought. If you use the arithmetic mean of all deaths, you include a great many very low ages from deaths of infants, while deaths of people in their twenties or thirties are very low as are the numbers living to extreme ages. Thus, the average age of death for a given year is not the best measure of when most people are likely to die. A report showing deaths by decade might be more useful as information than the single number that is the average. Similarly, for a single number, the median (half way between the top and the bottom) might be more meaningful.

Furthermore, in the past century the average length of life by any measure has tended to increase. Thus, the true life expectancy is greater for a person born in 1991 than the average age of all the people who died that year. The figures in the table below have been corrected for this so that they represent the average age at which people born in 1991 are expected to die, presuming that cancer and heart disease are not suddenly cured and that a very large asteroid does not strike the earth in, say, 1996.

Of course most people now living were not born in 1991. Another useful measure of life expectancy is based on the average taken after a certain number of people have already died. For example, if you consider people who are 50 years old in 1991 only, then you know that none of them died before 1991, so all of them will live to be at least 50. Thus, life expectancy of people who are 50 in 1991 is 79.2 years, almost four years more than for people born in 1991 (even though people born in 1991 might benefit from advances in medicine that take place after 2021, when the "average person" who was 50 in 1991 is "expected" to be dead).

Year	At birth all	At birth women all	At birth men all	At birth women black	At birth men black	At birth women white	At birth men white
1991	75.5	78.9	72.0	73.8	64.6	79.6	72.9

LIFE EXPECTANCIES IN INDUSTRIALIZED NATIONS

The latest estimate for the average life expectancy at birth for all humans everywhere is 65 years, but there is a wide discrepancy from nation to nation.

Country	Year of data	Life expectancy at birth (avg. of male/female)
Developed countries	1990	75
Japan	1990	78.9
Iceland	1989–90	78.0
Sweden	1990	77.6
Switzerland	1989–90	77.4
Australia	1990	77.0
Netherlands	1990	77.0
Norway	1990	76.6
Canada	1985–87	76.4
New Zealand	1987–89	74.6
France	1987	76.2
Germany (West)	1986–89	75.5
United States	1991	75.5
Finland	1989	75.0
United Kingdom	1985–87	74.8
Russia	1991	72

LIFE EXPECTANCIES IN
SELECTED DEVELOPING NATIONS

Country	Year of data	Life expectancy at birth (avg. of male/female)
Developing countries	1990	62
Cuba	1990	76
Singapore	1990	74
Panama	1990	73
Sri Lanka	1990	72
China	1990	71
Brazil	1991	67
Algeria	1990	66
Guatemala	1990	65
Indonesia	1990	63
Bolivia	1990	61
Egypt	1991	61
India	1990	60
Kenya	1990	59
Haiti	1990	57
Ghana	1990	56
Papua New Guinea	1990	56
Gabon	1990	54
Sudan	1990	52
Cambodia	1990	51
Angola	1990	46
Afghanistan	1990	43
Sierra Leone	1990	43
Uganda	1990	42

(Periodical References and Additional Reading: *Statistical Bulletin* 7/9-92, p 10; *New York Times* 9-1-93, p A13)

Appendices

APPENDIX A

ORGANIZATION OF THE HUMAN BODY

Biologists have long recognized that higher life forms have a number of levels of organization. Early humans were aware of the larger features of the system, but cells and their parts had to await the invention of the microscope. Although the larger features were recognized, their function was often unknown. The brain was once thought to be a kind of air conditioner, and even today people speak of the heart as the seat of the emotions, although science has relocated these functions to different features.

Systems The human body consists of nine main *systems:* the skeleton, the muscles, the nervous system, the hormonal system, the circulatory system, the digestive system, the respiratory system, the immune system, and the reproductive system.

Organs Each system is made up of a number of *organs*. An organ is a part of the body with a specific purpose. Some organs, such as the liver or the skin, have more than one function. A few organs, such as the eyes and ears, are not really part of a major system.

Tissues Organs are made from *tissues*. A tissue is a part of the organ made from similar cells and, in some cases, extracellular material (for example, bone tissue consists of bone cells and extracellular minerals).

Cells *Cells* are the fundamental components of all organisms. Even they are composed of several different parts—the nucleus, the cytoplasm, the cell membrane, and various smaller parts—that have different functions.

The Skeleton

A central feature of humans and their nearer relatives in the animal kingdom is an internal framework. Today scientists know that the bones that form this framework also have important roles besides the structural.

Bones There are 206 bones in the human body, or one or two more or less, depending on how you count. Their main function is to provide a structural support for everything else, but they also have other vital functions. Bones might be classified as part of the circulatory system, for example, since their marrow produces all of the body's blood cells. Bones are also part of the hormonal system in that they are an important reservoir for calcium, an element necessary for life. If the body's intake of calcium is too low, the bones make up the deficit. This weakens their role as structural support and can result in the condition osteoporosis, or fragile bone structure.

Cartilage   This is a flexible substance that precedes bone development in children and that is found in adults at *joints,* places where bones meet, as well as in the nose and ears.

Ligaments   Bones are attached to each other by flexible tissues called *ligaments.* A few bones, such as those in the skull, grow together, forming rigid attachments.

The Muscles

There are over 600 muscles in the body that have been named. They occur in three different systems.

Skeletal muscles   These muscles are used to move various parts of the body. They are what one normally thinks of when one thinks of muscles, and nearly all of them are attached to bones by *tendons,* long or flat sheets of tough tissue. They are made from fibers that are striped (or striated) in appearance under a microscope. Each fiber can contract or lengthen when the muscle receives a message from the brain. Because we control the use of these muscles, they are also called the *voluntary muscles.*

Smooth muscles   These are found in the walls of the stomach and intestines, in the walls of veins and arteries, and in various other internal organs. They are for the most part not controlled by the will, so they are also known as the *involuntary muscles.* People do have partial control over some of the "involuntary" muscle, however; for example, you can stop the smooth muscle of the diaphragm from causing you to breathe for a time.

Cardiac muscle   The muscles of the heart resemble the skeletal muscles in being striped and smooth muscles in their involuntary nature.

The Nervous System and Senses

While the nervous system is largely a single, large, interacting system that pervades the body and includes the brain, the sense organs are localized in various ways.

Brain   The organ that controls the rest of the body and undertakes thought is composed of three main parts. The *cerebrum* is the folded outer part of each half of the brain. It governs thought, the senses, and movement. The *cerebellum* controls balance and muscle coordination. Deep in the brain is the *brain stem,* which governs involuntary muscles. A small, but important, part of the human brain is the *hypothalamus,* which controls the hormonal system (see below). Located in the head, the brain is protected by the bones of the skull.

Spinal cord   Extending from the brain to the base of the torso and protected by the vertebrae, the spinal cord is the main highway for messages to and from the brain. The spinal cord can initiate actions on its own, which are known as *reflexes.*

Nerves   Twelve pairs of *cranial nerves* connect directly to the brain. Ten of these pairs are connected to parts of the head concerned with sight, sound, smell, and taste, such as the *optic nerves* to the eyes and the *auditory nerves* to the ears. The *vagus nerves* extend to various organs of the torso, where they control involuntary muscles.

The twelfth pair of cranial nerves are connected to the shoulder, where they are mostly involved in the sense of position.

Thirty-two pairs of *spinal nerves* connect to the spinal cord and are the nerves involved in touch and other sensations, in giving direction to and receiving information from skeletal muscles, and in controlling to some extent the other internal organs. For example, the *median nerve* connects from the spinal cord to the finger muscles. Some nerves connected to the cranial and spinal nerves form the *autonomic nervous system,* one set of nerves that handles stress and another set of nerves that directly control most of the organs of the body.

Sense organs Specialized organs mediate several of the senses—sight, sound, smell, and taste. The *eyes* each contain a lens that focuses light upon a part of the brain called the retina (the only part of the brain directly exposed to the outside environment); the retina sends signals induced by light to the interior of the brain along the optic nerves. Each *ear* consists of an outer (visible) ear that gathers sound, a middle ear with an ingenious arrangement for transmitting sound, and an inner ear that uses tiny hairs in a liquid to detect sound waves and to transmit them to the auditory nerve.

The Hormonal System

Hormones are chemicals produced in the body that control various body processes. The important chemicals used to regulate activity of the nervous system (such as dopamine and serotonin) and various other chemical messengers are not considered hormones, however. See the chart on p 602 for the main hormones and their purposes and the chart on p 308 for neurotransmitters.

Glands Many hormones are produced by organs called *glands.* Some hormones are produced by organs that have other purposes as well and are not considered glands. For example, the stomach, the heart, and the small intestine all produce important hormones. For the most part glands come in two varieties—those that release their hormones into the blood and those that release hormones through tubes called ducts. Those that release hormones into the bloodstream are called *endocrine glands,* while those that have ducts for hormone release are called *exocrine glands.* Some glands, such as the pancreas, have both endocrine and exocrine functions. The exocrine glands are all part of the digestive system, and, with the exception of the pancreas, are included there.

Major endocrine glands

- **Pineal** Responds to light and helps regulate reproduction. Located in the forehead.
- **Pituitary** Under control by the brain, this "master gland" produces hormones that control many other glands and also produces growth hormone. Located in the head, below the center of the brain.
- **Thyroid** Regulates metabolism, growth, and calcium uptake by bones. Located in the neck or just below it.
- **Parathyroids** Regulate the release of stored calcium from bones. Located on the thyroid gland.

- **Adrenals**   Help regulate blood pressure, blood sugar, and the sex drive and also partially control metabolism. Located in the abdomen.
- **Pancreas**   Controls blood sugar. The pancreas, located in the abdomen, is also a part of the digestive system, acting as an exocrine gland that releases chemicals that break down fats, carbohydrates, and proteins in the small intestine.
- **Ovaries**   Produce hormones that regulate pregnancy, induce female secondary sexual characteristics, and also help control calcium uptake into bones. Located in the groin in women.
- **Testes**   Produce sperm and secondary sexual characteristics in males. Located in a sack suspended below the penis in men.

The Circulatory System

Blood is mainly the messenger that carries chemicals throughout the body, although its white cells are essentially part of the immune system and are treated under that heading. If blood flow is cut off from any organ, that organ cannot obtain oxygen, it has no nutrients, and it cannot get rid of wastes. After a short time, the cells of the organ die.

Blood   This material is a complex substance that contains a number of different kinds of cells and extracellular substances. It can be described as the body's only liquid organ. The red color of blood comes from *erythrocytes,* commonly known as *red blood cells.* Unlike true cells, erythrocytes lack nuclei and internal structure. They are produced by true cells in the bone marrow (called *stem cells*) to carry oxygen needed by cells for metabolism and to remove carbon dioxide, which is produced when cells metabolize. Various *white blood cells* are also made by stem cells (*see* "The Immune System," below). Another component of blood made by stem cells are the *platelets,* which are even less like cells than erythrocytes. The platelets' function is to keep blood from flowing out of the body when there is a break in the circulatory system; in other words, they cause clotting. About half of blood is an extracellular mix of water and chemicals that is called either *plasma* or, when separated from proteins that, with the platelets, are involved in clotting, *serum.*

Blood vessels   Blood is carried throughout the body in a closed system of tubes known collectively as blood vessels. Vessels carrying blood away from the heart are called *arteries.* Arteries have strong, four-layered walls to maintain blood under pressure. Arteries connect to very tiny tubes with quite thin walls called *capillaries.* The walls are so thin that oxygen and nutrients pass through them to reach the cells, while carbon dioxide and wastes from the cells pass through the capillary walls into the blood. The waste-carrying blood then passes into vessels that lead back to the heart, the *veins.* Most of the blood pressure has been lost by this point, so the veins do not need the strong walls of the arteries. Instead, the veins need and have valves that make sure the blood does not travel in the wrong direction.

Heart   The heart is primarily a pump that pushes the blood through the blood vessels. It consists of four chambers. Blood from the body enters the chamber known as the right *atrium,* and is pumped through a valve to a larger chamber below the atrium called the right *ventricle*, which pumps the blood into an artery leading to the lungs. After picking up oxygen and leaving carbon dioxide behind, the blood returns to the heart, entering the left atrium. The blood is pumped through a valve to the left ventricle, which is the largest chamber (and therefore the most powerful pump). The left ventricle sends the blood into the arteries that lead to the body.

The heart is also an endocrine gland, secreting a hormone that helps regulate blood pressure.

Spleen   This organ is a cleaner and storehouse for blood. It especially removes damaged red blood cells or platelets. It also stores excess blood and red blood cells until they are needed. The spleen may have a role in the immune system. A person can live without a spleen.

Kidneys   The kidneys, along with the *bladder* and associated tubes, are often considered the *urinary* system. Kidneys are technically part of the circulatory system in the sense that they remove chemical wastes from blood. They act as an endocrine gland by secreting hormones that aid in regulating blood pressure. They also regulate the composition of blood, keeping it from becoming too acidic or alkaline. The wastes removed by the kidneys are dissolved in water as *urine,* which is stored in the bladder before passing through the *urethra* to leave the body.

The Digestive System

The digestive system consists largely of a pathway for food from the mouth to the anus with several ducted or exocrine glands that empty into it (the pancreas, one of these, is treated as part of the hormonal system).

Teeth   Thirty-two permanent teeth (if none have been lost) in an adult are used to chop food into small bits.

Salivary glands   These glands release saliva, the first of many *enzymes* (proteins that are chemically active) that are used to break down large molecules, such as carbohydrates, proteins, and fats, into smaller molecules that the body can then reassemble to meet its needs. Saliva breaks down some starches into sugars, as you can tell by seeing how much sweeter a cracker becomes if you chew it and then keep it in your mouth for a short while.

Tongue   While an important organ of speech in humans, the tongue is basically the part of the digestive system that moves food around and pushes it down the throat.

Esophagus   This is a tube through which food moves on its way to the stomach. Its opening to the stomach has a valve called the esophageal sphincter at its base to prevent food from traveling back up again.

Stomach   This organ produces enzymes (and therefore acts as a gland) and hydrochloric acid. These are mixed with the food by churning motions of the stomach, which also tend to further break the food into smaller particles, even as the stomach enzymes and acid are chemically changing the food. From this point forward, one can no longer call this soup of nutrients *food.*

Liver   The main chemical factory of the body and, after the skin, the largest organ in the body is the liver. As part of the digestive system, it acts as a ducted or exocrine gland that produces *bile,* a substance that helps reduce the acidity of the nutrient mixture and also helps break down fats. The liver is also part of the circulatory system, since it cleans poisons out of the blood and regulates blood's composition in various other ways. In many cases the liver scavenges unwanted chemicals from the blood, takes them apart, and reassembles the parts into needed chemicals.

Gall bladder   This organ simply stores bile from the liver until the body consumes food; it then releases bile into the small intestine.

Small intestine   Like the stomach, the 21-foot-long small intestine produces enzymes that further break down the nutrients that pass through it. The upper portion of the small intestine is also called the *duodenum*. As nutrients break down into small enough molecules, they are able to pass into the blood through projections in the wall of the small intestine.

Large intestine   With most of the nutrients gone, the remains of the food pass into the five-foot-long large intestine as a kind of soup. Water is extracted from the soup through the walls of the large intestine. Most of the large intestine is the section called the *colon,* which is between the opening of the small intestine and the rectum.

Rectum   A short tube collects the partially dehydrated waste in preparation for evacuation, which is through a valve called the *anus*.

The Respiratory System

The main purpose of the respiratory system is to get oxygen to the blood and to remove carbon dioxide. Along the way, the air is sampled for chemicals (smelled), partly cleaned, and frequently used to make sounds.

Nose   In addition to being an organ of smell, the nose is the place best designed to admit air into the body, for it can warm and moisten it, and hairs in the nose can filter out dust. Often there is a need for more air than can pass through the nose, however, and the mouth is used as a supplemental way to take in air. From either the nose or the mouth, air then passes through the throat (also called the *pharynx*). The *sinuses* are air-filled cavities in the skull that are connected to the nose.

Trachea   After passing through the throat, air goes into a tube called the trachea. A flap called the *epiglottis* closes the top of the trachea when food or water is being swallowed and opens to permit air to enter the trachea. The trachea branches into two tubes called *bronchi* (singular *bronchus*) that actually carry the air into the lungs.

Larynx   Near the top of the trachea is the larynx, or voice box. The main feature of the larynx is a pair of membranes that stretch across the air passageway. As air is exhaled, these membranes can be tightened across the passage to produce sound.

Lungs   The principal organs of respiration are the lungs, two large spongy masses located in the chest which are protected by the ribs. Air enters a lung through a bronchus. The bronchus proceeds to divide into smaller *bronchial tubes,* which continue to divide until they become very fine tubes called *bronchioles.* Each bronchiole ends in a cluster of tiny round bodies called an *air sac.* As small as air sacs are, each of the round bodies contains even smaller cavities called *alveoli.* It is in the thin-walled alveoli that the exchange of oxygen to and carbon dioxide from the blood actually takes place. The lungs contain about 300 million alveoli, and, although each alveolus is tiny, the total surface area they present is about 40 times the surface area of the skin.

Diaphragm   The reason that air moves in and out of the body is that the volume of the lungs is continually being changed. The principal agent of change is the diaphragm, a muscle stretched across the abdomen just below the lungs. When the diaphragm is pulled down, the volume of the chest cavity is increased, causing air to enter the lungs. Similarly, when the diaphragm is pulled up, it reduces the volume of the chest cavity and expels air. This process is aided by the muscles of the rib cage, which also expand and contract the size of the chest cavity.

The Immune System

The immune system was not recognized as a separate system until recently. Although evidence of immune protection was known in ancient times, the first inkling of how immunity is caused came in 1884, when macrophages were first observed. Since then, many different components of the system have been found. Much still remains to be learned about this system, however.

Skin   Although a part of the immune system, skin is often viewed as simply a barrier between the body and the outside world. The largest organ in the body, the skin is far more complex. Its immune functions include not only the barrier against invaders, but also production of oil and sweat, both of which kill or retard many bacteria and fungi. At the same time, the skin harbors millions of helpful bacteria that resist invasion by other bacteria. The skin even has a role in the development of some lymphocytes (white blood cells—see below).

Skin also helps regulate body temperature, helps produce cholesterol (a necessary body chemical, even though we do not want to have too much of it in our blood), and is the location of sensors for heat, cold, and pressure.

Thymus   The thymus is a medium-sized organ in the upper chest that looks as if it could be an endocrine gland (and was often identified as one in the past). It becomes smaller as a person ages. In some as-yet-unknown way, the thymus "trains" certain lymphocytes to be a part of the immune system. If the thymus is removed from a very young animal, it does not develop the immune response that causes transplant rejection, for example.

Lymphatic system   When blood passes through the capillaries, it loses some of its plasma, which becomes part of a liquid that is between the cells. This liquid is known as *lymph*. Lymph needs to be returned to the circulatory system to keep the blood volume fairly constant, so a system of tubes called the lymphatic system drains the lymph back into the blood. Along the way, lymph passes through masses of spongy tissue called *lymph nodes* that filter out any debris, including bacteria, from the lymph. Lymph nodes are made from *lymphoid tissue,* but they are not the only organs where lymphoid tissue is found; it is found everywhere that bacteria or other germs can easily invade the body, specifically in the linings of the parts of the body that are exposed to the outside, such as the respiratory system and parts of the digestive system. Much of the action of the immune system takes place in lymphoid tissue.

Lymphocytes   Although lymphocytes are known as *white blood cells,* they are found in the lymph as well as in the blood. Draining all the lymph from an animal's body will remove all the lymphocytes, suppressing immune reactions. Like red blood cells, lymphocytes are produced in the marrow of the bone, a very well-protected place, suggesting their importance to the body. Scientists have found and continue to find many distinct types of lymphocytes, but there are two main varieties (*see also* "Allergies and Asthma," p 431).

The *T lymphocytes* are those that must mature in the thymus before they can be involved in the immune response. The "T" is for *thymus*. They are the principal cells involved in graft rejection, but they also have a role in fighting bacteria and other invaders. The loss of one type of T cell is a major symptom of AIDS, although AIDS seems to affect the immune system in many other ways as well.

The *B lymphocytes* mature directly in the bone, but the "B" does not stand for *bone*. In birds, B lymphocytes mature in an organ that humans do not have, the bursa of Fabricius, and the "B" stands for *bursa*. B cells react to invaders by releasing chemicals called *antibodies*. An antibody is a chemical that is specific to a particular protein, sugar, nucleic acid, or fat, but the strongest reaction is with proteins. If, for example, a measles virus is in the blood or lymph, a B lymphocyte will release an antibody that attaches to a protein on the surface of the virus. One kind of T cell then stimulates the production of many B cells that release the same antibody. The next measles virus that comes along is met with great amounts of the antibody, causing immunity to measles.

Phagocytes   There are many other cells produced as part of the immune system by the bone marrow that were formerly grouped under the general heading "white blood cell," including *neutrophils, mast cells,* and *macrophages*. When an antibody binds to a protein, it attracts a macrophage, which proceeds to "eat" the protein and anything attached to it, such as a cell, thus removing the whole complex. The ability to ingest cells indicates that macrophages are *phagocytes,* or "eaters of cells." The macrophage, after eating a cell, pushes the original protein that triggered the antibody to the macrophage's surface, where the protein projects from the macrophage cell membrane and causes more B lymphocytes to make antibodies against it. Neutrophils are smaller phagocytes than macrophages, or "big eaters." Mast cells collect near a source of infection and release the chemical histamine, which causes phagocytes to gather and quell the infection.

The Reproductive System

The male and female reproductive systems differ in fundamental ways.

Male reproductive system   Sperm are formed in the two *testes* that hang below the groin; they hang so because human body temperature is too high for proper sperm formation. Sperm are stored in the *epididymis,* just above the testes. During sex, the sperm move through tubes and are mixed with secretions from the *prostate* and *Cowper's gland,* both ducted glands. The result is called *semen*. Semen exits the body through a tube in the *penis* called the *urethra,* which is otherwise used for the excretion of urine.

Female reproductive system   Corresponding to the testes in males, the *ovaries* produce eggs (also known as *ova*). Unlike sperm, eggs can be produced at human body temperature, so the ovaries are located inside the pelvis. Eggs pass through the *Fallopian tubes* to the *uterus,* or *womb,* which is sealed at the other end by the *cervix*. On the other side of the cervix is a muscular tube called the *vagina,* or *birth canal*.

Pregnancy and birth   Female physiology changes considerably during pregnancy, although the organs remain the same with one exception. Sperm that have been implanted in the vagina swim to the uterus, where they fertilize an egg. The egg gradually develops into an *embryo* attached to the new organ, which consists of the *placenta* and *cord*. The placenta has many functions, including the production of hormones, so it is an endocrine gland. It is formed from tissue both from the embryo and from the uterus. When the baby is fully formed, the cervix opens and the baby passes through the vagina, still attached to its mother by the cord, which is cut at the navel. The placenta also passes through the vagina and is discarded.

APPENDIX B

ELEMENTS OF THE HUMAN BODY

The normal human body contains almost all of the elements in small amounts, although not all are used by the body. Some elements found in tiny quantities in the body are poisonous, such as lead.

The elements that the body uses are necessary for health. For the body to grow it needs the large amounts of the elements found in the major nutrients—*proteins, carbohydrates, fats,* and *water*—as well as smaller amounts of other elements, known as *minerals* (*see* "Minerals UPDATE," p 168). When very small amounts are needed, the minerals are called *trace elements.* (Vitamins, the remaining nutrient, are needed compounds that the body cannot make itself in sufficient quantity; they are not elements. *See* "Vitamin UPDATE," p 160.)

In the following table, the amount of each element is given as the weight in pounds of that element in a 150-pound human.

Element	Weight	Use by the body
Oxygen	97.5	Oxygen is part of all the major nutrients, which make up the tissues of the body, but it is also vital to the production of energy in the form of elemental oxygen that is obtained from air.
Carbon	27.0	Carbon is considered the essential element for life—most compounds based on carbon are called *organic,* meaning "from life." Carbon is an essential part of proteins, carbohydrates, and fats, the building blocks of human cells.
Hydrogen	15.0	Like oxygen, hydrogen is a part of each of the major nutrients, and thus a building block of every cell. Unlike oxygen, hydrogen has no part in respiration.
Nitrogen	4.5	Nitrogen is an essential part of proteins, DNA, and RNA, the compounds that are most active in controlling the cells; most of the body's functions depend upon nitrogen compounds at one stage or another.
Calcium	3.0	While the bulk of calcium is locked into the hard compounds that form the nonliving parts of bone, another role for calcium is even more important. Calcium is one of the principal messengers between cells, telling them when to act and when to stay quiet.
Phosphorus	1.8	Phosphorus is also an important element in bone building, but, like calcium, it has another role. It is essential in producing energy in a cell.

Element	Weight	Use by the body
Potassium	0.3	Potassium, along with sodium, regulates the contraction of muscle cells (and some other cell functions). In general, potassium is involved with muscle contractions and the general maintenance of the pressure a cell exerts on its covering membrane.
Sulfur	0.3	Sulfur, like all of the elements above it in this list, is essential to almost all forms of life. It is an important constituent of proteins.
Chlorine	0.3	Chlorine, in the form of chloride ions, is used to transport messages from the body to cells and helps regulate electrical activity.
Sodium	0.165	Although sodium is not required by all living creatures, it is required by vertebrates, including humans. One of the principal reasons is that it is used (along with potassium) to control fluid pressure in cells.
Magnesium	0.06	Magnesium is required by both plants (it is in chlorophyll) and animals. In humans, it works with enzymes to speed chemical reactions, it is involved in transmission of messages between the nerves, and it has a role in bone structure.
Iron	0.006	Although found in a small amount, iron in the blood's red cells is essential for carrying oxygen to the cells and waste carbon dioxide away; lack of iron causes anemia.
Cobalt	0.00024	Cobalt is part of vitamin B_{12}, found in meats and dairy products, but its exact role in the body is not well understood.
Copper	0.00023	Copper helps form red blood cells, maintain the nervous system, and regulate cholesterol levels.
Manganese	0.00020	Manganese aids in bone formation, helps regulate the nervous system, and is a part of the sex hormones.
Iodine	0.00006	Iodine is part of the thyroid hormone that controls the rate at which food is burned for energy.
Zinc	trace	Zinc is needed for some enzymes, for proper sex development, in healing wounds, for the sense of taste, and for a normal sperm count.
Boron	trace	Low levels of boron are required by plants, and hence the element appears in the human body, but its role, if any, is not known.
Aluminum	trace	The role of aluminum in the body is not clear, but it is believed that too much aluminum may have a role in Alzheimer's disease or other neurological disorders.
Vanadium	trace	The role, if any, of vanadium in the body is poorly understood.
Molybdenum	trace	Various enzymes require molybdenum.
Silicon	trace	Since silicon is among the most abundant elements on the earth, it is not surprising to find it in the body, but it is not clear that it is necessary to any essential function.
Fluorine	trace	This element strengthens the teeth and bones.
Chromium	trace	Chromium is used in the metabolism of sugar and the regulation of fats.
Selenium	trace	It is believed that selenium in small amounts reduces cell damage and promotes growth.

APPENDIX C

HUMAN HORMONES

Hormones are chemicals made in the body that regulate body functions or achieve specific tasks. Some are fairly familiar, such as insulin and estrogen. Others, though less familiar, are easily recognized from their names, such as growth hormone, which regulates growth. Increasingly, hormones are available either as products of genetic engineering (human insulin and human growth hormone, for example) or as synthetics (the notorious *steroids* used for body building are synthetic testosterone and close analogs). Such manufactured hormones offer both the promise of relief from hormone-deficiency diseases and the possibility of hormone abuse.

Hormone	*Associated gland(s)*	*Function*
Adrenalin (epinephrine)	Adrenal medulla	Increases blood sugar, pulse, and blood pressure
Adrenocorticotropic hormone (ACTH)	Anterior pituitary	Stimulates adrenal cortex
Aldosterone	Adrenal cortex	Controls reabsorption of sodium and potassium by the kidneys
Calcitonin (thyrocalcitonin)	Thyroid gland	Lowers level of calcium in blood by inhibiting calcium release from bones
Cholecystokin (CCK)	Glands in the small intestine	Stimulates pancreatic secretions, contraction of the gall bladder, and intestinal motility
Chorionic gonadotropin	Placenta	Stimulates the ovaries to continue producing estrogens and progesterone during the early stages of pregnancy; hormone detected in a pregnancy test
Corticotropin releasing factor (CRF)	Hypothalamus	Causes the adrenals to produce hormones
Cortisol and related hormones	Adrenal cortex	Affects metabolism of proteins, carbohydrates, and lipids
Estrogens	Ovaries and placenta	Stimulate development of secondary sexual characteristics in females; help regulate the ovaries and uterus during the menstrual cycle and pregnancy
Follicle-stimulating hormone (FSH)	Anterior pituitary	Stimulates follicle development in females and sperm production in males

Hormone	Associated gland(s)	Function
Gastrin	Glands in the stomach	Stimulates the secretion of gastric juice
Glucagon	Pancreas (Islet cells)	Increases blood sugar level by stimulating the breakdown of glycogen
Growth hormone (somatropin or somatrophic hormone or STP)	Anterior pituitary	Stimulates bone and muscle growth
Insulin	Pancreas (Islet cells)	Lowers blood sugar level and increases the storage of glycogen
Luteinizing hormone (LH)	Anterior pituitary	Stimulates ovulation and formation of corpus luteum in females and testosterone production in males
Nerve Growth Factor (NGF, or p 75)	Brain	Needed for growth of brain cells
Norepinephrine	Adrenal medulla	Increases metabolic rate and constricts blood vessels
Oxytocin	Produced in hypothalamus, stored in posterior pituitary	Causes sex to be pleasurable; stimulates uterine contractions during childbirth and milk release; promotes bonding with children in females of some mammal species and may help regulate social interactions in human females
Parathormone (parathyroid hormone or PTH)	Parathyroid glands	Increases level of calcium in blood by increasing calcium release from bones; decreases blood phosphate
Progesterone	Ovaries and placenta	Helps regulate the uterus during the menstrual cycle and pregnancy level
Prolactin (lactogenic hormone or LTH)	Anterior pituitary	Stimulates milk production (lactation)
Secretin	Glands in the small intestine	Stimulates secretion of pancreatic digestive juices
Testosterone (androgens)	Testes	Stimulates development of male sex organs and secondary sexual characteristics; supports sperm production
Thyroid-stimulating hormone (TSH)	Anterior pituitary	Stimulates thyroid gland to produce and secrete thyroxin
Thyroxin (thyroxine)	Thyroid gland	Controls rate of metabolism and growth
Vasopressin	Produced in hypothalamus, stored in posterior pituitary	Controls reabsorption of water by the kidneys (antidiuretic); increases blood pressure; causes parental or sexual bonding in males of some mammals, and may affect social interaction in human males

(Periodical Sources and Further Reading: *New York Times* 7-20-93, p C3; *New York Times* 11-2-93, p C1)

APPENDIX D

THE NOBEL PRIZE FOR PHYSIOLOGY OR MEDICINE

Date	Name [Nationality]	Achievement
1993	Richard J. Roberts [U.K., U.S.: 1943-] Phillip A. Sharp [U.S.: 1944-]	Discovery that genes in higher organisms are not continuous; instead, they are fragmented by stretches of unrelated DNA known as introns.
1992	Edmond H. Fischer [U.S.: 1920-] Edwin G. Krebs [U.S.: 1918-]	Discovery of protein kinases and the key role they play in turning on cell switches through the process of phosphorylation.
1991	Erwin Neher [German: 1944-] Bert Sakmann [German: 1942-]	Analysis of ion channels in cells.
1990	Joseph E. Murray [U.S.: 1919-] E. Donnall Thomas [U.S.: 1920-]	First kidney transplant (Murray) and first successful bone-marrow transplant (Thomas).
1989	J. Michael Bishop [U.S.: 1936-] Harold E. Varmus [U.S.: 1939-]	Discovery of the cellular origin of cancer-causing genes found in retroviruses.
1988	Sir James W. Black [U.K.: 1924-] Gertrude B. Elion [U.S.: 1918-] George H. Hitchings [U.S.: 1905-]	Development of artificial variations on DNA that block cell replication, the basis for many new drugs.
1987	Susumu Tonegawa [U.S.: 1939-]	Discovery of the genetic principle of antibody diversity.
1986	Stanley Cohen [U.S.: 1922-] Rita Levi-Montalcini [Italian-U.S.: 1909-]	Discovery of growth factors.
1985	Michael S. Brown [U.S.: 1941-] Joseph L. Goldstein [U.S.: 1940-]	Discovery and analysis of cholesterol receptors.
1984	Niels K. Jerne [Danish: 1911-] Georges J. F. Köhler [German: 1946-] César Milstein [U.K.-Argentinian: 1927-]	Pioneering work in immunology (Jerne) and the invention of monoclonal antibodies (Köhler and Milstein).
1983	Barbara McClintock [U.S.: 1902-]	Discovery of mobile genes in chromosomes of corn.
1982	John R. Vane [U.K.: 1927-] Sune K. Bergstrom [Swedish: 1916-] Bengt I. Samuelsson [Swedish: 1934-]	Studies on formation and function of prostaglandins, hormonelike substances that combat disease.

Date	Name [Nationality]	Achievement
1981	Roger W. Sperry [U.S.: 1913-1994] David H. Hubel [U.S.: 1926-] Torsten N. Wiesel [U.S.: 1924-]	Studies on the organization and local functions of brain areas.
1980	George D. Snell [U.S.: 1903-] Baruj Benacerraf [U.S.: 1920-] Jean Dausset [French: 1916-]	Discovery of antigens useful for making the immune system accept transplanted organs.
1979	Allan MacLeod Cormack [U.S.: 1924-] Godfrey N. Hounsfield [English: 1919-]	Invention of computed axial tomography, or CAT scan.
1978	Daniel Nathans [U.S.: 1928-] Hamilton O. Smith [U.S.: 1931-] Werner Arber [Swiss: 1929-]	Use of restrictive enzymes in gene splicing to produce mutants in molecular genetics.
1977	Rosalyn S. Yalow [U.S.: 1921-] Roger C. L. Guillemin [U.S.: 1924-] Andrew V. Schally [U.S.: 1926-]	Advances in the synthesis and measurement of hormones.
1976	Baruch S. Blumberg [U.S.: 1925-] D. Carleton Gajdusek [U.S.: 1923-]	Identification of and tests for different infectious viruses.
1975	David Baltimore [U.S.: 1938-] Howard M. Temin [U.S.: 1934-] Renato Dulbecco [U.S.: 1914-]	Discovery of the interaction between tumor viruses and the genetic material of host cells.
1974	Albert Claude [U.S.: 1898-1983] George E. Palade [U.S.: 1912-] C. René de Duvé [Belgian: 1917-]	Advancement of cell biology, electron microscopy, and structural knowledge of cells.
1973	Karl von Frisch [German: 1886-1982] Konrad Lorenz [German: 1903-1989] Nikolaas Tinbergen [Dutch: 1907-1988]	Study of individual and social behavior patterns of animal species for survival and natural selection.
1972	Gerald M. Edelman [U.S.: 1929-] Rodney R. Porter [English: 1917-1985]	Determination of the chemical structure of antibodies.
1971	Earl W. Sutherland, Jr. [U.S.: 1915-1974]	Work on the action of hormones.
1970	Julius Axelrod [U.S.: 1912-] Ulf von Euler [Swedish: 1905-1983] Sir Bernard Katz [English: 1911-]	Discoveries in the chemical transmission of nerve impulses.
1969	Max Delbrück [U.S.: 1906-1981] Alfred D. Hershey [U.S.: 1908-] Salvador E. Luria [U.S.: 1912-1991]	Discoveries in the workings and reproduction of viruses in human cells.
1968	Robert Holley [U.S.: 1922-1993] Har Gobind Khorana [U.S.: 1922-] Marshall W. Nirenberg [U.S.: 1927-]	Understanding and deciphering the genetic code that determines cell function.
1967	Haldan K. Hartline [U.S.: 1903-1983] George Wald [U.S.: 1906-] Ragnar A. Granit [Swedish: 1900-]	Advanced discoveries in the physiology and chemistry of the human eye.
1966	Charles B. Huggins [U.S.: 1901-] Francis Peyton Rous [U.S.: 1879-1970]	Research on causes and treatment of cancer.
1965	François Jacob [French: 1920-] André Lwoff [French: 1902-1994] Jacques Monod [French: 1910-1976]	Studies and discoveries on the regulatory activities of human body cells.
1964	Konrad Bloch [U.S.: 1912-] Feodor Lynen [German: 1911-1979]	Work on cholesterol and fatty acid metabolism.
1963	Sir John C. Eccles [Australian: 1903-] Alan Lloyd Hodgkin [English: 1914-] Andrew F. Huxley [English: 1917-]	Study of mechanism of transmission of neural impulses along a single nerve fiber.

Date	Name [Nationality]	Achievement
1962	Francis H. C. Crick [English: 1916-] James D. Watson [U.S.: 1928-] Maurice Wilkins [English: 1916-]	Determination of the molecular structure of DNA.
1961	Georg von Békésy [U.S.: 1899-1972]	Study of auditory mechanisms.
1960	Sir Macfarlane Burnet [Australian: 1899-1985] Peter Brian Medawar [English: 1915-]	Study of immunity reactions to tissue transplants.
1959	Severo Ochoa [U.S.: 1905-1993] Arthur Kornberg [U.S.: 1918-]	Artificial production of nucleic acids with enzymes.
1958	George Wells Beadle [U.S.: 1903-1989] Edward Lawrie Tatum [U.S.: 1909-1975] Joshua Lederberg [U.S.: 1925-]	Beadle and Tatum for genetic regulation of body chemistry, Lederberg for genetic recombination.
1957	Daniel Bovet [Italian: 1907-]	Synthesis of curare.
1956	Werner Forssmann [German: 1904-1979] Dickinson Richards [U.S.: 1895-1973] André F. Cournand [U.S.: 1895-1988]	Use of catheter for study of the interior of the heart and circulatory system.
1955	Hugo Theorell [Swedish: 1903-1982]	Study of oxidation enzymes.
1954	John F. Enders [U.S.: 1897-1985] Thomas H. Weller [U.S.: 1915-] Frederick C. Robbins [U.S.: 1916-]	Discovery of a method for cultivating poliomyelitis virus in tissue culture.
1953	Fritz A. Lipmann [U.S.: 1899-1986] Hans Adolph Krebs [English: 1900-1981]	Discovery by Lipmann of coenzyme A and by Krebs of citric acid cycle.
1952	Selman A. Waksman [U.S.: 1888-1973]	Discovery of streptomycin.
1951	Max Theiler [S. Africa: 1899-1972]	Development of 17-D yellow fever vaccine.
1950	Philip S. Hench [U.S.: 1896-1965] Edward C. Kendall [U.S.: 1886-1972] Tadeusz Reichstein [Swiss: 1897-]	Discovery of cortisone and other hormones of the adrenal cortex and their functions.
1949	Walter Rudolf Hess [Swiss: 1881-1973] Antonio Egas Moniz [Portuguese: 1874-1955]	Hess for studies of middle brain function, Moniz for prefrontal lobotomy.
1948	Paul Müller [Swiss: 1899-1965]	Discovery of effect of DDT on insects.
1947	Carl F. Cori [U.S.: 1896-1984] Gerty T. Cori [U.S.: 1896-1957] Bernardo A. Houssay [Argentinian: 1887-1971]	Coris for discovery of catalytic metabolism of starch, Houssay for pituitary study.
1946	Hermann J. Muller [U.S.: 1890-1967]	Discovery of X-ray mutation of genes.
1945	Sir Alexander Fleming [English: 1881-1955] Sir Howard W. Florey [English: 1898-1968] Ernst Boris Chain [English: 1906-1979]	Discovery of penicillin and research into its value as a weapon against infectious disease.
1944	Joseph Erlanger [U.S.: 1874-1965] Herbert Spencer Gasser [U.S.: 1888-1963]	Work on different functions of a single nerve fiber.
1943	Henrik Dam [Danish: 1895-1976] Edward A. Doisy [U.S.: 1893-1986]	Dam for discovery and Doisy for synthesis of vitamin K.
1942	No award	

Date	Name [Nationality]	Achievement
1941	No award	
1940	No award	
1939	Gerhard Domagk [German: 1895-1964]	Discovery of first sulfa drug, prontosil (declined award).
1938	Corneille Heymans [Belgian: 1892-1968]	Discoveries in respiratory regulation.
1937	Albert Szent-Györgyi [Hungarian: 1893-1986]	Study of biological combustion.
1936	Sir Henry Dale [English: 1875-1968] Otto Loewi [Austria: 1873-1961]	Work on chemical transmission of nerve impulses.
1935	Hans Spemann [German: 1869-1941]	Discovery of the "organizer effect" in embryonic development.
1934	George R. Minot [U.S.: 1885-1950] William P. Murphy [U.S.: 1892-] George H. Whipple [U.S.: 1878-1976]	Discovery and development of liver treatment for anemia.
1933	Thomas H. Morgan [U.S.: 1866-1945]	Discovery of chromosomal heredity.
1932	Sir Charles Sherrington [English: 1857-1952] Edgar D. Adrian [U.S.: 1889-1977]	Multiple discoveries in the function of neurons.
1931	Otto H. Warburg [German: 1883-1970]	Discovery of respiratory enzymes.
1930	Karl Landsteiner [U.S.: 1868-1943]	Definition of four human blood groups.
1929	Christiaan Eijkman [Dutch: 1858-1930] Sir Frederick G. Hopkins [English: 1861-1947]	Eijkman for antineuritic vitamins, Hopkins for growth vitamins.
1928	Charles Nicolle [French: 1866-1936]	Research on typhus.
1927	Julius Wagner von Jauregg [Austria: 1857-1940]	Fever treatment, with malaria inoculation, of some paralyses.
1926	Johannes Fibiger [Danish: 1867-1928]	Discovery of Spiroptera carcinoma.
1925	No award	
1924	Willem Einthoven [Dutch: 1860-1927]	Invention of electrocardiograph.
1923	Sir Frederick Banting [Canadian: 1891-1941] John J. R. MacLeod [English: 1876-1935]	Discovery of insulin.
1922	Archibald V. Hill [English: 1886-1977] Otto Meyerhof [German: 1884-1951]	Hill for discovery of muscle heat production and Meyerhof for oxygen-lactic acid metabolism.
1921	No award	
1920	Shack August Krogh [Danish: 1874-1949]	Discovery of motor mechanism of blood capillaries.
1919	Jules Bordet [Belgian: 1870-1961]	Studies in immunology.
1918	No award	
1917	No award	
1916	No award	
1915	No award	
1914	Robert Bárány [Austrian: 1876-1936]	Studies of inner ear function and pathology.

Date	Name [Nationality]	Achievement
1913	Charles Robert Richet [French: 1850-1935]	Work on anaphylaxis allergy.
1912	Alexis Carrel [French: 1873-1944]	Vascular grafting of blood vessels and organs.
1911	Allvar Gullstrand [Swedish: 1862-1930]	Work on dioptrics, or refraction of light in the eye.
1910	Albrecht Kossel [German: 1853-1927]	Study of cell chemistry.
1909	Emil Theodor Kocher [Swiss: 1841-1917]	Work on the thyroid gland.
1908	Paul Ehrlich [German: 1854-1915] Elie Metchnikoff [Russian: 1845-1916]	Pioneering research into the mechanics of immunology.
1907	Charles L. A. Laveran [French: 1845-1922]	Discovery of the role of protozoa in disease generation.
1906	Camillo Golgi [Italian: 1843-1926] Santiago Ramón y Cajal [Spanish: 1852-1934]	Study of structure of nervous system and nerve tissue.
1905	Robert Koch [German: 1843-1910]	Tuberculosis research.
1904	Ivan P. Pavlov [Russian: 1849-1936]	Study of physiology of digestion.
1903	Niels Ryberg Finsen [Danish: 1860-1904]	Light ray treatment of skin disease.
1902	Sir Ronald Ross [English: 1857-1932]	Work on malaria infections.
1901	Emil von Behring [German: 1854-1917]	Discovery of diphtheria antitoxin.

APPENDIX E

ALBERT LASKER MEDICAL AWARDS

The Lasker Awards, presented by the Albert and Mary Lasker Foundation since 1944, have long been considered second only to a Nobel Prize in Medicine or Physiology and often a precursor to the Nobel—a total of 51 Lasker winners have gone on to win Nobels. Although the actual amount of each award is currently only $25,000 (and was less in the past), the prestige is enormous. The awards have been granted every year since 1944 except for 1960, 1990, and 1992.

Mary W. Lasker died on February 21, 1994 at the age of 93.

1993
Basic research

Gunter Blobel   Rockefeller University, New York City, New York

For techniques explaining how some proteins travel across cell membranes into the cell's cytoplasm.

Clinical medical research

Donald Metcalf   Walter and Eliza Hall Institute of Medical Research, Melbourne, Australia

Discovery of how to use colony-stimulating factors to increase production of leukocytes (white blood cells) in patients with cancer or blood diseases.

Public service

Paul Rogers   Former U.S. Representative (Democrat, Florida)

Championship of health legislation over a 24-year career in House of Representatives.

Nancy Wexler   Columbia University College of Physicians and Surgeons, New York City, New York

Direction of research into Huntington's disease, working with the Hereditary Disease Foundation.

1992
No awards

1991
Basic research

Edward B. Lewis   California Institute of Technology, Pasadena

Christiane Nüsslein-Volhard   Max-Plank Institute for Developmental Biology

For mapping out steps in the embryonic development of the fruit fly (*Drosophila spp.*).

Clinical medical research

Yuet Wai Kan   University of California in San Francisco

> Detection of the gene defect that causes thalassemia, a severe congenital anemia, and development of prenatal diagnosis of the defect.

Public service

Thomas P. O'Neill   Former Speaker of U.S. House of Representatives (Democrat, Massachusetts)

> Efforts to increase government funding of medical research, especially research in cancer.

Robin Chandler Duke   Population Crisis Committee

> Promotion of international steps to aid family planning.

1990
No awards

(Periodical Sources and Further Reading: *New York Times* 9-28-91, p 26; *New York Times* 10-1-93, p A24; *New York Times* 2-23-94, p A17)

APPENDIX F

OBITUARIES: 1990-1993

Ackerman, Lauren Vedder   [March 12, 1905-July 27, 1993] U.S. pathologist who wrote important textbooks that influenced a change of focus from anatomical to surgical pathology, including *Cancer: Diagnosis, Treatment and Prognosis* in 1947 with Juan del Regato and *Surgical Pathology* in 1953.

Anderson, Albert D.   [January 11, 1928-February 8, 1993] U.S. physician who, despite his loss of motor control due to a rare spinal-cord disease called syringomyelia, was founding director of the rehabilitation medicine department at Harlem Hospital Center in New York and president of the New York Society of Physical Medicine and Rehabilitation.

Ariel, Irving M.   [1911-October 16, 1993] U.S. surgeon and radiation specialist who used new techniques with isotopes to treat thyroid disease and to diagnose pulmonary embolisms; he was founding president of the Society of Nuclear Medicine.

Bacon, Selden Daskam   [September 10, 1908-December 6, 1992] U.S. sociologist who was director of Rutgers University's Center of Alcohol Studies, and worked with the center to open the Yale Plan Clinics, the first public clinics for alcoholics; these clinics were inspired by research he performed that indicated that most of the people in jails were there for alcohol abuse.

Bailey, Charles Philamore   [September 8, 1910-August 18, 1993] U.S. heart surgeon and lawyer whose daring approach to heart surgery was often controversial, but successful. He developed several new techniques and instruments, and demonstrated that the heart could withstand more manipulations than were previously thought possible.

Bergner, Marilyn Neufeld   [1933-December 12, 1992] U.S. researcher and professor who, while at the University of Washington School of Public Health from 1972 to 1986, helped develop the Sickness Impact Profile, a widely used system for evaluating the medical condition of patients by monitoring their level of functioning and progress during the course of an illness through questionnaires completed periodically by those patients.

Bland, Edward Franklin   [January 24, 1901-September 20, 1992] U.S. cardiologist who was known for his early research on rheumatic fever; he and T. Duckett Jones conducted ten- and 20-year follow-up studies of 1,000 patients from 1921 to 1931.

Blankenhorn, David Henry   [November 16, 1924-May 9, 1993] U.S. cardiologist and University of Southern California professor whose research showed that a material called plaque, visible through computer processing of X-ray pictures, contributes to the hardening of the arteries and causes most heart attacks; and that a cholesterol-lowering drug, lovastatin, along with a low-fat diet, can reverse heart disease.

Bodansky, Barbara Biber [1904-September 14, 1993] U.S. psychologist who, while at the Bank Street College in New York City, was driven by her belief in the importance of the emotional development of children to help establish teacher workshops in this area, as well as to devise the basic principles for federally funded day care and Head Start programs.

Bodian, David [May 15, 1910-September 18, 1992] U.S. medical scientist who in the 1940s and 1950s with Howard Howe and Isabel Morgan at the Johns Hopkins School of Public Health discovered that the polio virus was actually three distinct viruses, and that antibodies to polio were carried in the bloodstream; the team also worked to develop early vaccines against the disease.

Bordley, John Earle [November 8, 1902-July 12, 1993] U.S. otolaryngologist and Johns Hopkins researcher who, with William G. Hardy, devised a program to match speech pathology and audiology, a branch of science dealing with hearing defects, with medical care and screening. He also co-founded the Hearing and Speech Clinic at Johns Hopkins, the first clinic for audiology and speech pathology to be affiliated with a medical center.

Bowers, John Zimmerman [August 27, 1913-October 18, 1993] U.S. medical educator who from 1965 to 1980 was president of the Josiah Macy, Jr. Foundation, which instituted programs to help bring more minorities and women into the field of medicine.

Boyle, Joseph Francis [1924-July 16, 1992] U.S. internist who was president of the American Medical Association in 1984-1985, and who spoke out on medical issues such as abortion, testifying in 1981 against a bill attempting to overturn the 1973 *Roe v. Wade* Supreme Court decision that legalized abortion.

Bumpus, Francis Merlin [December 6, 1922-August 8, 1993] U.S. researcher who worked with Irvine H. Page to identify and isolate crucial compounds in the body that affect blood pressure, thus increasing the understanding of hypertension and providing evidence that it is not caused by a single agent. Bumpus and Page also led a team that synthesized angiotensin, a substance that causes rising blood pressure. Bumpus continued the research, discovering the function of the renin-angiotensin system in affecting blood pressure.

Burkitt, Denis Parsons [February 28, 1911-March 23, 1993] Missionary surgeon, born in Northern Ireland, who in the late 1950s and early 1960s discovered Burkitt's lymphoma, a form of cancer common in East African children, as well as a drug to treat the disease; he was one of the first specialists to suggest a link between viruses and cancer. His thesis that a high fiber diet could help prevent colon cancer changed the eating habits of millions of people.

Campbell, Charlotte Catherine [December 4, 1914-October 8, 1993] U.S. mycologist who wrote or co-wrote over 100 treatises, particularly on the causes and cures of histoplasmosis, or lung diseases caused by fungi; she was given the highest award of the International Society for Human and Animal Mycology in 1979.

Charny, Charles W. [November 8, 1902-November 10, 1992] U.S. urologist, born in Ostropol, Ukraine, who provided insight into the existence of male infertility by being the first in the United States to perform a testicle biopsy to diagnose the condition and show that varicose veins of the scrotum were a source of semen problems.

Cogan, David Glendenning [February 14, 1908-September 9, 1993] U.S. ophthalmologist and professor emeritus at Harvard University who in 1949, with Dr. Forrest Martin, discovered cataracts caused by radiation in the survivors of the atomic bomb explosions at Hiroshima and Nagasaki. He is also credited for founding neuro-ophthalmology, a subspecialty of ophthalmology.

Cohen, Philip Pacy [September 26, 1908-October 25, 1993] U.S. researcher who studied the process by which the human body converts ammonia into urea for passage out of the digestive system, which led to an understanding of acidosis caused by diabetes and the body's functioning during fasting or starvation. His work in the late 1960s inspired a phylogenetic tree in which animals were classified according to how they converted nitrogen into urea after digestion.

Cohn, Zanvil Alexander [November 16, 1926-June 28, 1993] U.S. cell biologist and immunologist whose research on T cells and macrophages provided insights into white-blood-cell functions, helping investigations of leprosy, tuberculosis, and AIDS. He also used hormone-like products of the immune system to increase patients' resistance to microbial infections.

Collins, John A. [1934-September 21, 1992] U.S. medical educator who led an Army research team during the Vietnam War that discredited the traditional practice of using alkalizing solution in blood transfusions in order to balance accumulated acidity in stored blood; they discovered that the human body on its own could neutralize acid in the blood and that alkalizing solution was more harmful.

Cooney, James Patrick [March 17, 1903-July 6, 1993] U.S. Army major general and radiologist who, at the end of World War II, was medical director of a special mission to Japan to study the effects of the atomic bomb on the survivors of the Hiroshima and Nagasaki explosions. He also served as the Deputy Surgeon General of the Army in 1955 and chief surgeon of the United States forces in Europe in 1959.

Crawford, E. Stanley [1922-October 27, 1992] U.S. heart surgeon whose development of techniques for treating extensive aneurysm of the aorta included co-inventing the Baylor Rapid Autologus Transfusion System, which recycles a patient's red blood cells to cut down on the amount of transfused blood needed during chest and aneurysm surgery.

Crile, George Washington, Jr. [November 3, 1907-September 11, 1992] U.S. surgeon who led a controversial battle against surgical procedures he viewed as unnecessary, particularly radical mastectomies on breast cancer patients when lumpectomies would have been sufficient. His own work on less radical medical solutions included the development of treatments for thyroid diseases using radioactive iodines instead of surgery.

Davis, Hallowell [August 31, 1896-August 22, 1992] U.S. physician whose accomplishments included being the first to have an EEG, or electroencephalograph, of brain waves recorded (in the 1930s by his students) and his physiological studies of the inner ear and the auditory nerve's electrical responses. The latter led to his research on electrical-response audiometry to diagnose hearing impairment in the early stages of infancy. He was awarded the National Medal of Science by President Gerald Ford in 1976.

Dembo, Tamara [May 28, 1902-October 17, 1993] U.S. psychologist, born in Russia, who developed a method in Gestalt psychology that involved provoking anger in patients to demonstrate that anger depends more on situations than personality.

Donahue, Wilma Thompson [1901-August 17, 1993] One of the first clinical psychologists in the U.S., who started her career at the University of Michigan in 1935. She was known as an expert in the psychology of aging, participated in White House Conferences on Aging in 1961, 1971, and 1981, and was a member of several related policy boards for five presidents, from Harry S. Truman to Jimmy Carter.

Druss, Joseph George [1898-November 14, 1992] U.S. otolaryngologist whose work in histopathology of the ear, the study of microscopic changes in tissues caused by disease, led to his discovery of petrositis, which is an inflammation of the petrous portion of the temporal bone, the skull bone that encases and protects the inner ear.

Duane, Thomas David [October 10, 1917-June 20, 1993] U.S. ophthalmologist and two-time recipient of the Howe Medal, ophthalmology's highest award, whose achievements included the discovery of the cause of blackouts suffered by Korean War pilots, which was a reduction in the blood supply to the eye's retina. Also, he was one of the first researchers to describe valsalva hemorrhages in the eye, caused by unusual chest pressure.

Eberhart, Howard Davis [August 16, 1906-July 18, 1993] U.S. civil engineer and amputee who with Verne Inman founded the Biomechanics Laboratory, where they conducted studies on human locomotion muscle action and joint movement and foot pressure that led to principles used to develop artificial lower limbs and braces.

Echols, Harrison "Hatch" [May 1, 1933-April 11, 1993] U.S. biologist who was known for his research on viruses that infect bacteria, which demonstrated how viral DNA transports itself into and out of a bacterium's DNA; he also helped discover how complexes that include DNA manage to control a cell's activities. He was a member of the U.S. National Academy of Sciences.

English, Oliver Spurgeon [September 27, 1901-October 4, 1993] U.S. psychotherapist who was one of the first to make the connection between mental health problems, including stress, and physical ailments. He co-wrote *Psychosomatic Medicine,* the first medical text covering this area. His work furthered the development of hypnosis, family therapy, and marriage counseling.

Fineberg, Seymour Koeppel [1915-August 15, 1993] U.S. internist who was known as one of the first researchers to recognize obesity as a disease; he also evaluated the effects of drugs used to combat anorexia, drug treatments for obesity, and oral drugs for diabetics.

Gaynor, Florence Small [October 29, 1921-September 16, 1993] U.S. nurse who became the first African American woman to head a major teaching hospital when she was chosen as executive director of the Sydenham Hospital in Harlem, New York, in 1971.

Gibbs, Frederic Andrew [February 9, 1903-October 18, 1992] U.S. neurologist whose significant contributions to the treatment of epilepsy included: establishing in 1944 the oldest clinic devoted to the condition of epilepsy in the U.S., the University of Illinois Clinic for Epilepsy; being one of the first U.S. doctors to apply electroencephalographic technology, including encephalography, or X-rays of the brain; matching electroencephalograph patterns to a particular seizure or neurological disturbance; and identifying and describing nearly every EEG wave form known. This research made it easier to detect epilepsy and predict attacks.

Gillespie, David Hutton [January 22, 1940-December 19, 1993] U.S. genetic researcher who contributed to the understanding of AIDS and cancers by developing a test to analyze disease-causing genes and monitor genetic changes in blood, bone marrow, and tumor cells during treatment. In his research, he also searched for "footprints" in human and animal cancer tumors, and reported that it was possible to find genetic clues of high cancer risk in people.

Goldstein, Ira M. [March 30, 1942-December 2, 1992] U.S. rheumatologist who was an expert on inflammation. He identified patients with systemic lupus erythematosus, or SLE, a connective tissue disorder in which white blood cells lack the structure necessary for appropriate immune responses, which can lead to chronic, severe swelling affecting many systems in the human body.

Gordon, Mildred Kobrin [1920-August 24, 1993] U.S. cell biologist whose work in molecular biology provided insight on human reproduction and aided development of *in vitro* fertilization. Her work provided further knowledge of the elemental structures of human sperm and endometrium, or inner lining of the uterus, and of calcium's role in the function of the spermatocyte, a stage in the growing male sex cell.

Hardy, Harriet Louise [September 23, 1905-October 13, 1993] U.S. physician who in 1971 was the first woman to become a full professor of medicine at Harvard University. She was known for her work in occupational medicine, and particularly for the discovery of berylliosis, an often fatal disease caused by exposure to the light metal beryllium, in factory workers in Lynn and Salem, Massachusetts, in the 1940s; this led to more research and precautions regarding the use of this metal.

Harley, John H. [1916-July 25, 1993] U.S. researcher who was director of the Environmental Measurements Laboratory of the United States Department of Energy, and whose work on environmental radioactivity included the development of methods and systems that analyzed airborne materials and biological samples. These systems were used to measure occupational exposures to radiation wastes left in production plants after the Manhattan Project, which produced the first atomic bomb.

Harrington, William Fields [September 25, 1920-October 31, 1992] U.S. biologist whose research on the structure and function of collagen, a fibrous protein in connective tissue, and myosin, responsible for muscle contractions, increased knowledge about the origins of the flexing force of muscle and how chemical energy of the body is converted into the mechanical energy of muscle flexing.

Harrington, William J. [September 21, 1923-September 5, 1992] U.S. blood specialist who performed experiments on himself involving injection of the blood of a patient suffering from idiopathic thrombocytopenia purpura (ITP), a disorder in which the number of platelets in the blood becomes low enough to cause black and blue marks in the skin; as a result of his work, ITP became the first known autoimmune disease, caused in part by antibodies produced against a normal component of an individual's own platelets.

Hellerstein, Herman Kopel [June 6, 1916-August 17, 1993] U.S. cardiologist and emeritus professor at Case Western Reserve University whose research, carried out in the 1950s, used dietary controls and exercise to restore the health and postpone early retirement of heart attack patients. He also served on the International Olympic Committee's medical commission and the scientific committee of the International Federation of Sports Medicine.

Hobby, Gladys Lounsbury   [November 19, 1910-July 4, 1993] U.S. microbiologist who advocated the widespread production and use of penicillin for the treatment of infections during World War II, helped develop streptomycin and other antibiotics while working for Pfizer, and performed early research on the broad-spectrum antibiotic Terramycin, contributing to the understanding of the function of antibiotics.

Holley, Robert William   [January 28, 1922-February 11, 1993] U.S. biologist who shared the Nobel Prize for Medicine in 1968 for his work in unraveling the genetic code for ribonucleic acid, or RNA.

Holtfreter, Johannes Friedrich Karl   [January 9, 1901-November 13, 1992] U.S. zoologist, born in Richtenberg, Germany, whose groundbreaking work in the study of embryo development included his invention of the Holtfreter solution for growing embryonic cells and tissue outside the body in test tubes for research purposes.

Horn, Daniel   [May 28, 1916-October 7, 1992] U.S. psychologist who was better known for his advocacy against smoking; while assistant director of statistical research at the American Cancer Society in the 1950s, he and E. Cuyler Hammond demonstrated through studies that there was a link between cigarette smoking and lung cancer.

Horowitz, Leonard N.   [November 21, 1947-May 21, 1992] U.S. cardiologist who was a pioneer in the treatment of a potentially fatal fast-heartbeat condition called ventricular tachycardia. He had been director of several cardiological units in Philadelphia, including the Heart Institute at the Presbyterian Medical Center, and a University of Pennsylvania School of Medicine professor.

Hungerford, David A.   [May 7, 1927-November 3, 1993] U.S. researcher who, while a graduate student, worked with Dr. Peter C. Nowell to discover the Philadelphia chromosome; a shortened arm of this uninherited chromosome is linked to a blood cancer called chronic granulocytic leukemia.

Jacobson, Leon Orris   [December 16, 1911-September 20, 1992] U.S. physician who was chief doctor for the research team of the Manhattan Project to develop the first atomic bomb. He had been chosen because he was one of the first doctors to treat blood disorders with radioactive phosphorus, and during the project his team tested the first forms of radiation therapy to fight cancer.

Kean, Benjamin Harrison   [December 2, 1912-September 24, 1993] U.S. physician who with Sherwood Gorbach identified the symptoms of turista, or travelers' diarrhea, and the role of *E. coli* bacteria in causing this ailment. He also worked with Edward Goldsmith to discover a treatment for schistosomiasis, a tropical disease also known as bilharziasis, by filtering parasitic worms from the blood.

Kellner, Aaron   [September 24, 1914-December 11, 1993] U.S. medical doctor who with Lindsley F. Kimball founded the New York Blood Center, the largest blood bank and blood research institution in the U.S., established in 1964. He served as executive director and president of the Center.

Kirkpatrick, Paul   [July 21, 1894-December 27, 1992] U.S. researcher and retired Stanford University professor who with Albert Baez developed the X-ray reflection microscope, still used today in astronomy to take pictures of galaxies and in medicine to examine living cells.

Langmuir, Alexander Duncan   [September 22, 1910-November 22, 1993] U.S. public health official who in 1949 formed and was chief epidemiologist of the

Epidemic Intelligence Service, a corps of epidemiologists at what is now known as the U.S. Centers of Disease Control and Prevention; this "disease detective service" conducted investigations that discovered the bacterium that causes Legionnaire's disease and identified toxic shock syndrome, among other successes.

Lehfeldt, Hans M. [1900-June 18, 1993] U.S. gynecologist, born in Berlin, who was known for his early support of family planning. He co-founded and directed the Clinic for Birth Control and Family Planning at Berlin's Friedrich Wilhelm University in 1928 and the Family Planning Clinic at New York's Bellevue Hospital in 1958; worked with Margaret Sanger, leader of the birth control movement in the U.S.; performed research on intrauterine contraceptive devices, or IUDs; and invented a cervical cap.

Leopold, Irving H. [April 19, 1915-August 2, 1993] U.S. ophthalmologist whose patients included Presidents Lyndon Johnson and Richard Nixon and who was an expert on treatments of eye diseases, particularly those involving antibiotics and chemotherapy; he was a past chairman of the American Board of Ophthalmology and other panels, and was also vice president of the National Society to Prevent Blindness.

Lowey, Hans [1907-August 4, 1993] U.S. researcher, born in Vienna and self-taught in the area of pharmaceuticals, who developed the concept of time-release pills; his first product was salt tablets coated with cellulose, developed in the 1950s for Korean War soldiers suffering from nausea; later he created a material that bonds with the stomach wall until medicine is absorbed, enabling drug release to be longer than 12 hours.

Man, Evelyn Brower [October 7, 1904-September 3, 1992] U.S. biochemist who with John P. Peters and Herman Yannet developed the protein-bound iodine test to help identify people with abnormal thyroid functions; a low thyroid level can be treated with supplements to prevent mental retardation.

Manuelidis, Elias Emmanuel [August 15, 1918-November 11, 1993] Internationally known pathologist, born in Constantinople, who performed research on Alzheimer's disease and the polio virus, as well as on Creutzfeldt-Jacob disease, the degenerative disease of the nervous system that eventually caused his own death. He showed that people can be infected with Creutzfeldt-Jacob disease from contaminated blood or from tissue transplants.

Marble, Alexander [February 2, 1902-September 13, 1992] U.S. physician who was president emeritus of the Joslin Diabetes Center in Boston and president of the American Diabetes Association.

Mayer, Jean [February 19, 1920-January 1, 1993] U.S. nutritionist, born in Paris, France, who was Chancellor of Tufts University after serving 16 years as president. He advised three U.S. presidents, including Richard Nixon, under whom he organized the 1969 White House Conference on Food, Nutrition and Health, which established the first food stamp programs for the poor in 307 countries and expanded school lunch programs for needy children. His research on obesity shed light on how high phosphorus levels, insulin production, and the hypothalamus contribute to this condition.

McClintock, Barbara [June 16, 1902-September 2, 1992] U.S. geneticist who won many awards, including the Nobel Prize for Physiology or Medicine in 1983, for her research, including her discoveries of the crossing-over process, in which chromosomes break and recombine to create genetic changes, and of the nuclear organizer of the chromosome, which orders genetic material during cell division. Her work, performed using kernels of corn, provided insight into the patterns of inheritance.

Morris, John McLean [September 1, 1914-April 8, 1993] U.S. gynecologic researcher, born and raised in Kuling, China, who in the 1960s with Gertrude Van Wagenen developed the first "morning after" birth control pill, which used estrogen compounds to prevent a fertilized egg from being implanted in the womb; he also discovered a sexual disorder known as Morris's syndrome, in which children that produce male hormones develop nevertheless as females due to insensitivity to testosterone.

Ochoa, Severo [September 24, 1905-November 1, 1993] U.S. biochemist, born in Luarca, Spain, who shared the Nobel Prize with Arthur Kornberg in 1959 for work on synthesizing RNA by using a bacterial enzyme; this development shed light on how RNA turns DNA's genetic information into instructions for making proteins.

Oldendorf, William H. [March 27, 1925-December 14, 1992] U.S. medical researcher who developed a device for cross-sectional scanning of the brain with X rays in the early 1960s which led to the development of the CT scan in 1972. He received the Albert and Mary Lasker Award in 1975 with Godfrey Hounsfield (who won the Nobel Prize for the CT scan), for their work on magnetic resonance imaging techniques.

Paiva, Apolinario Souza [1888-October 17, 1993] Well-known Brazilian medicine man who treated thousands of patients for all kinds of illnesses using roots, herbs, and teas from a variety of Amazon rain forest plants.

Palmer, Walter Lincoln [June 29, 1896-October 28, 1993] U.S. internist who was one of the first to practice gastroenterology, performing research on ulcers that included the discovery that acid secretions, instead of gastric contractions, caused the pain of peptic ulcers.

Paul, Howard A. [1933-February 10, 1993] U.S. veterinarian who developed Robodoc, a five-foot robotic arm that used a high-speed drill and complex imaging technology to increase the accuracy of surgeons. At the time of Paul's death, Robodoc was undergoing successful FDA testing, and it was hoped that the arm could become standard equipment for many procedures, including hip and knee replacements, ligament repairs, and brain tumor removal.

Pomerantzeff, Oleg [1910-October 7, 1993] U.S. biomedical engineer and physicist who, while working at the Schepens Eye Research Institute in Boston, developed several innovative optical instruments and devices, including an indirect binocular ophthalmoscope, which improved surgery on the retina by providing a three-dimensional perspective within the eye.

Ralston, Henry James [February 10, 1906-January 2, 1993] U.S. physiologist whose research and book *Human Walking*, written and compiled with Verne Inman, led to the development of improved artificial limbs for World War II veterans and other amputees that functioned more naturally and caused fewer cardiovascular problems.

Ramsey, Elizabeth Mapelsden [February 17, 1906-July 2, 1993] U.S. embryologist who in the 1930s helped discover a 14-day-old embryo known as the Yale embryo, believed to be the youngest studied embryo at the time. This sparked a career of research on embryos that included work with Martin Donner using radioactive dyes and X rays to reveal that the human embryo and placenta have a similar circulation system.

Resnekov, Leon [March 20, 1928-August 17, 1993] U.S. cardiologist and University of Chicago professor of medicine, born in Cape Town, South Africa, who performed early research in using electrical shock to restore normal heart beat after rhythm disturbances; helped develop the use of nuclear medicine in imaging the heart; and catalogued prosthetic heart valves by their radiological contours and the sounds they produce.

Rimington, Claude   [November 17, 1902-August 8, 1993] British biochemist who, after investigating the research on the death of George III by psychiatric historians, developed the theory that the king suffered from an inherited abnormality of porphyrin metabolism referred to as variegate porphyria, in which porphyrins, pigments that are vital components of the blood's hemoglobin, build up in the body, which can cause delirium and psychotic behavior.

Roe, Daphne A.   [January 4, 1923-September 22, 1993] British-born U.S. dermatologist, nutrition expert, and professor emeritus at Cornell University who performed research that shed light on the role of carotenoids such as beta carotene (a nutrient that the human body converts to vitamin A) in protecting the immune systems of older people. She also proposed that the recommended daily allowance of riboflavin for women who exercise be doubled.

Sabin, Albert Bruce   [August 26, 1906-March 3, 1993] U.S. researcher, born in Bialystok, Poland, who was well-known as an expert on viruses and viral diseases. His most famous development was a polio vaccine containing "live" but harmless polio viruses, which is taken orally. Sabin also shed light on the nature of polio by establishing that the virus attacks the human body through the digestive system and later moves into the nerve tissue.

Salk, Lee   [December 27, 1926-May 2, 1992] Well-known U.S. child psychologist who wrote eight books on family relationships, including *What Every Child Would Like His Parents to Know,* appearing frequently on television talk shows to discuss social issues affecting families. In the early days of his career, he developed a theory that a mother's heartbeat has a calming effect on her newborn infant.

Sawyer, George C., Sr.   [1926-July 2, 1992] U.S. chemical engineer and drug researcher who helped develop and patent streptokinase, the main clot-busting medication used during heart attacks.

Sebrell, William Henry   [September 11, 1901-September 29, 1992] U.S. nutritionist and expert on vitamin B complex, who helped discover the use of B vitamins to prevent and cure pellagra, an illness caused by a deficiency of niacin. While he was director of the National Institutes of Health and Assistant Surgeon General between 1950 and 1955, he proposed that niacin, thiamine, and riboflavin be added to flour and bread in order to eradicate pellagra, beriberi, and other ailments.

Selikoff, Irving John   [January 15, 1914-May 20, 1992] U.S. researcher who was the founding director of the first environmental and occupational medicine department, at New York's Mt. Sinai Hospital. In 1952, he and Edward H. Robitzek proved that isoniazid, still used widely today, was an effective tuberculosis medicine, and he later reported the connection between exposure to asbestos and lung cancer.

Selverstone, Bertram   [March 2, 1917-March 20, 1993] U.S. neurosurgeon who performed research in radiotherapy to localize brain tumors and in surgery to control cerebral aneurysms, the bulging of the wall of a blood vessel due to the hardening of the arteries or high blood pressure. He also devised the Selverstone Carotid Clamp to control the flow of blood through the carotid artery.

Sheehan, George   [1918-November 1, 1993] U.S. cardiologist who became an advocate for the recreational running movement; he ran in 21 consecutive Boston Marathons, and although he fought his own cancer since 1986, he continued running as well as writing and lecturing on the subject of recreational running.

Sherry, Sol [December 8, 1916-January 28, 1993] U.S. medical researcher and professor emeritus at Temple University whose research on blood-clotting drugs led to the development of streptokinase and urokinase, which are used widely to treat heart attacks because of their ability to dissolve clots, thus allowing the return of normal blood flow.

Sleeper, Ruth [1899-December 10, 1992] U.S. nursing educator who was past president of the National League of Nursing Education and the National League for Nursing, and while director of the School of Nursing at Massachusetts General Hospital, developed an innovative curriculum that combined nine months of training with 28 months of academic classes.

Srole, Leo [October 8, 1908-May 1, 1993] U.S. sociologist who was known for directing the controversial Midtown Manhattan Study, a mental health survey that found in 1962 that only 18.5 percent of 1660 New York City residents who participated in the study were in good mental health; this provided evidence of the harmful effects of city life, although later Srole and other researchers found that the subjects' mental health improved with age.

Stellar, Eliot [November 1, 1919-October 12, 1993] U.S. physiological psychologist whose work on human and animal behavior and motivation provided insight into how the physiological processes of the brain affect behavior; he also wrote and cowrote many books, including *Physiological Psychology,* an important textbook on the subject.

Stinchfield, Frank E. [August 12, 1910-December 1, 1992] U.S. orthopedic surgeon who was one of the first to restore normal functioning to arthritic hips by replacing diseased bone with a metal joint. He was past president of the American College of Surgeons and other organizations.

Thomas, Lewis [November 25, 1913-December 3, 1993] U.S. medical doctor, former president of the Memorial Sloan-Kettering Cancer Center, and dean of the medical schools at New York University and Yale, who was best known for biology essays and other publications that helped non-specialists understand the subject; one of his books, *The Lives of a Cell,* earned him a National Book Award in 1974.

Toolan, Helene Wallace [1912-November 29, 1992] U.S. cancer researcher whose achievements included directing a team that in 1960 linked viruses to eight types of human cancer, a connection previously only made for leukemia. She also conducted award-winning research on the transplantation of human tumors and tissues into laboratory animals.

Volwiler, Ernest H. [August 22, 1893-October 3, 1992] U.S. medical chemist who with Dr. Donalee Tabern developed Nembutal in 1930 and Pentothal in 1936. He was a former president and general manager of Abbott Laboratories, where he worked his entire life, and he was inducted into the National Inventors Hall of Fame in 1985.

Voorhees, Arthur B., Jr. [1921-May 12, 1992] U.S. physician whose accidental discovery of a silk suture in a laboratory animal led to his developing the first artificial arteries; he performed the first implant with success in 1952, using a tube made of vinyon-N cloth, and his invention is still used by other surgeons, who have adopted newer materials.

Wallerstein, Harry [December 11, 1906-June 26, 1993] U.S. hematologist who was an authority on leukemia and an advocate of establishing blood banks in the early 1930s. He performed the first exchange transfusion, replacing an infant's blood to save the lives of babies born to parents whose blood is Rh incompatible, and trained hundreds of physicians in this now common procedure.

Wang, Shih-Chun   [January 25, 1910-June 6, 1993] U.S. neuroscientist and Columbia University pharmacology professor, born in Tientsin, China, whose research provided insight on the mechanisms by which the brain regulates functions such as blood circulation, breathing, temperature control, and bodily reactions to motion, thereby increasing understanding of motion sickness and leading to the development of drugs that prevent vomiting and other adverse reactions.

Warner, Robert   [February 16, 1912 May 17, 1992] U.S. pediatrician and specialist in treating disabled children, including those with phenylketonuria, or PKU, a genetic disorder causing abnormal brain development due to decreased metabolism of phenylalanine; he helped simplify testing procedures by having his institution, the Children's Hospital Rehabilitation Center in Buffalo, become the first to perform a test developed by Robert Guthrie, now given to all American babies, that required only a drop of blood instead of the large amounts previously used.

Wesolowski, Sigmund Adam   [February 6, 1923-August 8, 1993] U.S. chest specialist, also known as Dr. Adam Wesolow, who played a role in devising a heart pump in the early days of open-heart surgery and in developing the use of prostheses to replace diseased arteries.

Wolfe, Samuel   [June 25, 1923-December 10, 1993] Canadian-born professor emeritus at Columbia University's School of Public Health, who in the 1960s was an early advocate for Canada's national health insurance plan, which provides universal health insurance. He also opened a large community health center in a poor section of Nashville in 1968 as a part of his efforts toward increasing access to medical care for the poor.

Woolsey, Theodore D.   [1913-November 27, 1992] U.S. health statistician who was former director of the National Center for Health Statistics, the federal government's principal health statistics agency; he also helped write the National Health Survey Act of 1956.

Zarowitz, Harold   [1923-September 28, 1993] U.S. physician who was known for his early advocacy of the rigid-control concept for treating diabetes, which involves encouraging the body's own insulin production through monitoring insulin levels and supplying smaller doses instead of a large single dose that lasts all day.

Zeppa, Robert   [September 17, 1924-September 2, 1993] U.S. surgeon who worked with Dean Warren in the 1960s to develop the distal splenorenal shunt, a life-saving treatment for cirrhosis of the liver that involved diverting blood away from the damaged liver to prevent bleeding that may lead to death.

Zizmor, Judah   [1909-February 26, 1993] U.S. physician whose research in computerized tomography and magnetic resonance imaging to diagnose and treat trauma, cancer, and other head and neck disorders led to his being considered one of the founders of the field of otolaryngologic radiology.

Zwerling, Israel   [June 12, 1917-November 12, 1993] U.S. psychologist who was an advocate of community-based outpatient care for the mentally ill and was the first to demonstrate that day treatment was a healthy alternative. He established measures such as allowing patients to come and go through unlocked doors at the Bronx Psychiatric Center, where he served as director in the 1960s.

Index

Index

2/4/95